Infection and Haematology

Infection and Haematology

G.C. Jenkins PhD, MB, BS, FRCPath, FRCP(Edin.)
Emeritus Professor of Haematology
The London Hospital Medical College
London, UK

J.D. Williams BSc, MD, FRCPath, MRCP, DCP
Professor of Medical Microbiology
The London Hospital Medical College
London, UK

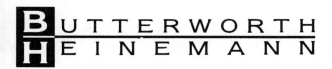

BUTTERWORTH
HEINEMANN

Butterworth-Heinemann Ltd
Linacre House, Jordan Hill, Oxford OX2 8DP

A member of the Reed Elsevier plc group

OXFORD LONDON BOSTON
MUNICH NEW DELHI SINGAPORE SYDNEY
TOKYO TORONTO WELLINGTON

First published 1994

British Library Cataloguing in Publication Data

A catalogue record for this book is available from the British Library
ISBN 0 7506 1622 9

Library of Congress Cataloguing in Publication Data

A catalogue record for this book is available from the Library of Congress

Typeset by EJS Chemical Composition, Midsomer Norton, Bath
Printed and bound in Great Britain by the Bath Press, Avon

Contents

Part Four Infection and the Blood

Contributors

C. Aitken MSc, MB, MRCP
Senior Registrar
Department of Virology
St. Bartholomews' Hospital Medical College
London

B.A. Bannister MSc, FRCP
Consultant
Royal Free Department of Infectious Diseases
Coppetts Wood Hospital, London

E.J. Bow MD, MSc, DBact, FRCP(C)
Associate Professor
Departments of Internal and
Medical Microbiology, University of Manitoba
Winnipeg, Manitoba, Canada

J.P. Burnie MA, MSc, MD, PhD, MRCP,
MRCPath
Professor
Division of Bacteriology
Department of Pathological Sciences
Medical School
Manchester

B.T. Colvin MA, MB, FRCP, FRCPath
Senior Lecturer and Consultant
Department of Haematology
The London Hospital Medical College
London

A.G. Dalgleish BSc, MD, MRCP, FRCP(A),
MRCPath
Professor
Department of Virology, Division of Oncology
St. George's Hospital Medical School
London

L.R. Davis TD, MD, MRCS, AKC, FRCPath
Formerly Consultant
King's College Hospital Medical School
London

J.K.M. Duguid MB, MRCPath
Consultant
Mersey Regional Transfusion Centre
Liverpool

C.A. Facer BSc, MSc, PhD, FIBiol, FLS
Reader
Department of Haematology
The London Hospital Medical College
London

L.E. Fenelon MB, MRCPI, MRCPath
Consultant
Department of Microbiology
St. Vincent's Hospital, Dublin

P. Flanagan MRCP, MRCPath
Consultant Haematologist
Yorkshire Regional Blood Transfusion Centre
Leeds

H. Gaya MB, FRCPath
Consultant
Department of Microbiology
Brompton Hospital, London

P.G.R. Godwin BSc, MB, ChB, MRCPath
Department of Medical Microbiology
University of Leeds Old Medical School
Leeds

C.N. Gutteridge BA, MB, MRCP, MRCPath
Department of Haematology
Senior Lecturer and Consultant
The London Hospital Medical College
London

C. Haworth BSc, MB, MRCP, FRCPath
Consultant Paediatric Haematologist
Leicester Royal Infirmary Children's Hospital
Leicester

G.C. Jenkins PhD, MB, FRCPE, FRCPath
Professor Emeritus
Department of Haematology
The London Hospital Medical College
London

S.M. Kelsey BSc, MB, MRCP, MRCPath
Senior Lecturer and Consultant
Department of Haematology
The London Hospital Medical College
London

R.W. Lacey MA, MD, PhD, DCH, FRCPath
Professor
Department of Medical Microbiology
University of Leeds, Old Medical School
Leeds

A.C. Newland MA, MB, FRCP, FRCPath
Professor
Department of Haematology
The London Hospital Medical College
London

C.D. Overholser DDS, MSD
Department of Oral Diagnosis
Baltimore College of Dental Surgery
University of Maryland, USA

S. Ramskill FIMLS
Scientific Head
Microbiology Department
Yorkshire Regional Blood Transfusion Centre
Leeds

J.D.M. Richards MA, MD, FRCP, FRCPE,
FRCPath
Consultant
Department of Haematology
University College Hospital, London

E.A.E. Robinson MB, FRCPath
Medical Director
Yorkshire Regional Blood Transfusion Centre
Leeds

T.R.F. Rogers MSc, MRCPI, FRCPath
Reader
Department of Infectious Diseases and
Bacteriology
Hammersmith Hospital, London

A.R. Ronald BSc(Med), MD, FRCP(C), FACP
Distinguished Professor
Departments of Internal Medicine
Medical Microbiology and Community
Health Sciences
University of Manitoba
Winnipeg, Manitoba, Canada

D. Samson BSc, MD, MRCP, FRCPath
Senior Lecturer and Consultant
Department of Haematology
Charing Cross and Westminster Medical School
London

S.A. Schey MB, MRCP, FRACP, MRCPath
Senior Lecturer and Consultant
Department of Haematology
Guy's Hospital, London

G.M. Scott MD, MRCP, MRCPath, DTM&H
Consultant
Department of Microbiology
University College Hospital
London

S. Selwyn BSc, MD, FIBiol, FRCPath
Professor
Department of Medical Microbiology
Charing Cross and Westminster Medical School
London

J.A. Wedzicha MD, MRCP
Consultant
Department of Thoracic Medicine
The London Chest Hospital, London

J.D. Williams BSc, MD, FRCPath,
MRCP, DCP
Professor of Medical Microbiology
The London Hospital Medical College
London

M.E. Wood MB, MRCP, MRCPath
Consultant
Department of Haematology
Colchester General Hospital, Essex

A.J. Zuckerman MD, DSc, FRCP, FRCPath
Dean of the School of Medicine and
Professor of Medical Microbiology
Royal Free School of Medicine, London

Part One

The Blood and Infections

1

Infection and the bone marrow

Diana Samson and Catherine Haworth

Anaemia and changes in white cell and platelet counts are common features of infection, anaemia and leucocytosis frequently accompanying bacterial infection, while neutropenia and thrombocytopenia are more common in viral infections. Except in the case of immune-mediated peripheral destruction such as the auto-immune haemolysis or thrombocytopenia which can follow viral infections, these changes result largely from alteration in the function of the bone marrow. The underlying mechanisms are as yet incompletely understood, although much of the available evidence suggests that macrophages and T-lymphocytes may be closely involved in many of the changes seen in bacterial infection, while in viral infection direct damage to bone marrow cells may be important. Some of these effects can now be attributed directly to the pleomorphic effects of the mediators of the immune response including lymphokines, interleukins and colony stimulating factors.

The marrow in bacterial infection

The anaemia of chronic disorders

It was Cartwright and his co-workers who over the years from 1945 to 1966 established that in many chronic disease states there was a characteristic type of anaemia associated with abnormalities of iron metabolism, which he termed the anaemia of chronic disorders (Cartwright, 1966). The anaemia of chronic disorders can be defined as a non-progressive mild to moderate anaemia characterized by reduced plasma and erythroblast iron in the presence of normal or increased reticulo-endothelial iron stores. Interestingly, it was the anaemia and disturbance of iron metabolism in infection which were his first interest and field of study, and it was later that it became clear from his own work and that of others (Cartwright and Lee, 1971) that the same disturbances are present in chronic inflammatory states, malignancy and other forms of chronic tissue damage. The anaemia develops gradually and is not seen in infections lasting less than two weeks, so is unusual in viral infections which are generally transient, and is classically associated with chronic bacterial infections such as tuberculosis, sub-acute bacterial endocarditis and osteomyelitis.

Laboratory features and diagnosis

Peripheral blood

The anaemia is normally of moderate severity and the haemoglobin rarely falls below 8.0 g/dl unless additional factors are present. Anaemia develops gradually over the first month of the illness and does not tend to worsen thereafter, and in general there is an inverse relationship between the haemoglobin level and the height of the ESR. The anaemia is often said to be normochromic normocytic but experience with electronic counters has shown that it is commonly slightly microcytic with the mean corpuscular volume (MCV) in the range 70–80 fl

(Chernow and Wallner, 1978). An MCV of below 70 fl suggests accompanying iron deficiency, though it does occasionally occur in the presence of adequate iron stores. The lower the haemoglobin, the more likely is the presence of microcytosis. Similarly, though the cells may be normochromic, mild hypochromia is common, as shown by a reduction in mean corpuscular haemoglobin concentration (MCHC) (Bainton and Finch, 1964; Chernow and Wallner, 1978). The absolute reticulocyte count is usually within normal limits, i.e., it is not appropriately raised for the degree of anaemia, implying an inadequate marrow response. There is often an elevated white cell count with a neutrophil leucocytosis in bacterial infection and monocytosis may be seen in more chronic infections. The platelet count may also be raised. In chronic viral infections, on the other hand, neutropenia and thrombocytopenia are more common.

On the basis of the haemoglobin and red cell indices alone it is not usually possible to distinguish between the anaemia of chronic disorders and mild iron deficiency anaemia, and the use of newer technology in contributing to the diagnosis has been investigated in two areas, digital image processing and measurement of the red cell distribution width (RDW). The RDW is a measure of the heterogeneity of red cell size (being the coefficient of variation of the red cell volume) and is routinely calculated in addition to the MCV by modern electronic counters. It is the equivalent of anisocytosis as seen on the blood film but is more sensitive and more quantitative than a visual assessment. Bessman, Gilmer and Gardner (1983) reported improved classification of anaemias by looking at RDW and MCV together. They found that whereas in 67 patients with iron deficiency anaemia there was a low MCV and high RDW, in 215 patients with the anaemia of chronic disorders both these values were normal. These results are surprising as one would have expected a significant reduction in MCV in such a large study, and assuming iron deficient erythropoiesis is an integral part of the anaemia of chronic disorders, one would also expect at least some change in RDW. Bessman's classification was challenged in several areas by McDonald *et al.* (1984), who found that only four of 31 patients with anaemia of chronic disorders had normal values for MCV and RDW. Baynes *et al.* (1986) noted that the patients with

chronic disorders in Bessman's study were a very heterogeneous group and therefore undertook a similar study with a more homogeneous group of 102 patients with prove tuberculosis and compared the results with normal subjects and patients with iron deficiency anaemia. They found that in untreated patients with tuberculosis the haemoglobin and MCV were reduced and the RDW was elevated, and these abnormalities returned to normal during treatment. The values for RDW were almost identical to those seen in iron deficiency anaemia though the iron deficient patients were more microcytic. Baynes *et al.* concluded first that it was not possible to distinguish between the anaemia of chronic disorders and iron deficiency anaemia on the basis of the RDW, and second that as there was no evidence for any other factor, such as folate deficiency, affecting the RDW in the patients with tuberculosis and that the increase in RDW was the result of iron-deficient erythropoiesis.

Digital image processing of erythrocytes is a technique in which a blood film is analysed by an image processor to separate morphological sub-populations of red cells. On the basis of shape and degree of central pallor, cells are divided into spherocytes, target cells, elongated cells, irregular cells and biconcave cells and the probability of certain diagnoses can be calculated by comparison with reference data. Westerman, O'Donnell and Bacus (1980) studied 18 patients with the anaemia of chronic disease and found that this method was 83% correct (15 of 18 patients) in making the diagnosis, whereas MCV and MCHC were normal in all their patients and serum iron and iron-binding capacity and ferritin levels were diagnostic in less than half the cases. Indeed, it is questionable as to whether the accepted diagnostic criteria of the anaemia of chronic disorders were fulfilled in all their patients. In this study the disorder most closely resembling anaemia of chronic disorders was β thalassaemia trait, which was listed as the most likely diagnosis in two of the patients and second most likely in twelve, whereas iron deficiency was listed as the second most likely diagnosis in only two patients. The authors did not comment on this aspect and it was not stated whether the reference iron deficiency anaemia samples were from severely or mildly anaemic patients. Although the authors felt that digital image processing would be of value in the diagnosis of anaemia of chronic disease, it remains to be seen if this will prove to be the case where distinction from mild iron deficiency is concerned.

The bone marrow

The bone marrow shows normal or increased stainable iron within the macrophages, but the percentage of sideroblasts, i.e. erythroblasts with granules of iron in the cytoplasm, is reduced (Bainton and Finch, 1964). The erythroblasts often show poor haemoglobinization and minor dyserythropoietic features such as ragged cytoplasm and an indistinct nuclear outline. In chronic infections there is often an increase in plasma cells, histiocytes (macrophages) and mononuclear cells, and in chronic viral infections atypical large lymphoid cells may be seen.

Serum iron, iron-binding capacity and ferritin

Serum iron is reduced in the anaemia of chronic disorders and in those patients with microcytic hypochromic anaemia is in the same range as in patients with iron deficiency anaemia (Bainton and Finch, 1964). However, in contrast to iron deficiency anaemia the total iron binding capacity (TIBC), i.e. the transferrin level, is not elevated and may be reduced, though not as reliably as the serum iron. The more anaemic the patient, i.e., the more active the disease, the lower is the transferrin level (Kurnick, Ward and Pickett, 1972). The combination of the two measurements gives the percentage saturation of transferrin which will therefore be reduced, though not to the same extent as in iron deficiency anaemia. Transferrin saturation in the anaemia of chronic disorders generally falls in the range 10–20% (normally greater than 25%) while in iron deficiency anaemia it is commonly below 10% (Bainton and Finch, 1964). If iron deficiency is superimposed on the anaemia of chronic disorders the TIBC will tend to rise, although not to supranormal levels; in one series of patients with rheumatoid arthritis (Williams *et al.*, 1982) those with absent marrow iron stores had TIBC values significantly higher ($74.2 + 5.2$ μmol/l) than those with adequate marrow iron stores ($51.5 + 9.1$ μmol/l). However, other authors have not found a correlation of TIBC with iron stores in rheumatoid arthritis (Blake *et al.*, 1980) or other chronic disorders (Kurnick, Ward and Pickett, 1972) and although the combination of serum iron and TIBC may give strong clues as to iron status, in a patient with a chronic disorder it is often difficult to be certain whether or not iron stores are present without obtaining a bone marrow sample. In recent years the assay of serum ferritin has been increasingly used to assess iron status. Not only is it free from the problems surrounding the assay of serum iron such as diurnal variation, but it has been shown to be in equilibrium with the tissue ferritin and to give an accurate indication of tissue iron stores in normal subjects and in patients with iron deficiency and iron overload, levels in iron deficiency being below 12 μg/l (Jacobs *et al.* (1972). However, in acute and chronic inflammation (as well as in liver disease) ferritin levels tend to rise. Lipschitz, Cook and Finch (1974) showed that in patients with inflammation, identified on the basis of fever, leucocytosis and a raised ESR, ferritin levels correlated with marrow iron stores but at each grade of marrow iron the ferritin levels were much higher than in control subjects. They also observed an overall negative correlation between serum ferritin and TIBC in the patients with inflammation, i.e. the lower the TIBC the higher the serum ferritin. Hence, a raised ferritin in the context of a reduced iron and TIBC is confirmatory evidence of anaemia of chronic disorders. However, where a patient is iron deficient and may therefore be expected to have a low ferritin, the effect of inflammation may be to raise the ferritin into the normal range. Of the patients studied by Lipschitz, Cook and Finch, only two out of five with absent iron stores had a low ferritin level, and various studies on the relation between serum ferritin and iron stores in rheumatoid arthritis also suggest that the normal lower limit of around 12–15 μg/l for serum ferritin is inappropriate in the presence of inflammation. Bentley and Williams (1974) found that although there was a close correlation between serum ferritin and storage iron in patients with rheumatoid arthritis (confirming the observations of Lipschitz, Cook and Finch in acute inflammation) the mean ferritin in 13 patients with absent iron stores was 38 μg/l and only three had values below 12 μg/l. Similar results were obtained by Smith *et al.* (1977) while Koerper, Stempel and Dallman (1978) found that in children with arthritis all those with a serum ferritin of below 25 μg/l responded to iron therapy and Davidson *et al.* (1984) in a study of adults with rheumatoid arthritis found that those with microcytosis and serum ferritin below 25 μg/l all responded to iron. For practical purposes, in a patient with acute or chronic inflammation or infection, a ferritin of below 25 μg/l indicates probable iron deficiency, a level of over 50 μg/l makes iron deficiency unlikely and values in between 25 and 50 μg/l may be found in patients with or without iron stores. Even these guidelines will be inappropriate for patients with acute or chronic liver damage where ferritin levels may increase out of proportion to other features of the inflammation; Lipschitz, Cook and Finch (1974) found a mean ferritin level of 516 μg/l in alcoholic liver disease, 471 μg/l in viral hepatitis and 801 μg/l in patients with both liver dysfunction and an inflammatory process. Where there is doubt over the interpretation of serum ferritin levels a bone marrow aspirate should be stained for iron. Alternatively, a therapeutic trial of iron can be undertaken. Where a patient has both anaemia of chronic disorders and iron deficiency, treatment with oral iron will partly correct the anaemia and there will usually be some rise in the MCV and fall in the TIBC without a significant change in the serum iron (Table 1.1).

Other biochemical changes

Apart from the characteristic change in serum iron, TIBC and ferritin, there are other consistent biochemical alterations associated with the anaemia of chronic disorders, most of which are part of the acute phase response. For example,

there is increased synthesis of fibrinogen, von Willebrand factor (Factor VIII RAg), caeruloplasmin, haptoglobin, serum amyloid A (SAA) protein and C-reactive protein (CRP) (Dinarello, 1984; Kushner, 1982; Morley and Kushner, 1982). The raised fibrinogen level is largely responsible for the raised ESR, while the increase in caeruloplasmin results in elevated serum copper levels (Cartwright, 1966). On the other hand, albumin levels are reduced. The level of transferrin, like albumin, is reduced in proportion to the degree of anaemia (Kurnick, Ward and Pickett, 1972). This may be the result of inhibition of transferrin synthesis by IL-1 (see Dinarello, 1984 for review). Unrelated to the acute phase response is a rise in red cell protoporphyrin levels to values similar to those in iron deficiency anaemia (Kurnick, Ward and Pickett, 1972), consistent with reduced iron supply to the developing erythroblast.

The aetiology of the anaemia of chronic disorders

There is good evidence that very similar pathogenetic mechanisms are responsible for producing the anaemia of chronic disorders in the various different disease states in which it occurs (Cartwright, 1966) and although we cannot be certain that the changes causing anaemia in infection are exactly the same as those operative in, for example, rheumatoid arthritis, it is therefore reasonable to look at evidence gained from studies in patients with diseases other than infection, particularly as relatively little work has actually been done on patients with infection.

Table 1.1 Comparison of laboratory data in the anaemia of chronic disorders and iron deficiency anaemia

	Anaemia of chronic disorders	*Uncomplicated iron deficiency*	*Combined iron deficiency chronic disorders*
Hb	Usually over 9 g/dl Rarely below 8 g/dl	Variable	Variable
MCV and MCHC	Normal or slightly low	Always low	Always low
Serum iron	Low	Low	Low
TIBC	Normal or slightly low	Always high	Variable but often upper end of normal range
Ferritin	Over 25 μg/l, usually over 50 μg/l	Below 12 μg/l	Usually below 12 μg/l
Marrow iron stores	Normal or increased	Absent	Absent
% Sideroblasts	Reduced	Markedly reduced	Markedly reduced
Response to iron	None	Full	Partial

Red cell survival

Although early work using the Ashby technique (differential red cell agglutination) suggested a modest decrease in red cell survival in patients with rheumatoid arthritis (Freireich *et al.*, 1957b) later studies using chromium labelling failed to show any significant alterations in red cell survival (Lewis and Porter, 1966; Mongan and Jacox, 1964). Both of these techniques are, however, not sensitive enough to detect modest shortening of red cell lifespan. Figures for red cell lifespan obtained from computer analysis of ferrokinetic data have shown normal or modest reduction in red cell survival in the majority of patients with chronic inflammatory disease (Cavill, Ricketts and Napier, 1977b), rheumatoid arthritis (Dinant and de Maat, 1978; Cavill and Bentley, 1982) and Hodgkin's Disease (Al-Ismail *et al.*, 1979). For example, Cavill, Ricketts and Napier found mean cell survival in rheumatoid arthritis to be 81 + 36 days compared with 98 + 23 days in normal subjects. Similar studies have not been done in patients with infection although in rabbits with experimental *S. viridans* endocarditis red cell survival was reduced to less than 50% of normal (Joyce and Sande, 1975). This was associated with splenomegaly and prevented by splenectomy prior to infection. These rabbits had raised reticulocyte counts and very large spleens and appear to have had a haemolytic anaemia of increasing severity rather than uncomplicated anaemia of chronic disorders. However, there is no doubt that whenever the spleen is enlarged by infection there will be an effect on red cell survival. Activation of macrophages by infection even without splenic enlargement will enhance their ability to phagocytose red cells. Endotoxin injection produces a marked and rapid increase in phagocytic activity of the reticuloendothelial system in the rat (Arredondo and Kampschmidt, 1963) and Atkinson and Frank (1974) showed that in guinea pigs injected with BCG the clearance of antibody-coated erythrocytes was greatly enhanced by day 3 after injection, at which time splenomegaly had not yet occurred. Overwhelming red cell destruction by macrophages can occur in infection, producing overt haemolytic anaemia (see p. 29).

There is also experimental animal work showing that fever *per se* can cause increased red cell destruction, as described in a series of papers by Karle. It is well known that red cells are haemolysed at temperatures of over 45 °C but he showed that increasing the body temperature of rabbits by only 1 to 3 °C by injection of bacterial pyrogen or heated milk, or by external heat caused a reduction in red cell survival, a fall in haemoglobin and a reticulocytosis (Karle, 1968a). The average reduction of red cell mass was 15% and the maximum 35% (Karle, 1969a). The haemolysis affected predominantly the older red cells and took place mainly in the spleen (Karle, 1968b; Karle, 1968c) suggesting a change in membrane structure or metabolic function. He later showed that heating rabbit red cells to 38 °C or 41.5 °C for long periods of time produced a distinct increase in osmotic fragility and spontaneous haemolysis and when such heated cells were labelled and re-injected, their survival was greatly reduced (Karle, 1969b). Further studies indicated a change in the red cell membrane detectable by an increased permeability to cations and a reduction in deformability (Karle, 1974; Karle and Hansen, 1970). Human red cells show similar changes after heat exposure in vitro though their susceptibility is less than that of rabbit cells (Karle, 1969b; Karle and Hansen, 1970).

Extrapolating from this work to the human situation it appears likely that both fever and macrophage activation may contribute to a reduced red cell lifespan which may therefore be expected to be a more significant factor in the anaemia of chronic disorders associated with infection than with non-infective conditions. However, the normal bone marrow should be able to respond to this haemolysis and the fact that it is incapable of increasing red cell supply to meet demand implies failure of production as the major problem. The major factors limiting the marrow response include inadequate erythropoietin synthesis, inadequate iron supply to the marrow and abnormal regulation and development of erythroid precursors.

Iron and iron metabolism

One of the earliest changes to occur in infection and inflammation is the fall in serum iron (Cartwright, Lauritzen and Jones, 1946; Cartwright, 1966; Roeser, 1980). In experimental infection of humans with Francisella tularensis, Pekarek *et al.* (1969) showed significant decreases in serum iron by the

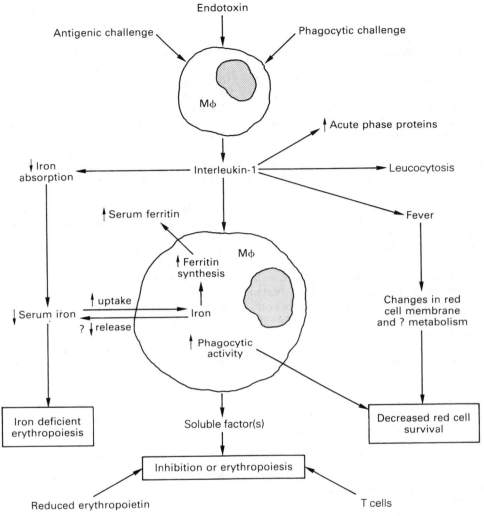

Figure 1.1 The role of the macrophage in the production of the anaemia of chronic disorders. Mφ = Macrophage

second day after exposure, before any clinical symptoms had appeared; thereafter, serum iron continued to fall and reached a nadir on the fifth day coinciding with the onset of fever and a peak in neutrophil count. Hypoferraemia was more marked in those who were most ill and fell as low as 25% of baseline levels in this group. Similar changes in serum iron were shown to follow the injection of bacterial endotoxin in rats, with a fall in serum iron approximately 16 hours after a single injection (Kampschmidt and Schultz, 1961). Furthermore, plasma from the rats who had been given endotoxin two hours previously, when injected into other rats,

produced hypoferraemia in the recipients (Kampschmidt and Upchurch, 1962). This effect was abolished by heating the plasma. The time course of production of this factor and its heat lability suggests it was what was then called endogenous pyrogen (now interleukin-1) and further studies showed that the same effect could be produced by leucocyte extracts (Kampschmidt and Upchurch, 1969). A similar fall in serum iron was observed in human volunteers with experimental fever produced by injection of endotoxin or aetiocholanolone (Elin, Wolff and Finch, 1977).

Transferrin-bound iron is only a small

fraction of total body iron, about half being in the plasma and half in the extravascular fluid. This pool is turning over very rapidly from 10–20 times a day even in normal subjects (Cavill *et al.*, 1977a). In this situation changes in the rate of removal of iron from transferrin or the rate of entry of iron into the plasma from the reticuloendothelial system or from absorption can produce rapid change in the plasma iron level. There is evidence both for increased iron uptake and diminished iron release by macrophages in infection and inflammation. The increased uptake of iron by macrophages appears to be closely linked to an increased rate of ferritin synthesis with a resulting increase in storage iron.

The *in vivo* clearance of iron bound to transferrin is increased in inflammatory states (Roberts *et al.*, 1963) and this may be due to increased uptake by the reticuloendothelial system rather than by the bone marrow, as the clearance rate of colloidal gold is also increased (Reizenstein, Gheorghescu and Wiklund-Hammarstrom, 1975). In the studies of Elin, Wolff and Finch (1977) on experimental fever in man, the fall in serum iron was followed by a slower and more sustained rise in serum ferritin and similar observations were made by Birgegard *et al.* (1978). In a longitudinal study of serum iron and ferritin in patients with infection, they found that the rise in ferritin persisted for up to five weeks following the resolution of fever, and the changes in ferritin levels correlated closely with those of serum haptoglobin. These observations suggested that the cause of the rise in serum ferritin was an increase in iron stores rather than release from damaged tissues, and the fact that the ferritin in the serum during infection is of the glycosylated form normally present rather than the non-glycosylated form characteristic of intracellular ferritin, supports this interpretation.

Both the rate of uptake of iron from transferrin and the rate of ferritin synthesis by mouse peritoneal macrophages are markedly increased in animals with experimental inflammation (Birgegard and Caro, 1984). The same results were obtained whether the infection was local or systemic, indicating a humoral mechanism. In addition, hepatocytes from endotoxin treated rats were shown to take up iron from transferrin three times as fast as controls, and parallel *in vitro* studies indicated that this was not due to a direct effect of endotoxin on the hepatocyte, i.e. it was mediated by an extra-hepatic factor (Potter, Blades and Rand, 1986). There is also increased incorporation of iron into ferritin *in vivo* in the liver and spleen of endotoxin-treated rats, although not in the marrow (Mazur, Carleton and Carlsen, 1961; Mazur and Carleton, 1963) and ferritin synthesis by liver and spleen tissue *in vitro* was increased in animals with inflammation (Konijn and Hershko, 1977; Konijn *et al.*, 1981). The cells involved were not identified and it is not clear whether the increased ferritin synthesis was occurring only in macrophages or also in the hepatocytes. In contrast to this data indicating increased iron uptake and ferritin synthesis in macrophages and hepatocytes in infection, Summers and Jacobs (1976) failed to show any increase in either iron uptake or ferritin synthesis by peripheral blood monocytes from patients with the anaemia of chronic disease, even though the ferritin content of these cells was significantly increased.

There is some evidence that lactoferrin, which is released by neutrophils in response to endotoxin (Hansen, Karle and Valerius, 1978) is involved in the increased iron uptake by macrophages. Lactoferrin takes up iron from transferrin and the lactoferrin-bound iron is then taken up by reticuloendothelial cells (which have lactoferrin receptors) and stored as ferritin van Snick, Masson and Heremans, 1974). Transferrin-iron complexes are also taken up by macrophages from rats with experimental inflammation and this may contribute both to the hypoferraemia and to a reduction in serum transferrin level, since transferrin synthesis by hepatocytes was found to be normal (O'Shea, Kershenobich and Tavill, 1973). Potter, Blades and Rand (1986) in their study on the effects of endotoxin in rats also observed increased uptake of transferrin by hepatocytes and reduced transferrin synthesis.

In addition to the increased rate of uptake of iron from the plasma in infection there is also indirect evidence for a reduction in the rate of return of iron by macrophages to the plasma, the so-called reticuloendothelial iron block. The existence of such a block was first suggested by the combination of low serum iron levels with normal or increased reticuloendothelial iron stores in the anaemia of chronic disorders. This failure of iron release would result in reduced iron supply for erythropoiesis and the haematological features of mild iron deficiency.

Virtually all the iron used for haemoglobin synthesis is derived from the breakdown of senescent red cells. After the reticuloendothelial cells have broken down the haemoglobin, the iron is released onto plasma transferrin which delivers it to the developing erythroblasts via receptor-mediated endocytosis. It is possible that a small amount of iron can be directly transferred from the reticuloendothelial cell to erythroblasts as ferritin, but the majority has to be released onto transferrin before it is available to the erythroblast. In the normal situation, it appears that almost all the iron derived from red cell breakdown is released from the reticuloendothelial cell and very little mixing with storage iron takes place. Thus, when a very small amount of heat damaged labelled red cells was injected into human volunteers, 81–88% of the label was subsequently incorporated into newly formed red cells (Noyes, Bothwell and Finch, 1960), which is the same as the utilization of labelled iron given as transferrin-bound iron. The labelled iron was detectable in the plasma bound to transferrin by 80 minutes after injection of the labelled cells, showing that at least part of the iron is very rapidly released. When larger amounts of iron as damaged red cells are given, there was retention of up to half of the iron in the reticuloendothelial tissue at two weeks and only a small amount of the iron which was stored subsequently appeared in red cells, indicating that under normal circumstances the iron stores are relatively stable. Gradual mixing with the stores does, however, occur because after red cells are labelled *in vivo* the radioactivity declines by 50% over the first year, consistent with the mixing of the labelled iron with storage iron after its release from successive generations of red cells (Green *et al.*, 1968).

Conventional ferrokinetic studies measuring the incorporation into red cells of ^{59}Fe given as ^{59}Fe-transferrin have shown normal percentage incorporation of the dose in patients with the anaemia of chronic disorders, including patients with chronic infection and animals with experimental inflammation (Beamish *et al.*, 1971; Bush, Ashenbrucker and Cartwright, 1956; Freireich *et al.*, 1957a; Freireich *et al.*, 1957b; Kumar, 1974, Roberts *et al.*, 1963). These observations are unexpected in view of the fact that red cell production is obviously impaired and may be an artefact resulting from a reduction in the miscible iron pool (Kumar, 1974, Kumar, 1979) but still imply a failure of erythropoiesis to increase in response to the anaemia. When the utilisation of iron for red cell production is calculated as the daily erythrocyte iron turnover (EIT) which takes into account the serum iron level, then EIT is found to be increased, although not to the extent predicted for the degree of anaemia (Cavill *et al.*, 1977b; Douglas and Adamson, 1975). The EIT is correlated with the serum iron level and Douglas and Adamson interpreted this as indicating that erythropoiesis is as effective as can be expected on the basis of the serum iron level supply (Hillman and Henderson, 1969). If the labelled iron is administered in the form of labelled haemoglobin or heat damaged red cells then the iron must be removed by the reticuloendothelial cells and released onto transferrin before it can be used, more accurately reflecting the *in vivo* situation. Studies of this nature have shown defective re-utilisation of iron in animals with experimental inflammation and in patients with anaemia associated with chronic disorders including patients with infections such as tuberculosis and subacute bacterial endocarditis (Freireich *et al.*, 1957a; Haurani, Burke and Martinez, 1965; Haurani, Young and Tocantins, 1963). Subsequently, Beamish, *et al.* (1971) developed a method of simultaneously comparing iron utilisation and iron re-utilisation by using a double isotope technique in which ^{59}Fe-transferrin was used to measure utilisation of plasma iron and ^{55}Fe-labelled dextran was used to measure iron re-utilisation, the dextran-bound iron needing to be released by the reticuloendothelial system in the same way as haemoglobin iron. Comparison of the incorporation of the two isotopes into red cells enabled calculation of the amount of dextran-bound iron which has been returned to the plasma. Using this method reduced re-utilisation of dextran-bound iron compared with transferrin bound iron, i.e. reduced reticuloendothelial iron release was demonstrated in patients with anaemia of chronic disorders associated with rheumatoid arthritis, lymphoma and uraemia (Davies, Beamish and Jacobs, 1971; Beamish *et al.*, 1972; Bennett, Holt and Lewis, 1974) though no patients with infection were included in these studies. In contrast, Zarrabi *et al.* (1977) found normal re-utilisation of iron in rats with turpentine abscesses (and also in tumour-bearing rats) when very small amounts of damaged red cells were used and felt that the earlier results may have been affected by the use of unphysiologically large amounts of iron.

Ferrokinetic studies in animals during sterile inflammation and after injection of endotoxin also suggested that the hypoferraemia observed is due to a slower return of iron from recently destroyed erythrocytes to plasma, consistent with the hypothesis of the reticuloendothelial iron block (Freireich *et al.*, 1957b; Kampschmidt and Arredondo, 1963; Kampschmidt, Upchurch and Johnson, 1965; Quastel and Ross, 1966). Studies looking directly at the reappearance in the plasma of ^{59}Fe given as labelled damaged red cells showed reduced iron release in rats with turpentine abscesses (Lipschitz *et al.*, 1971) and in dogs injected with entotoxin (Fillet, Cook and Finch, 1974; Hershko, Cook and Finch, 1974). In man reticuloendothelial iron release has been studied directly by looking at the appearance of labelled transferrin-bound iron following injection of labelled iron-dextran (Kanakakorn, Cavill and Jacobs, 1973). This method was used to study patients with the anaemia of chronic disorders associated with rheumatoid arthritis (Williams, Cavill and Kanakakorn, 1974). In these patients, no difference was found from normal subjects in either the clearance of the iron dextran, the rate of reappearance of the label on transferrin or the total amount of labelled iron which reappeared. These results contradicted the data discussed above showing that the re-utilisation for haemoglobin synthesis of iron given as iron dextran is reduced in rheumatoid arthritis (Beamish *et al.*, 1971) and it was suggested that the dose of iron in the latter studies might have affected the results. Subsequently, a similar method of looking directly at reticuloendothelial iron release was developed using tracer doses of ^{59}Fe-hydroxide colloid (Bentley, Cavill and Ricketts, 1979). In seven of nine patients with rheumatoid arthritis the fraction of labelled iron reappearing in the plasma within the first six hours of injection was normal although it was considerably reduced in the other two patients who subsequently showed reduced incorporation of the injected dose of iron into red cells. More extensive studies with either of these methods have not been reported and there is no published data pertaining to patients with infection.

In summary therefore, the evidence for a failure in reticuloendothelial iron release as a limiting factor in erythropoiesis is conflicting. The early work on the re-utilisation of labelled haemoglobin solutions and labelled red cells which supported this concept has been criticised (Bentley, Cavill and Ricketts, 1979; Zarrabi *et al.*, 1977) because the doses of iron often exceeded physiological doses and might be expected to disturb reticuloendothelial iron metabolism and also because haemoglobin in solution is cleared by hepatocytes and not by macrophages, while more recent work on re-utilisation of small amounts of red cell iron and on direct measurement of reticuloendothelial iron release has failed to confirm the earlier results. However, at present the data are not sufficient to disprove the hypothesis of the reticuloendothelial iron block. Moreover, this is the only way to explain satisfactorily the iron-deficient erythropoiesis in the presence of adequate iron stores and the normal utilisation of labelled transferrin-bound iron in a situation where red cell production is evidently reduced.

If failure of iron release is important, why does it occur? Unfortunately, little is known about how iron is normally released from macrophages – at what stage it is bound to transferrin and whether there is another carrier molecule transporting it from the site of haemoglobin breakdown onto transferrin. There is evidence that the rate of release is dependent on the number of free binding sites on transferrin, i.e. the percentage saturation (Fillet, Cook and Finch, 1974; Lipschitz *et al.*, 1971). Thus the rate of release is inhibited by raising the serum iron, which may be due to stimulation of ferritin synthesis within the reticuloendothelial iron stores. The increased rate of ferritin synthesis by macrophages in infection has already been referred to and it is possible that this may result in inhibition of iron release; infusion of caeruloplasmin results in a rapid shift of iron from stores to transferrin (Ragan, Nacht and Lee, 1969). This effect may be due to oxidation of iron by the caeruloplasmin from the ferrous to the ferric form in which it is bound to transferrin (Freiden and Osaki, 1974). However, lack of caeruloplasmin cannot be invoked as a reason for reduced iron release in the anaemia of chronic disorders as caeruloplasmin levels are generally increased.

Over the past few years, studies of the effects of individual cytokines produced by recombinant DNA technology, both *in vivo* and *in vitro*, have identified some of the immune mediators which may influence iron metabolism, in the whole animal and at the single cell level. Interleukin-1 (IL-1) given to rats produced a fall in serum iron by six hours after injection as the result of increased iron clearance (Uchida *et al.*, 1991). At the single cell level many cytokines induce transferrin receptor expression (which is widely regarded as a marker of cell activation) on a wide variety of target cells, including T-lymphocytes (IL-2 and PMA) (Plana, *et al.*, 1991), B-lymphocytes (Interferon) (Lomo, *et al.*, 1991), macrophages and fibroblasts. In the last two cell types, TNF and IL-1 have also been shown to induce ferritin H chain synthesis (Tsuji *et al.*, 1991). As H chain is the rate limiting step in ferritin synthesis this would enhance ferritin production by these cell types.

Many experiments have shown that iron depletion *in vitro* inhibits lymphocyte activation (Polson, *et al.* 1990; Keyna, *et al.* 1991). It is therefore possible that the immune response may divert iron from haemopoietic tissues to activated immune effector cells which have been induced to express high levels of transferrin receptor.

There is also evidence that iron absorption is reduced in infection and inflammation. Roberts *et al.* (1963) found that patients with anaemia of rheumatoid arthritis had reduced iron absorption unless they were also iron deficient and Haurani, Green and Young (1965) found similarly reduced iron absorption in patients with anaemia associated with malignancy and inflammation, including two patients with tuberculosis. The reduced iron absorption occurs quite rapidly after the onset of inflammation; Beresford, Neale and Brooks (1971) found that iron absorption was markedly depressed during acute febrile episodes in children while animal studies have shown reduced absorption within hours of injection of bacterial endotoxin or induction of sterile inflammation (Cortell and Conrad, 1967; Schade, 1972). The block appears to be in the transfer of iron from the cell to the plasma rather than in iron uptake from the lumen; although Schade found no increase in mucosal ferritin after endotoxin injection occurring over the same time scale as the increase in serum ferritin observed by Elin, Wolff and Finch (1977).

In summary, reduced iron absorption, increased uptake by macrophages and possibly other cells, and failure of iron release from stores may all contribute to hypoferraemia and hence reduced availability of iron for erythropoiesis.

Erythropoietin

In most forms of anaemia erythropoietin levels increase progressively as the haemoglobin falls (Cotes, 1982). Low or inadequately raised levels of erythropoietin have been observed in patients with infection and inflammation and in animals with experimental inflammation (Douglas and Adamson, 1975; Lukens, 1973; Ward, Kurnick and Pisarczyk, 1971; Wallner *et al.*, 1977; Zucker, Friedman and Lysik, 1974) as well as in patients with rheumatoid arthritis or malignant disease (Douglas and Adamson, 1975; Firat and Banzon, 1971; Mahmood *et al.*, 1977; Pavlovic-Kentera *et al.*, 1979; Ward, Gordon and Pickett, 1969; Ward, Kurnick and Pisarczyk, 1971; Zucker, Friedman and Lysik, 1974). In experimental studies, Schade and Fried (1976) found that injection of endotoxin in rats resulted in a fall in urinary excretion of erythropoietin. However, these results were all obtained using bioassay methods for erythropoietin which are not reliable and not sensitive enough to measure erythropoietin levels within the normal range, and more work is needed using the newer radio-immunoassay methods to confirm the earlier data. For example, measurements of erythropoietin using radio-immunoassay have found most patients with rheumatoid arthritis to have appropriately elevated erythropoietin levels (Cotes, 1982; Samson and Evans, unpublished observations). The further use of radio-immunoassay and the availability of recombinant erythropoietin which could be used for metabolic studies will assist in the further clarification of erythropoietin metabolism in chronic disease.

Normally, the bone marrow responds to erythropoietin by increasing the proliferation of committed erythroid progenitors and increasing their rate of maturation and differentiation. The rate of haem biosynthesis increases in response to anaemia as the result of stimulation of the rate-limiting enzyme δ-aminolaevulinic acid synthase (ALA-S). The rate of haem synthesis in marrow from patients with chronic infection was however, found to be reduced compared with both normal controls and marrows from patients with iron deficiency anaemia and this was not due to a reduction in the amount of iron taken up by the cells (Kumar, 1979). Campbell, *et al.* (1978) measured the major enzymes of the haem biosynthetic pathway in patients with anaemia of rheumatoid arthritis and found that there was a failure of ALA-S to increase in response to the anaemia, but there is no similar data on patients with chronic infection.

Zucker, Friedman and Lysik (1974) studied the effect of erythropoietin on iron incorporation into haem in marrow cultures, in an attempt to determine whether reduced erythropoietin production or marrow unresponsiveness to erythropoietin was more important in anaemia of chronic disorders. In patients with infection, in whom they observed lower than expected levels of erythropoietin, the marrow responded normally to added erythropoietin by increasing the amount of haem synthesized, although the absolute amounts of haem synthesized were not determined. Similar results were obtained in patients with rheumatoid arthritis but in their study patients with malignancy had appropriately elevated levels of erythropoietin and the response of the marrow to added erythropoietin was markedly reduced. Reissman and Udupa (1978) studied the effects of *in vivo* injections of erythropoietin on the number of erythroid precursors in the marrow and on iron incorporation into haem in rats with turpentine abscesses, now known to induce production of TNF. After the abscesses were induced there was a fall in the number of marrow CFU-E and morphologically recognizable erythroblasts and a reduction in iron incorporation into haem *in vitro* (although they did not relate the iron incorporation to the numbers of erythroblasts present). Injections of erythropoietin failed to restore normal numbers of erythroid precursors. Further studies showed that endotoxin suppresses the CFU-E numbers and the incorporation of ^{59}Fe into red cells *in vivo* and this is not reversed by erythropoietin even when large doses are given (Schade and Fried, 1976; Udupa and Reissman, 1977). However, other workers have found that injection of erythropoietin, or cobalt or hypoxia, which stimulate erythropoietin synthesis, can correct the anaemia associated with experimental abscess formation (Gutnitsky and Van Dyke, 1963; Lukens, 1973; Robinson, James and Kark, 1949; Wintrobe, *et al.*, 1947) and Zarrabi, *et al.* (1977) found that erythropoietin treatment of such animals increased the incor-

poration of iron into red cells to the same extent as in control animals. As yet, there are no reported studies of the effects of erythropoietin treatment in patients with the anaemia of chronic disease.

Abnormalities of erythroid progenitor cells

Morphological assessment of the bone marrow and studies of haem biosynthesis and iron incorporation can give some idea of the numbers and function of morphologically recognizable erythroblasts but information about the more primitive erythroid cells can only be obtained by culturing erythroid progenitor cells *in vitro*. Two main types of erythroid progenitors give rise to colonies in agar, collagen and cellulose, the more primitive burst forming unit (BFU-E) which gives rise to large colonies of erythroblasts or 'bursts' after 10–14 days in culture and the more mature erythroid colony forming unit (CFU-E) which develops into small colonies after 7 days. The BFU-E were initially found to be dependent for early proliferation on burst promoting activity (BPA), now identified as interleukin-3, a glycoprotein produced by activated T-cells but do not require erythropoietin until the cells have developed to the stage corresponding to the CFU-E. Erythropoietin is essential for the terminal differentiation including haemoglobin synthesis from the CFU-E stage onwards and is an essential requirement in all culture systems. BFU-E growth also appears to be regulated in a very complex way by T-lymphocytes and monocytes. Several groups of workers have found that T lymphocytes stimulate the growth of BFU-E (see Lipton and Nathan, 1983), although others have found removal or addition of T cells to have no effect on burst formation (Nomdedeu *et al.*, 1980). Torok-Storb, Martin and Hansen (1981) found that the two major subsets of T cells had opposing actions on erythroid burst formation, the CD4+ helper T cells producing stimulation while the CD8+ cytotoxic T cells were inhibitory and proposed that the net effect of T cells results from the balance between these opposing actions. Mangan *et al.* (1982) found that T-cells were merely less actively stimulatory than T helper cells and Haq, Rinehart and Balcerzak (1983) found that the two populations were equally stimulatory. In clinical practice there have been several reports of patients with erythroid hypoplasia due to an expansion of the CD8+ subset (Hoffman *et al.*, 1978; Nagasawa, Abe and Nakagawa, 1981) and it seems likely that an imbalance of T cells, such as occurs in viral and fungal infections (Blumberg and Schooley, 1985; Stobo *et al.*, 1976) can cause disturbances of erythropoiesis. Similar opposing actions of T-helper and cytotoxic cells have been observed in the regulation of granulopoiesis (Bagby, 1981).

Monocytes and macrophages have also been found to exert an influence on BFU-E and CFU-E proliferation and again, they appear to be able to stimulate or inhibit erythropoiesis depending on the *in vivo* situation and on experimental conditions. The morphological observation that erythroblasts develop in close association with macrophages in the marrow, suggests a direct involvement of macrophages in erythroid maturation. Although terminal differentiation of erythroblasts in the steady state appear to be regulated by erythropoietin, little is known about the control of steady state haemopoiesis in general, including that of the early erythroid progenitor cells in normal marrow. Most authors have found that adherent cells from marrow (macrophages) and peripheral blood monocytes stimulate proliferation of erythroid progenitors (Eaves and Eaves, 1978; Kurland, Meyers and Moore, 1980; Reid, Baptista and Chanarin, 1981; Roodman, Horadam and Wright, 1983) although Rinehart *et al.* (1978) found that peripheral blood monocytes in large numbers were inhibitory and Zanjani, *et al.* (1982) also found large numbers of marrow adherent cells to be inhibitory. Reid, Baptista and Chanarin (1981) demonstrated a synergistic effect of peripheral blood monocytes and T-cells on erythroid burst formation and a similar synergistic effect appears likely in the differentiation of granulocyte precursors (Bagby, *et al.*, 1981). The effects of macrophages on erythropoiesis have been shown to be mediated at least partly, via a secretory product of these cells (Aye, 1977; Gordon *et al.*, 1980; Kurland, Meyers and Moore, 1980) as discussed below.

Reissman and Udupa (1978) found that numbers of bone marrow CFU-E, but not BFU-E, were reduced in mice with turpentine abscesses and that this was not reversed by *in vivo* erythropoietin treatment, suggesting a block at the stage between BFU-E and CFU-E. This did not appear to be due to unresponsiveness to erythropoietin because the numbers of CFU-E in the spleen increased markedly in response to the erythropoietin injections. They therefore postulated a decrease in numbers of progenitors of CFU-E due to either humoral or cell-mediated suppression, or possibly as a result of the increased granulopoiesis in the marrow. This now appears to be secondary to IL-1 and/or TNF (Furmanski and Johnson, 1979). A similar shift in erythropoiesis from the marrow to the spleen in rats and mice injected with endotoxin has been observed by other workers (Day Werts, Gibson and Degowin, 1979; Fruhman, 1967; Mazur and Carleton, 1963; Mazur, Carleton and Carlsen, 1961; Twentyman, 1972) but its relevance to man is uncertain. Further experiments studying the effects of the injection of endotoxin on the response of erythroid progenitors injected with erythropoietin (Udupa and Reissman, 1977) showed that endotoxin given at the same time as, or shortly before or after erythropoietin, abolished the increase in bone marrow CFU-E normally observed 24 hours after erythropoietin injection. However, there was no direct effect of endotoxin on CFU-E growth *in vitro*, as it did not directly damage the CFU-E growth *in vitro*, i.e. it did not directly damage the CFU-E or inhibit the erythropoietin present in the culture system. These experiments indicate that infection or endotoxin are inhibitory to the development of erythroid progenitors via erythropoietin-independent mechanisms.

Since macrophage function is known to be altered in infection and inflammation (Stobo, 1977; Stobo *et al.*, 1976) it is tempting to postulate a role for abnormal macrophage function in affecting erythroid progenitor cell development. Zanjani *et al.* (1982) first demonstrated such an effect in a study of BFU-E and CFU-E growth in marrow from patients with disseminated fungal infection. They observed reduced growth in five out of 10 cases, but when the marrow was depleted of macrophages prior to culture, there was normal growth of erythroid precursors, in contrast to their results for normal subgroups in whom removal of the macrophages resulted in diminished colony growth. Macrophages from the infected patients also suppressed the growth of erythroid precursors from normal marrow. Further studies using macrophage-conditioned medium or macrophage underlayers suggested that the inhibition was mediated via a soluble product. Roodman, Horadam and Wright (1983) observed similar effects of macrophages on erythroid colony formation in marrow from patients with anaemia of chronic disease, most of whom had malignancy or connective tissue disease but one of whom had tuberculosis. Although numbers of colonies in unfractionated marrow were not significantly decreased compared with normal, there was a significant increase in colony numbers when the adherent cells were removed prior to culture. Again they observed that removal of the macrophages from normal marrow depressed colony formation. Since their cultures were done in a plasma clot system over adherent cell underlayers they felt it very likely that the macrophages were exerting their effect by release of soluble products rather than by direct cellular interaction. However, in contrast to the findings of Zanjani *et al.* (1982) they did not find that the adherent cells from the anaemic patients suppressed colony formation by normal marrow. Direct evidence for a soluble macrophage mediator producing suppression of erythropoiesis came from a study in which conditioned medium from mouse macrophages incubated with endotoxin inhibited the growth and differentiation of erythroleukaemia cells, endotoxin itself having no effect (Sassa, Kawakami and Cerami, 1983).

In a study of patients with anaemia of renal failure (Lamperi, Carrozzi and Nasini, 1986) both peripheral blood monocytes and peritoneal macrophages were found to suppress growth of peripheral blood BFU-E. The peritoneal macrophages were found to release greater than normal amounts of prostaglandin E2 but less interleukin-1 than control macrophages when stimulated, which does not explain their effects on erythroid colony growth. Stimulation *in vitro* may well not mirror the *in vivo* state. Increased prostaglandin E (PGE) synthesis has also been observed in macrophages from tumour-bearing mice (Pelus and Bockman, 1979) and it was suggested that this might be responsible for the immune suppression observed in this situation. The enhancing effects of PGE on normal erythroid colony growth are dependent on T cells (Lu and Broxmeyer, 1985) and also alterations in B cell function could modify the effects of increased PGE production by macrophages in infection.

Studies of the effect of T-cells on erythroid progenitor developments in patients with anaemia of chronic disorders due to infection have not yet been reported.

Although the inhibitory effects of macrophages are almost certainly mediated by a secretory product, there is no evidence at present for a detectable inhibitor in the serum of patients with infection. In one study, Wallner *et al.* (1976) serum from patients with anaemia of renal disease inhibited erythropoietin-stimulated haem synthesis by normal marrow but serum from patients with chronic diseases, including some patients with chronic infection, had no effect.

Ineffective erythropoiesis

The role of ineffective erythropoiesis, i.e. the death of erythroblasts within the bone marrow, has been studied in the anaemia of chronic disorders associated with rheumatoid arthritis and malignancy and conflicting results obtained according to the techniques used (Samson, 1983). Quantitative data is available for only two patients with anaemia associated with chronic infection (Williams *et al.*, 1982). In this study, which was primarily looking at patients with rheumatoid arthritis, ineffective erythropoiesis was assessed using the release of haem from a labelled cohort of erythroblasts in culture as an index of cell death. Significant increases in haem release were observed in the patients with anaemia of rheumatoid arthritis but in none of 10 patients with anaemia of chronic disorders associated with other diseases, including the two with chronic bacterial infection, who had chronic osteomyelitis and infected varicose ulcers. However, other evidence suggests that ineffective erythropoiesis may be a factor in infective disease. An autoradiographic study of proliferation and maturation of erythropoiesis indicated normal relative production rates of early erythroblasts but a significant reduction in the production rate of late erythroblasts, i.e. a significant rate of premature cell death in the erythroid lineage (Dormer *et al.*, 1990). Wickramasinghe *et al.* (1989) found electron microscopic evidence of dyserythropoiesis in anaemic patients with *P. vivax* malaria which appeared to result from the infection itself and which was associated with macrophage hyperplasia. Further work is therefore needed to evaluate ineffective erythropoiesis as a contributing factor in the anaemia of infection.

Cytokines, the immune response and erythropoiesis

There is a considerable amount of data on the effect on erythroid progenitor cells of cytokines produced during the immune response. These cytokines are likely to be involved in the pathogenesis of the anaemia of chronic infection; however it is difficult to produce conclusive experimental data in all cases. Pure cytokines tested individually on non-purified haemopoietic cells may have differing effects, depending on the sub-populations within the haemopoietic cells which respond and the induction of other cytokine mediators. In addition, the outcome *in vivo* may be modified by co-existing (possibly as yet unidentified) cytokines. Some cytokines play a more dominant role in the further induction of cytokines than others. Thus, TNFα and IL-1 are the most dominant inducers, whereas other cytokines e.g. IL-6 and GM-CSF are weak by comparison. In addition, cytokines such as IL-6 and IL-4 have no effect in isolation but are co-stimulatory with specific haemopoietic growth factors *in vivo* and the net effect will therefore depend on the combination of cytokines present and their relative concentrations.

Erythropoiesis may be influenced by cytokines acting on committed erythroid progenitors or pluripotent stem cells. Cytokines so far implicated in the uncommitted stem cells and erythroid progenitors include IL-1, TNFα, TNFβ (LT), IL-4, IL-6, IL-3, interferonγ, type 1 interferons, TGFβ, MIP-1α (in mouse (Graham *et al.*, 1990)) and possibly GM-CSF (Donahue *et al.*, 1985) and IL-9 (Yang *et al.*, 1991). TGFβ and MIP-1α are inhibitory to the proliferation of early haemopoietic progenitor cells and IL-6 and IL-4 are co-stimulatory for a wide variety of haemopoietic cells. IL-6 has been shown to be co-stimulatory with IL-3 to early progenitor cells including CFU-S in mouse (Okano *et al.*, 1989) and also in human marrow. It is considered to be important as a mediator of the haemopoietin 1 action of IL-1. IL-4 (previously known as BSF-1) is recognized as a cofactor with IL-3 for mast cell development but is synergistic with GM-CSF and G-CSF (Rennick *et al.*, 1987; Ohara and Paul, 1987; Broxmeyer *et al.*, 1988) for haemo-

poietic colony growth. There is little evidence that IL-3 (synonymous with BPA) is produced in significant amounts in response to chronic bacterial infections. Both IL-1 and TNF have significant effects on enhancing haemopoietic stem cell proliferation directly and also indirectly, e.g. via the induction of IL-6 and the myeloid colony stimulating factors: GM-, G-, M-CSFs. IL-1 enhances stem cell survival (Moore and Warren, 1987) and synergizes with IL-3 and GM-CSF in colony formation (Zsebo *et al.*, 1988) thus it might be expected that the early progenitor cell pool would be expended in chronic infections when significant amounts of these proinflammatory mediators are produced, and that erythropoiesis might also be enhanced as a consequence of this. However, both IL-1 and TNF inhibit the later stages of erythropoiesis (Gasparetto *et al.*, 1989) leading to reduced red cell production. In the case of IL-1 at least, this block in erythroid maturation can be overcome by increased erythropoietin (Johnson *et al.*, 1989). This may explain some of the previously reported data and provides a rationale for the use of erythropoietin in the management of anaemia of chronic disease. Interferon, which is a major macrophage activating molecule and stimulator of HLA Class II expression and therefore is considered to play a major role in the maintenance of the immune response in some disease states, has been shown to be an inhibitor of erythropoiesis by several workers (Toretsky *et al.*, 1986; Zoumbos *et al.*, 1984).

Thus, in chronic bacterial infections, the sustained production of the inflammatory mediators IL-1, TNF and interferon is likely to be associated with anaemia which may be partially overcome by enhanced erythropoietin levels.

Granulopoiesis in bacterial infection

The initial leucocytosis of bacterial infection is due to mobilisation of neutrophils from the bone marrow storage pool. A wide variety of cytokines influence the distribution of neutrophils within the body depending on mobilisation from the marrow by, e.g. IL-1 (Ulich *et al.*, 1987), adhesion to endothelial cells due to enhanced expression of adhesion molecules, e.g. ICAM-1 on these cells induced by proinflammatory mediators (Dustin *et al.*, 1986), and migration into the tissues under the influence of other regulatory molecules, e.g. IL-8 and TGFβ (Brandes *et al.*, 1991; Matsushima *et al.*, 1989). Thereafter high counts are maintained by increased proliferation of myeloid precursor cells. However, in some cases of overwhelming bacterial infection the mature cells are mobilized from the marrow faster than the proliferation of new cells can occur and the patient may be neutropenic with a bone marrow showing a 'maturation arrest' picture with few mature myeloid cells and an increased proportion of blasts and promyelocytes. This can be marked enough to be mistaken for acute myeloid leukaemia. In addition, typhoid fever is characteristically associated with neutropenia, the reason being unknown. Neutropenia may also be seen in association with tuberculosis, as discussed further below.

Marrow granulopoiesis and monocytopoiesis are enhanced by haemopoietic stimulating factors which are produced by immune effector cells in response to pro-inflammatory cytokines, particularly IL-1 and TNF (Kaushansky *et al.*, 1988; Seelantag *et al.*, 1987). The haemopoietic growth factors – GM-CSF, G-CSF and M-CSF may be produced by fixed cells local to the site of inflammation including fibroblasts, endothelial cells and fixed macrophages. In addition migratory cells, particularly T-cells produce GM-CSF and IL-3 on activation. These cytokines act on committed progenitor cells in the bone marrow to enhance proliferation and production of mature cells (see Metcalf, 1986 for review). IL-3, which has a short half-life, probably has no effect except adjacent to the site of production. It may recruit blood-borne haemopoietic progenitor cells to proliferate locally, but its role in enhancing haemopoiesis is currently little understood. Not only do these haemopoietic growth factors induce proliferation of target progenitor cells (which express the appropriate receptor molecules) they also stimulate the activation of the mature cells and therefore are directly involved in the activation of bacterial cell killing. As yet there is little understanding of the role, if any, of these molecules in the determination of the commitment of multipotential haemopoietic progenitor cells along specific pathways of differentiation. In addition to the specific haemopoietic growth factors myelopoietic activity in the marrow may be modified by other pleomorphic cytokines. Thus IL-1, TNF, IL-6 and IL-4 may synergize with the haemo-

poietic growth factors to enhance haemopoiesis (see above). It is possible that combinations of one or more of the above cytokines together with the haemopoietic growth factors may favour granulocytopoiesis versus monocytopoiesis. For example, as mentioned previously, it has been shown that IL-4 inhibits M-CSF dependent colony proliferation in humans.

In addition to proliferation and activation it is necessary for migratory cells to be directed to the site of inflammation. This involves adhesion to the vascular endothelium and migration through the vessel wall. In the past few years a considerable amount of information has become available on the mechanism of adhesion with many of the pairs of molecules in the migratory cells and the endothelial cells being identified, and the importance of the upregulation on both cell types by pro-inflammatory molecules being recognized (see Springer, 1990 for review; von Andrian *et al.*, 1991; Smith *et al.*, 1989; Lawrence and Springer, 1991). Cytokines are known to be important chemotactic agents in addition to the classically identified chemotactic factors. In the recent past attention has been focused on the role of IL-8 (formerly identified as monocyte-derived neutrophil chemotactic factor – MDNCF; Matsushima *et al.*, 1989) (see van Damme, 1991 for review) which is rapidly induced in endothelial cells by IL-1. High concentrations of IL-8 lead to non-directed neutrophil movement (Hechtman *et al.*, 1991). It is therefore likely that at least one other cytokine, probably TGFβ which is known to be a potent chemotactic agent (Fava *et al.*, 1991) is involved as a second factor to enhance the specificity of neutrophil migration adjacent to the site of inflammation. Thus the initial changes in neutrophil count enhanced migratory stimulus from the peripheral blood and from the bone marrow into the circulation.

The initiation of transcription of specific haemopoietic growth factor mRNA takes 6–24 hours, therefore it is only after some time that increased marrow stimulation takes place. During acute extracellular bacterial infections enhanced phagocytic activity together with antibody production (stimulated in response to the cytokine produced by activated T helper cells) leads to resolution of the infection. The stimulus to myelopoiesis is reduced, although it is not known whether this is due to a reduction of the production of stimulatory factors concomitant with reduced lymphocyte stimulation or whether there is a positive switch-off mechanism.

In contrast to the extracellular bacteria, facultative intracellular organisms including *Listeria* and *Mycobacterium* spp. are killed by the activation of the phagocytic macrophages in which they survive. This depends to a great degree on T-cell produced cytokines. In the mouse T-cell cloning experiments have shown that although there are T-cells which produce the wide repertoire of T-cell cytokines (T H[0]) prolonged stimulation can lead to the two distinct subsets of T-cells with different cytokine profiles evolving under different conditions (Mosmann and Coffman, 1989). TH[1] cells produce IL-2, interferon γ, IL-3, GM-CSF and TNF. These cells are associated with enhanced delayed type hypersensitivity (DTH).

The second group identified as TH[2] also produce IL-3, GM-CSF and TNF but to a lesser degree than TH[1] cells, and also produce IL-5, IL-4 and IL-10 (initially identified as cytokine synthesis inhibiting factor – CSIF because of its ability to inhibit interferon γ production by TH[1] cells (Fiorentino *et al.*, 1989). The TH[2] subset are associated with enhanced IgE production and are important in parasitic infections and in allergy. In addition IL-4 and IL-10 are important in downregulating macrophage function including HLA Class II expression (de Waal Malefyt *et al.*, 1991) and IL-4 inhibits the growth of haemopoietic colonies dependent on M-CSF (Rennick, *et al.*, 1989). Therefore inappropriate production of these cytokines may have an adverse effect on the outcome of some intracellular infections and conversely failure to produce the appropriate cytokine may lead to decreased resistance to infection. Studying T cell clones in humans has not yet led to the recognition of such definitive subpopulations of T-helper cells. However there is evidence accumulating to suggest that restriction of cytokine repertoire does occur in disease states (Yssel *et al.*, quoted by de Waal Malefyt *et al.*, 1991; Haanen *et al.*, 1991). It is therefore possible that the anaemia associated with some chronic infections and other disease states, e.g. autoimmunity, reflects the repertoire of cytokines produced in these conditions, e.g. the inhibitory interferon γ which may synergize with TNF in this inhibitory effect (Broxmeyer *et al.*, 1986) versus the co-stimulatory effect (at least *in vitro*) of IL-4 and IL-6.

The marrow in specific bacterial (and fungal) infections

Tuberculosis

Secondary anaemia is common in patients with tuberculosis, and occult tuberculosis should be specifically sought for in a patient without an evident cause for anaemia of chronic disease. Changes in white cells and platelets are also well described. In a series of 265 patients with pulmonary TB, anaemia was present in 60%, neutrophilia in 40%, a raised platelet count in 52% and lymphopenia in 17% (Morris, Bird and Nell, 1989). These abnormalities resolved with treatment and failure to return to normal was invariably associated with persistent infection. Onwubalili (1990) observed the same changes in untreated patients; lymphocyte counts returned to normal within two weeks of starting therapy and normal ranges for all parameters were restored by six months. In this series and in a further series reported by Morris (1989) monocytosis was reported whereas in the series of Morris, Bird and Nell (1989) a low monocyte count was seen in half the patients.

In miliary tuberculosis lymphopenia is more frequent and neutropenia and thrombocytopenia rather than raised neutrophil and platelets counts may be seen. In a study of 109 patients with miliary tuberculosis (Maartens *et al.*, 1990), 87% were lymphopenic, 15% were leucopenic and 23% were thrombocytopenic, while pancytopenia was observed in six patients, three of whom died. Lymphopenia and thrombocytopenia were among the factors found to predict for mortality.

Little is known about any changes in bone marrow function which may be responsible for the cytopenias observed in tuberculosis. Experimental infection of mice with *M. lepraemurium* results in accumulation of monocyte precursors and macrophages in the bone marrow with a reduction in normal haemopoietic elements, accompanied by extramedullary haemopoiesis in the spleen (Resnick *et al.*, 1988a, 1988b). However, in man there is no evidence of extramedullary haemopoiesis during infection with *M. tuberculosis*. Evidence of T-cell-mediated suppression of granulopoiesis was observed in two patients with disseminated tuberculosis (Bagby and Gilbert, 1981); one was treated with prednisolone but failed to respond (Bagby *et al.*, 1983).

More profound disturbances in haemopoiesis including 'leukaemoid reactions' and aplastic anaemia have been described in association with tuberculosis (Proudfoot *et al.*, 1969; Twomey and Leavell, 1965). In the earlier literature the tuberculosis was considered to be the cause of the haematological abnormalities, but as the patients died this was not proved and there is no report of a patient with a so-called leukaemoid reaction or aplastic anaemia having recovered from infection with disappearance of the haematological abnormalities. More recently it has become clear that in the majority of cases it is the haematological disorder which is the primary factor and that cases described as leukaemoid reactions were almost certainly true leukaemia while pancytopenic patients may have underlying aplasia or myelodysplasia (Coburn *et al.*, 1973; Hunt *et al.*, 1987). The failure of cell-mediated immunity associated with leukaemia and other severe haematological disorders appears to predispose to tuberculous infection or reactivation even in the absence of immunosuppressive therapy. Coburn *et al.* (1973) showed an incidence of active tuberculous infection of 4.6% in patients with haematological disorders compared with 0.2% in all other hospital admissions, and the frequency of tuberculosis in large series of patients with leukaemia has been reported as between 6.4% and 12.8% (Muller, 1943; Lowther, 1959; Oswald, 1963). Patients with haematological disease tend to have nonreactive tuberculosis with enormous numbers of bacilli and lack of inflammatory response on tissue sections and the Mantoux test is typically negative.

Atypical mycobacteria

Mycobacterium avium intracellulare (MAI) is now well recognized in patients with AIDS (see below) and is typically associated with hypoplasia particularly affecting red cell precursors. MAI has also been described following allogeneic bone marrow transplantation (Ozkaynak *et al.*, 1990). One patient has also been reported who developed aplasia due to MAI in the absence of immunosuppression; this

MAI-associated aplastic anaemia resolved following anti-mycobacterial therapy (Fox *et al.*, 1989).

Fungal infection

Disseminated fungal infection, which usually occurs in immunosuppressed patients, is almost always associated with haematological abnormalities. Disseminated histoplasmosis in particular usually produces anaemia, leucopenia and thrombocytopenia (Goodwin *et al.*, 1980; Sarosi *et al.*, 1971). The bone marrow typically shows myeloid hyperplasia but hypoplasia of the erythroid and megakaryocyte series. The marrow is involved to a variable extent with parasitized macrophages and is one of the best sources of material for culture, being positive in approximately 50% of cases (Sarosi *et al.*, 1971). However, the severity of the haematological abnormalities correlates better with the overall severity of the infection than with the degree of involvement of the marrow itself and the changes in the marrow do not appear to result from replacement of haemopoietic cells by macrophages (Goodwin *et al.*, 1980). The inhibition of erythropoiesis by macrophages from patients with fungal infection has been discussed above.

Viral infection and the bone marrow

Viral infection and anaemia

Acute viral illnesses are not characteristically associated with the biochemical features of the acute phase response and the anaemia of chronic disorders is not a feature. However, in chronic viral illness, e.g. in immunosuppressed patients, the characteristic changes in serum iron and iron-binding capacity together with anaemia may be observed. In contrast to bacterial infection, however, there is a clear association between some viral infections and aplastic anaemia or pure red cell aplasia. Pure red cell aplasia, as its name implies, selectively affects the erythroid precursors, whereas in aplastic anaemia, the production of all cell lines is affected, implying a defect at stem cell level. The aetiology and pathogenesis of virus-induced bone marrow failure have recently been reviewed by Rosenfeld and Young (1991).

Hepatitis-associated aplastic anaemia

Clinical features

The infection most clearly associated with aplastic anaemia is hepatitis, usually non-A non-B (Camitta, Storb and Thomas, 1982). Aplastic anaemia following infectious hepatitis was first described in 1955 (Lorenz and Quaisar, 1955) and since then several hundred cases have been reported (Ajouni and Doeblin, 1974; Camitta *et al.*, 1974; Hagler, Pastore and Bergin, 1975). From 0.3 to 5.0% of cases of aplastic anaemia follow viral hepatitis (Camitta, Storb and Thomas, 1982) but only 0.1 to 0.2% of patients with hepatitis develop aplastic anaemia (Camitta, 1979). Infection with hepatitis B virus has been demonstrated only rarely in association with aplasia (Casciato *et al.*, 1978). A few cases associated with hepatitis A have been reported (Aoyagi *et al.*, 1987) but most cases are associated with non-A non-B (NANB) hepatitis (Camitta, Storb and Thomas, 1982). Earlier cases reported as being due to hepatitis A on the basis of negative results for hepatitis B antigen or antibody were probably also due to non-A non-B hepatitis. As yet there is insufficient data to indicate whether all these NANB infections are hepatitis C or whether yet another type of virus may be involved. The association of aplastic anaemia with hepatitis viruses may be under-estimated because hepatitis virus infection may occur in the absence of obvious hepatic disturbance (Kurtzman and Young, 1989).

The time from the infectious illness to the diagnosis of pancytopenia can be as long as 36 weeks, but the mean time is 8–9 weeks (Camitta *et al.*, 1974; Hagler, Pastore and Bergin, 1975), by which time liver function tests or liver biopsy usually indicate sub-acute or resolving disease. The hepatitis itself in patients who subsequently develop aplasia is not more severe than usual and there is no difference in age, sex or frequency of the HLA B8 tissue type in these patients compared with other patients with hepatitis (Camitta, 1979; Camitta *et al.*, 1974). However, nine of 32 patients undergoing liver transplant for NANB hepatitis developed aplasia which appeared to be related to the hepatitis rather than the transplant process (Tzakis *et al.*, 1988). The development of aplastic anaemia after hepatitis carries an extremely poor prognosis. This is because the degree of aplasia is usually severe, and it is the neutrophil count which is the major prognostic factor in aplastic anaemia. The overall mortality rate without marrow transplantation is over 85% (Camitta *et al.*, 1974; Hagler, Pastore and Bergin, 1975). Most of the few patients who have survived without marrow transplantation have shown evidence of improvement within two months (Camitta *et al.*, 1974; Dhingra *et al.*, 1988). On the other hand, the results of marrow transplantation for hepatitis-associated aplasia do not appear to differ from overall results from aplastic anaemia in general, which at present show 60–80% long-term survival depending largely on how early in the disease the procedure is carried out (Camitta, Storb and Thomas, 1982). The implication of these findings is that any patient who develops aplastic anaemia after hepatitis should be considered for bone marrow transplantation without delay. In the mean time, transfusion support should theoretically be kept to the minimum to avoid antigen stimulation which will increase the chances of graft rejection. However, it is even more important that the patient is in the best possible condition at transplant and in practice, this means giving platelet and red cell support; the best way to minimize transfusions is to transplant as early as possible (Gordon-Smith, 1983). If no compatible sibling donor is available the choice of treatment is between a transplant from a less than perfectly matched relative or a matched unrelated donor, or immunosuppressive therapy. Recovery following antilymphocyte globulin (ALG) has been reported (Speck, *et al.*, 1977), but the likelihood of response appears to be only about 35% which is significantly lower than that of idiopathic aplastic anaemia (Bacigalupo, 1989). This may reflect the proportion of cases with very severe aplasia rather than any aetiological factor.

Pathogenesis and aetiology

The pathogenesis of hepatitis-associated aplastic anaemia is unknown, although several possible mechanisms have been proposed (Editorial, 1965; Editorial, 1971; Alter, Potter and Li, 1978; Camitta, 1979). The subject has recently been reviewed by Kurtzman and Young (1989) and Rosenfeld and Young (1991). Liver damage *per se* is almost certainly not the cause as the hepatitis is often mild and aplasia does not follow other causes of liver damage including hepatitis B infection. The virus might infect and damage haemopoietic stem cells themselves or the accessory stromal cells of the bone marrow microenvironment. The latter seems unlikely in view of the success of marrow transplantation in curing the aplasia (although bone marrow stromal elements are capable of engraftment) and focuses attention on the stem cells themselves. These might be directly destroyed by viral infection or damaged so as to impair their capacity for self-renewal, e.g. as a result of damage to the chromosomal DNA. Inoculation of human marrow cultures with hepatitis A produces dose-dependent suppression of CFU-GM, BFU-E and CFU-GEMM (Busch *et al.*, 1987), and serum taken during the viraemic stage of NANB hepatitis infection in monkeys inhibits the growth of erythroid and granulocyte-macrophage progenitor cells from normal human bone marrow (Zeldis *et al.*, 1989). Hepatitis B infection will also suppress erythropoiesis *in vitro* (Zeldis *et al.*, 1988). Serum from hepatitis patients has been reported to produce chromosomal damage and inhibition of mitosis of leucocytes in culture (El-Alfi, Smith and Biesele, 1965; Mella and Lang, 1967). However, gross chromosome changes are infrequent in the marrow cells of patients with post-hepatitis aplasia (Hagler, Pastore and Bergin, 1975), although more studies are needed with newer banding techniques to see whether minor chromosome changes are present. Viral infection of stem cells could also induce damage directly by triggering an auto-immune response. There is no clear cut evidence for this although the response of some patients to immunosuppressive therapy would be consistent with such a hypothesis.

Suppression of marrow colony formation by lymphocytes from patients with aplastic anaemia in general has been reported, but is rare if the patient has not been sensitized by prior transfusion (Singer *et al.*, 1978). However, lymphocytes capable of suppressing bone marrow colony formation have been implicated in cases of hepatitis and infectious mononucleosis-associated aplastic anaemia (O'Reilly *et al.*, 1977; Shadduck *et al.*, 1979; Wilson, *et al.*, 1980). Other cases of aplasia with infectious mononucleosis have apparently responded to steroids (Lazarus and Baehner, 1981). Kojima *et al.* (1989) found a relative increase in activated T suppressor lymphocytes in children with hepatitis-associated aplastic anaemia, which was not seen in children with idiopathic aplasia nor in children with hepatitis who did not develop AA. Inhibitory factors in serum have been observed in patients with post-hepatitis aplasia (Burke, Karp and Schachter, 1977); serum from such patients, but not from patients with idiopathic or drug-induced aplastic anaemia, inhibited myeloid colony growth. The possible role of interferon in virus-associated aplasia is suggested by the observation of high interferon levels in patients with aplastic anaemia (Zoumbos *et al.*, 1985). Profound bone marrow suppression occurs in mice with acute lymphocyte choriomeningitis at the same time as appreciable titres of interferon are detectable in the serum and spleen extracts (Bro-Jorgensen and Knudtzon, 1977). Anaemia and a fall in leucocyte and platelet counts are common in patients being treated with either alpha- or gamma-interferon (α-IFN and γ-IFN), and both α-IFN and γ-IFN and more significantly recombinant γ-IFN, which is free of impurities, will suppress the proliferation and development of erythroid, myeloid and mixed colonies *in vitro* (Broxmeyer *et al.*, 1983, 1986; Coutinho, Testa and Dexter, 1986; Greenberg and Mosny, 1977; Lutton and Levere, 1980; Neumann and Fauser, 1982; Ortega *et al.*, 1979; Raefsky *et al.*, 1984; Verma *et al.*, 1979). However, Busch *et al.* (1987) found that inhibition of haemopoiesis by HAV was independent of IFN-α, β, γ and TNF.

Progress in understanding the aetiology of virus-associated aplasia is hampered by our lack of understanding of the pathogenesis of aplastic anaemia in general. Perhaps the most interesting unanswered question is whether as yet unidentified viruses are implicated in the pathogenesis of idiopathic aplastic anaemia.

Parvovirus B19 and pure red cell aplasia

Transient arrest of erythropoiesis (aplastic crisis) is well recognized in patients with chronic haemolytic anaemia, especially those with sickle cell disease. An infectious cause always seemed probable because of the association with symptoms such as fever and malaise, the occurrence of clusters of cases, and the absence of any recurrence after a single attack, but it was only recently that the B19 virus was identified as the infectious agent involved. This virus was first identified by chance during the routine screening of blood donor sera for hepatitis B surface antigen (Cossart *et al.*, 1975). Electron microscopy revealed small virus particles with a diameter of 22 nm and the morphological appearances of parvoviruses, a group of viruses known to cause disease in animals but not previously identified as human pathogens. The virus was initially called serum parvovirus-like virus because of its similarity to the animal parvoviruses. As further evidence has confirmed that the virus is a true parvovirus it was subsequently referred to as human parvovirus (HPV), but has now been officially designated B19 virus, B19 being the name given to the virus originally identified in one of the sera studied by Cossart. No other type of parvovirus has been implicated so far in causing disease in man.

In 1981 investigation of six children with sickle cell disease and aplastic crises showed that they either had B19 antigen in the serum or had developed B19 antibody (Pattison *et al.*, 1981). Since then several further reports have confirmed that the B19 virus is the cause of aplastic crises in children and adults with sickle cell disease and hereditary spherocytosis (Anderson *et al.*, 1982; Evans *et al.*, 1984; Goldstein *et al.*, 1987; Kelleher *et al.*, 1983; Lefrere *et al.*, 1985; Rappaport *et al.*, 1987; Saarinen *et al.*, 1986; Serjeant *et al.*, 1981) and Lefrere *et al.* (1986) described six patients with hereditary spherocytosis in whom the diagnosis was only made after they had presented with an HPV-associated aplastic crisis. There are also a few reports of B19-associated aplastic crises in patients with other types of haemolytic anaemia including thalassaemia, pyruvate kinase deficiency, paroxysmal nocturnal haemoglobinuria, and dyserythropoietic anaemia, and auto-immune haemolysis (Duncan *et al.*, 1983; Lakhani *et al.*, 1987; Rao *et al.*, 1983; Smith *et al.*, 1989; West *et al.*, 1989).

The bone marrow in B19 associated aplasia shows a marked decrease in the total number of erythroid precursors but with characteristic giant pronormoblasts. These are unusually large (up to 100 μ diameter), have deep blue cytoplasm, often vacuolated, and large nuclei which may contain multiple nucleoli or inclusion bodies. Viral proteins can be demonstrated in the cytoplasm and nucleoli of these cells using immunofluorescence techniques. Usually the diagnosis is suggested by the clinical context and can be confirmed by finding IgM antibody to B19 in the serum. Following sero-

conversion the infection normally resolves rapidly and reticulocytes reappear within the circulation, usually within a week of the clinical presentation.

More recently it has been recognized that in patients who are immunosuppressed, B19 infection can persist and cause chronic anaemia (see Frickhofen and Young, 1989 for review). This has been reported in patients with HIV, children with congenital immunodeficiency or acute lymphoblastic leukaemia in remission and patients receiving cancer chemotherapy (Kurtzman *et al.*, 1987, 1988; Graeve *et al.*, 1989; Koch *et al.*, 1990; Rao *et al.*, 1990; Mitchell *et al.*, 1990). In these patients the infection may respond to treatment with immunoglobulin (Kurtzman *et al.*, 1987; Morinet and Perol, 1990; Frickhofen *et al.*, 1990).

B19 infection is common and usually occurs during childhood; antibody is present in the serum of 30–60% of blood donors depending on the method used for detection (Cohen, Mortimer and Pereira, 1983; Cossart *et al.*, 1975). Infection may be asymptomatic or may produce fever, rashes and joint pains, a syndrome known as erythema infectiousum or 'fifth disease' (Anderson *et al.*, 1983). In a small proportion of patients purpura may be a feature, and although this is usually non-thrombocytopenic (Lefrere *et al.*, 1985), a few cases of thrombocytopenic purpura have also been recorded (Mortimer *et al.*, 1983) and careful monitoring of the platelet count in individuals infected with B19-associated red cell aplasia shows that the platelet count frequently falls although not necessarily to subnormal levels (Anderson *et al.*, 1985). Neutropenia accompanying B19 infection has also been reported (Doran and Teall, 1988) and has recently been implicated in benign infantile neutropenia.

The recognition of B19 virus as a common human pathogen raises the question of whether transient arrest of erythropoiesis occurs during infection in normal subjects but is unrecognized because it would not result in a significant fall in haemoglobin, or whether the hyperplastic marrow of patients with chronic haemolysis is particularly vulnerable. Transient red cell aplasia in patients without previous blood disorders is occasionally recognized (Bauman and Swisher, 1967; Chanarin *et al.*, 1964; Gasser, 1957) and it is possible that such cases are due to B19 infection. Studies in which normal human volunteers inoculated intranasally with B19 virus (Anderson *et al.*, 1985) showed that a short-lived but intense viraemia occurred about one week after inoculation, and in the week after the viraemia reticulocytes disappeared from the peripheral blood and there was a fall in haemoglobin of 1–2 g/dl. In addition, there was also a significant drop in neutrophil, lymphocyte and platelet counts. Culture studies of bone marrow showed that at the time of reticulocytopenia there was a virtual absence of erythroid progenitors (Potter *et al.*, 1987). It is therefore clear that the B19 virus does produce transient red cell aplasia in normal individuals and it is only the high steady state haemoglobin, the long lifespan of the normal red cells, and the transient nature of the erythroid arrest which prevent this from being clinically apparent. B19 infection has been considered as a possible cause of transient erythroblastopenia of childhood but there is no serological evidence for B19 infection in these patients (Young *et al.*, 1984), nor in adults with pure red cell aplasia or aplastic anaemia.

Serum containing B19 virus inhibits the growth of erythroid colonies *in vitro* (BFU-E and CFU-E) but not the growth of myeloid or mixed colonies (CFU-GM or CFU-GEMM), indicating that the virus affects committed erythroid progenitors rather than stem cells (Humphries *et al.*, 1983; Mortimer *et al.*, 1983; Srivastava and Lu, 1988; Young *et al.*, 1982) and the more mature CFU-E are more sensitive than the BFU-E (Saarinen *et al.*, 1986; Takahashi *et al.*, 1990; Young *et al.*, 1984). After culture in the presence of virus, B19 virus has been demonstrated within the erythroid cells by electron microscopy and specific immunofluorescence (Young *et al.*, 1984). Parvoviruses require the host cell to pass through the S-phase of the mitotic cycle for vital replication to proceed (Siegl, 1984) and this may explain why B19 virus preferentially affects the rapidly dividing erythroid cells.

Other viruses and aplastic anaemia

Dengue and similar viruses may cause aplastic anaemia although selective megakaryocyte depression is more common (Bierman and Nelson, 1965) and dengue type 4 can be propagated in human haemopoietic cells especially in BFU-E derived colonies and in erythroid cell lines (Nakao, Lai and Young, 1989). Aplastic anaemia has been described in association with infectious mononucleosis (Lazarus and Baehner, 1981; Mir and Delamore, 1973; van Doornik *et al.*, 1978). A case of aplasia associated with adenovirus infection in a child with congenital immunodeficiency has been reported (Tuvia *et al.*, 1988).

Thrombocytopenia and neutropenia in viral infection

Thrombocytopenia in viral infections appears in two main settings, first as an almost universal feature of disseminated infection in the neonate or immunosuppressed patient and second as a rare complication of acute transient infection in previously healthy subjects. There are probably two main mechanisms of thrombocytopenia which can be involved: either immune-mediated platelet destruction with or without immune-mediated megakaryocyte damage, or alternatively, direct toxicity to megakaryocytes resulting from viral infection of these cells (Fig. 1.2).

Acute viral infections often produce a mild neutropenia and are the most common cause of neutropenia in children. Influenza, infectious mononucleosis, rubella, varicella, measles and infectious hepatitis are among the viral infections frequently associated with neutropenia. Unlike the thrombocytopenia associated with viral infections, the neutropenia is mild and causes no problems, and hence its cause remains uninvestigated. However, as the neutropenia tends to occur early in the disease, before the antibody response has occurred it seems more likely to be due to an effect on neutrophil production or distribution than to immune-mediated destruction. In chronic or overwhelming viral infections, particularly with CMV and HIV, neutropenia may be more severe.

Acute idiopathic thrombocytopenic purpura (ITP)

About 80% of cases of acute ITP (that is ITP which resolves within 6–8 weeks) are preceded by a viral illness, particularly in children (Lusher and Zuelzer, 1966). The majority of such infections are non-specific upper respiratory tract infections but acute ITP has been specifically associated with measles (Fisher and Krasewski, 1952; Hudson, Weinstein and

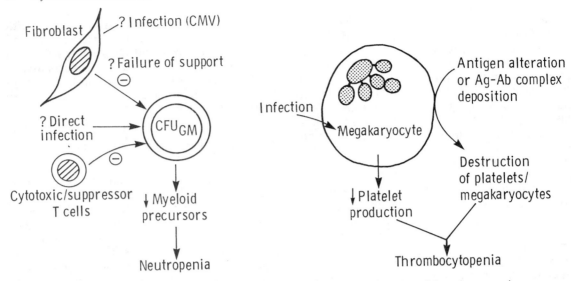

Figure 1.2 Possible pathogenetic mechanisms in virus associated neutropenia and thrombocytopenia.

Chang, 1956), rubella (Ferguson, 1960; Morse, Zinkham and Jackson, 1966; Myllyla *et al.*, 1969; Wallace, 1963), chickenpox (Welch, 1956), mumps (Fama, Paton and Bostock, 1964; Kolars and Spink, 1958), infectious mononucleosis (Carter, 1965; Clarke and Davis, 1964; Radel and Schorr, 1963), cytomegalovirus infection (Fiala and Kattlove, 1973; Chanarin and Walford, 1973; Harris, Meyer and Brody, 1975; Sahud and Bachelor, 1978), hepatitis (Woodward, 1943), cat scratch disease (Jim, 1961) and Colorado tick fever (Markovitz, 1963) and has also been reported after smallpox vaccination (Meindersma and de Vries, 1962) and vaccination with live attenuated measles virus (Alter, Scanlon and Schechter, 1968; Oski and Naiman, 1966). A more chronic form of ITP is associated with HIV infection (see below). These cases of post-viral acute ITP typically show increased numbers of megakaryocytes in the bone marrow, indicating increased peripheral destruction. The time of onset of the purpura, usually one to six weeks after the acute infection, its transient nature in most cases, and the rapid response to steroids, splenectomy or intravenous immunoglobulin are all supportive of an immune-mediated mechanism for destruction, as is the occurrence of acquired immune haemolytic anaemias in association with infec-

tions with the same viruses (Kantor *et al.*, 1970; Horowitz *et al.*, 1977; Petz and Garratty, 1980; Zuelzer *et al.*, 1966). Platelet-bound immunoglobulin can be demonstrated in approximately 60% of cases in both childhood and adult ITP (Dixon and Rosse, 1975; Luiken *et al.*, 1977; Lightsey *et al.*, 1979). Immune-mediated platelet destruction may result from non-specific adsorption onto platelets of antigen-antibody complexes rather than antibodies against the platelets themselves, because the amount of bound IgG is greater than can be accounted for by binding to platelet antigens (Lightsey *et al.*, 1979), as has been demonstrated in the case of rubella (Myllyla *et al.*, 1969) and more recently in the case of chronic ITP associated with HIV infection (Walsh, Nardi and Karpatkin, 1984).

Congenital rubella

The congenital infections which are particularly associated with thrombocytopenia are rubella and CMV, which both also produce hepatosplenomegaly and variable anaemia and leucopenia. Herpes simplex infection is in many respects similar but does not usually cause thrombocytopenia in the absence of disseminated intravascular coagulation.

In congenital rubella, thrombocytopenia is

present in about 50% of cases and may be low enough to cause purpura or bleeding; the purpura may also have a vascular component as it may occur without thrombocytopenia (Banatvala, 1965; Bayer, Sherman and Michaels, 1965; Cooper *et al.*, 1965; Rausen *et al.*, 1967; Rudolph *et al.*, 1965; Zinkham, Medearis and Osborn, 1967). Anaemia and leucopenia are also common and the anaemia appears to be at least partly haemolytic in origin (Zinkham, Medearis and Osborn, 1967). The bone marrow is usually reported as being hypocellular with decreased numbers of megakaryocytes, but this is extremely difficult to assess in neonates and in some cases which showed hypocellular aspirates, post-mortem sections of marrow revealed normal cellularity (Zinkham, Medearis and Osborn, 1967).

Rubella virus can be cultured from the bone marrow in affected babies and ability to isolate virus from the marrow is correlated with the severity of the thrombocytopenia. As the infection resolves, the thrombocytopenia improves and the temporal relation of the thrombocytopenia to the presence of virus suggests direct megakaryocyte damage rather than an immune mechanism as in the case of post-rubella ITP.

The thrombocytopenia is usually mild and self-limiting, resolving by one to four months of age. Severe bleeding including intracranial haemorrhage is rare, in contrast to neonatal immune thrombocytopenia. Platelet concentrates are not normally required, but if needed their effectiveness should be assessed on an individual basis.

CMV

In previously healthy adults with CMV infection, there is some indirect evidence for immune destruction as a cause of the thrombocytopenia. First there is an association of immune haemolytic anaemia with CMV infection. Kantor *et al.* (1970) observed transient anaemia in five of 10 patients with post-transfusion mononucleosis, with evidence of haemolysis in three cases, two of which had a positive direct antiglobulin test (DAT), while Zuelzer *et al.* (1966) described an association between transient haemolytic anaemia and CMV infection of 22 children aged 0–12 years, in 18 of whom the DAT was positive. None of these patients apparently had thrombocytopenia but Harris, Meyer and Brody (1975)

described a patient with both thrombocytopenia and haemolytic anaemia. Second, the reported patients with isolated thrombocytopenia have had normal or increased numbers of megakaryocytes in the marrow and third, they have responded to prednisolone or to splenectomy (Fiala and Kattlove, 1973; Chanarin and Walford, 1973; Harris, Meyer and Brody, 1975; Sahud and Bachelor, 1978). However, it must be said that the relation of the platelet recovery to the prednisolone therapy or splenectomy in these cases is not entirely clear and it may have been more closely related to the duration of the infection. In addition, although megakaryocyte numbers were normal, in at least one of these patients (Chanarin and Walford, 1973) the megakaryocytes showed morphological abnormalities.

In the neonate the clinical features of intra-uterine CMV infection are very similar to those of congenital rubella, although the two viruses are unrelated. Thrombocytopenia is common and a purpuric rash is seen in about 50% of severely affected infants. The thrombocytopenia may resolve rapidly or persist for several months, but significant bleeding is rare (Hanshaw, 1976). A decrease in megakaryocyte numbers with intranuclear inclusions was reported in one child with congenital CMV infection (Chesney *et al.*, 1978), suggesting a direct effect of the virus on the bone marrow.

In disseminated CMV infection in immunosuppressed patients the evidence also favours marrow toxicity as the main cause of thrombocytopenia. Thrombocytopenia is common and usually accompanied by anaemia and neutropenia (Fiala *et al.*, 1975; Ho, 1982), the latter being a poor prognostic sign (Rubin *et al.*, 1977). In bone marrow transplant recipients, CMV infection is particularly likely to cause pancytopenia and may result in graft failure. The bone marrow in patients with disseminated CMV infections shows a variable reduction in both granulopoietic precursors and megakaryocytes with toxic features such as cytoplasmic vacuolation and variable numbers of large basophilic lymphoid cells.

In experimental murine CMV (MCMV) infection, Osborn and Shahidi (1973) observed significant thrombocytopenia in all animals by day 4 after infection. The megakaryocytes showed cytoplasmic and intranuclear vacuolation and a shift towards earlier forms, suggesting increased megakaryocyte turnover, and immunofluorescent staining revealed MCMV antigen within the megakaryocytes. This evidence favoured impaired platelet production due to infection of megakaryocytes with CMV as the main factor in the thrombocytopenia. CMV infection *in vitro* also affects granulopoiesis but it is not clear whether this is a direct effect or via other cells. Forman *et al.* (1985) studied myeloid colony growth (CFU-GM) in marrow infected *in vitro* with CMV. They found that infection of the haematopoietic precursors did not affect growth, but when precursors were co-cultured with CMV-infected lymphocytes then colony growth was inhibited. Apperley, *et al.* (1989) found that incubation of progenitor cells with CMV had no effect on myeloid colony formation and CMV mRNA was not detectable in these colonies; infection of stromal monolayers however produced specific cytopathic effects and reduced the capacity of these layers to support proliferation of uninfected myeloid progenitor cells. They concluded that CMV infection impaired haemopoiesis via an effect on the marrow stroma. Simmons, Kaushansky and Torok-Storb (1990) also found that CMV inhibited colony formation in long-term cultures which in the majority of cases was associated with infection of stromal elements but in a minority of cases this was correlated with infection of the developing granulocytes. Sing and Ruscetti (1990) found that granulocyte colonies from marrow infected with CMV *in vitro* contained CMV-specific mRNA and immediate-early antigens. Thus both direct infection of myeloid precursors and secondary effects mediated by stromal cells may be present, though the balance of the current evidence favours stromal cell infection as the more important. This would be consistent with the fact that the cell which best supports CMV infection is the fibroblast (Matthews, 1979).

Megakaryocyte damage in other viral infections

In experimental animals, several viruses in addition to CMV have been found to produce morphological abnormalities of the megakaryocytes with evidence of intracellular virus. Friend leukaemia virus infection of mice produces virus particles in megakaryocytes whether or not the mice become thrombocytopenic (Dalton *et al.*, 1961). Guinea-pig megakaryocytes infected *in vitro* with Newcastle disease virus showed failure of granulation with positive immunological staining for viral antigen (Jerushalmy *et al.*, 1963) and when infected *in vitro* with encephalomyocarditis virus (which causes progressive, fatal thrombocytopenia), a similar feature of granulation and also vacuolation were observed (Modai *et al.*, 1967). Observations in patients also suggest that megakaryocyte damage may be common in virus infection. Chesney *et al.* (1978) showed intranuclear inclusions in the megakaryocytes of a child with a congenital CMV infection and thrombocytopenia and intranuclear viral particles have also been seen in the megakaryocytes of a patient with varicella and thrombocytopenia (Espinoza and Kuhn, 1974), while influenza and myxo viruses have been demonstrated within the platelets after incubation of platelets with these viruses *in vitro* (Danon, Jerushalmy and de Vries, 1959). Oski and Naiman (1966), in their study of thrombocytopenia after measles vaccination, observed a decrease in megakaryocyte numbers with vacuolation of the cytoplasm and nucleus and presented some evidence for impaired platelet production rather than increased production. Thrombocytopenia only occurred with live vaccine, showing it was not immune-mediated.

In a study of 681 patients with dengue and related diseases in Thailand (Bierman and Nelson, 1965), thrombocytopenia was found to be associated with early suppression of megakaryopoiesis and persistence of abnormal megakaryocytes in the marrow long after the blood had returned to normal. Abnormalities included loss of nuclear definition, agranular cytoplasm, vacuolation and abnormal nuclei. There was an associated but later depression of granulopoiesis.

It seems probable that overwhelming viral infection is likely to produce thrombocytopenia mainly by damage to megakaryocytes while acute transient infections with adequate antibody responses are more likely to produce thrombocytopenia via immune complex-mediated destruction. It is also possible, though there is no direct evidence for this, that initial infection of megakaryocytes may result in antigenic change which stimulates auto-antibody production.

HIV and the bone marrow

Thrombocytopenic purpura in HIV infection

A chronic form of thrombocytopenic purpura is frequent in patients with serological evidence of HIV infection (Treacy *et al.*, 1987; Karpatkin, 1984; Morris *et al.*, 1982; Walsh, Nardi and Karpatkin, 1984; Walsh *et al.*, 1985). Many of these patients are otherwise asymptomatic while others may have progressive generalized lymphadenopathy, AIDS-related complex or CDC-defined AIDS. In those with isolated thrombocytopenia who are relatively well the haematological features are identical to those of chronic autoimmune thrombocytopenia. The marrow shows normal or increased numbers of megakaryocytes and antibodies have been found on the platelets or in the serum in the majority of cases tested (Walsh, Nardi and Karpatkin, 1984). Most workers consider that these represent adsorbed antigen-antibody complexes because complement is also present on the platelet surface and the eluted immunoglobulin does not react with platelets (Walsh, Nardi and Karpatkin, 1984) although Stricker (1985) produced data suggesting that the antibody was specific for a platelet antigen. The response of these patients shows no major differences from that of chronic ITP in adults, in other words steroids and high dose intravenous immunoglobulin are both effective but the response is usually transient and splenectomy is more likely to induce a lasting remission (Abrams *et al.*, 1983; Treacy *et al.*, 1987; Walsh *et al.*, 1985). However, it is not known whether splenectomy in HIV-positive patients carries a higher than usual risk of post-splenectomy infection or whether the use of steroids or splenectomy influences the chance of progression to AIDS (Walsh *et al.*, 1985).

The bone marrow in AIDS

Several reviews have now appeared describing the changes in the peripheral blood and bone marrow in patients with AIDS (Abrams *et al.*, 1984; Castella *et al.*, 1985; Franco, Hendrix and Lokey, 1984; Spivak, Bender and Quinn, 1984; Spivak, Selonick and Quinn, 1983; Geller, Muller and Greenberg, 1985; Namiki, Boone and Meyer, 1987; Shenoy and Lin, 1986; Treacy *et al.*, 1987; Costello, 1988; Zon, Arkin and Groopman, 1987). Many of these patients by definition have had other infections in

addition to HIV, particularly CMV and *Mycobacterium avium intracellulare* (MAI) and the effect of these infections on the marrow is hard to separate from the effect of the HIV virus. The interpretation of the data is further complicated by the fact that many patients are receiving treatment with drugs known to have haematological side-effects, including zidovudine (AZT), cotrimoxazole (Septrin), pentamidine, ganciclovir and foscarnet and also by the poor nutritional status of some of these patients.

Nevertheless, a fairly clear picture emerges of peripheral blood cytopenias, in most cases with a cellular marrow showing increased histiocytes, plasma cells and atypical lymphoid cells and commonly an increase in reticulin fibrils. Over 80% of patients are anaemic (Castella *et al.*, 1985; Treacy *et al.*, 1986). Although a few patients have megaloblastic marrows, this is usually explained by folate deficiency or treatment with cotrimoxazole or AZT. More commonly anaemia shows the features of the anaemia of chronic disorders with morphological evidence of reticuloendothelial iron block in the marrow aspirate and the characteristic changes in serum iron and ferritin (Blumberg *et al.*, 1984; Castella *et al.*, 1985; Treacy *et al.*, 1987) and the degree of anaemia correlates with increases in levels of TNFα and IL-1β (Maury and Lahdevirta, 1990). Leucopenia is also common – lymphopenia is *a priori* an almost universal feature and will not be discussed further here, but neutropenia is also common, being reported in 40–60% of patients in most series (Abrams *et al.*, 1984; Castella *et al.*, 1985; Treacy *et al.*, 1987). Monocytopenia has also been observed, but more characteristic is vacuolation of the monocytes (Spivak, Bender and Quinn, 1984; Spivak, Selonick and Quinn, 1983; Treacy *et al.*, 1987). Thrombocytopenia appears to be somewhat less frequent than neutropenia in patients with AIDS, being found in 20–30% of patients. About 20% of patients show decreases in all cell types, i.e. pancytopenia, and these patients are more likely to have a hypocellular bone marrow, which in turn is usually associated with additional infection with CMV or MAI. The majority of bone marrow samples are, however, normocellular or hypercellular (83% in the largest series of 55 marrows, Castella *et al.*, 1985) and show normal numbers of erythroid and myeloid precursors with apparently normal maturation. Similarly, in the majority of patients megakaryocyte numbers are normal or increased, including in those patients with thrombocytopenia (Castella *et al.*, 1985). These findings suggest peripheral destruction as the cause of cytopenias in the majority of patients. The immunomediated platelet destruction has already been referred to and antibodies against neutrophils have also been demonstrated in some neutropenic patients (Abrams *et al.*, 1984; Murphy *et al.*, 1985). There may also be an element of hypersplenism in patients with Kaposi's sarcoma involving the spleen (Abrams *et al.*, 1984). Haemophago-cytosis with ingestion of red cells, neutrophils and platelets has been consistently observed in a variable proportion of patients and may also contribute to cytopenia (Abrams *et al.*, 1984; Castella *et al.*, 1985; Spivak, Bender and Quinn, 1984; Spivak, Selonick and Quinn, 1983; Garcia-Diaz *et al.*, 1989; Lortholary *et al.*, 1990; Sasadeusz *et al.*, 1990). Haemophago-cytosis may or may not be associated with con-current infection with CMV or Herpes simplex virus. As far as the anaemia is concerned, failure of production is more important in most cases as shown by the lack of reticulo-cytosis (Spivak, Bender and Quinn, 1984).

Numerous studies have demonstrated a reduction in numbers of myeloid and erythroid progenitors, megakaryocyte progenitors and the earlier CFU-GEMM (Lunardi-Iskander *et al.*, 1989; Ganser *et al.*, 1990; Bagnara *et al.*, 1990; Groopman, 1990). As with CMV infec-tion, there is evidence both for direct infection of haemopoietic progenitor cells and bone marrow stromal cells including fibroblasts and histiocytes (Folks *et al.*, 1988; Scadden *et al.*, 1990; Stutte *et al.*, 1990). It has been suggested that the abnormal ratio of T helper to T sup-pressor lymphocytes in the marrow may result in inhibition of erythropoiesis, but while this is an attractive hypothesis there is no direct evidence to support it. There are certainly alterations in the lymphoid population of the marrow and abnormal aggregates of lymphoid cells as well as atypical lymphocytes are fre-quently observed (Castella, *et al.*, 1985; Franco, Hendrix and Lokey, 1984; Spivak, Bender and Quinn, 1984). However, Lunardi-Iskander *et al.* observed no improvement in erythroid or myeloid colony growth following depletion of the marrow lymphocytes or macrophages or addition of normal cells. They also failed to

demonstrate *in vitro* response to addition of erythropoietin or colony stimulating factors. However, in clinical studies both anaemia and neutropenia have been shown to respond to pharmacological doses of recombinant erythro-poietin and G-CSF respectively (Miles *et al.*, 1990).

Other alterations in the bone marrow are increased numbers of plasma cells, an increase in reticulin, and the presence of granulomata. Increased numbers of plasma cells, varying from 4–16% of total nucleated cells, have been observed in the majority of patients in most series (Castella *et al.*, 1985; Franco, Hendrix and Lokey, 1984; Spivak, Bender and Quinn, 1984). An increase in reticulin was observed in 27 of 55 cases by Castella *et al.* (1985) and in 10 of 11 cases by Spivak, Bender and Quinn (1984) but in a series of British patients no increase in reticulin was observed in 20 cases although marrow was often difficult to aspirate (Treacy *et al.*, 1987). There seems to be a similar vari-ability in the frequency with which granulomata have been observed. Castella *et al.* (1985) found granulomata in eight out of 55 patients. The granulomata were mostly small and poorly formed, non-caseating and composed mainly of epitheloid histiocytes; in four cases culture of the marrow was positive for MAI and MAI was cultured at post-mortem in three of the other four cases in whom culture of the marrow proved negative. In addition, MAI was cultured from six patients in whom no granulomata was seen and in two of whom, however, AFB stains were positive, showing that some patients with MAI fail to form granulomata at all. Spivak, Bender and Quinn (1984) observed no granulo-mata in their 12 patients and no positive cultures for bacteria or fungi and Treacy *et al.* (1987) observed no granulomata in their 20 British patients including one patient in whom culture grew MAI from which the patient died.

Castella *et al.* (1985) observed a clear associ-ation of MAI infection with hypocellularity of the marrow; nine of their 55 patients had hypo-cellular marrows and five of these had MAI infection. Pure red cell hypoplasia was observed in six of 10 AIDS patients with MAI infection and MAI was cultured from the marrow in all six cases (Gardener *et al.*, 1988). Castella *et al.* concluded first that MAI should be suspected in a patient with granulomas in the marrow, even if these are poorly formed, second that AFB staining should be done routinely as this identified some culture negative patients who subsequently died with MAI, and third that hypocellularity of the marrow in AIDS patients was strongly suggestive of MAI infection even in the absence of granulomata. Persistent B19 infection should also be considered as a cause of anaemia in AIDS patients, as discussed above.

Examination of the bone marrow in patients with AIDS may show morphological evidence of other infections, particularly Leishmaniasis, toxoplasmosis, cryptococcosis and histoplasmosis, and *Pneumocystis carinii* organisms have also been identified in the bone marrow (Heymann and Rasmussen, 1987). Culture of the bone marrow is particularly useful in diagnosis of systemic opportunistic infection in these patients (Bisnburg *et al.*, 1986).

Infection-associated haemophagocytic syndrome

The increased phagocytic activity of macrophages in infections has already been referred to as an element in decreasing red cell survival and as one of the possible causes of virus-associated thrombocytopenia. In some cases the macrophage proliferation and phagocytosis of red cells, neutrophils and platelets can be so marked as to produce pancytopenia and overt haemolytic anaemia and the morphological appearances of the bone marrow can be confused with those of a malignant histiocytic proliferation. Histiocytic proliferation with haemophagocytosis was originally termed histiocytic medullary reticulosis (HMR) by Robb-Smith (1938) and subsequently this term was used synonymously with the term malignant histiocytosis. Over the past few years, however, it has become apparent that some cases reported as HMR in association with infections do not have features of the malignant disorder and represent a reactive process which can resolve with recovery of the infection (Editorial, 1983; Chandra *et al.*, 1975; Risdall *et al.*, 1979, 1984).

The haemophagocytic syndrome has been most frequently described in association with viral infections, particularly CMV and other herpes viruses including EBV and human herpes virus 6 (Adlan *et al.*, 1990; Cohen *et al.*, 1980; Mills, 1982; Risdall *et al.*, 1979; Wilson *et al.*, 1981; Huang *et al.*, 1990), but has also

been reported in association with HIV, parvovirus (B-10), coxsackie A9, adenovirus and para-influenza (Boruchoff *et al.*, 1990; Guérin *et al.*, 1989; Liu Yin *et al.*, 1983; Risdall *et al.*, 1979). Haemophagocytic syndrome has also been described in bacterial infections including tuberculosis (Chandra *et al.*, 1975; Browett *et al.*, 1988), *M. lepraemurium* infection in mice (Resnick *et al.*, 1988a), typhoid fever (Fernandez-Costa and Eintracht, 1979), *Salmonella enteritidis* (Gutierrez-Rave-Pecero *et al.*, 1990), brucellosis (Andreo *et al.*, 1988; Zuazu, Duran and Julia, 1979), Gram-negative septicaemia (Manoharan and Painter, 1982; Risdall *et al.*, 1984) and pneumococcal infection (Risdall *et al.*, 1984). It has also been seen in association with Leishmaniasis (Broeckaert-van Orshoven, Michielsen and Vandepitte, 1979; Matzner *et al.*, 1979), trichosporosis (del Palacio *et al.*, 1990) and histoplasmosis (Cooperberg and Schwartz, 1964). In both the virus- and bacteria-associated syndrome patients show severe constitutional symptoms, high fever, pancytopenia, abnormal liver function tests and evidence of disseminated intravascular coagulation. Hepatomegaly, splenomegaly, pneumonitis and skin rashes are common in virus-associated haemophagocytic syndrome but have not been features of the reported cases associated with bacterial infection (Risdall *et al.*, 1984). In some patients a source of infection is obvious but in others it has only been documented in a search for an underlying aetiology for the haemophagocytic process.

In many of the reported cases, the patients were immunosuppressed by previous chemotherapy for malignant disease (Manoharan and Painter, 1982; Liu Yin *et al.*, 1983; Risdall *et al.*, 1984) or were receiving immunosuppressive therapies following renal transplantation (Brockhaert-van Orshoven, Michielsen and Vandepitte, 1979; Risdall *et al.*, 1979). In addition, as discussed above, haemophagocytosis is a characteristic of the bone marrow in patients with AIDS. Thus infection-associated haemophagocytic syndrome may be a phenomenon of overwhelming infection, usually occurring in immunosuppressed patients but rarely also in previously healthy individuals.

Although most patients with infection-associated haemophagocytic syndrome recover, it can be fatal and requires extensive supportive care and appropriate antibiotic or anti-viral therapy. It is obviously very important to distinguish infection-associated haemophagocytic syndrome from malignant histiocytosis so as to prevent inappropriate cytotoxic chemotherapy. A search for an infective agent and careful examination of the morphology of the histiocytes will enable a correct diagnosis in most cases. The morphological differences were well described by Risdall *et al.* (1979) in their study of 19 cases of virus-associated haemophagocytic syndrome (VAHS). Both bone marrow samples and lymph node biopsies from patients with VAHS showed histiocytic hyperplasia with marked haemophagocytosis. The histiocytes had a mature appearance with a low nuclear-cytoplasmic ratio, a mature nuclear chromatin pattern, inconspicuous nuceoli and abundant cytoplasm whereas in malignant histiocytosis, the histiocytes tend to be large with a high nuclear cytoplasmic ration, a reticular chromatin pattern and variably prominent nucleoli. In VAHS the histiocytes almost all contained large numbers of ingested cells whereas in malignant histiocytosis the number of cells showing phagocytosis was much smaller. The lymph node biopsies in VAHS frequently showed histiocytes in the cortical areas but the architecture was preserved. In addition, the bone marrow from most patients with VAHS was hypocellular, though with increased megakaryocytes (Risdall *et al.*, 1979) suggesting that, as in other situations, overwhelming viral infection can damage haemopoietic precursor cells.

Abbreviations

IL-1–10	Interleukin 1–10
TNF	Tumor necrosis factor
LT	Lymphotoxin
GM-CSF	Granulocyte macrophage CSF
M-CSF	Monocyte CSF
G-CSF	Granulocyte CSF
CSF	Colony stimulating activity
BPA	Burst promoting activity
MIP	Macrophage inflammatory protein

References

Abrams, D.I., Chinn, E.K., Lewis, B.J., Volberding, P.A., Conant, M.A. and Townsend, R.M. (1984) Hematologic manifestations in homosexual men with Kaposi's sarcoma. *American Journal of Clinical Pathology*, **81**, 13–18

Abrams, D., Volberding, P., Linker, C., Kiprov, D., Moss, A., Sperling, J. and Enbury, S. (1983) Immune thrombocytopenia in homosexual men – clinical manifestations and treatment results. *Blood*, **62**, Suppl, 198a (abstract)

Adlan, K., Malnick, S.D.H. and Shattner, A. (1990) Human herpes virus 6 associated with fatal haemophagocytic syndrome. *Lancet*, **2**, 60–61 (letter)

Ajouni, K. and Doeblin, T.D. (1974) The syndrome of hepatitis and aplastic anaemia. *British Journal of Haematology*, **27**, 345–355

Al-Ismail, S., Cavill, I., Evans, I.H., Jacobs, A., Ricketts, C., Trevett, D. and Whittaker, J.A. (1979) Erythropoiesis and iron metabolism in Hodgkin's disease. *British Journal of Cancer*, **40**, 365–370

Alter, B.P., Potter, N.U. and Li, F.P. (1978) Classification and aetiology of the aplastic anaemias. *Clinics in Haematology*, **7**, 431–466

Alter, H.J., Scanlon, R. T. and Schechter, G.P. (1968) Thrombocytopenic purpura following vaccination with attenuated measles virus. *American Journal of Diseases of Children*, **115**, 111–113

Anderson, M.J., Davis, L.R., Hodgson, J., Jones, S.E., Murtaza, L., Pattison, J.R., Stroud, C.E. and White, J.M. (1982) Occurrence of infection with a parvovirus-like agent in children with sickle cell anaemia during a two year period. *Journal of Clinical Pathology*, **35**, 744–749

Anderson, M.J., Higgins, P.G., Davis, L.R., *et al.* (1985) Experimental parvoviral infections in humans. *Journal of Infectious Diseases*, **152**, 257–265

Anderson, M.J., Jones, S.E., Fischer-Hoch, S.P., Lewis, E., Hall, S.M., Bartlett, C.L.R., Cohen, B.J., Mortimer, P.P. and Pereira, M.S. (1983) Human parvovirus, the cause of erythema infectiousum (fifth disease)? *Lancet*, **1**, 1978 (letter)

Andreo, J.A., Vidal, J.B., Hernandez, J.E., Serrano, P., Lopez, V.M. and Soriano, J. (1988) Hemophagocytic syndrome associated with brucellosis. *Medical Clinics Barcelona*, **90**, 502–505

Aoyagi, K., Ohhara, N., Okamura, S., Otsuka, T., Shibuya, T., Yamano, Y. and Tsuda, Y. (1987) Aplastic anaemia associated with type A viral hepatitis – possible role of T lymphocytes. *Japan Journal of Medicine*, **26**, 348–352

Apperley, J.F., Dowding, C., Hibbin, J., Buiter, J., Matutes, E., Sissons, P.J., Gordon, M. and Goldman, J.M. (1989) The effect of cytomegalovirus on hemopoiesis: in vitro evidence for selective infection of bone marrow stromal cells. *Experimental Haematology*, **17**, 38–45

Arredondo, M.I. and Kampschmidt, R.F. (1963) Effect of endotoxins on phagocytic activity of the reticulo-endothelial system of the rat. *Proceedings of the Society for Experimental Biology and Medicine*, **112**, 78–81

Atkinson, J.P. and Frank, J.M. (1974) The effect of bacillus Calmette-Guerin-induced macrophage activation on the *in vivo* clearance of sensitised erythrocytes. *Journal of Clinical Investigation*, **53**, 1742–1749

Aye, M.T. (1977) Erythroid colony formation in cultures of human marrow: effect of leucocyte conditioned medium. *Journal of Cell Physiology*, **91**, 96–101

Bacigalupo, A. (1989) Treatment of severe aplastic anaemia. *Baillière's Clinical Haematology*, **2**(1), 19–36

Bagby, G.C. Jr. (1981) T-lymphocytes involved in inhibition of granulopoiesis in two neutropenic patients are of the cytotoxic/suppressors (T3+ T8+) subset. *Journal of Clinical Investigation*, **68**, 1597–1600

Bagby, G.C. Jr. and Gilbert, D.N. (1981) Suppression of granulopoiesis by T-lymphocytes in two patients with disseminated mycobacterial infection. *Annals of Internal Medicine*, **94**, 478–481

Bagby, G.C. Jr., Lawrence, J. and Neerhout, R.C. (1983) T-lymphocyte-mediated granulopoietic failure. In vitro identification of prednisolone responsive patients. *New England Journal of Medicine*, **309**, 1073–1078

Bagnara, G.P., Zauli, G., Giovannini, M., Re, M.C., Furlini, G. and La Placa, M. (1990) Early loss of circulating hemopoietic progenitors in HIV-infected subjects. *Experimental Haematology*, **18**, 426–430

Bainton, D.F. and Finch, C.A. (1964) The diagnosis of iron deficiency anaemia. *American Journal of Medicine*, **37**, 62–70

Banatvala, J.E. (1965) Rubella syndrome and thrombocytopenic purpura in newborn infants. *New England Journal of Medicine*, **273**, 474–478

Bauman, A.W. and Swisher, S.N. (1967) Hyporegenerative processes in hemolytic anemia. *Seminars in Haematology*, **4**, 265–272

Bayer, E.L., Sherman, F.E. and Michaels, R.H. (1965) Purpura in congenital and acquired rubella. *New England Journal of Medicine*, **273**, 1362–1366

Baynes, R.D., Flax, H., Bothwell, T.H., Bezwoda, W.R., Atkinson, P. and Mendelow, B. (1986) Red blood cell distribution width in the anaemia secondary to tuberculosis. *American Journal of Clinical Pathology*, **85**, 226–229

Beamish, M.R., Davis, A.G., Eakins, J.D., Jacobs, A. and Trevett, D. (1971) The measurement of reticuloendothelial iron release using iron-dextran. *British Journal of Haematology*, **21**, 617–622

Beamish, M.R., Jones, P.A., Trevett, D., Evans, I.H. and Jacobs, A. (1972) Iron metabolism in Hodgkin's disease. *British Journal of Cancer*, **26**, 444–452

Bennett, R.M., Holt, P.J. and Lewis, S.M. (1974) Role of the reticuloendothelial system in the anaemia of rheumatoid arthritis. A study using the 59-Fe-labelled dextran model. *Annals of Rheumatic Disease*, **33**, 147–152

Bentley, D.P., Cavill, I. and Ricketts, C. (1979) A method for the investigation of reticuloendothelial iron kinetics in man. *British Journal of Haematology*, **43**, 619–624

Bentley, D.P. and Williams, P. (1974) Serum ferritin concentration as an index of storage iron in rheumatoid arthritis. *Journal of Clinical Pathology*, **27**, 786–788

Beresford, C.H., Neale, R.J. and Brooks, O.G. (1971) Iron absorption and pyrexia. *Lancet*, **1**, 568–575

Bessman, J.D., Gilmer, P.T. and Gardner, F.H. (1983) Improved classification of anaemias by MCV and RDW. *American Journal of Clinical Pathology*, **80**, 322–326

Bierman, H.R. and Nelson, E.R. (1965) Hematodepressive virus diseases of Thailand. *Annals of Internal Medicine*, **62**, 867–884

Birgegard, G., Hallgren, R., Killander, A., Stromberg, A., Venge, P. and Wide, L. (1978) Serum ferritin during infection: a longitudinal study. *Scandinavian Journal of Haematology*, **21**, 333–340

Birgegard, G. and Caro, J. (1984) Increased ferritin synthesis and iron uptake in inflammatory mouse macrophages. *Scandinavian Journal of Haematology*, **33**, 43–48

Bisnburg, E., Eng, R.H.K., Smith, S.M. and Kapila, R. (1986) Yield of bone marrow culture in the diagnosis of infectious disease in patients with acquired immunodeficiency syndrome. *Journal of Clinical Microbiology*, **24**, 312–314

Blake, D.R., Scott, D.G., Eastham, E.J. and Rashid, H. (1980) Assessment of iron deficiency in rheumatoid arthritis. *British Medical Journal*, **280**, 527

Blumberg, R.S. and Schooley, R.T. (1985) Lymphocyte markers and infectious diseases. *Seminars in Haematology*, **22**, 81–114

Boruchoff, S.E., Woda, B.A., Pihan, G.A., Durbin, W.A., Burstein, D. and Blacklow, N.R. (1990) Parvovirus B19-associated hemophagocytic syndrome. *Archives of Internal Medicine*, **150**, 987–899

Brandes, M.E., Mai, U.E., Ohura, K. and Wahl, S.M. (1991) Type 1 transforming beta receptors on neutrophils mediate chemotaxis to transforming growth factor beta. *Journal of Immunology*, **147**, 1600–1606

Broeckaert-van Orshoven, A., Michielsen, P. and Vendepitte, J. (1979) Fatal leishmaniasis in renal transplant recipient. *Lancet*, **2**, 740–741

Bro-Jorgensen, K. and Knudtzon, S. (1977) Changes in haemopoiesis during the course of acute LCM virus infection in mice. *Blood*, **49**, 47–58

Browett, P.J., Varcoe, A.R., Fraser, A.G. and Ellis-Pegler, R.B. (1988) Disseminated tuberculosis complicated by the hemophagocytic syndrome. *Australian and New Zealand Journal of Medicine*, **18**, 79–80

Broxmeyer, H.E., Lu, L., Cooper, S., Tushinski, R., Mochizuki, D., Rubin, B.Y., Gillis, S. and Williams, D.Z. (1988) Synergistic effects of purified recombinant human and murine B cell growth factor/IL-4 on colony formation *in vitro* by haematopoietic progenitor cells – multiple actions. *Journal of Immunology*, **141**, 3852–3862

Broxmeyer, H.E., Platzer, E., Feit, C., Juliano, L. and Rubin, B.V. (1983) Comparative analysis of the influences of human gamma, alpha and beta interferons on human multipotential (CFU-GEMM), erythroid (BFU-E) and granulocyte-macrophage (CFU-GM) progenitor cells. *Journal of Immunology*, **131**, 1300–1305

Broxmeyer, H.E., Williams, D.E., Lu, L., Cooper, S.,

Anderson, S.L. *et al.* (1986) The suppressive influence of human tumor necrosis factors on bone marrow hematopoietic progenitor cells. *Journal of Immunology*, **136**, 4487–4495

Burke, P.J., Karp, J.E. and Schachter, L.P. (1977) Evidence for an etiologic role of serum inhibitor factors in patients with hepatitis related aplastic anaemia. *Experimental Haematology*, **5** (suppl. 2), 103 (abstract)

Bush, A., Ashenbrucker, H. and Cartwright, G.E. (1956) The anaemia of infection. XX. The kinetics of iron metabolism in the anaemia associated with chronic infection. *Journal of Clinical Investigation*, **35**, 89–97

Busch, F.W., de Vas, S., Flehmig, B., Herrman, F., Sandler, C. and Valbracht, A. (1987) Inhibition of *in vitro* haematopoiesis by hepatitis A virus. *Experimental Haematology*, **15**, 978–982

Camitta, B.M. (1979) The role of viral infections in aplastic anaemia. *Hematologie und Bluttransfusion*, **24**, 39–46

Camitta, B.M., Nathan, D.G., Forman, E.N., Parkman, R., Rappeport, J.M. and Orelland, T.D. (1974) Post-hepatitic severe aplastic anaemia: an indication for early bone marrow transplatation. *Blood*, **43**, 473–483

Camitta, B.M., Storb, R. and Thomas, E.D. (1982) Aplastic anaemia: pathogenesis, diagnosis, treatment and prognosis. *New England Journal of Medicine*, **306**, 645–652, 712–718

Campbell, B.C., Rennie, N., Thompson, G.G., Moore, M.R. and Goldberg, A. (1978) Haem biosynthesis in rheumatoid disease. *British Journal of Haematology*, **40**, 563–569

Carter, R.L. (1965) Platelet levels in infectious mononucleosis. *Blood*, **25**, 817–821

Cartwright, G.E. (1966) The anaemia of chronic disorders. *Seminars in Haematology*, **3**, 351–375

Cartwright, G.E. and Lee, G.R. (1971) The anaemia of chronic disorders. *British Journal of Haematology*, **21**, 147–152

Cartwright, G.E., Lauritzen, P.J. and Jones, I.M. (1946) The anaemia of infection. I. Hypoferraemia, hypercupraemia and alterations in porphyrin metabolism in patients. *Journal of Clinical Investigation*, **25**, 65–80

Casciato, D.A., Klein, C.A., Kaplowitz, N. and Scott, J.L. (1978) Aplastic anaemia associated with type B viral hepatitis. *Archives of Internal Medicine*, **138**, 1557–1558

Castella, A., Croxson, T.S., Mildvan, D., Witt, D.H. and Zalusky, R. (1985) The bone marrow in AIDS. A histologic, haematologic and microbiologic study. *American Journal of Clinical Pathology*, **84**, 425–432

Cavill, I. and Bentley, D.P. (1982) Erythropoiesis in the anaemia of rheumatoid arthritis. *British Journal of Haematology*, **50**, 583–590

Cavill, I., Ricketts, C. and Napier, J.A.F. (1977a) Ferrokinetics and erythropoiesis in man: red cell production and destruction in normal and anaemic subjects. *British Journal of Haematology*, **135**, 33–40

Cavill, I. Ricketts, C. and Napier, J.A.F. (1977b) Erythropoiesis in the anaemia of chronic disease. *Scandinavian Journal of Haematology*, **19**, 509–512

Chanarin, I., Barkhan, P., Peacock, M. and Stamp, T.C.B. (1964) Acute arrest of haematopoiesis. *British Journal of Haematology*, **10**, 43–49

Chanarin, I. and Walford, D.M. (1973) Thrombocytopenic purpura in cytomegalovirus mononucleosis. *Lancet*, **2**, 238–239

Chandra, P., Chaudhery, S.A., Rosner, F. and Kagen, M. (1975) Transient histiocytosis with striking phagocytosis of platelets, leucocytes and erythrocytes. *Archives of Internal Medicine*, **135**, 989–991

Chernow, B. and Wallner, S.F. (1978) Is the anaemia of chronic disorders normocytic-normochromic? *Military Medicine*, **143**, 345–346

Chesney, P.J., Taher, A., Gilbert, E.M.F. and Shahidi, N.T. (1978) Intranuclear inclusions in megakaryocytes in congenital cytomegalovirus infection. *Journal of Paediatrics*, **92**, 957–958

Clarke, B.F. and Davies, S.H. (1964) Severe thrombocytopenia in infectious mononucleosis. *American Journal of Medical Science*, **248**, 703–708

Coburn, R.J., England, J.M., Samson, D.M., Walford, D.M., Blowers, R., Chanarin, I., Levi, A.J. and Slavin, G. (1973) Tuberculosis and blood disorders. *British Journal of Haematology*, **25**, 793–799

Cohen, B., Mortimer, P.P. and Pereira, M.S. (1983) Diagnostic assays with monoclonal antibodies for the human serum parvovirus-like virus. *Journal of Hygiene*, **91**, 113–130

Cohen, R.A., Hutter, J.J., Boxer, M.A. and Goldman, D.S. (1980) Histocytic medullary reticulosis associated with acute Epstein-Barr virus infection. *American Journal of Pediatric Hematology and Oncology*, **2**, 245–248

Cooper, L.Z., Green, K.H., Krugman, S., Giles, J.P. and Mirick, G.S. (1965) Neonatal thrombocytopenic purpura and other manifestations of rubella contracted *in utero*. *American Journal of Diseases of Childhood*, **110**, 416–427

Cooperberg, A.A. and Schwartz, J. (1964) The diagnosis of disseminated histoplasmosis from marrow aspiration. *Annals of Internal Medicine*, **61**, 289–295

Cortell, S. and Conrad, M.E. (1967) Effect of endotoxin on iron absorption. *American Journal of Physiology*, **213**, 43–47

Cossart, Y.E., Field, A.M., Cant, N. and Widdon, S.D. (1975) Parvovirus-like particles in human sera. *Lancet*, **1**, 72–73

Costello, C. (1988) Haematological abnormalities in human immunodeficiency virus (HIV) disease. *Journal of Clinical Pathology*, **41**, 711–715

Cotes, P.M. (1982) Immunoreactive erythropoietin in human serum. *British Journal of Haematology*, **50**, 427–438

Coutinho, L.H., Testa, N.G. and Dexter, T.M. (1986) The myelosuppressive effect of recombinant interferon in short-term and long-term marrow cultures. *British Journal of Haematology*, **63**, 517–524

Dalton, A.J., Law, L.W., Moloney, J.B. and Manaker, R.A. (1961) Electron microscope studies of series of murine neoplasms. *Journal of the National Cancer Institute*, **27**, 747–791

Danon, D., Jerushalmy, Z. and de Vries, A. (1959) Incorporation of influenza virus in human blood platelets *in vivo*: Electron microscopical observation. *Virology*, **9**, 719–722 (letter)

Davidson, A., Van der Weyden, M.B., Fong, H., Breidahl, M.J. and Ryan, P.F.J. (1984) Red cell ferritin content: a re-evaluation of indices for iron-deficiency in the anaemia of rheumatoid arthritis. *British Medical Journal*, **289**, 648–650

Davies, A.G., Beamish, M.R. and Jacobs, A. (1971) Utilisation of iron-dextran. *British Medical Journal*, **1**, 146–147

Day Werts, E., Gibson, P. and DeGowin, R.L. (1979) Chronic inflammation suppresses bone marrow stromal cells and medullary erythropoiesis. *Journal of Laboratory and Clinical Medicine*, **93**, 995–1003

del Palacio, A., Perez-Revilla, A., Albanil, R., Sotelo, T. and Kalter, D.C. (1990) Disseminated neonatal trichosporosis associated with the hemophagocytic syndrome. *Pediatric Infectious Diseases Journal*, **9**, 520–522

de Waal Malefyt, Haanen, J., Smits, H., Roncarolo, M.G., te Velde, A., Figdor, G. *et al.* (1991) IL-10 and viral IL-10 strongly reduce antigenic specific human T cell proliferation. *Journal of Experimental Medicine*, **174**, 915–924

Dhingra, K., Michels, S.D., Winton, E.F. and Gordon, D.S. (1988) Transient bone marrow aplasia associated with non-A non-B hepatitis. *American Journal of Hematology*, **29**, 168–171

Dinant, J.H. and de Maat, C.E.M. (1978) Erythropoiesis and mean cell life span in normal subjects and in patients with the anaemia of active rheumatoid arthritis. *British Journal of Haematology*, **39**, 437–444

Dinarello, C.A. (1984) Interleukin-1 and the pathogenesis of the acute-phase response. *New England Journal of Medicine*, **311**, 1413–1418

Dixon, R. and Rosse, W. (1975) Platelet antibody in auto-immune thrombocytopenia. *British Journal of Haematology*, **31**, 129–134

Donahue, R.E., Emerson, S.G., Wang, E.A., Wong, G.G., Clark, S.C. and Nathan, D.G. (1985) Demonstration of burst promoting activity of recombinant human GM-CSF on circulating erythroid progenitors using an assay involving the delayed addition of erythropoietin. *Blood*, **66**, 1479–1481

Doran, J.M. and Teall, A.J. (1988) Neutropenia accompanying erythroid aplasia in human parvovirus infection. *British Journal of Haematology*, **69**, 287–288

Dormer, P., Huttner, L. and Mergenthaler, H.G. (1990) Proliferation and maturation of human bone marrow cells in infectious diseases. *Pathology Research and Practice*, **186**, 145–149

Douglas, S.W. and Adamson, J.W. (1975) The anaemia of chronic disorders: studies of marrow regulation and iron metabolism. *Blood*, **45**, 55–65

Duncan, J.R., Capellini, M.D., Anderson, M.J., Potter,

C.G., Kurtz, J.B. and Weatherall, D.J. (1983) Aplastic crisis due to parvovirus infection in pyruvate kinase deficiency. *Lancet*, **2**, 14–16

Dustin, M.L., Rothlein, R., Bhan, A.K., Dinarello, C.A. and Springer, T.A. (1986) Induction by IL-1 and inter-feron gamma: tissue, distribution, biochemistry and function of a natural adherence molecule (ICAM-1). *Journal of Immunology*, **137**, 245–254

Eaves, C.J. and Eaves, A.C. (1978) Erythropoietin (Ep) dose-response curves for three classes of progenitors in normal human marrow and in patients with poly-cythaemia vera. *Blood*, **52**, 1196–1210

Editorial (1965) Aplastic anaemia after hepatitis. *New England Journal of Medicine*, **273**, 1165–1166

Editorial (1971) Infectious hepatitis and aplastic anaemia. *Lancet*, **1**, 844–845

Editorial (1983) Histiocytic medullary reticulosis. *Lancet*, **1**, 455–456

El-Alfi, O.S., Smith, P.M. and Biesele, J.J. (1965) Chromosome breaks in human leucocyte cultures induced by an agent in the plasma of infectious hepatitis patients. *Hereditas*, **52**, 285–294

Elin, R.J., Wolff, S.M. and Finch, C.A. (1977) Effect of induced fever on serum iron and ferritin concentrations in man. *Blood*, **49**, 147–153

Espinoza, C. and Kuhn, C. (1974) Viral infection of megakaryocytes in varicella with purpura. *American Journal of Clinical Pathology*, **61**, 203–208

Evans, J.P.M., Rossiter, M.A., Kumaran, T.O., March, G.W. and Mortimer, P.P. (1984) Human parvovirus aplasia: case due to cross-infection in a ward. *British Medical Journal*, **228**, 681

Fama, P.G., Paton, W.B. and Bostock, M.I. (1964) Thrombocytopenia purpura complicating mumps. *British Medical Journal*, **2**, 1244

Fava, R.A., Olsen, N.J., Postlethwaite, A.E., Broadley, K.N., Davidson, J.M., Nonney, L.B., Lucas, C. and Townes, A.S. (1991) Transforming growth factor $\beta1$ (TGF$\beta1$) induced neutrophil recruitment to synovial tissues. *Journal of Experimental Medicine*, **173**, 1121–1132

Fernandez-Costa, F. and Eintracht, I. (1979) Histocytic medullary reticulosis. *Lancet*, **2**, 204–205

Ferguson, A.W. (1960) Rubella as a cause of thrombo-cytopenic purpura. *Paediatrics*, **25**, 400–408

Fiala, M. and Kattlove, H. (1973) Cytomegalovirus mono-nucleosis with severe thrombocytopenia. *Annals of Internal Medicine*, **79**, 450–451

Fiala, M., Payne, J.E., Berne, T.V., Moore, T.L., Henk, W., Montgomerie, J.Z., Chatterjee, S.N. and Guze, L.B. (1975) Epidemiology of cytomegalovirus after transplantation and immunosuppression. *Journal of Infectious Diseases*, **132**, 421–433

Fillet, G., Cook, J.D. and Finch, C.A. (1974) Storage iron kinetics. VIII. A biologic model for reticuloendothelial iron transport. *Journal of Clinical Investigation*, **53**, 1527–1533

Fiorentino, D.F., Bond, M.W. and Mosmann, T.R. (1989)

Two types of mouse T helper cell. IV: Th2 clones secrete a factor that inhibits cytokine production by Th1 cells. *Journal of Experimental Medicine*, **170**, 2081–2095

Firat, D. and Banzon, J. (1971) Erythropoietic effect of plasma from patients with advanced cancer. *Cancer Research*, **31**, 1355–1359

Fisher, O.D. and Kraszewski, Y.M. (1952) Thrombocytopenic purpura following measles. *Archives of Diseases of Childhood*, **27**, 144–146

Folks, T.M., Kessler, S.W., Orenstein, J.M., Justement, J.S., Jaffe, E.S. and Fanci, A.S. (1988) Infection and replication of HIV-1 in purified progenitor cells of normal human bone marrow. *Science*, **242**, 919–922

Forman, S.J., Zaia, J.A., Racklin, B.C., Wright, C.L. and Blume, K.G. (1985) *In vitro* suppression of bone marrow growth by human cytomegalovirus antigen-stimulated mononuclear cells and supernatant. *Blood*, **66**, Suppl. 1 259A (abstract)

Fox, B.L., Ross, D.D., Huang, A.B., Gabrielson, E.W. and Furth, P.A. (1989) Mycobacterial disease associated with aplastic anaemia. *Journal of Infection*, **19**, 157–165

Franco, C.M., Hendrix, L.E. and Lokey, T.L. (1984) Bone marrow abnormalities in the acquired immunodeficiency syndrome. *Annals of Internal Medicine*, **101**, 275–276 (letter)

Freiden, E. and Osaki, S. (1974) Ferroxidases and ferri-reductases: their role in iron metabolism. *Advances in Experimental Biology and Medicine*, **48**, 235–265

Freireich, E.J., Miller, A., Emerson, C.P. and Ross, J.F. (1957a) The effect of inflammation on the utilisation of erythrocyte- and transferrin-bound radioiron for red cell production. *Blood*, **12**, 972–983

Freireich, E.J., Ross, J.F., Bayles, T.B., Emerson, E.P. and Finch, S.C. (1957b) Radioactive iron metabolism and erythrocyte survival studies of the anaemia associated with rheumatoid arthritis. *Journal of Clinical Investigation*, **36**, 1043–1058

Frickhofen, N., Abkowitz, J.L., Safford, M. *et al.* (1990) Persistent B19 parvovirus infection in patients infected with human immunodeficiency virus-1: a treatable cause of anaemia in AIDS. *Annals of Internal Medicine*, **113**, 926–933

Frickhofen, N. and Young, N.S. (1989) Persistent parvovirus B19 infections in humans. *Microbial Pathogenesis*, **7**, 319–327

Fruhman, G.J. (1967) Endotoxin induced shunting of erythropoiesis in mice. *American Journal of Physiology*, **212**, 1095–1098

Furmanski, P. and Johnson, C.S. (1990) Macrophage control of normal and leukemic erythropoiesis: identification of the macrophage-derived erythroid suppressing activity as interleukin-1 and the mediator of its action as tumor necrosis factor. *Blood*, **75**, 2328–2334

Ganser, A., Ottman, O.G., von Briesen, H., Volkers, B., Rubsamen-Waigman, H. and Hoelzer, D. (1990) Changes in the haematopoietic progenitor cell compartment in the acquired immunodeficiency syndrome. *Research in Virology*, **141**, 185–193

Garcia-Diaz, J.D., Guillen-Camargo, V. and Alonso-Navas, F. (1989) Recurrent haemophagocytic syndrome and immunodeficiency virus infection. *Medical Clinics (Barcelona)*, **91**, 359

Gardener, T.D., Flanagan, P., Dryden, M.S., Costello, C., Shanson, D.C. and Gazzard, B.G. (1988) Disseminated *Mycobacterium avium-intracellulare* infection and red cell hypoplasia in patients with the acquired immune deficiency syndrome. *Journal of Infection*, **16**, 135–140

Gasparetto, C., Laver, J., Abboud, M., Gillio, A., Smith, C., O'Reilly, R.J. and Moore, M.A.S. (1989) Effects of interleukin 1 of haematopoietic progenitors: evidence of stimulatory and inhibitory activities in a primate model. *Blood*, **74**, 747–750

Gasser, C. (1957) Aplasia of erythropoiesis. *Pediatric Clinics of North America*, **4**, 445–468

Geller, S.A., Muller, R. and Greenberg, M.L. (1985) Acquired immunodeficiency syndrome: distinctive features of bone marrow biopsies. *Archives of Pathology and Laboratory Medicine*, **109**, 138–141

Goldstein, A.K., Anderson, M.J. and Serjeant, G.R. (1987) Parvovirus associated aplastic crisis in homozygous sickle cell disease. *Archives of Diseases of Childhood*, **62**, 585–588

Goodwin, R.A., Shapiro, J.L., Thurman, S.S. and Des Press, R.M. (1980) Disseminated histoplasmosis: clinical and pathological correlations. *Medicine*, **59**, 1–33

Gordon, L.I., Miller, W.J., Brandra, R.F., Zanjani, E.D. and Jacobs, H.S. (1980) Regulation of erythroid colony formation by bone marrow macrophages. *Blood*, **55**, 1047–1050

Gordon-Smith, E.C. (1983) Clinical annotation: the management of aplastic anaemia. *British Journal of Haematology*, **53**, 185–188

Graeve, J.L., de Alarcon, P.A. and Naides, S.J. (1989) Parvovirus B19 infection in patients receiving cancer chemotherapy: the expanding spectrum of disease. *American Journal of Pediatric Hematology and Oncology*, **11**, 441–444

Graham, G.J., Wright, E.S., Hewick, R., Wolpe, S.D., Wilkie, N.M., Donaldson, D., Lorimore, S. and Pragnell, I.D. (1990) Identification and characterisation of an inhibitor of haemopoietic stem cell proliferation. *Nature*, **344**, 442–444

Green, R., Charlton, R., Seftel, H., Bothwell, T., Mayet, M., Adams, B. and Finch, S.C. (1968) Body iron excretion in man, a collaborative study. *American Journal of Medicine*, **45**, 336–353

Greenberg, P.L. and Mosny, S.A. (1977) Cytotoxic effects of interferon on granulocytic progenitor cells. *Cancer Research*, **37**, 1794–1799

Groopman, J.E. (1990) Retroviral infection and haemopoiesis. *Ciba Foundation Symposium*, **148**, 173–180; discussion 180–185

Guerin, C., Pozzetto, B. and Berthoux, F. (1989) Hemophagocytic syndrome associated with coxsackie virus A9 infection in a non-immunosuppressed adult. *Intensive Care Medicine*, (letter) **15**, 547–548

Gutnitsky, A. and van Dyke, D. (1963) Normal response to erythropoietin or hypoxia in rats made anaemic with turpentine abscesses. *Proceedings of the Society for Experimental Biology and Medicine*, **112**, 75–78

Guttierez-Rave-Pecero, V., Luque-Marquez, R., Ayerza-Lerchundi, M., Canavate-Illescas, M. and Prados-Madrona, D. (1990) Reactive haemophagocytic syndrome: analysis of a series of seven cases. *Medical Clinics (Barcelona)*, **94**, 130–134

Haanen, J.B.A.S., de Waal Malefyt, R., Res, R.C.M., Kraakman, E.M., Otlenhof, T.H.M., de Vries, R.R.P. and Spits, H. (1991) Selection of human Th1 like T cell subsets by mycobacteria. *Journal of Experimental Medicine*, **174**, 583–592

Hagler, L., Pastore, R.A. and Bergin, J.V. (1975) Aplastic anaemia following viral hepatitis: report of two fatal cases and literature review. *Medicine (Baltimore)*, **54**, 139–164

Hansen, N.E., Karle, H. and Valerius, N.H. (1978) Neutrophil turnover in acute bacterial infection. *Acta Medica Scandinavica*, **204**, 407–412

Hanshaw, J.B. (1976) Cytomegalovirus. In: Remington, J.S. and Klein, J.O. (eds) *Infectious Diseases of the Fetus and Newborn Infant*. Philadelphia, W.B. Saunders & Co.

Haq, A.U., Rinehart, J.J. and Balcerzak, S.P. (1983) T cell subset modulation of blood erythroid burst-forming unit proliferation. *Journal of Laboratory and Clinical Medicine*, **101**, 53–57

Harris, A.I., Meyer, R.J. and Brody, E.A. (1975) Cytomegalovirus-induced thrombocytopenia and haemolysis in an adult. *Annals of Internal Medicine*, **83**, 670–671

Haurani, F.J., Burke, W. and Martinez, E.J. (1965) Defective iron re-utilisation in the anaemia of inflammation. *Journal of Laboratory and Clinical Medicine*, **65**, 560–570

Haurani, F.J., Green, D. and Young, K. (1965) Iron absorption in hypoferraemia. *American Journal of Medical Science*, **249**, 537–547

Haurani, F.J., Young, K. and Tocantins, L.M. (1963) Re-utilisation of iron in anaemia complicating malignant neoplasms. *Blood*, **22**, 73–81

Hechtman, D.H., Cybulsky, M.I., Fuchs, H.J., Baker, J.B. and Gimbrone, M.A. (1991) Intravascular IL-8 inhibitor of polymorphonuclear leucocyte accumulation at sites of inflammation. *Journal of Immunology*, **147**, 883–892

Hershko, C., Cook, J.D. and Finch, C.A. (1974) Storage iron kinetics. VI. The effect of inflammation on iron exchange in the rat. *British Journal of Haematology*, **28**, 67–75

Heymann, M.R. and Rasmussen, P. (1987) *Pneumocystis carinii* involvement in acquired immuno-deficiency syndrome. *American Journal of Clinical Pathology*, **87**, 780–783

Hillman, R.S. and Henderson, P.A. (1969) Control of marrow production by the level of iron supply. *Journal of Clinical Investigation*, **48**, 454–460

Ho, M. (1982) Human cytomegalovirus infections in immunosuppressed patients. In: Cytomegalovirus: Biology and Infection. Current Topics in Infectious Disease. Series eds W.B. Greenough, T.C. Merigan. New York, Plenum Medical, pp. 171–204

Hoffman, R., Kopel, S., Hsu, S.D., Dainiak, N. and Zanjani, E.D. (1978) T cell chronic lymphocytic leukaemia: presence in bone marrow and peripheral blood cells that suppress erythropoiesis in vitro. *Blood*, **52**, 255–260

Horowitz, C.A., Moulds, J., Henle, W., Henle, G., Polesky, H., Balfour, H.H., Schwart, B. and Hoff, T. (1977) Cold agglutinins in infectious mononucleosis and heterophil antibody-negative mononucleosis-like syndromes. *Blood*, **50**, 195–202

Huang, L.M., Lee, C.Y., Lin, K.H., Chau, W.M., Lee, P.I., Chen, R.L., Chen, J.M. and Lin, D.T. (1990) Human herpesvirus-6 associated with fatal haemophagocytic syndrome (letter). *Lancet*, **336**, 60–61

Hudson, J.B., Weinstein, L. and Chang, T.W. (1956) Thrombocytopenic purpura in measles. *Journal of Paediatrics*, **48**, 48–56

Humphries, R.K., Mortimer, P.P., Moore, J.G. and Young, N.S. (1983) Characterisation of a human virus causing transient aplastic crisis and inhibition of in vitro haemopoiesis. *Experimental Haematology*, **11**, (suppl. 4), 2a

Hunt, B.J., Andrews, V. and Pettingale, K.W. (1987) The significance of pancytopenia in miliary tuberculosis. *Postgraduate Medical Journal*, **63**, 801–804

Jacobs, A., Miller, F., Worwood, M., Beamish, M.R. and Wardrop, C.A. (1972) Ferritin deficiency and iron overload. *British Medical Journal*, **4**, 206–208

Jerushalmy, Z., Kaminski, E., Kohn, A. and de Vries, A. (1963) Interaction of Newcastle disease virus with megakaryocytes in cell cultures of guinea-pig bone marrow. *Proceedings of the Society for Experimental Biology and Medicine*, **114**, 687–690

Jim, R.T.S. (1961) Thrombocytopenic purpura in cat-scratch disease. *Journal of the American Medical Association*, **176**, 1036–1037

Johnson, C.S., Keckler, D.J., Topper, M.I., Braunschweiger, P.G. and Furmanski, P. (1989) In vivo hematopoietic effects of recombinant interleukin 1α in mice. *Blood*, **73**, 678–683

Joyce, R.A. and Sande, M.A. (1975) Mechanism of anaemia in experimental bacterial endocarditis. *Scandinavian Journal of Haematology*, **15**, 306–311

Kampschmidt, R.F. and Arredondo, M.I. (1963) Some effects of endotoxin on plasma iron turnover in the rat. *Proceedings of the Society for Experimental Biology and Medicine*, **113**, 142–145

Kampschmidt, R.F. and Schultz, G.A. (1961) Hypoferraemia in rats following injection of bacterial endotoxin. *Proceedings of the Society for Experimental Biology and Medicine*, **106**, 870–871

Kampschmidt, R.F. and Upchurch, H.F. (1962) Effects of bacterial endotoxin on plasma iron. *Proceedings of the Society for Experimental Biology and Medicine*, **110**, 191–193

Kampschmidt, R.F. and Upchurch, H.F. (1969) Lowering of plasma iron concentration in the rat with leucocytic extracts. *American Journal of Physiology*, **216**, 1287–1291

Kampschmidt, R.F., Upchurch, R.F. and Johnson, H.L. (1965) Iron transport after injection of endotoxin in rats. *American Journal of Physiology*, **208**, 68–72

Kanakakorn, K., Cavill, I. and Jacobs, A. (1973) The metabolism of intravenously administered iron dextran. *British Journal of Haematology*, **25**, 637–643

Kantor, G.L., Goldberg, L.S., Johnson, B.L. Jr., Derechin, M.M. and Barnett, E.V. (1970) Immunologic abnormalities induced by post-perfusion cytomegalovirus infection. *Annals of Internal Medicine*, **73**, 553–558

Karle, H. (1968a) Elevated body temperature and the survival of red blood cells. A study on experimental pyrexia in rabbits. *Acta Medica Scandinavica*, **183**, 587–592

Karle, H. (1968b) Significance of red cell age to red cell destruction during experimental pyrexia. *British Journal of Haematology*, **15**, 221–229

Karle, H. (1968c) The site of abnormal erythrocyte destruction during experimental fever. *British Journal of Haematology*, **15**, 475–485

Karle, H. (1969a) Destruction of erythrocytes during experimental fever. Quantitative aspects. *Acta Medica Scandinavica*, **186**, 349–359

Karle, H. (1969b) Effect on red cells of a small rise in temperature. *In vitro* studies. *British Journal of Haematology*, **16**, 409–419

Karle, H. (1974) The pathogenesis of the anaemia of chronic disorders and the role of fever in erythrokinetics. *Scandinavian Journal of Haematology*, **13**, 81–86

Karle, H. and Hansen, N.E. (1970) Changes in the red cell membrane induced by a small rise in temperature. *Scandinavian Journal of Clinical and Laboratory Investigation*, **26**, 169–174

Karpatkin, S. (1984) Idiopathic thrombocytopenic purpura in homosexual men. *Annals of the New York Academy of Science*, **437**, 58–64

Kaushansky, K., Broudy, V.C., Harlan, J.M. and Adamson, J.W. (1988) TNFα and TNFβ (LT) stimulate the production of GM-CSF, M-CSF and IL-1 *in vivo*. *Journal of Immunology*, **141**, 3410–3415

Kelleher, L.F., Luban, N.L.C., Mortimer, P.P. and Kanimura, T. (1983) Human serum 'parvovirus': a specific cause of aplastic crisis in children with hereditary spherocytosis. *Journal of Paediatrics*, **102**, 720–722

Keyna, U., Musslein, I., Rohwer, P., Kalden, J.R. and Manger, B. (1991) The role of transferrin receptor for the activation of human lymphocytes. *Cell Immunology*, **132**, 411–422

Koch, W.C., Massey, G., Russel, C.E. and Adler, S.P. (1990) Manifestations and treatment of human parvovirus B19 infection in immunocompromised patients. *Journal of Paediatrics*, **116**, 355–359

Koerper, M.A., Stempel, D.A. and Dallman, P.R. (1978)

Anaemia in patients with juvenile rheumatoid arthritis. *Journal of Paediatrics*, **92**, 930–933

Kojima, S., Matsuyama, K., Kodera, Y. and Okada, J. (1989) Circulating activated suppressor T-lymphocytes in hepatitis-associated aplastic anaemia. *British Journal of Haematology*, **71**, 147–151

Kolars, C.P. and Spink, W.W. (1958) Thrombocytopenic purpura as a complication of mumps. *Journal of American Medical Association*, **168**, 2213–2215

Konijn, A.M. and Herschko, C. (1977) Ferritin synthesis in inflammation. I. Pathogenesis of impaired iron release. *British Journal of Haematology*, **37**, 7–15

Konijn, A.M., Carmel, N., Levy, R. and Herschko, C. (1981) Ferritin synthesis in inflammation. II. Mechanism of increased ferritin synthesis. *British Journal of Haematology*, **49**, 361–370

Kumar, R. (1974) Ferrokinetic studies – red cell iron utilisation and red cell iron turnover – in the anaemia of chronic infection. *Indian Journal of Medical Research*, **62**, 53–64

Kumar, R. (1979) Mechanism of anaemia of chronic infection – estimation of labile iron pool and interpretation of ferrokinetic data. *Indian Journal of Medical Research*, **70**, 455–462

Kurland, J.J., Meyers, P.A. and Moore, M.A.S. (1980) Synthesis and release of erythroid colony and burst-potentiating activities by purified populations of murine peritoneal macrophages. *Journal of Experimental Medicine*, **151**, 839–852

Kurland, J. and Moore, M.A.S. (1977) Modulation of haemopoiesis by prostaglandins. *Experimental Haematology*, **5**, 357–373

Kurnick, M.J.E., Ward, H.P. and Pickett, J.C. (1972) Mechanism of the anaemia of chronic disorders. Correlation of haematocrit value with albumin, vitamin B12, transferrin and iron stores. *Archives of Internal Medicine*, **130**, 323–326

Kurtzman, G.J., Ozawa, K., Cohen, B., Hanson, G., Oseas, R. and Young, N.S. (1987) Chronic bone marrow failure due to persistent B19 parvovirus infection. *New England Journal of Medicine*, **317**, 287–294

Kurtzman, G.J., Cohen, B., Meyers, P., Amunallah, A. and Young, N.S. (1988) Persistent B19 parvovirus infection as a cause of severe chronic anaemia in children with acute lymphocytic leukaemia. *Lancet*, **2**, 1159–1162

Kurtzman, G. and Young, N. (1989) Viruses and bone marrow failure. *Baillières Clinical Haematology*, **2**(1), 51–67

Kushner, I. (1982) The phenomenon of the acute phase response. *Annals of the New York Academy of Sciences*, **389**, 39–48

Lamperi, S., Carozzi, S. and Nasini, M.G. (1986) Monocyte-macrophage mediated suppression of erythropoiesis in renal anaemia. Book of Abstracts XXI Congress of the International Society of Haematology, Sydney, p. 551 (abstr.)

Lakhani, A.K., Malkovska, V., Bevan, D.H. and Anderson, M.J. (1987) Transient pancytopenia associated with parvovirus infection in paroxysmal nocturnal haemoglobinuria. *Postgraduate Medical Journal*, **63**, 483–484

Lawrence, M.B. and Springer, T.A. (1991) Leucocytes role on a selection at physiologic flow rates distinction from and prerequisite for adhesion through integrins. *Cell*, **65**, 859–873

Lazarus, K.H. and Baehner, R.L. (1981) Aplastic anaemia complicating infectious mononucleosis: a case report and review of the literature. *Paediatrics*, **67**, 907–910

Lefrere, J.J., Courouce, A-M., *et al.* (1985) Aplastic crisis and erythema infectiosum (fifth disease) in a familial human parvovirus (HPV) infection. *British Medical Journal*, **290**, 1112

Lefrere, J.J., Courouce, A-M., Girot, R., Bertrand, Y. and Soulier, J-P. (1986) Six cases of hereditary spherocytosis revealed by human parvovirus infection. *British Journal of Haematology*, **62**, 653–658

Lewis, S.M. and Porter, I.H. (1960) Erythrocyte survival in rheumatoid arthritis. *Annals of the Rheumatic Diseases*, **19**, 54–58

Lightsey, A.L., Koenig, H.M. and McMillan, R. (1979) Platelet-associated immunoglobulin G in childhood idiopathic thrombocytopenic purpura. *Journal of Paediatrics*, **94**, 201–204

Lipschitz, D.A., Cook, J.D. and Finch, C.A. (1974) A clinical evaluation of serum ferritin as an index of iron stores. *New England Journal of Medicine*, **290**, 1213–1216

Lipschitz, D.A., Simon, M.O., Lynch, S.R., Dugard, J., Bothwell, T.H. and Charlton, R.W. (1971) Some factors affecting the release of iron from reticuloendothelial cells. *British Journal of Haematology*, **21**, 289–303

Lipton, J.M. and Nathan, D.G. (1983) Annotation: cell-cell interaction in the regulation of erythropoiesis. *British Journal of Haematology*, **53**, 366–367

Liu Yin, J.A., Kumaran, T.O., Marsh, G.W., Rossiter, M. and Catovsky, D. (1983) Complete recovery of histiocytic medullary reticulosis-like syndrome in a child with acute lymphoblastic leukaemia. *Cancer*, **51**, 200–202

Lomo, J., Smeland, E.B., Stokke, T., Holte, H., Funderud, S. and Blomhoff, H.K. (1991) Differential effects of interferon and low molecular weight BCGF on growth of human B lymphocytes. *Scandinavian Journal of Immunology*, **33**, 365–373

Lorenz, E. and Quaisar, K. (1955) Panmyelopathie nach Hepatitis epidemica. *Wien Medizine Wochenschrift*, **105**, 19–22

Lortholary, A., Raffi, F., Aubertin, P., Barrier, J.H., Boibeux, A. and Peyramond, D. (1990) HIV-associated haemophagocytic syndrome. *Lancet*, **2**, 1128 (letter)

Lowther, C.P. (1959) Leukaemia and tuberculosis. *Annals of Internal Medicine*, **51**, 52–56

Lu, L. and Broxmeyer, H.E. (1985) Comparative influences of phytohaemagglutinin-stimulated leucocyte conditioned medium, hemin, prostaglandin E, and low oxygen tension on colony formation by erythroid progenitors in normal human bone marrow. *Experimental Haematology*, **13**, 989–993

Luiken, G.A., McMillan, R., Lightsey, A.L., Gordon, P., Zevely, S., Schulman, I., Gribble, T.J. and Longmire, R.L. (1977) Platelet-associated IgG in immune thrombocytopenic purpura. *Blood*, **50**, 317–325

Lukens, J.N. (1973) Control of erythropoiesis in rats with adjuvant induced chronic inflammation. *Blood*, **41**, 37–44

Lunardi-Iskandar, V., Georgouolias, V., Bertoli, A.M., Augery-Bourget, Y., Ammar, A., Vitticoq, D., Rosenbaum, W., Meyer, P. and Jasmin, C. (1989) Impaired *in vitro* proliferation of haemopoietic precursors in HIV-1 infected subjects. *Leukaemia Research*, **13**, 573–581.

Lusher, J.M. and Zuelzer, W.W. (1966) Idiopathic thrombocytopenic purpura in childhood. *Journal of Paediatrics*, **68**, 971–979

Lutton, J.D. and Levere, R.D. (1980) Suppressive effect of human interferon on erythroid colony growth in disorders of erythropoiesis. *Journal of Laboratory and Clinical Medicine*, **96**, 328–333

Maartens, G., Willcox, P.A. and Benatar, S.R. (1990) Miliary tuberculosis: rapid diagnosis, hematologic abnormalities, and outcome in 109 treated adults. *American Journal of Medicine*, **89**, 291–296

Mahmood, T., Robinson, W.A., Kurnick, J.E. and Vautrin, R. (1977) Granulopoietic and erythropoietic activity in patients with anaemias of iron deficiency and chronic disease. *Blood*, **50**, 449–455

Mangan, K.F.G., Chikkappa, G., Bieler, L.Z., Scharfman, W.B. and Parkinson, D.R. (1982) Regulation of human blood erythroid burst-forming unit (BFU-E) proliferation by T-lymphocyte subpopulations defined by Fc receptors and monoclonal antibodies. *Blood*, **59**, 990–996

Manoharan, A. and Painter, D. (1982) Histocytic medullary reticulosis. *Lancet*, **2**, 881 (letter)

Markman, S., Ali, M., Walker, I. and Sauder, D.N. (1984) Induction of anaemia of chronic disease by chronic administration of IL-1. *Blood*, **64**, suppl. 1, 45a (abstr.)

Markowitz, A. (1963) Thrombocytopenia in Colorado tick fever. *Archives of Internal Medicine*, **111**, 307–308

Matsushima, K., Larsen, C.G., DuBois, G.C. and Oppenheim, J.J. (1989) Purification and characterisation of a novel monocyte chemotactic and activating factor produced by a human myelomonocytic cell line. *Journal of Experimental Medicine*, **169**, 1485–1490

Matthews, R.E.W. (1979) Classification and nomenclature of viruses. Third Report of the International Committee on Taxonomy of Viruses. *Intervirology*, **12**, 132–296

Matzner, Y., Behar, A., Beeri, E., Gunders, A.E. and Herschko, C. (1979) Systemic leishmaniasis mimicking malignant histiocytosis. *Cancer*, **43**, 398–402

Maury, C.P. and Lahdevirta, J. (1990) Correlation of serum cytokine levels with haemotological abnormalities in human immunodeficiency virus infection. *Journal of Internal Medicine*, **227**, 253–257

Mazur, A. and Carleton, A. (1963) Relation of ferritin iron to heme synthesis in marrow and reticulocytes. *Journal of Biological Chemistry*, **238**, 1817–1824

Mazur, A., Carleton, A. and Carlsen, A. (1961) Relation of oxidative metabolism on the incorporation of plasma iron into ferritin *in vivo. Journal of Biological Chemistry*, **236**, 1109–1116

McDonald, M.E., Smyrk, T.C., Payne, B.A. and Pierre, B.V. (1984) Evaluation of the concept of the classification of anaemia by use of the RDW/MCV. *Blood*, **64**, (suppl), 45a (abstract)

Meindersma, T.C. and de Vries, S.I. (1962) Thrombocytopenic purpura after smallpox vaccination. *British Medical Journal*, **1**, 226–228

Mella, B. and Lang, D.J. (1967) Leukocyte mitosis: suppression *in vitro* associated with acute infectious hepatitis. *Science*, **155**, 80–81

Metcalf, D. (1986) The molecular biology and functions of the granulocyte macrophage colony stimulating factors. *Blood*, **67**, 257–267

Miles, S.A., Mitsuyasu, R.T., Lee, K., Moreno, J., Alton, K., Egrie, J.C. and Souza, L. (1990) Recombinant human granulocyte colony-stimulating factor increases circulating burst-forming unit erythron and red blood cell production in patients with severe human immunodeficiency virus infection. *Blood*, **75**, 2137–2142

Mills, J. (1982) Post-viral haemophagocytic syndrome. *Journal of the Royal Society of Medicine*, **75**, 555–557

Mir, M.A. and Delamore, I.W. (1973) Aplastic anaemia complicating infectious mononucleosis. *Scandinavian Journal of Haematology*, **11**, 314–318

Mitchell, A., Welch, J.M., Weston-Smith, S., Nicholson, F. and Bradbeer, C.S. (1990) Parvovirus infection and anaemia in a patient with AIDS. Case report. *Genitourinary Medicine*, **66**, 95–96

Modai, Y., Oren, R., de Vries, A. and Kohn, A. (1967) Thrombocytopenia in guinea-pigs infected by encephalomyocarditis virus (EMC). *Thrombosis et Diathesis Hemorrhagica*, **18**, 686–690

Mongan, E.S. and Jacox, R.F. (1964) Erythrocyte survival in rheumatoid arthritis. *Arthritis and Rheumatism*, **7**, 481–486

Moore, M.A.S. and Warren, D.J. (1987) Synergy of interleukin 1 and granulocyte macrophage colony stimulating factor *in vivo. Proceedings of the National Academy of Sciences USA*, **84**, 7134–7138

Morinet, F. and Perol, Y. (1990) B19 chronic bone marrow failure: a persistent parvovirus infection of humans. *Nouv. Rev. Fr. Hematol.*, **32**(1), 91–94

Morley, J.J. and Kushner, I. (1982) Serum C-reactive protein levels in disease. *Annals of the New York Academy of Sciences*, **389**, 406–418

Morris, C.D. (1989) The radiography, haematology and biochemistry of pulmonary tuberculosis in the aged. *Quarterly Journal of Medicine*, **71**, 529–536

Morris, C.D., Bird, A.R. and Nell, H. (1989) The haematological and biochemical changes in severe pulmonary tuberculosis. *Quarterly Journal of Medicine*, **73**, 1151–1159

Morris, L., Distenfeld, A., Amorosi, E. and Karpatkin, S. (1982) Autoimmune thrombocytopenic purpura in homosexual men. *Annals of Internal Medicine*, **96**, 714–717

Morse, E.E., Zinkham, W.H. and Jackson, D.P. (1966) Thrombocytopenic purpura following rubella infections in children and adults. *Archives of Internal Medicine*, **117**, 573–579

Mortimer, P.P., Humphries, R.K., Moore, J.G., Purcell, R.H. and Young, N.S. (1983) A human parvovirus-like virus inhibits haemopoietic colony formation *in vitro. Nature*, **302**, 426–429

Mosmann, T.R. and Coffman, R.L. (1989) TH1 and TH2 cells, different patterns of lymphokine secretion lead to different functional properties. *Annals of Reviews of Immunology*, **7**, 145–173

Muller, G.L. (1943) Clinical significance of blood in tuberculosis. *Commonwealth Fund, New York*

Murphy, M.F., Metcalfe, P. and Waters, A.H. (1985) Immune neutropenia in homosexual men. *Lancet*, **1**, 217–218 (letter)

Myllyla, C., Vaheri, A., Vesikari, T. and Penttinen, K. (1969) Interaction between human blood platelets, viruses and antibodies: IV post-rubella antigen-antibody interaction. *Clinical and Experimental Immunology*, **4**, 323–332

Nagasawa, T., Abe, T. and Nakagawa, T. (1981) Pure red cell aplasia and hypogammaglobulinaemia associated with T cell chronic lymphocytic leukaemia. *Blood*, **57**, 1025–1031

Nakao, S., Lai, C.J. and Young, N.S. (1989) Dengue virus, a flavivirus, propagates in human bone marrow progenitors and hemopoietic cell lines. *Blood*, **74**, 1235–1240

Namiki, T.S., Boone, D.C. and Meyer, P.R. (1987) A comparison of bone marrow findings in patients with acquired immunodeficiency syndrome (AIDS) and AIDS-related conditions. *Haematology and Oncology*, **5**, 99–106

Neumann, H.A. and Fauser, C.A.A. (1982) Effect of interferon on pluripotent haemopoietic progenitors (CFU-GEMM) derived from human bone marrow. *Experimental Haematology*, **10**, 587–590

Nomdedeu, B., Gormus, B.J., Banisadre, M., Rinehart, J.J., Kaplan, M.E. and Zanjani, E.D. (1980) Human peripheral blood burst-forming units (BFU e): evidence against T lymphocyte requirement for proliferation *in vitro. Experimental Haematology*, **8**, 845–852

Noyes, W.D., Bothwell, T.H. and Finch, C.A. (1960) The role of the reticuloendothelial cell in iron metabolism. *British Journal of Haematology*, **6**, 43–55

Ohara, J. and Paul, W.E. (1987) Receptors for B cell stimulatory factor expressed as cells of haematopoietic lineage. *Nature*, **325**, 537–540

Okano, A., Suzuki, C., Takatsuki, F., Akiyama, Y., Koike, K., Ozawa, K., Hirano, T., Kishimoto, T., Nakahata, T. and Asano, S. (1989) *In vitro* expansion of the murine pluripotent haemopoietic stem cell population in response to interleukin 3 and interleukin 6. Application to bone marrow transplantation. *Transplantation*, **48**, 495–498

Onwubalili, J.K. (1990) Untreated tuberculosis may be associated with lymphopaenia not lymphocytosis.

African Journal of Medicine and Medical Science, **19**, 181–183

O'Reilly, R.J., Pahwa, R., Kagan, W., Kapoor, N., Sorrell, M., Meyers, P. and Good, R.A. (1977) Reconstitution of haematopoietic aplasia following high dose cyclophosphamide and allogenic foetal liver. *Experimental Haematology*, **5**, (suppl. 2), 46, (abstr.)

Ortega, J.A., Ma, A., Shore, N.A., Dukes, P.P. and Merigan, T.C. (1979) Suppressive effect of interferon on erythroid cell proliferation. *Experimental Haematology*, **7**, 145–150

Osborn, J.H. and Shahidi, N.T. (1973) Thrombocytopenia in murine cytomegalovirus infection. *Journal of Laboratory and Clinical Medicine*, **81**, 53–63

O'Shea, M.J., Kershenobich, D. and Tavill, A.S. (1973) Effects of inflammation on iron and transferrin metabolism. *British Journal of Haematology*, **25**, 707–714

Oski, F.A. and Naiman, J.L. (1966) Effect of live measles vaccine on the platelet count. *New England Journal of Medicine*, **275**, 352–356

Oswald, N.C. (1963) Acute tuberculosis and granulocytic disorders. *British Medical Journal*, **2**, 1489–1496

Ozkaynak, M.F., Lenarsky, C., Kohn, D., Weinberg, K. and Parkman, R. (1990) *Mycobacterium avium-intracellulare* infections after allogeneic bone marrow transplantation in children. *American Journal of Pediatric Hematology and Oncology*, **12**, 220–224

Pattison, J.R., Jones, S.E., Hodgson Davis, L.R., White, J.M., Stroud, C.E. and Murtaza, L. (1981) Parvovirus infection and hypoplastic crisis in sickle-cell anaemia. *Lancet*, **1**, 664–665

Pavlovic-Kentera, V., Ruvidivic, R., Milenkovic, P. and Marinkovic, D. (1979) Erythropoietin in patients with anaemia in rheumatoid arthritis. *Scandinavian Journal of Haematology*, **23**, 131–145

Pekarek, R.S., Bostian, K.A., Bartelloni, P.J., Calia, F.M. and Beisel, W.R. (1969) The effects of Francisella tularensis infection on iron metabolism in man. *American Journal of Medical Science*, **258**, 14–25

Pelus, L.M. and Bockman, R.W. (1979) Increased prostaglandin synthesis by macrophages from tumour-bearing mice. *Journal of Immunology*, **123**, 2118–2125

Petz, L.D. and Garratty, G. (1980) Classification and clinical characteristics of auto-immune haemolytic anaemias. In: *Acquired Immune Haemolytic Anaemias*, Churchill Livingstone, New York, pp. 26–63

Plana, M., Vinas, O., de la Calle-Martin, O., Lozano, F., Ingles-Esteve, J. and Romero, M. (1991) Induction of interleukin 2, interferon and enhancement of IL-2 receptor expression by a CD26 monoclonal antibody. *European Journal of Immunology*, **21**, 1085–1088

Polson, R., Jenkins, R., Lombard, M., Williams, A.C., Roberts, S., Nouri-Aria, K., Williams, R. and Bomford, A. (1990) Mechanisms of inhibition of mononuclear cell activation by the iron chelating agent desferrioxamine. *Immunology*, **71**, 176–181

Potter, B.J., Blades, B. and Rand, J.H. (1986) The role of the hepatocyte in endotoxin-induced hypoferraemia.

Book of Abstracts XXI Congress of the International Society of Haematology, Sydney, p. 469 (abstr.)

Potter, C.G., Potter, A.C., Hatton, C.S.R., Anderson, M.J., Pattison, J.R., Tyrell, D.A.J., Higgins, P.G., Willman, A.J., Cotes, P.M., Parry, H.F. and Chapel, H.M. (1987) Variation of erythroid and myeloid precursors in the marrow and peripheral blood of volunteer subjects infected with human parvovirus B19. *Journal of Clinical Investigation*, **79**, 1486–1492

Proudfoot, A.T., Akhtar, A.J., Douglas, A.C. and Horne, N.W. (1969) Miliary tuberculosis in adults. *British Medical Journal*, **2**, 273–276

Quastel, M.R. and Ross, J.F. (1966) The effect of acute inflammation on the utilisation and distribution of transferrin-bound and erythrocyte radioiron. *Blood*, **28**, 738–757

Radel, E.G. and Schorr, J.B. (1963) Thrombocytopenic purpura with infectious mononucleosis. *Journal of Paediatrics*, **63**, 46–60

Raefsky, E., Platamas, L., Zoumbos, N. and Young, N. (1984) Recombinant gamma interferon acts synergistically with alpha-interferon and interferons complete with colony stimulating factor to regulate bone marrow progenitor cell proliferation. *Blood*, **63**, 134a (abstr.)

Ragan, H.A., Nacht, S. and Lee, G.R. (1969) Effect of caeruloplasmin on plasma iron in copper deficient swine. *American Journal of Physiology*, **217**, 1320–1323

Rao, K.R.P., Patel, A.R., Anderson, M.J., Hodgson, J., Jones, S.E. and Pattison, J.R. (1983) Infection with a parvovirus-like agent and aplastic crisis in chronic haemolytic anaemia. *Annals of Internal Medicine*, **98**, 930–932

Rao, S.P., Miller, S.T. and Cohen, B.J. (1990) Severe anaemia due to B19 parvovirus infection in children with acute leukaemia in remission. *American Journal of Pediatric Hematology and Oncology*, **12**, 194–197

Rappaport, E.S., Quick, G., Ransom, D., Helbert, B. and Frankel, L.S. (1987) Aplastic crisis in occult hereditary spherocytosis caused by human parvovirus (HPV B19). *Southern Medical Journal*, **82**, 247–251

Rausen, A.R., Richter, P. and Tallal, L. (1967) Hematologic effects of intra-uterine rubella. *Journal of The American Medical Association*, **199**, 75–78

Reid, C.D.L., Baptista, L.C. and Chanarin, I. (1981) Erythroid colony growth in vitro from human peripheral blood null cell: evidence for regulation by T lymphocytes and monocytes. *British Journal of Haematology*, **48**, 155–164

Reissman, K.R. and Udupa, K. (1978) Effect of inflammation on erythroid precursors (BFU-E and CFU-E) in bone marrow and spleen of mice. *Journal of Laboratory and Clinical Medicine*, **92**, 22–29

Reizenstein, P., Gheorghescu, B. and Wiklund-Hammerstrom, B. (1975) Secondary anaemia (XII) and reticuloendothelial uptake in inflammatory disease. *Medikon (Ghent)*, **4**, 7–11

Rennick, D., Yang, G., Muller-Sieburg, C., Smith, C., Arai, A., Takabe, Y. and Gemmel, L. (1987) Interleukin

4 (B cell stimulating factor) can enhance or antagonize the factor dependent growth of haemopoetic progenitor cells. *Proceedings of the National Academy of Science USA*, **84**, 6889–6893

Rennick, D., Jackson, J., Yang, G., Wideman, J., Lee, F. and Hadak, S. (1989) Interleukin 6 interacts with interleukin 4 and other haematopoietic growth factors to selectively enhance the growth of megakaryocytic, erythroid, myeloid and multipotential progenitor cells. *Blood*, **73**, 1828–1835

Resnick, M., Ben-Ishay, Z., Mor, N., Levy, L. and Bercovier, H. (1988a) Haemophagocytosis and other haematological aspects of *Mycobacterium lepraemurium* disease of mice. *Journal of Comparative Pathology*, **99**, 65–75

Resnick, M., Fibach, E., Lebastard, M., Levy, L. and Bercovier, H. (1988b) Response of the murine haemopoietic system to chronic infection with *Mycobacterium lepraemurium*. *Infection and Immunology*, **56**, 3145–4151

Rinehart, J.J., Zanjani, E.D., Nomdedeu, B. and Gormus, B.J. (1978) Cell-cell interaction in erythropoiesis. Role of human monocytes. *Journal of Clinical Investigation*, **62**, 979–986

Risdall, R.J., Brunning, R.D., Hernandez, J.I. and Gordon, D.H. (1984) Bacteria-associated haemophagocytic syndrome. *Cancer*, **54**, 2968–2972

Risdall, R.J., McKenna, R.W. and Nesbit, M.E. (1979) Virus-associated haemophagocytic syndrome: A benign histiocytic proliferation distinct from malignant histiocytosis. *Cancer*, **44**, 993–1002

Robb-Smith, A.H.T. (1938) Reticulosis and reticulosarcoma: a histological classification. *Journal of Pathology and Bacteriology*, **47**, 457–480

Roberts, R.D., Hagedorn, A.B., Slocumb, C.H. and Owen, C.A. (1963) Evaluation of the anaemia of rheumatoid arthritis. *Blood*, **21**, 470–478

Robinson, J.C., James, G.W. and Kark, R.M. (1949) The effect of oral cobaltous chloride therapy on the blood of patients suffering with chronic suppurative infection. *New England Journal of Medicine*, **240**, 749–754

Roeser, H.P. (1980) Iron metabolism in inflammation and malignant disease. In: Jacobs, A. and Worwood, M. (eds) *Iron in Biochemistry and Medicine II*, New York, Academic Press, pp. 605–640

Roodman, G.D., Horadam, V.W. and Wright, T.L. (1983) Inhibition of erythroid colony formation by autologous bone marrow adherent cells from patients with the anaemia of chronic disease. *Blood*, **62**, 406–412

Rosenfeld, S.J. and Young, N.S. (1991) Viruses and bone marrow failure. *Blood Reviews*, **5**, 71–77

Rubin, R.H., Cosimi, A.B., Tolkoff-Rubin, N.E., Russell, P.S. and Hirsch, M.S. (1977) Infectious disease symptoms attributable to cytomegalovirus and their significance among renal transplant patients. *Transplantation*, **24**, 458–464

Rudolph, A.J., Yow, M.D., Phillips, C.A., Desmond, M.M., Blattner, R.J. and Melnick, J.L. (1965) Transplacental rubella infection in newly born infants. *Journal of the American Medical Association*, **191**, 843–845

Saarinen, U.M., Chorba, T.L., Tattersall, P., Young, N.S., Anderson, L.J., Palmer, E. and Coccia, P.F. (1986) Human parvovirus B19-induced epidemic and acute red cell aplasia in patients with hereditary haemolytic anaemia. *Blood*, **67**, 1411–1717

Sahud, M.A. and Bachelor, M.M. (1978) Cytomegalovirus-induced thrombocytopenia. An unusual case report. *Archives of Internal Medicine*, **138**, 573–575

Samson, D. (1983) Review: The anaemia of chronic disorders. *Postgraduate Medical Journal*, **549**, 543–550

Sarosi, G.A., Voth, D.W., Dahl, B.A., Doto, I.L. and Tosh, F.E. (1971) Disseminated histoplasmosis: results of long-term follow-up. *Annals of Internal Medicine*, **75**, 511–516

Sasadeusz, J., Buchanan, M. and Speed, B. (1990) Reactive haemophagocytic syndrome in human immunodeficiency virus infection. *Journal of Infection*, **20**, 65–68

Sassa, S., Kawakami, M. and Cerami, A. (1983) Inhibition of the growth and differentiation of erythroid precursor cells by an endotoxin-induced mediator from peritoneal macrophages. *Proceedings of the National Academy of Science USA*, **50**, 1717–1720

Scadden, D.T., Zeira, M., Woon, A., Wang, Z., Schieve, L., Ikeuchi, K., Lim, B. and Groopman, J.E. (1990) Human immunodeficiency virus infection of human bone marrow stromal fibroblasts. *Blood*, **76**, 317–322

Schade, S.G. (1972) Normal incorporation of oral iron into intestinal ferritin in inflammation. *Proceedings of the Society of Experimental Biological Medicine*, **139**, 620–622

Schade, S.G. and Fried, W. (1976) Suppressive effect of endotoxin on erythropoietin-responsive cells in mice. *American Journal of Physiology*, **231**, 73–76

Seelentag, W.K., Mermod, J.J., Montesano, R. and Vassali, P. (1987) Additive effects of interleukin 1 and tumor necrosis factor-alpha on the accumulation of the three granulocyte and macrophage colony stimulating factor mRNAs in human endothelial cells. *EMBO Journal*, **6**, 2261–2265

Sergeant, G.R., Tople, J.M., Mason, K., Sergeant, B.E., Pattison, J.R., Jones, S.E. and Mohamed, R. (1981) Outbreak of aplastic crisis in sickle cell anaemia associated with parvovirus-like agent. *Lancet*, **2**, 595–597

Shadduck, R.K., Winkelstein, A., Ziegler, Z., Lichter, J., Goldstein, M., Michaels, M. and Rabin, B. (1979) Aplastic anaemia following infectious mononucleosis: possible immune aetiology. *Experimental Haematology*, **7**, 264–271

Shenoy, C.M. and Lin, J.L. (1986) Bone marrow findings in acquired immunodeficiency syndrome (AIDS). *American Journal of Medical Sciences*, **292**, 372–375

Siegl, G. (1984) Biology and pathogenicity of autonomous parvoviruses. In: *The Parvoviruses*. Ed Berns, K.I. New York, Plenum Press, p. 297

Simmons, P., Kaushansky, K. and Torok-Storb, B. (1990) Mechanism of cytomegalovirus-mediated myelosuppression: perturbation of stromal cell function versus direct infection of myeloid cells. *Proceedings of the National Academy of Sciences*, **87**, 1386–1390

Sing, G.K. and Ruscetti, F.W. (1990) Preferential suppression of myelopoiesis in normal human bone marrow cells after *in vitro* challenge with human cytomegalovirus. *Blood*, **75**, 1965–1973

Singer, J.W., Brown, J.E., James, M.C., Doney, K., Warren, R.P., Storb, R. and Thomas, E.D. (1978) The effect of peripheral blood lymphocytes from patients with aplastic anaemia or granulocytic colony growth from HLA matched and mismatched marrows: the effect of transfusion sensitisation. *Blood*, **52**, 37–46

Smith, C.W., Marlin, C.D., Rothlein, R., Toman, C. and Anderson, D.C. (1989) Co-operative interactions of LFA-1 and Mac 1 with ICAM-1. *Journal of Clinical Investigation*, **83**, 2008–2017

Smith, R.J., Davis, P., Thomson, A.B., Wadsworth, C.D. and Fackre, P. (1977) Serum ferritin levels in the anaemia of rheumatoid arthritis. *Journal of Rheumatology*, **4**, 389–392

Smith, M.A., Shah, N.S. and Lobel, J.S. (1989) Parvovirus B19 infection associated with reticulocytopenia and chronic autoimmune haemolytic anaemia. *American Journal of Pediatric Hematology and Oncology*, **11**, 167–169

Speck, B., Gluckman, E., Haak, V.L. van Rood, J.J. (1977) Treatment of aplastic anaemia by antithymocyte globulin with and without allogenic bone marrow infusions. *Lancet*, **2**, 1145–1148

Spivak, J.L., Bender, B.S. and Quinn, T.C. (1984) Hematologic abnormalities in the acquired immune deficiency syndrome. *American Journal of Medicine*, **77**, 224–228

Spivak, J.L., Selonick, S.E. and Quinn, T.C. (1983) Acquired immune deficiency syndrome and pancytopenia. *Journal of the American Medical Association*, **250**, 3084–3087

Springer, T.A. (1990) Adhesion receptors of the immune system. *Nature*, **346**, 425–434

Srivastava, A. and Lu, L. (1988) Replication of B19 parvovirus in highly enriched hemopoietic progenitor cells from normal human bone marrow. *Journal of Virology*, **62**, 3059–3063

Stobo, J.D. (1977) Immunosuppression in man: suppression by macrophages can be mediated by interactions with regulatory T cells. *Journal of Immunology*, **119**, 918–924

Stobo, L.D., Paul, S., van Scoy, R.E. and Herman, P.E. (1976) Suppressor thymus-derived lymphocytes in fungal infection. *Journal of Clinical Investigation*, **57**, 319–328

Stricker, R.B., Abrams, D.I., Corash, L. and Shuman, M.A. (1985) Target platelet antigen in homosexual men with immune thrombocytopenia. *New England Journal of Medicine*, **313**, 1375–1380

Stutte, H.J., Muller, H., Falk, S. and Schmidt, H.L. (1990) Pathophysiological mechanisms of HIV-induced defects in haematopoiesis: pathology of the bone marrow. *Research in Virology*, **141**, 195–200

Summers, M.R. and Jacobs, A. (1976) Iron uptake and ferritin synthesis by peripheral blood leucocytes from normal subjects and patients with iron deficiency and the anaemia of chronic disease. *British Journal of Haematology*, **34**, 221–229

Takahashi, T., Ozawa, K., Takahashi, K., Asono, S. and Takaku, K. (1990) Susceptibility of human erythropoietic cells to B19 parvovirus in *in vitro* increases with differentiation. *Blood*, **75**, 603–610

Toretsky, J., Shahidi, N.T. and Finlay, J.L. (1986) Effects of recombinant human interferon gamma on haematopoietic progenitor cell growth. *Experimental Haematology*, **14**, 182–186

Torok-Storb, B.J., Martin, P.J. and Hansen, J.A. (1981) Regulation of *in vitro* erythropoiesis by normal T cells: evidence for two T cell subsets with opposing functions. *Blood*, **58**, 171–174

Torrance, J.D., Charlton, R.W., Simon, M.O., Lynch, S.R. and Bothwell, T.H. (1978) The mechanism of endotoxin-induced hypoferraemia. *Scandinavian Journal of Haematology*, **21**, 403–410

Treacy, M., Lai, L., Costello, C. and Clark, A. (1987) Peripheral blood and bone marrow abnormalities in patients with HIV-related disease. *British Journal of Haematology*, **65**, 289–294

Tsuji, V., Miller, L.L., Miller, S.C., Torti, S.V. and Torti, S.M. (1991) Tumour necrosis factor α and interleukin 1α regulate transferrin receptor in human diploid fibroblasts. Relationship to the induction of ferritin heavy chain. *Journal of Biological Chemistry*, **266**, 7257–7261

Tuvia, J., Weisselberg, B., Shif, I. and Keren, G. (1988) Aplastic anaemia complicating adenovirus infection in di George syndrome. *European Journal of Paediatrics*, **147**, 643–644

Twentyman, P.R. (1972) The effect of repeated doses of bacterial endotoxin on erythropoiesis in the normal and splenectomised mouse. *British Journal of Haematology*, **22**, 169–177

Twomey, J.J. and Leavell, S.S. (1965) Leukaemoid reaction to tuberculosis. *Archives of Internal Medicine*, **116**, 21–28

Tzakis, A.G., Arditi, M., Whitington, P.F., Yanaga, K., Esqvivel, C., Andrews, W.A., Makowka, L., Malatak, J., Freese, D.K. and Stock, P.G. (1988) Aplastic anaemia complicating orthotopic liver transplantation from non-A non-B hepatitis. *New England Journal of Medicine*, **319**, 393–396

Uchida, T., Yamagiwa, A. and Nakamura, K. (1991) The effect of interleukin 1 on iron metabolism in rats. *European Journal of Haematology*, **46**, 1–5

Udupa, K.B. and Reissman, K.R. (1977) *In vivo* and *in vitro* effect of bacterial endotoxin on erythroid precursors (CFU-E and ERL) in the bone marrow of mice. *Journal of Laboratory and Clinical Investigation*, **89**, 278–283

Ulich, T.R., del Castillo, J., Keys, M., Granger, G.A. and Ni, R.X. (1987) Kinetics and mechanisms of recombinant human interleukin 1 and tumor necrosis factor alpha induced changes in circulating numbers of neutrophils and lymphocytes. *Journal of Immunology*, **139**, 3406–3415

Van Damme, J. (1991) Interleukin 8 and related molecules. in, *The Cytokine Handbook*. Thompson, A. (ed.), Academic Press, London, pp. 201–214

Van Doornik, M.C., van'T Veer-Korthof, E.T. and Wierenga, H. (1978) Fatal aplastic anaemia complicating infectious mononucleosis. *Scandinavian Journal of Haematology*, **20**, 52–56

Van Snick, J.L., Masson, P.L. and Heremans, J.F. (1974) The involvement of lactoferrin in the hyposideraemia of acute inflammation. *Journal of Experimental Medicine*, **140**, 1068–1084

Verma, D.S., Spitzer, G., Gutterman, J.U., Zander, A.R., McCredie, K.B. and Dicke, K.A. (1979) Human leucocyte interferon preparation blocks granulopoietic differentiation. *Blood*, **54**, 1423–1427

Von Andrian, U.H., Chambers, D.J., McEvoy, L.M., Bargatze, R.F., Arfors, K.E. and Butcher, E.C. (1991) Two step model of leukocyte endothelial interaction in inflammation. *Proceedings of the National Academy of Science USA*, **88**, 7538–7542

Wallace, S. (1963) Thrombocytopenia purpura after rubella. *Lancet*, **1**, 139–141

Wallner, S.F., Kurnick, J.E., Vautrin, R.M., White, M.J., Chapman, R.J. and Ward, H.P. (1977) Levels of erythropoietin in patients with the anaemia of chronic diseases. *American Journal of Haematology*, **3**, 37–44

Wallner, S.F., Kurnick, J.E., Ward, H.P., Vautrin, R.M. and Alfrey, A.C. (1976) The anaemia of chronic renal failure and chronic diseases: *in vitro* studies of erythropoiesis. *Blood*, **47**, 561–569

Walsh, M., Krigel, R., Lennette, E. and Karpatkin, S. (1985) Thrombocytopenia in homosexual patients: prognosis, response to therapy and prevalence of antibody to the retrovirus associated with the acquired immunodeficiency syndrome. *Annals of Internal Medicine*, **103**, 542–545

Walsh, C.M., Nardi, M.A. and Karpatkin, S. (1984) On the mechanism of thrombocytopenia in sexually active homosexual men. *New England Journal of Medicine*, **311**, 635–639

Ward, H.P., Gordon, B. and Pickett, J.C. (1969) Serum levels of erythropoietin in rheumatoid arthritis. *Journal of Laboratory and Clinical Medicine*, **74**, 93–97

Ward, H.P., Kurnick, J.E. and Pisarczyk, M.J. (1971) Serum levels of erythropoietin in anaemias associated with chronic infections, malignancy and primary haematopoietic disease. *Journal of Clinical Investigation*, **50**, 332–335

Welch, R.G. (1956) Thrombocytopenic purpura and chickenpox. *Archives of Diseases of Childhood*, **31**, 38–41

West, N.C., Meign, R.E., Mackie, M. and Anderson, M.J. (1986) Parvovirus infection associated with aplastic crisis in a patient with HEMPAS. *Journal of Clinical Pathology*, **39**, 1019–1020

Westerman, M.P., O'Donnell, J. and Bacus, J.W. (1980) Assessment of anaemia of chronic disease by digital image processing of erythrocytes. *American Journal of Clinical Pathology*, **74**, 163–166

Wickramasinghe, S.N., Looareesuwan, S.S., Nagachinta, B. and White, N.J. (1989) Dyserythropoiesis and ineffective erythropoiesis in *Plasmodium vivax* malaria. *British Journal of Haematology*, **72**, 91–99

Williams, P., Cavill, I. and Kanakakorn, K. (1974) Iron kinetics and the anaemia of rheumatoid arthritis. *Rheumatology and Rehabilitation*, **13**, 17–20.

Williams, R.A., Samson, D., Tikerpae, J., Crowne, H. and Gumpel, J.M. (1982) In vitro studies of ineffective erythropoiesis in the anaemia of rheumatoid arthritis. *Annals of Rheumatic Disease*, **41**, 502–507

Wilson, E.R., Malluhk, A., Stagno, S. and Crist, W.M. (1981) Fatal Epstein-Barr virus-associated haemophagocytic syndrome. *Journal of Paediatrics*, **98**, 260–262

Wilson, H.A., Maclaren, G.D., Dworken, H.J. and Tebbi, K. (1980) Transient pure red cell aplasia: cell-mediated suppression of erythropoiesis associated with hepatitis. *Annals of Internal Medicine*, **92**, 196–198

Wintrobe, M.M., Grinstein, M., Dubash, J.J., Humphreys, S.R., Ashenbrucker, H. and Worth, W. (1947) The anaemia of infection. VI. The influence of cobalt on the anaemia associated with inflammation. *Blood*, **2**, 323–331

Woodward, T.E. (1943) Thrombocytopenic purpura complicating acute catarrhal jaundice: Report of a case, review of the literature, a review of 48 cases of purpura at University Hospital. *Annals of Internal Medicine*, **19**, 799–805

Yang, Y-C., Ricciadri, S., Ciarletta, A., Calvetti, J., Kelleher, K. and Clark, S.C. (1989) Expression of a cDNA encoding a novel human haemopoietic growth factor-human homologue of murine T-cell growth factor. *Blood*, **74**, 1880–1884

Young, N., Humphries, R.K., Moore, J., Purcell, R. and Mortimer, P. (1982) A human virus inhibits haematopoiesis in vitro. *Blood*, **60** (suppl. 1) 42a (abstract)

Young, N.S., Mortimer, P.P., Moor, J.G. and Humphries, R.L. (1984) Characterisation of a virus that causes transient aplastic crisis. *Journal of Clinical Investigation*, **73**, 224–230

Zanjani, E.D., McGlave, P.B., Davies, S.F., Banisadre, M., Kaplan, M.E. and Sarosi, G.A. (1982) *In vitro* suppression of erythropoiesis by bone marrow adherent cells from some patients with fungal infection. *British Journal of Haematology*, **50**, 479–490

Zarrabi, M.H., Lysik, R., Di Stefano, J. and Zucker, S. (1977) The anaemia of chronic disorders. Studies of iron re-utilisation in the anaemia of experimental malignancy and chronic inflammation. *British Journal of Haematology*, **35**, 647–658

Zeldis, J.B., Boender, P.J., Hellings, J.A. and Steinberg, H. (1989) Inhibition of human haemopoiesis by non-A non-B hepatitis virus. *Journal of Medical Virology*, **27**, 34–38

Zeldis, J.B., Farraye, F.A. and Steinberg, H.N. (1988) In vitro hepatitis B suppression of erythropoiesis is dependent on the multiplicity of infection and is reversible with anti-HBs antibodies. *Hepatology*, **8**, 755–759

Zinkham, W.H., Medearis, O.N. Jr. and Osborn, J.E.

(1967) Blood and bone marrow in congenital rubella. *Journal of Paediatrics*, **71**, 512–524

Zon, L.I., Arkin, C. and Groopman, J.E. (1987) Haematological manifestations of the human immune deficiency virus (HIV). *British Journal of Haematology*, **66**, 251–256

Zoumbos, N.C., Gascon, P., Djeu, J.Y. and Young, N.S. (1985) Interferon is a mediator of hematopoietic suppression in aplastic anemia *in vitro* and possibly *in vivo*. *Proceedings of the National Academy of Science USA*, **82**, 188–192

Zsebo, K.M., Yurschenkoff, V.N., Schiffer, S., Chong, D., McCall, E., Dinarello, C.A. *et al.* (1988) Effects of hematopoietin 1 and interleukin 1 activities on early progenitor cells of the bone marrow. *Blood*, **71**, 99–103

Zuazu, J.P., Duran, J.W. and Julia, A.F. (1979) Hemophagocytosis in acute brucellosis (Letter). *New England Journal of Medicine*, **301**s, 1185–1186

Zucker, S., Friedman, S. and Lysik, R. (1974) Bone marrow erythropoiesis in the anemia of infection, inflammation and malignancy. *Journal of Clinical Investigation*, **53**, 1132–1138

Zuelzer, W.W., Stulberg, C.S., Page, R.H., Teruya, J. and Brough, A.J. (1966) Etiology and pathogenesis of acquired hemolytic anemia. *Transfusion*, **6**, 438–460

2

Iron and infection

C.N. Gutteridge

Introduction

Micro-organisms and higher species compete for iron because of the limited bioavailability of soluble forms of iron. Animals have no mechanisms for obtaining inorganic iron and depend on pre-solubilized iron from plants, foodstuffs, micro-organisms or other animals for their source of iron. Bacteria and fungi, on the other hand, have low affinity and high affinity systems for obtaining inorganic iron from the environment. In the low affinity systems, iron is passively absorbed across the cell membrane, whereas active transport pathways and receptor molecules which may be induced by low iron levels define the high affinity systems. Competition for iron may select for micro-organisms that have developed high affinity mechanisms for obtaining iron from mammalian iron storage proteins or from intracellular pools of low molecular weight iron. In this way, host iron status and microbial iron scavenging mechanisms may be important virulence factors in infection (Weinberg, 1978; Neilands, 1980; Herschko, et al., 1988).

The mammalian host response to infection is characterized by the development of hypoferraemia. It has been argued over the last 30 years that hypoferraemia may represent an early defence mechanism to infectious organisms by inhibiting bacterial growth through iron deprivation. Kochan (1973) proposed the term 'nutritional immunity' to underscore the potential importance of iron deprivation in the initial response to bacterial invasion. There is considerable experimental data that confirms the importance of iron for bacterial growth in in vitro systems. However, clinical data supporting the concept of 'nutritional immunity' in intact hosts remains elusive. Host iron status has yet to be shown to be an important determinant in the severity and prevalence of human infectious disease. In the intact host, protection against infectious disease is provided by a variety of mechanisms. Redundancy in the immune response ensures the greatest level of protection and may result in a selective advantage. It is then, perhaps, not surprising that clinical data correlating iron status alone with outcome of infectious disease is often contradictory and confusing. This is emphasized by the fact that any disturbance of iron balance may have a deleterious effect on the immune system. Here we examine the question of iron as a virulence factor in infection by considering microbial and host requirements for iron, and examining the relationship of iron and the immune system in human studies of infection.

Iron metabolism: implications for infectious disease

Mammalian iron transport proteins

The mucosal and internal iron transport system of humans consists of transferrin, a glycoprotein with two binding sites for iron. Transferrin is approximately 30% bound with iron under normal conditions and in normal balance the concentration of free iron salts in the blood plasma is close to zero (Hershko, *et al.*, 1978; Gutteridge, *et al.*, 1981; Hershko, 1987). Similarly the iron chelating protein, lactoferrin, is present at most mucosal surfaces and in body fluids such as milk and maintains minimal free iron levels at these sites. The absence of non-chelated iron at mucosal surfaces and in the plasma has two biological consequences. First, efficient iron chelation by transferrin and lactoferrin maintains a low iron environment that inhibits bacterial growth. Second, little iron is available to catalyse oxygen radical induced tissue and microbial damage. The catalytic activity of iron in one-electron transfer reactions is reduced by the high affinity binding of iron to transferrin (Aisen, 1980; Hershko, 1987). Although lactoferrin (Winterbourn, 1983; Arouma and Halliwell, 1987) and transferrin can act as catalysts of hydroxyl radical formation, most authors have concluded that neither protein chelate is as effective as simple iron chelates (Baldwin, *et al.*, 1984; Winterbourn and Sutton, 1984). These proteins act as antioxidants in biological fluids and may be important in preventing cellular damage that would allow bacterial invasion and the release of the non-protein bound iron for bacterial use. For example, oxidative damage to neutrophil complement receptors may contribute to the pathogenesis of chronic infection in cystic fibrosis by preventing the effective phago-cytosis of opsonized micro-organisms such as *Pseudomonas aeruginosa* (Berger, *et al.*, 1989). The efficacy of transferrin and lactoferrin in preventing oxidative damage is similar at physiological pH. However at low pH values (<5–6) iron is released from transferrin and may thus become available both for microbial use and for one electron redox reactions. Lactoferrin on the other hand (Groves, 1960; Johansson, 1960) continues to bind iron at much lower pH values. The release of lactoferrin by activated adherent phagocytic cells may bind iron released from transferrin at inflammatory sites by low pH stress (Halliwell, *et al.*, 1985), and inhibit bacterial growth by iron deprivation.

Regulation of intracellular and plasma iron levels

As excess serum iron is potentially so dangerous to the host, transferrin bound iron is rapidly transferred to intracellular storage sites. Cellular uptake of iron begins with the binding of the transferrin iron complexes to specific transferrin receptors and ends with the storage of intracellular iron as ferritin or haemo-siderin. Iron procurement from the reticulo-endothelial system or by intestinal iron absorption is regulated by the erythron which has the greatest transferrin receptor mass (Huebers and Finch, 1984). Transferrin receptor density appears to be a major mechanism for controlling intracellular iron levels (Testa, *et al.*, 1989). Intracellular iron release from transferrin is an energy dependent process (Nunez, *et al.*, 1990) and results in a small intracellular pool of 'free iron' (Jacobs, 1977). The free iron pool may act as a source of iron for intracellular organisms such as the malarial parasite. *P. falciparum* obtains iron from extraerythrocytic transferrin (Pollack and Fleming, 1984) and from intracellular sources of iron (Pollack, 1987). Chelation of this source of iron markedly inhibits growth of Plasmodium species *in vitro* and *in vivo* (Hershko and Peto, 1988; Pollack, 1987; Yinnon, *et al.*, 1989). Similarly Byrd and Horwitz (1989) have shown that intracellular monocyte iron deprivation pro-duced by down regulating transferrin receptor expression may be a host defence mechanism in *Legionella pneumophilia* infections.

Failure of the regulatory system maintaining normal plasma iron levels results in iron over-load. Release of stored iron may continue in states of complete iron saturation. In this situa-tion iron exists as low molecular weight chelates which are effective in the formation of toxic oxygen species and may be available for micro-bial iron metabolism (Hershko, *et al.*, 1978; Gutteridge, *et al.*, 1985).

Iron response to inflammation

Profound changes in iron metabolism take place in response to inflammatory stress. Brief inflammatory episodes induce serum hypo-ferraemia with transient changes in trans-ferrin and ferritin levels. Prolonged inflamma-tory change produces complex changes in iron turnover and iron storage which result in dyserythropoiesis and anaemia. It is often argued that the hypoferraemic response to inflammation and infection is a protective mechanism that limits the severity of the inflammation and infection by iron deprivation.

Macrophage activation, following phago-cytosis, is an early response to bacterial invasion. Macrophages are potent producers of Interleukin 1 in response to bacterial endotoxin and other stimuli, secreting IL protein within three hours of stimulation (Windle, *et al.*, 1984). IL mediates a wide range of pro-inflammatory and immune responses that include the hypoferraemic response to infection (Dinarello, 1984). Similarly, Interleukin 6 regulates iron and transferrin levels in inflammation (Castell, *et al.*, 1989). The rapid fall in serum iron is accompanied by a reduced release of iron from tissue stores. The reduction in plasma iron turnover is accompanied by a rise in ferritin synthesis (Lipschitz, *et al.*, 1975). The rise in ferritin is an early response detectable within 24 hours of an inflammatory stress and precedes the block in iron release (Konijn and Hershko, 1977). At present it appears that IL and IL6 induce the cellular sequestration of iron and the hyperferritinaemia which characterize an inflammatory reaction although the precise mechanism by which this occurs remains unresolved.

IL$_1$ and other inflammatory mediators may alter the expression of transferrin receptors on storage cells and thus reduce serum iron and transferrin levels. Gamma interferon down-regulates the expression of transferrin receptors on human monocytes which may explain the mechanism of intracellular iron deprivation in *Legionella pneumophilia* infections (Byrd, *et al.*, 1989). However, other workers have shown that gamma interferon may stimulate the expression of transferrin receptors in human monocyte and macrophages (Taetle and Honeysett, 1988; Hirata, *et al.*, 1986). Yet in experimental *Neisseria meningitidis* infection in mice, there does not appear to be an accelerated removal of iron from the plasma transferrin pool during the hypoferraemic phase of infection (Letendre and Holbein, 1983). The kinetics of iron release during experimental *Neisseria meningitidis* infections suggest that there is impaired release of haem derived iron from the reticulo-endothelial system to the plasma trans-ferrin iron pool (Letendre and Holbein, 1984). Iron is incorporated into ferritin with very little iron being released to the transferrin plasma pool. Other studies confirm that macrophage activation may affect macrophage iron release (McGowan, *et al.*, 1986; Alvarez-Hernandez, *et al.*, 1986; Testa, *et al.*, 1989) have recently suggested that intracellular iron levels exert a negative feedback on transferrin receptor expression on cells requiring iron for pro-liferation, whereas iron levels exert a positive feedback on macrophages and iron storage cells.

Although the hypoferraemic response to infection may represent a protective mechanism whereby iron deprivation limits the severity of infection, it is uncertain whether serum iron levels reflect iron availability at inflamed or infected sites. Low molecular weight iron com-plexes in the form of bleomycin detectable iron can be demonstrated in knee joint synovial fluid from arthritic patients (Gutteridge, *et al.*, 1981; Rowley, *et al.*, 1984). Iron scavenged at local sites by bacterial siderophores may participate in the generation of hydroxyl radicals and may propagate tissue damage in this way (Coffman, *et al.*, 1990). The availability of iron in the microenvironment of an infected site with low antioxidant protection may be a key factor in determining the extent and severity of an infection. Iron enriched *Staphylococcus aureus* is more susceptible to killing by oxygen radicals and phagocytic cells (Repine, *et al.*, 1981; Hoepelman, *et al.*, 1990). Hydroxyl radical generation catalysed by bacterial iron may be important in microbial killing and inflammatory tissue injury. Control of this general mechanism may be important in preventing a self-perpetuating cycle of infection and tissue destruction. It is, perhaps, an over-simpli-fication to propose that bacterial iron depriva-tion is the main function of the hypoferraemic response to infection. The hypoferraemic response may also reduce tissue damage by limiting the oxidation potential of the extra-cellular tissue fluid. The price which the host may pay for reducing the extracellular fluid iron content is to induce the elaboration of bacterial siderophores thereby increasing microbial virulence.

Bacterial iron metabolism and virulence

The virulence of a large number of pathogens is increased if iron is administered at the time of infection (Bullen, 1981; Neilands, 1980; Finkel-stein, *et al.*, 1983). Bacterial growth has an absolute requirement for iron, and growth can be inhibited by the presence of iron binding proteins such as transferrin and lactoferrin. Most organisms have developed means of extracting iron from the host by low or high affinity pathways depending on the availability of iron in the tissue under study. The high affinity pathway is characterized by the presence of specific iron carrier molecules and bacterial membrane receptors. The specific iron carrier molecules, siderophores, compete successfully for iron with mammalian iron transport proteins. High affinity iron binding systems have been described in the majority of organisms pathogenic to man. In the low affinity pathway iron is incorporated from solution in the form of iron salts or haem iron. Bacterial mutants with no high affinity systems can proliferate as successfully as wild type cells as long as iron is available in solution at micromolar quantities. However, it seems likely that in the low iron environment of the host, successful bacterial iron scavenging due to a high affinity iron acquisition system will act as a virulence factor.

The molecular basis for the regulation of one of the high affinity iron uptake systems is now relatively well understood. In a high iron environment, iron and a gene named fur (ferric uptake regulation gene) repress the transcription of the operons of a number of iron transport proteins by inhibiting the action of RNA polymerase (Bagg and Neilands, 1987a, 1987b). The promotor regions of the genes for these transport proteins have closely related base sequences which appear to be recognized by the ferrous fur complex. The product of the fur gene is necessary for repression of the iron uptake systems of *Escherichia coli* and *Salmonella typhimurium* (Schaffer, *et al.*, 1985; Murphy, *et al.*, 1990). Fur gene product also controls the expression of receptors for colicins and phages such as the cir gene product (Griggs, *et al.*, 1990) and metalloproteins classified as superoxide dismutases (Neiderhoffer, *et al.*, 1990). In addition, the inability of fur mutants to grow in certain media independent of iron concentration (Hantke, 1987) suggests that the fur protein may provide a link between iron metabolism and the general metabolism of the organism. At present it is not known how far the principle of iron regulated protein synthesis can be applied to other bacterial species. However, it is clear that iron deprivation has a pronounced effect on bacterial metabolism and the structure of the cell envelope in pathogenic bacteria and may be important in determining bacterial virulence.

Siderophores

The iron binding proteins enterobactin and aerobactin are the best characterized bacterial siderophores. Both proteins compete with human iron transport proteins for iron. However, in physiological media, enterobactin deferrates iron from transferrin at a slower rate than aerobactin and also binds to circulating proteins such as albumin (Konopka and Neilands, 1984). Direct evidence that enterobactin is a virulence factor *in vivo* is contradictory. An association of enterobactin with virulence has been demonstrated by Rogers (1973) and Kochan (1977). Yancey (1979) isolated enterobactin deficient mutants of *Salmonella typhimurium* which showed markedly reduced virulence in a murine model of infection. However Miles and Khimji (1975) were unable to demonstrate a correlation between enterobactin production and virulence in *E. coli* and *Klebsiella* species. Similarly Benjamin, *et al.* (1985) were unable to confirm that enterobactin deficient *Salmonella* species were less virulent than enterobactin producing parent strains in the mouse typhoid model.

Aerobactin production, on the other hand, does appear to be a true virulence factor. Aerobactin deficient mutants are less virulent than their aerobactin producing parents (Miles and Khimji, 1975; Crosa, 1984). In animal models aerobactin is a virulence factor in *Klebsiella* infections of mice, *Escherichia coli* infections in chickens (Nassif and Sonsetti, 1986; Lafont, *et al.*, 1987) and *Shigella* infections of chicken embryos (Lawlor, *et al.*, 1987). Griffiths, *et al.* (1985) have suggested that aerobactin synthesis is a virulence factor for *Shigella flexneri* and *Escherichia coli* after demonstrating that aerobactin genes are found in clinical isolates of the bacteria.

Non-siderophore producing organisms may scavenge for iron by expressing surface receptors for transferrin or lactoferrin. Such receptors have been demonstrated for *Neisseria gonorrhoea* (Blanton, *et al.*, 1990), *Neisseria meningitidis* (Mickelsen and Sparling, 1981), *Haemophilus influenzae* (Schryvers, 1988), *Trichomonas vaginalis* (Petersen and Aderete, 1984), *Bordetella pertussis* (Redhead, *et al.*, 1987) and *Mycoplasma pneumoniae* (Tyron and Baseman, 1987). The transferrin receptors appear to be critical to iron scavenging: transferrin receptor low mutants are unable to grow when transferrin is the only source of iron (Blanton, *et al.*, 1990). These mutants retain the ability to use citrate iron and haem iron. The expression of transferrin receptors in Neisseria is repressed by iron (Archibald and DeVere, 1980; Simonson, *et al.*, 1982) in a manner analogous to the iron repression of siderophore production. As far as Neisseria species are concerned the presence of bacterial transferrin receptors appears to be critical for pathogenesis as no transferrin receptor negative mutant has ever been isolated *in vivo* (Holbein, 1980, 1981). The importance of lactoferrin receptors to pathogenesis is not clearly established as lactoferrin receptor negative mutants have been cultured in clinical isolates. It may be that these species obtain iron from haem iron sources, from leaked serum transferrin or by competition for siderophores produced by other microorganisms (West and Sparling, 1987).

Iron repression of the genes controlling toxin production may also be important in determining the virulence of some pathogens (Betley, *et al.*, 1986). Several investigators have shown that exotoxin A production by *Pseudomonas aeruginosa* is repressed by the presence of iron in the culture medium (Chen, *et al.*, 1987; Grant and Vasil, 1986). The production of exotoxin A is controlled by a gene designated tox A. Insertion of copies of the tox A gene do not relieve the iron inhibition of Exotoxin A production (Hindahl, *et al.*, 1987). The tox A gene is controlled by a repressor protein transcribed from a positive regulatory gene reg A (Frank, *et al.*, 1989). Comparison of the base sequences of the operon that is iron regulated with the highly conserved *E. coli* promoters for fur shows limited homology. The same *Pseudomonas* sequence, however, has perfect homology with the iron-regulated promotor sequence for diptheria toxin. Similar sequences have also been demonstrated in the regulatory genes of cholera toxin (Miller, *et al.*, 1987). Iron levels also control the production of *Clostridium tetani* (Bullen, *et al.*, 1978), *Clostridium perfringens* and *Shigella* toxins (Murphy, *et al.*, 1974). Thus, it may be that a common mechanism of regulating toxin production exists that is determined by environmental iron levels and with iron deficiency leading to the emergence of greater virulence.

Other forms of iron may reverse serum bacteriostasis (Schade and Caroline, 1944).

Haemoglobin and haem iron released during haemolysis, tissue trauma or by bacterial haemolysins can be an important source of iron for invading pathogens. Salmonellosis may accompany outbreaks of malaria and salmonella infections may be particularly severe in patients with malarial infection (Kaye, *et al.*, 1967; Weinberg, 1978). In bartonellosis, the incidence of salmonellosis may be as high as 40% (Cuadra, 1956). Intraperitoneal haemoglobin may be a virulence factor in the development of peritonitis in animal models (Burnside, *et al.*, 1968). Haptoglobin binding of free haemoglobin provides protection against *E. coli* peritonitis in rats and mice (Lee, *et al.*, 1979; Eaton, *et al.*, 1982). Haemoglobin also enhances infection with *Neisseria meningitidis* in mice (Schryvers and Gonzalez, 1989). Free haemoglobin may be an important source of iron for *Pasturella* species (Bullen and Rogers, 1968; Paerry and Brubaker, 1979). These observations suggest that there is a case for associating increased susceptibility to infection with clinical situations where haemoglobin is released which overcomes the iron deprivation imposed by host iron binding proteins. Similarly the administration of iron, sufficient to saturate plasma transferrin, enhances experimental infections with *Listeria* (Sword, 1966), *Corynebacterium* (Henderson, *et al.*, 1978), *Pseudomonas* (Forsberg and Bullen, 1972) and *E. coli* (Bullen, *et al.*, 1968). The degree of enhancement varies with both the species of bacterium and animal (Miles, *et al.*, 1979; Fletcher and Goldstein, 1970).

There are much less data examining the effect of iron deprivation on clinical infections in animal models. Reducing serum iron levels by the injection of endotoxin may improve survival in experimental infections with *Candida albicans* or *Salmonella typhimurium* (Elin and Wolff, 1974; Kampschmidt and Pulliam, 1975). However, nutritionally induced iron deficiency produces different results. Mice with nutritional iron deficiency have a lower mortality following infection with *Salmonella typhimurium* (Puschmann and Ganzoni, 1977). Moderate to severe iron deficiency had no effect on outcome in experimentally induced peritonitis with *Escherichia coli* and *Staphylococcus aureus* in guinea-pigs (Peck, *et al.*, 1989). In contrast, there was higher mortality in animals with severe iron deficiency infected with *Strepto-*

coccus pneumoniae or *Salmonella gallinarum* (Chu, *et al.*, 1976; Smith, *et al.*, 1977). Iron deficiency may exacerbate infection with ascaris in a mouse model (Laubach, 1989). Apparently contradictory results have been demonstrated in experimental malaria infections. Harvey, *et al.*, 1985) showed that iron deficiency reduced the severity of *Plasmodium chabaudi* infection in mice. However, varying iron status had no effect in changing outcome in *Plasmodium berghei* infections in rats (Hershko and Peto, 1988).

These data demonstrate that there is no simple relationship between iron availability and bacterial virulence in animal models of infection. The severity of infection may be as clinically dependent on the effect of iron on the immune status of the host as it is on bacterial iron scavenging mechanisms.

Effect of iron status on immune function

Tissue iron stores in inflammation and infection are either normal or increased, so that it is likely that sufficient intracellular iron is available to maintain cellular immune responses in the face of extracellular hypoferraemia. However, immune function may be compromised in iron deficiency states. Evidence of dysfunction has been observed in both the innate and adaptive compartments of the immune system.

Bacterial killing by neutrophils is dependent on chemotaxis, adherence, phagocytosis, the oxidative burst and degranulation. The bactericidal capacity of iron deficient neutrophils has been shown to be reduced in most studies (Chandra, 1973; Yetgin, *et al.*, 1979; MacDougall, *et al.*, 1975; Srikantia, *et al.*, 1976; Walter, *et al.*, 1986). Normal function is restored by iron supplementation although different rates of recovery have been observed. Adherence, chemotaxis and phagocytosis are generally normal (Chandra and Saraya, 1975; Walter, *et al.*, 1986), although Likhite, *et al.*, 1976) detected depressed phagocytic function in iron deficient rabbit neutrophils. Phagocytosis of *Candida albicans* is slightly reduced in iron deficient rat neutrophils (Moore and Humbert, 1984). Reduced levels of myeloperoxidase have been demonstrated in iron deficient neutrophils (Prasad, 1979; Mackler, *et al.*, 1984; Murakawa, 1987), although the clinical relevance of this is uncertain as it is thought that bacterial killing is primarily dependent on the

oxidative burst. There is disagreement as to whether iron deficient neutrophils generate a normal respiratory burst. Human neutrophils have decreased activity in some studies (Chandra and Saraya, 1975), and normal activity in others (MacDougall, *et al.*, 1975; Yetgin, *et al.*, 1979). Iron reversible defects in the respiratory burst have been consistently shown in neutrophils from iron deficient rats (Mackler, *et al.*, 1984; Murakawa, *et al.*, 1987). It is likely that many of these contradictory findings can be attributed to methodological problems in handling neutrophils.

Defective cell mediated immunity and lymphocyte function have also been demonstrated in iron deficiency. Expression of transferrin receptors on B and T lymphocytes is an early event following antigen recognition or mitogen stimulation (Bomford, *et al.*, 1983). Transferrin binding to these receptors is required for lymphocyte transformation and proliferation (Galbraith, *et al.*, 1980; Bomford, *et al.*, 1986). Hypoferraemia may reduce skin reactions to *Candida* and PPD and *in vitro* responses of lymphocytes to mitogens (Joynson, *et al.*, 1972; Chandra and Saraya, 1975; Krantman, 1982). B cell function does not appear to be affected by iron deficiency as total immunoglobulin levels and antibody response to immunization are normal (Chandra and Saraya, 1975; MacDougall, 1975). However, antibody response to diptheria and tetanus toxoid were depressed in rat experiments (Mac-Dougall and Jacobs, 1978; Kochanowski and Sherman, 1985). In conclusion, there is evidence to suggest that iron deficiency may diminish the immune response to antigenic stimuli although the precise mechanism of this remains under investigation.

Immunity in iron overload states also appears to be compromised. Excess iron may damage immune effector cells through oxygen radical mediated lipid peroxidation of cell membranes. Many of the studies examining immunity in clinical iron overload are based on studies of patients with β-thalassaemia major. Thus blood transfusion may be a contributory factor in the immune disturbance that is observed in this group of patients.

The permissive effect of iron on bacterial growth is correlated to the degree of saturation of iron binding plasma proteins. This suggests that bacteria compete more successfully for iron at high saturation resulting in a corresponding growth advantage. Neutrophils in human plasma markedly increase the bacteriostatic action of plasma. This effect can be abrogated by the addition of iron or haem compounds (Ward, *et al.*, 1986). In addition, neutrophil function is impaired in patients with iron overload (De Souza, 1989). Iron, added *in vitro*, inhibits certain neutrophil functions: chemotaxis (Baggs and Miller, 1973), bactericidal activity (Walton and Gladstone, 1976), and phagocytic activity (Van Asbeck, *et al.*, 1984; Hoepelman, *et al.*, 1988). This impairment may be mediated by lipid peroxidation of neutrophil membrane structures (Heopelman, *et al.*, 1989). Impaired oxygen metabolism and myeloperoxidase activity were demonstrated in studies of neutrophil function in iron overloaded haemodialysis patients (Flament, *et al.*, 1986; Waterlot, *et al.*, 1985). The severity of the defect was related to the serum ferritin. The same authors and others have revealed similar defects in neutrophil function in patients with β-thalassaemia major and transfusional iron overload (Cantinieaux, *et al.*, 1987; Martino, *et al.*, 1984). The defects in neutrophil function can be reversed by iron chelation therapy with desferrioxamine (Waterlot, *et al.*, 1985).

Lymphocyte function and numbers are also altered by iron overload states. Iron added *in vitro* reduces the expression of CD4 on lymphocytes (Bryan, *et al.*, 1986). The proportion of CD4 positive cells is reduced in patients with thalassaemia intermedia (Guglielmo, *et al.*, 1984) and in thalassaemia major (Grady, *et al.*, 1985; Dwyer, *et al.*, 1987). Similarly increases in the numbers of CD8+ cells have been reported in thalassaemia major (Grady, *et al.*, 1985). The patients reported by Guglielmo (1984) had not received multiple blood transfusions and thus perhaps implicated iron overload more strongly as a factor in the altered CD4 subsets. However, altered lymphocyte subset populations have not been reported in haemachromatosis.

Changes in lymphocyte function have been reported in patients with β-thalassaemia and iron overload. Reduced natural killer activity can be re-established by treating effector cells with desferrioxamine. However, the mechanism of action of desferrioxamine in this setting is unclear, as independent immunomodulatory actions have been postulated for desferrioxamine (Carotenuto, *et al.*, 1986). Altered natural killer activity has not been found in patients with iron overload due to haemochromatosis (Good, *et al.*, 1988) which suggests that multiple transfusions and other factors may contribute to the altered natural killer activity in β-thalassaemia patients. The mixed lymphocyte reaction can be repressed by iron and this effect appears to be partially determined by HLA-A loci (Bryan, *et al.*, 1981). Diminished mixed lymphocyte reactions have also been demonstrated in patients with β-thalassaemia major (Dwyer, *et al.*, 1987). There is, therefore, evidence suggesting that iron both *in vitro* and *in vivo* modulates the immune system. Both iron deficiency and iron overload states may diminish the immune response and leave the host in a state of relative immune deficiency. To see if host iron status and bacterial iron requirements are determinants of the severity of infection, it is necessary to examine clinical studies of infection in populations with pathological iron status.

The relationship of iron stores and infection in disease

Iron overload

The incidence and severity of infection should be increased in iron overload states as the host immune response is diminished and iron is available for bacterial growth. Iron overload states induced by blood transfusion appear to be associated with an increased incidence and severity of infection. Severe bacterial infections are an important cause of mortality and morbidity in patients with thalassaemia major (Caroline, *et al.*, 1969a; Weatherall and Clegg, 1981). Modell and Berkdoukas (1984) reported 48 episodes of serious infection in a group of patients with thalassaemia major and intermedia. Severe infection was reported to be the cause of death in 10 out of 55 patients who died. Splenectomy is an additional risk factor for infection in most of these patients. Splenectomy may cause abnormalities of opsonization, neutrophil function and B-cell function (Westerhausen, 1981; Amlot, 1985; Polhill and Johnson, 1975). 25% of asplenic thalassaemic patients may develop serious infections, of which approximately half may be fatal (Wilson and Johnson, 1980). However, the risk of infection in thalassaemia cannot solely be attributed to splenectomy as the risk in this group is approximately 200 times greater than patients who have undergone splenectomy for trauma. Direct evidence that iron overload is a cause of these infections is lacking. There is no relationship between measurements of iron overload and the risk of infection. Similarly there is no relationship between age and risk of infection (Modell and Berdoukas, 1984). However, an increased susceptibility to infection with Listeria and Salmonella species has been demonstrated in a murine model of β-thalassaemia that is not complicated by either splenectomy or blood transfusion (Ampel, et al., 1989). Thus it appears that infection is more common in β-thalassaemia than in unaffected individuals and that the increased risk may in part be attributed to iron overload.

Bacterial infections continue to be a major threat to patients undergoing renal dialysis. Iron overload frequently complicates the clinical course of these patients as a result of multiple blood transfusions. Waterlot, et al. (1985) reported an increased number of infections and particularly genitourinary infections in uraemic patients with raised ferritin values compared to patients with normal serum ferritins. A more recent study has confirmed that the risk of bacterial infection in haemodialysed patients is correlated to serum ferritin values (Tidemans, et al., 1989). Treating these patients with desferrioxamine significantly reduced the incidence of infection, which returned to the previous infection rate when iron chelation was stopped.

Excessive iron stores are also a feature of sickle cell disease partly as a result of blood transfusion and partly as a result of increased intestinal iron absorption. Tissue damage secondary to iron overload is unusual in sickle cell disease whereas susceptibility to infection is well established (Serjeant, 1985). There is a greater incidence of *Salmonella typhii* infections and septicaemia with pneumococcus species and *Haemophilis influenza* B. The mechanism of susceptibility to infection is complex but may be related to functional hyposplenism, chronic complement activation, abnormal neutrophil function, increased iron levels and free haemoglobin. The frequency and risk of infection is greatest during the first decade of life (Robinson and Watson, 1966; Powars, 1983), whereas iron accumulates with increasing years. Thus the risk of infection in sickle cell disease

is most strongly related to the functional hyposplenism and possibly the presence of free haemoglobin.

Although serum iron levels and iron stores may be very high in idiopathic haemachromatosis there is no increased risk of infection in patients with uncomplicated disease (Finch and Finch, 1955). There have been occasional reports of unusual infections in patients with cirrhosis secondary to iron overload. Marlon, et al. (1971) and Yamashiro (1971) reported cases of *Pasturella septicaemia* and Rabson, et al. (1975) documented a case of *Yersinia enterocolitica*. However, in spite of increased transferrin saturations and raised tissue iron stores, an increased infection risk has not been reported in patients with uncomplicated haemochromatosis.

The effect of iron on susceptibility to infection appears to be particularly marked where iron induced tissue damage has occurred or where the underlying disease predisposes to immune dysfunction. Infection remains one of the leading causes of death in patients with acute leukaemia. Caroline, et al. (1969b) showed that serum from patients with acute leukaemia had a markedly reduced capacity to inhibit the growth of yeasts such as Candida. Growth of *Candida albicans* in the leukaemic sera was approximately 1000 times greater than in normal serum. Transferrin saturation experiments implicated the availability of iron as a key factor in the growth of Candida. However, there were no clinical data to show whether individuals who were normoferraemic had lower rates of infection with fungi, although serum from normoferraemic leukaemia patients failed to support fungal growth. More recently, Towns, et al. (1989) have demonstrated that leukaemic sera have a reduced capacity to inhibit the growth of an antibiotic resistant strain of *Pseudomonas aeruginosa*. In addition, these sera had higher serum iron levels and higher transferrin saturation values than did normal controls. The same authors have suggested that serum transferrin levels may be a prognostic factor in predicting outcome in acute leukaemia and following bone marrow transplantation (Hunter, et al., 1984a, 1984b). Low levels of serum transferrin were associated with death from sepsis. However, the number of patients in these studies was small, and it remains to be seen whether serum iron levels are an important determinant of outcome of infection in patients with neutropenia and acute leukaemia.

It is concluded, therefore, that iron overload is not associated with a markedly increased risk of infection in patients with a normal immune system. Although iron levels may be a factor in situations where the immune system is compromised, other factors usually assume greater clinical importance.

Iron deficiency

If iron is important in determining the incidence and severity of infection, then iron deficiency should result in some degree of protection from infection. This, of course, will only be true if the effects of iron deficiency on the immune system are clinically negligible. There are few studies that have satisfactorily explored the relationship of iron deficiency and infection. In one animal experiment, mice with nutritional iron deficiency were shown to have reduced mortality associated with *Salmonella typhimurium* infection (Puschman and Ganzoni, 1977). However, other studies have shown increased mortality in iron deficient animals infected with *Salmonella typhimurium* (Baggs and Miller, 1974), *Streptococcus pneumoniae* (Chu, *et al.*, 1976) and *Salmonella gallinarum* (Smith, *et al.*, 1977).

Mackay (1928) reported a reduced number of respiratory and gastrointestinal infections in a group of children given iron supplements. Most commentators have taken this to imply that iron deficiency may predispose to infection in children. Similarly iron supplementation appeared to reduce the prevalence of infection in a more recent study (Andelman and Sered, 1966). The incidence of bacterial infections in iron deficient patients was 7% compared to 65% in a group of patients with non-iron deficient anaemias in a report by Masawe, *et al.* (1974). The incidence of malaria contradicted this apparently simple relationship since it was higher – 24% as against 5% – in the deficiency anaemias. Herschko (1987) has pointed out that refractory anaemia and megaloblastic anaemia cannot be regarded as appropriate controls for comparison with the incidence of infection in iron deficiency anaemia in this study. It is also not clear how many patients had been treated with iron prior to the study and thus whether the results actually demonstrated an infection response to iron replacement therapy.

Iron supplementation may result in an increased incidence of infection when given by either the parenteral or oral route. Barry and Reeve (1977) reported an increased incidence of fatal neonatal sepsis with *Escherichia coli* in Polynesian infants given intramuscular iron dextran as part of a programme to prevent iron deficiency. Infections occurred 4 to 10 days following iron administration and the incidence of infection was 22 per 1000 during the treatment period which dropped to 1.8 per 1000 when the supplementation programme was stopped. Oppenheimer, *et al.* (1986a, 1986b) have reported an increase in the prevalence of malaria in a group of infants in Papua New Guinea treated with iron dextran compared to a placebo treated group. Death rates were similar in the two groups and there does not appear to have been an increase in bacterial sepsis. Increased bacterial sepsis has not been reported as a complication in adults given iron dextran either by total dose infusion or by intramuscular injection (Hamstra, *et al.*, 1980). Iron dextran was implicated in the flare-up of malaria following total dose infusions in 917 pregnant women in Tanzania (Byles and D'sa, 1970). However, there was no untreated control group in this study and thus the background incidence of malaria in this population was not known.

Similarly oral iron supplementation may predispose to infection in situations where plasma transferrin levels are very low. Iron therapy in children with severe malnutrition may be associated with infection because of the rapid saturation of any available transferrin by pharmacological doses of iron. Macfarlane, *et al.* (1970) reported on a group of 29 children with severe kwashiorkor who were treated with iron and protein supplementation. Children who survived had a mean transferrin level of 1.3 mg/ml whereas those who died had a mean level of 0.3 mg/ml, and it is argued that iron supplementation in this group may have been harmful because of the very low iron binding capacity. However, the exact relationship of survival to iron therapy is not clear in this group as the very low transferrin values in the non-survivors may simply have been a marker for more severe malnutrition.

The potential dangers of iron supplementation in iron deficient individuals is also demonstrated in the studies of Murray, *et al.* (1975 and 1978) in Somalia. Iron supplements were given to a group of Somali nomads with iron deficiency anaemia for one month. A control group received placebo of aluminium hydroxide. Serum iron levels and mean haemoglobin rose in the iron-treated group as expected. However, during the final two weeks of treatment, a marked increase in infectious episodes with malaria, brucellosis and tuberculosis was observed in the iron supplemented group. Although there were deficiencies in the design of the study, it is an indication that in certain situations iron supplementation may be harmful by making iron available for microbial proliferation.

Organisms capable of using foreign iron chelates as a source of iron may give rise to unusual infections in humans. Such chelated iron is implicated in the development of *Yersinia sepsis* in patients receiving desferrioxamine for iron overload (Gallant, 1986). A similar link has been proposed for Rhizopus infections in desferrioxamine treated haemodialysis patients (Windus, *et al.*, 1987; Veis, *et al.*, 1986) and in a case of *Pneumocystis carinii* pneumonia in a patient with β-thalassaemia major (Kouides, *et al.*, 1990). *In vitro*, however, desferrioxamine is able to suppress the growth of a wide variety of micro-organisms (Van Asbeck, 1983) and in clinical practice the use of desferrioxamine has not been associated with an increased number of infections. Similarly newer synthetic iron chelates appear to have little risk in promoting bacterial infection (Brock, *et al.*, 1988). In protozoal infections desferrioxamine may have a therapeutic role by chelating intracellular pools of low molecular weight iron. For example, growth of *Plasmodium falciparum*, cultured *in vitro*, is inhibited by desferrioxamine. Novel iron chelators are also active in inhibiting *in vitro* malarial growth and may prove to be useful as antimalarial compounds (Yinnon, *et al.*, 1989).

plasmic proteins, are regulated by the availability of iron. In many pathogens, iron transport genes are activated during iron deficiency as exemplified by the expression of the fur gene product. It now appears that the fur system has been widely conserved amongst bacterial species and may be a general mechanism by which bacteria respond to changing environmental iron levels (Staggs and Perry, 1991). The fur gene product also appears to be important in controlling expression of other virulence determinants such as the toxins of *Escherichia coli* and *Corynebacterium diptheria*. Therapeutic strategies aimed at interrupting bacterial iron transport or exploiting the activity of iron regulated protein synthesis may thus become a reality. Already, useful antimalarial activity has been demonstrated for drugs that deprive Plasmodium species of iron by intraerythrocytic iron chelation (Yinnon, *et al.*, 1989; Heppner, *et al.*, 1988). Further novel approaches to bacterostasis can be anticipated.

The effect on infection rates by host limitation of bacterial iron supply is difficult to gauge. It is unlikely that host measurements of general iron stores accurately reflect the availability of iron at common portals of entry for bacteria. Experimentally, it is clear that manipulating the availability of iron at specific tissue sites influences the outcome of infection. However, the relationship between microbial iron requirements and host iron levels remains obscure. In human infections, it seems likely that, in the presence of normal cellular and humoral immunity, the contribution that host iron-withholding mechanisms make to limiting bacterial invasion is minimal. Conversely, the availability and supply of iron may be a determinant of virulence in situations of immune deficiency or damage.

Summary

Iron is an essential growth requirement for microorganisms and their hosts. Successful competition for iron or iron-containing compounds is an important determinant of virulence. Bacteria, fungi and protozoa have developed an array of mechanisms to exploit host sources of iron. These transport systems, which are energy dependent and often require membrane receptors, periplasmic and cyto-

References

Aisen, P. and Listowsky, I. (1980) Iron transport and storage proteins. *Annual Review of Biochemistry*, **49**, 357–393

Akbar, A.N., Fitzgerald-Bocarsly, P.A., Giardina, P.J., Hilgartner, M.W. and Grady, R.W. (1987) Modulation of the defective natural killer activity seen in thalassaemia major with desferrioxamine and γ-interferon. *Clinical and Experimental Immunology*, **70**, 345–353

Alvarez-Hernandez, X., Felstein, M.V. and Bock, J.H. (1986) The relationship between iron release, ferritin synthesis and intracellular iron distribution in mouse peritoneal macrophages. Evidence for a reduced level of metabolically available iron in elicited macrophages. *Biochimica et Biophysica Acta*, **886**, 214–222

Amlot, P. and Hayes, A.E. (1985) Impaired human antibody response to the thymus independent antigen, DND-Ficoll after splenectomy: implications for postsplenectomy infections. *Lancet*, **i**, 1008–1011

Ampel, N.M., Van Wyck, D.B., Aguirre, M.L., Willis, D.G. and Popp, R.A. (1989) Resistance to infection in murine B-thalassaemia. *Infection and Immunity*, **57**, 1011–1017

Andelman, M.B. and Sered, B.R. (1966) Utilization of dietary iron by term infants: a study of 1048 infants from a low socioeconomic population. *American Journal of Diseases of Childhood*, **11**, 45–55

Archibald, F.S. and DeVere, I.W. (1980) Iron acquisition by *Neisseria meningitidis in vitro*. Infection and Immunity, **27**, 322–334

Arouma, J.I. and Halliwell, B. (1987) Superoxide-dependent and ascorbate dependent formation of hydroxyl radicals from hydrogen peroxide in the presence of iron. Are lactoferrin and transferrin promoters of hydroxyl-radical generation? *Biochemical Journal*, **241**, 273–278

Bagg, A. and Neilands, J.B. (1987a) The ferric uptake regulation protein acts as a repressor, employing iron as a cofactor to bind the operator of an iron transport operon in *Escherichia coli*. *Biochemistry*, **26**, 5471–5477

Bagg, A. and Neilands, J.B. (1987b) Molecular mechanism of regulation of siderophore-mediated iron assimilation. *Microbiological Reviews*, **51**, 509–518

Baggs, R.B. and Miller, S.A. (1973) Nutritional iron deficiency as a determinant of host resistance in the rat. *Journal of Nutrition*, **103**, 1554–1560

Baggs, R.B. and Miller, S.A. (1974) Defect in resistance to *Salmonella typhimurium* in iron deficient rats. *Journal of Infectious Diseases*, **130**, 409–411

Baldwin, D.A., Jenny, E.R. and Aisen, P. (1984) The effect of human serum transferrin and milk lactoferrin on hydroxyl radical formation from superoxide and hydrogen peroxide. *Journal of Biological Chemistry*, **259**, 13391–13394

Barry, D.M.J. and Reeve, A.W. (1977) Increased incidence of gram negative neonatal sepsis with intramuscular iron administration. *Paediatrics*, **60**, 908–912

Benjamin, W.H. Jnr., Turnbough, C.L. Jnr., Posey, B.S. and Briles, D.E. (1985) The ability of *Salmonella typhimurium* to produce the siderophore enterobactin is not a virulence factor in mouse typhoid. *Infection and Immunity*, **50**, 392–397

Berger, M., Sorensen, R.U., Tosi, M.F., Dearbourn, D.G. and Doring, G. (1989) Complement receptor expression on neutrophils at an inflammatory site, pseudomonas-infected lung in cystic fibrosis. *Journal of Clinical Investigation*, **84**, 1302–1313

Betley, M.J., Miller, V.L. and McKalanoc, J.J. (1986) Genetics of bacterial enterotoxins. *Annual Review of Microbiology*, **40**, 577–605

Blanton, K.J., Biswas, G.D., Tsai, T., Adams, J., Dyer,

D.W., Davis, S.M., Koch, G.C., Sen, D.K. and Sparling, P.F. (1990) Genetic evidence that *Neisseria gonorrhoeae* produces specific receptors for transferrin and lactoferrin. *Journal of Bacteriology*, **172**, 5225–5235

Bomford, A., Young, S.P., Nouri-Aria, K. and Williams, R. (1983) Uptake and release of transferrin and iron by mitogen stimulated human lymphocytes. *British Journal of Haematology*, **55**, 93–101

Bomford, A., Young, S. and Williams, R. (1986) Intracellular forms of iron during transferrin iron uptake by mitogen stimulated human lymphocytes. *British Journal of Haematology*, **62**, 487–494

Brock, J.H., Liceaga, J. and Kontoghiorghes, G.J. (1988) The effect of synthetic iron chelators on bacterial growth in human serum. *FEMS Microbiology and Immunology*, **1**, 55–60

Bryan, C.F., Nishiya, K., Pollack, M.S., Dupont, B. and de Souza, M. (1981) Differential inhibition of the MLR by iron: association with HLA phenotype. *Immunogenetics*, **12**, 129–140

Bryan, C.F., Leech, S.H. and Bozelka, B. (1986) The immunoregulatory nature of iron II Lymphocyte surface marker expression. *Journal of Leukocyte Biology*, **40**, 589–593

Bullen, J.J., Leigh, L.C. and Rogers, H.J. (1968) The effect of iron compounds on the virulence of *Escherichia coli* for guinea pigs. *Immunology*, **15**, 581–588

Bullen, J.J. and Rogers, H.J. (1968) Effect of haemoglobin on experimental infections with *Pasturella septia* and *Escherichia coli*. *Nature*, **217**, 86

Bullen, J.J., Rogers, H.J. and Griffiths, E. (1978) Role of iron in bacterial infection. *Current Topics in Microbiology and Immunology*, **80**, 1–35

Bullen, J.J. (1981) The significance of iron in infection. *Review of Infectious Diseases*, **3**, 1127–1114

Burnside, G.H., Boris, P.J. and Cohn, I. (1968) Haemoglobin and *Escherichia coli*, a lethal intraperitoneal combination. *Journal of Bacteriology*, **95**, 1567–1571

Byles, A.B. and D'sa, A. (1970) Reduction of reaction to iron dextran infusion using chloroquine. *British Medical Journal*, **3**, 625–627

Byrd, T.F. and Horwitz, M.A. (1989) Interferon gamma activated human monocytes downregulate transferrin receptors and inhibit the intracellular multiplication of *Legionella pneumophilia* by limiting the availability of iron. *Journal of Clinical Investigation*, **83**, 1457–1465

Cantineaux, B., Hariga, C., Ferster, A., De Maertelaere, E., Toppet, M. and Fondu, P. (1987) Neutrophil dysfunctions in thalassaemia major: the role of cell iron overload. *European Journal of Haematology*, **39**, 28–34

Caroline, L., Kozinn, P.J., Feldman, F., Stiefel, F.H. and Lichtman, H. (1969a) Infection and iron overload in thalassaemia. *Annals of the New York Academy of Sciences*, **165**, 148–155

Caroline, L., Rosner, F. and Kozinn, P.J. (1969b) Elevated serum iron, low unbound transferrin and candidiasis in acute leukaemia. *Blood*, **34**, 441–451

Carotenuto, P., Pontesilli, O., Cambior, J.C. and

Hayward, A.R. (1986) Desferrioxamine blocks IL2 receptor expression on human T lymphocytes. *Journal of Immunology*, **136**, 2342–2347

Castell, J.V., Gomez-Lechon, M.J., David, M., et al. (1989) Interleukin 6 is the major regulator of acute phase protein synthons in adult human hepatocytes. *FEBS Letters*, **242**, 237–239

Chandra, R.K. (1973) Reduced bactericidal capacity of polymorphs in iron deficiency. *Archives of Diseases in Childhood*, **48**, 864–866

Chandra, R.K. and Saraya, A.K. (1975) Impaired immunocompetence associated with iron deficiency. *Journal of Pediatrics*, **86**, 899–902

Chen, S.T., Jordan, E.M., Wilson, R.B., Draper, R.K. and Clowes, R.C. (1987) Transcription and expression of the exotoxin A gene of *Pseudomonas aeruginosa*. *Journal of General Microbiology*, **133**, 3081–3091

Chu, S.W., Welsh, K.J., Murray, F.S. and Hegted, D.M. (1976) Effect of iron deficiency on the susceptibility to *Streptococcus pneumoniae* infection in the rat. *Nutrition Reports International*, **14**, 605–609

Coffman, T.J., Cox, C.D., Edeker, B.L. and Britigan, B.E. (1990) Possible role of bacterial siderophores in inflammation. Iron bound to the Pseudomonas siderophore pyochelin can function as a hydroxyl radical catalyst. *Journal of Clinical Investigation*, **86**, 1030–1038

Crosa, J.H. (1984) The relationship of plasmid mediated iron transport and bacterial virulence. *Annual Review of Microbiology*, **38**, 69–89

Cuadra, M. (1956) Salmonella complications in human bartonellosis. *Texas Reports in Biology and Medicine*, **14**, 97–113

De Souza, M. (1989) Immune cell functions in iron overload. *Clinical and Experimental Immunology*, **75**, 1–6

Dinarello, C.A. (1984) Interleukin-1. *Review of Infectious Diseases*, **6**, 51–95

Dwyer, J., Wood, C., McNamara, J., Williams, A., Andiman, W., Rink, L., O'Connor, T. and Pearson, H. (1987) Abnormalities in the immune system of children with Beta-thalassaemia. *Clinical and Experimental Immunology*, **68**, 621–629

Eaton, J.W., Brandt, P., Mahoney, J.R. and Lee, J.T. (1982) Haptoglobin: a natural bacteriostat. *Science*, **215**, 691–693

Elin, R.J. and Wolff, S.M. (1974) The role of iron in non-specific resistance to infection induced by endotoxins. *Journal of Immunology*, **112**, 737–745

Finch, S.C. and Finch, C.A. (1955) *Idiopathic haemochromatosis*, an iron storage disease. *Medicine (Baltimore)*, **34**, 381–430

Finkelstein, R.A., Sciolino, C.V. and Mcintosh, M.A. (1983) Role of iron in microbe-host interactions. *Review of Infectious Diseases*, **5**, 8759–8777

Flament, J., Goldman, M., Waterlot, Y., Dupont, E., Nybrau, J. and Van Werbergen, J. (1986) Impairment of phagocyte oxidative metabolism in haemodialysed patients with iron overload. *Clinical Nephrology*, **25**, 227–230

Fletcher, J. and Goldstein, E. (1970) The effect of parenteral iron preparations on experimental pyelonephritis. *British Journal of Experimental Pathology*, **81**, 280–285

Forsberg, C.M. and Bullen, J.J. (1972) The effect of passage and iron on the virulence of *Pseudomonas aeruginosa*. *Journal of Clinical Pathology*, **25**, 65–68

Frank, D.W., Storay, D.G., Hindahl, M.S. and Iglewski, B.H. (1989) Differential regulation by iron of regA and toxA transcript accumulation in *Pseudomonas aeruginosa*. *Journal of Bacteriology*, **171**, 5304–5313

Galbraith, R.M., Werner, P., Arnaud, P. and Galbraith, G.M.P. (1980) Transferrin binding to peripheral blood lymphocytes activated by phytohemagglutinin involves a specific receptor-ligand interaction. *Journal of Clinical Investigation*, **66**, 1135–1143

Gallant, T., Freedman, M.H., Villend, H. and Francombe, W.H. (1986) *Yersinia sepsis* in patients with iron overload treated with desferrioxamine. *New England Journal of Medicine*, **314**, 1643

Good, M.F., Powell, L.W. and Halliday, J.W. (1988) Iron status and cellular immune competence. *Blood Reviews*, **2**, 43–49

Grady, R.W., Akbar, A.N., Giardina, P.J., Hilgartner, M.W. and de Souza, M. (1985) Disproportionate lymphoid cell subsets in thalassaemia major: the relative contributions of transferrin and splenectomy. *British Journal of Haematology*, **59**, 713–724

Grant, C.C.R. and Vasil, M.L. (1986) Analysis of transcriptions of the exotoxin-A gene of *Pseudomonas aeruginosa*. *Journal of Bacteriology*, **168**, 1451–1456

Griffiths, E., Stevenson, P., Hale, T.L. and Formal, S.B. (1985) The synthesis of aerobactin and a 76000 dalton iron-regulated outer membrane protein by *Escherichia coli* K12-Shigella hybrids and by enteroinvasive strains of *Escherichia coli*. *Infection and Immunity*, **49**, 67–71

Griggs, D.W., Kafka, K., Nan, C.D. and Konisky, J. (1990) Activation of expression of the *Escherichia coli* cir gene by an iron independent regulatory mechanism involving cyclic AMP-cyclic AMP receptor protein complex. *Journal of Bacteriology*, **172**, 3529–3533

Groves, M.L. (1960) The isolation of a red protein from milk. *Journal of the American Chemical Society*, **82**, 3345–3350

Guglielmo, P., Cunsolo, F., Lombardo, T., Sortino, G., Giustolisi, R. and Cacciola, E. (1984). T-subset abnormalities in thalassaemia intermedia: possible evidence for thymus functional deficiency. *Acta Haematologica*, **72**, 361–367

Gutteridge, J.M.C., Rowley, D.A. and Halliwell, B. (1981) Superoxide dependent formation of hydroxyl radicals in the presence of iron salts. Detection of 'free iron' in biological systems by using bleomycin-dependent degradation of DNA. *Biochemical Journal*, **199**, 259–261

Gutteridge, J.M.C., Rowley, D.A., Griffiths, E. and Halliwell, B. (1985) Low-molecular weight iron complexes and oxygen radical reactions in idiopathic haemachromatosis. *Clinical Science*, **68**, 463–467

Halliwell, D. and Gutteridge, J.M.C. (1985) The

importance of free radicals and catalytic metal ions in human diseases. *Molecular Aspects of Medicine*, **8**, 89–193

Hamstra, R.D., Block, M.H. and Schoket, A.L. (1980) Intravenous iron dextran in clinical medicine. *Journal of the American Medica*, **243**, 1726–1731

Hantke, K. (1987) Selection procedure for deregulated iron transport mutants fur in *Escherichia coli* K-12. *Molecular and General Genetics*, **210**, 135–139

Harvey, D.N., Bell, R.G. and Nesheim, M.C. (1985) Iron deficiency protects inbred mice against infection with *Plasmodium chabaudi*. *Infection and Immunity*, **50**, 932–934

Henderson, L.L., Solomon, K. and Chapman, W.L. Jnr. (1978) Influence of iron on *Corynebacterium renale* induced pyelonephritis in a rat experimental model. *Infection and Immunity*, **21**, 540–545

Heppner, D.G., Halloway, P.E., Kontoghiroghes, G.J. and Eaton, J.W. (1988) Antimalarial properties of orally active iron chelators. *Blood*, **72**, 358–361

Hershko, C., Graham, G., Bates, G.W. and Rachmilewitz, E.A. (1978) Non-specific serum iron in thalassaemia: an abnormal serum iron fraction of potential toxicity. *British Journal of Haematology*, **40**, 255–263

Hershko, C. (1987) Non-transferrin plasma iron. *British Journal of Haematology*, **66**, 149–151

Hershko, C., Peto, T.E.A. and Wetherall, P.J. (1988) Iron and Infection. *British Medical Journal*, **296**, 660–664

Hershko, C. and Peto, T.E.A. (1988) Deferoxamine inhibition of malaria is independent of host iron status. *Journal of Experimental Medicine*, **168**, 375–387

Hindahl, M.S., Frank, D.W. and Iglewski, B.H. (1987) Molecular studies of a positive regulator of toxin A synthesis in *Pseudomonas aeruginosa*. *Antibiotics and Chemotherapy*, **39**, 279–289

Hirata, T., Bitterman, P.B., Mernex, J.F. and Crystal, R.G. (1986) Expression of the transferrin receptor gene during the process of mononuclear phagocyte maturation. *Journal of Immunology*, **136**, 1339–1345

Hoepelman, I.M., Jaarsma, E.Y., Verhoef, J. and Marx, J.J.M. (1988) Effect of iron on polymorphonuclear granulocyte (PMN) phagocytic capacity: role of oxidative state and ascorbic acid. *British Journal of Haematology*, **70**, 495–500

Hoepelman, I.M., Bezemer, W.A., van Doormalen, E., Verhoef, J. and Marx, J. (1989) Lipid peroxidation of human granulocytes (PMN) and monocytes by iron complexes. *British Journal of Haematology*, **72**, 584–588

Hoepelman, I.M., Bezena, W.A., Vandenbroucke-Grands, C.M.J.E. and Marx, J. (1990) Bacterial iron enhances oxygen radical mediated killing of *Staphylococcus aureus* by phagocytes. *Infection and Immunity*, **58**, 26–31

Holbein, B.E. (1980) Iron controlled infection with *Neisseria meningitidis* in mice. *Infection and Immunity*, **29**, 886–891

Holbein, B.E. (1981) Enhancement of *Neisseria meningitidis* infection in mice. *Infection and Immunity*, **54**, 120–125

Huebers, H.A. and Finch, C.A. (1984) Transferrin: physiological behavior and clinical implications. *Blood*, **64**, 763–767

Hunter, R.L., Bennett, B., Garrison, C., Winton, E.F. and Vogler W.R. (1984a) Transferrin in disease. A prognostic indicator in patients undergoing bone marrow transplantation. *American Journal of Clinical Pathology*, **81**, 581–585

Hunter, R.L., Bennett, B., Towns, M. and Vogler, W.R. (1984b) Transferrin in disease. II Defects in the regulation of transferrin saturation with iron contribute to susceptibility to infection. *American Journal of Clinical Pathology*, **81**, 748–753

Jacobs, A. (1977) Low molecular weight intracellular iron transport compounds. *Blood*, **50**, 433–439

Johansson, B.C. (1960) Isolation of crystalline lactoferin from human milk. *Acta Chemica Scandinavica*, **14**, 510–512

Joynson, D.H.M., Jacobs, A., Walker, D.M. and Dolby, A.E. (1972) Defect of cell mediated immunity in patients with iron deficiency anaemia. *Lancet*, **ii**, 1058–1059

Kampschmidt, R.F. and Pulliam, L.A. (1975) Stimulation of antimicrobial activity in the rat with leucocytic endogenous mediator. *Journal of the Reticuloendothelial Society*, **17**, 162–169

Kaye, D., Gill, F. and Hook, E.W. (1967) Factors influencing host resistance to Salmonella infections: the effect of haemolysis and erythrophagocytosis. *American Journal of Medical Science*, **254**, 205–215

Kochan, I. (1973) The role of iron in bacterial infections with special consideration of host-tubercle bacillus interaction. *Current Topics in Microbiology and Immunology*, **60**, 1–30

Kochan, I., Kvach, J.T. and Wiles, T.I. (1977) Virulence associated acquisition of iron in mammalian serum by *Escherichia coli*. *Journal of Infectious Diseases*, **135**, 623–632

Kochanowski, B.A. and Sherman, A.R. (1985) Decreased antibody formation in iron deficient rat pups – effect of iron repletion. *American Journal of Clinical Nutrition*, **41**, 278–284

Konijn, A.M. and Herschko, C. (1977) Ferritin synthesis in inflammation 1. Pathogenesis of impaired iron release. *British Journal of Haematology*, **37**, 7–16

Konopka, K. and Neilands, J.B. (1984) Effect of serum albumin on siderophore mediated utilisation of transferrin iron. *Biochemistry*, **23**, 2122–2127

Kouides, P.A., Slapak, C.A., Rosenwasser, L.J. and Miller, K.B. (1988) *Pneumocystis carinii* pneumonia as a complication of desferrioxamine therapy. *British Journal of Haematology*, **70**, 383–384

Krantman, H.J., Young, S.R., Ank, B.J., O'Donnell, C.M., Rachelfsky, G.S. and Steihm, E.R. (1982) Immune function in pure iron deficiency. *American Journal of Diseases of Children*, **136**, 840–844

Lafont, J., Dho, M., D'hauteville, H.M., Bree, A. and Sonsonetti, P.J. (1987) Presence and expression of aerobactin genes in virulent avian strains of *Escherichia coli*. *Infection and Immunity*, **55**, 193–197

Laubach, H.E. (1989) Alterations in *Ascaris suum* larval burdens, eosinophil number and lysophospholipase activity associated with low levels of dietary iron. *Journal of Parasitology*, **75**, 317–320

Lawlor, K.M., Daskaleros, P.A., Robinson, R.E. and Payne, S.M. (1987) Virulence of iron transport mutants of *Shigella flexneri* and utilization of host iron compounds. *Infection and Immunity*, **55**, 594–599

Lee, J.T., Ahrenholz, D.H., Nelson, R.D. and Simmons, R.L. (1979) Mechanism of the adjuvant effect of haemoglobin in experimental peritonitis V. The significance of the co-ordinated iron component. *Surgery*, **86**, 41–48

Letendre, E.D. and Holbein, B.E. (1983) Turnover in the transferrin iron pool during the hypoferraemic phase of experimental *Neisseria meningitidis* infection in mice. *Infection and Immunity*, **39**, 50–59

Letendre, E.D. and Holbein, B.E. (1984) Mechanism of impaired iron release by the reticuloendothelial system during the hypoferraemic phase of experimental *Neisseria meningitidis* infection in mice. *Infection and Immunity*, **44**, 320–325

Likhite, V., Rodrian, R. and Crosby, W.H. Jnr. (1976) Depressed phagocytic function exhibited by polymorphonuclear leucocytes from chronically iron deficient rabbits. *British Journal of Haematology*, **34**, 251–255

Lipschitz, D.A., Cook, J.D. and Finch, C.A. (1975) Ferritin in formed blood elements. *Proceedings of the Society of Experimental Biology and Medicine*, **148**, 358–364

Macdougall, L.G. and Jacobs, M.R. (1978) The immune response in iron deficient children. Isohaemagglutin titres and antibody response to immunisation. *South African Medical Journal*, **53**, 405–407

Macdougall, L.G., Anderson, R., McNab, G.M. and Katz, J. (1975) The immune response in iron-deficient children: impaired cellular defense mechanisms with altered humoral components. *Journal of Paediatrics*, **86**, 833–843

Macfarlane, H., Reddy, S., Adcock, K.J., Adeshina, H., Cooke, A.R. and Akene (1970) Immunity, transferrin and survival in kwashiorkor. *British Medical Journal*, **4**, 268–270

Mackay, H.M. (1928) Anaemia in pregnancy: its prevalence and prevention. *Archives of Disease in Childhood*, **3**, 117–147

Mackler, B., Person, R., Ochs, H. and Finch, C.A. (1984) Iron deficiency in the rat: effects on neutrophil activation and metabolism. *Pediatric Research*, **18**, 549–551

Marlon, A., Gentry, L. and Merigan, T.C. (1971) Septicaemia and *Pasturella pseudotuberculosis* and liver disease. *Archives of Internal Medicine*, **127**, 947–949

Martino, M., Rossi, M.E., Resti, M., Vullo, C. and Vierucci, A. (1984) Changes in superoxide anion in neutrophils from multitransfused B-thalassaemia patients: correlation with ferritin levels and liver damage. *Acta Haematologica (Basel)*, **71**, 289–291

Masawe, A.E.J., Muindl, J.M. and Swai, G.B.R. (1974) Infections in iron deficiency and other types of anaemia in the topics. *Lancet*, **ii**, 314–317

McGowan, S.E., Murray, J.J. and Parrish, M.G. (1986) Iron binding, internalisation and fate in human alveolar macrophages. *Journal of Laboratory and Clinical Medicine*, **108**, 587–595

Mickelson, P.A. and Sparling, P.F. (1981) Ability of *Neisseria gonorrhoeae*, *Neisseria meningitidis* and commensal Neisseria species to obtain iron from lactoferrin. *Infection and Immunity*, **33**, 555–564

Miles, A.A. and Khimji, P.L. (1975) Enterobacteria chelators of iron; their occurrence, detection and relation to pathogenicity. *Journal of Medical Microbiology*, **8**, 477–490

Miles, K.A., Khimji, P.L. and Maskell, J. (1979) The variable response of bacteria to excess ferric iron in host tissues. *Journal of Medical Microbiology*, **12**, 17–28

Miller, K.L., Taylor, R.K. and McKalanos, J.J. (1987) Cholera toxin transcriptional activator toxR is a transmembrane DNA binding protein. *Cell*, **48**, 271–279

Modell, B. and Berdoukas, V. (1984) In The clinical approach to thalassaemia. London: Grune and Stratton

Moore, L.L. and Humbert, J.R. (1984) Neutrophil bactericidal dysfunction towards oxidant radical sensitive microorganisms during experimental iron deficiency. *Pediatric Research*, **18**, 684–687

Murakawa, H., Bland, C.E., Willis, W.T. and Dallman, P.R. (1987) Iron deficiency and neutrophil function: different rates of correction of the depressions in oxidative burst and MPO activity after iron treatment. *Blood*, **69**, 1464–1468

Murphy, C.K., Kalve, V.I. and Klebba, P.E. (1990) Surface topology of the *Escherichia coli* K-12 ferric enterobacter receptor. *Journal of Bacteriology*, **172**, 2736–2746

Murphy, J.R., Pappenheimer, A.M. Jnr. and Tayart de Borms, S. (1974) Synthesis of Diptheria tox-gene products in *Escherichia coli* extracts. *Proceedings of the National Academy of Sciences*, **71**, 11–15

Murray, M.J., Murray, A.B., Murray, M.B. and Murray, C.J. (1975) Refeeding malaria and hyperferraemia. *Lancet*, **i**, 653–654

Murray, M.J., Murray, A.B., Murray, M.B. and Murray, C.J. (1978) The adverse effect of iron repletion on the course of certain infections. *British Medical Journal*, **2**, 1113–1115

Nassif, X. and Sansoneti, P.J. (1986) Correlation of the virulence of *Klebsiella pneumoniae* KI and K'' with the presence of a plasmid encoding aerobactin. *Infection and Immunity*, **54**, 603–608

Neiderhoffer, E.C., Nuranjo, C.M., Bradley, K.L. and Fee, J.A. (1990) Control of Escherichia coli superoxide dismutase (SodA and SodB) genes by the ferric uptake regulation (fur) locus. *Journal of Bacteriology*, **172**, 1930–1938

Neilands, A.B. (1980) Microbial metabolism of iron. In *Iron in Biochemistry and Medicine*, **II**, edited by A. Jacobs and M. Worwood, pp. 529–572. London and New York: Academic Press

Nunez, M-T., Gaete, V., Watkins, J.A. and Glass, J. (1990) Mobilization of iron from endocytic vesicles. The effects of acidification and reduction. *Journal of Biological Chemistry*, **265**, 6688–6692

Oppenheimer, S.J., Gibson, F.D. and Macfarlane, S.B. (1986a) Iron supplementation increases prevalence and effects of malaria; report on clinical studies in Papua New Guinea. *Transactions of the Royal Society of Tropical Medicine and Hygiene*, **80**, 603–612

Oppenheimer, S.J., MacFarlane, S.P.J., Moody, J.B., Bunari, O. and Hendrickse, R.G. (1986b) Effect of iron prophylaxis on morbidity due to infectious disease. *Transactions of the Royal Society of Tropical Medicine and Hygiene*, **80**, 596–602

Paerry, R.D. and Brubaker, R.R. (1979) Accumulation of iron by Yersinia. *Journal of Bacteriology*, **137**, 1290–1298

Peck, M.D., Gonce, S.J., Alexander, J.W. and Miskell, P.W. (1989) Dietary iron and recovery from peritonitis in guinea pigs. *American Journal of Clinical Nutrition*, **50**, 524–527

Peterson, E.M. and Alderete, J.F. (1984) Iron uptake and increased intracellular enzyme activity follows host lactoferrin binding by *Trichomonas vaginalis* receptors. *Journal of Experimental Medicine*, **160**, 398–410

Peto, T.E. and Hershko, C. (1989) Iron and infection. In *Iron Chelating Therapy, Bailliere's Clinical Haematology*, edited by C. Hershko, pp. 435–458. London: Bailliere Tindall

Polhill, R.B. Jnr. and Johnson, R.B. Jnr. (1975) Diminished complement activity after splenectomy. *Pediatric Research*, **9**, 333

Pollack, S. and Fleming, J. (1984) *Plasmodium falciparum* takes up iron from transferrin. *British Journal of Haematology*, **58**, 289–293

Pollack, S. (1987) Effects of iron and desferrioxamine on the growth of *Plasmodium falciparum in vitro*. *British Journal of Haematology*, **65**, 256–257

Powars, D., Overturf, G. and Turner, E. (1983) Is there an increased risk of *Haemophilus influenza* septicemia in children with sickle cell anaemia? *Pediatrics*, **71**, 927–931

Prasad, S.J. (1979) Leukocyte function in iron deficiency anaemia. *American Journal of Clinical Nutrition*, **32**, 550–552

Puschman, M. and Ganzoni, A.M. (1977) Increased resistance of iron deficient mice to Salmonella infection. *Infection and Immunity*, **17**, 663–664

Rabson, A.R., Hallott, A.F. and Kornhof, H.J. (1975) Generalised *Yersinia enterocolitica* infection. *Journal of Infectious Diseases*, **131**, 447–451

Redhead, K., Hill, T. and Chart, H. (1987) Interaction of lactoferrin and transferrin with the outer membrane of *Bordetella pertussis*. *Journal of General Microbiology*, **133**, 891–898

Repine, J.E., Fox, R.B. and Berger, E.M. (1981) Hydrogen peroxide kills *Staphylococcus aureus* by reacting with staphylococcal iron to form hydroxyl radical. *Journal of Biological Chemistry*, **256**, 7094–7096

Robinson, M.G. and Watson, R.J. (1966) Pneumococcal meningitis in sickle cell anaemia. *New England Journal of Medicine*, **274**, 1006–1008

Rogers, H.J. (1973) Iron binding catechols and virulence in *Escherichia coli*. *Infection and Immunity*, **7**, 445–456

Rowley, P.A., Gutteridge, J.M.C., Blake, D., Farr, H. and

Halliwell, B. (1984) Lipid peroxidation in rheumatoid arthritis: thiobarbituric acid reactive material and catalytic iron salts in synovial fluid from rheumatoid patients. *Clinical Science*, **66**, 691–695

Schade, A.L. and Caroline, L. (1944) Raw hen egg white and role of iron in growth inhibition of *Shigella dysenteriae, Staphylococcus aureus, Escherichia coli* and *Saccharomyces cerevisiae*. *Science*, **100**, 14–15

Schaffer, S., Hantker, K. and Brown, V. (1985) Nucleotide sequence of the iron regulatory gene fur. *Molecular and General Genetics*, **200**, 110–113

Schryvers, A.B. (1988) Characterisation of the human transferrin and lactoferrin receptors in *Haemophilus influenzae*. *Molecular Microbiology*, **2**, 467–472

Schryvers, A.B. and Gonzalez, G.C. (1989) Comparison of the abilities of different protein sources of iron to enhance *Neisseria meningitidis* infection in mice. *Infection and Immunity*, **57**, 2425–2429

Serjeant, G.R. (1985) *In Sickle cell disease*, 1st edn, p. 105, Oxford University Press

Sigel, S.P., Stoebner, J.A. and Payne, S.M. (1985) Iron vibriobactin transport system is not required for virulence of *Vibrio cholerae*. *Infection and Immunity*, **47**, 360–362

Simonson, C., Brener, D. and DeVoc, I.W. (1982) Expression of a high affinity mechanism for acquisition of transferrin iron by *Neisseria meningitidis*. *Infection and Immunity*, **36**, 107–113

Smith, J.M., Hill, R. and Licencee, S.T. (1977) Enhancement of survival in acute experimental Salmonella typhoid in chicks by the administration of iron dextran. *Research in Veterinary Science*, **22**, 151–157

Srikantia, S.G., Prasad, J.S., Bhaskaram, C. and Krishnamachari, K.A.V.R. (1976) Anaemia and immune response. *Lancet*, **ii**, 1307–1309

Staggs, T.M. and Perry, R.D. (1991) Identification and cloning of a fur regulatory gene in *Yersinia pestis*. *Journal of Bacteriology*, **173**, 417–425

Sword, C.P. (1966) Mechanisms of pathogenesis in *Listeria monocytogenes* infection. *Journal of Bacteriology*, **92**, 536–542

Taetle, R. and Honeysett, J.M. (1988) Gamma interferon modulates human monocyte/macrophage transferrin receptor expression. *Blood*, **71**, 1590–1595

Testa, U., Petrini, M., Quaranta, M.T., et al. (1989) Iron upmodulates in expression of transferrin receptors during monocyte-macrophage maturation. *Journal of Biological Chemistry*, **264**, 13181–13187

Tidemans, C.L., Lenclud, C.M., Wens, R., Collart, F.E. and Dratwa, M. (1989) Critical role of iron overload in the increased susceptibility of haemodialysis patients to bacterial infections. Beneficial effects of desferrioxamine. *Nephrology Dialysis Transplantation*, **4**, 883–887

Towns, M.L., Bennett, B., Check, I.J. and Hunter, R.L. (1989) An improved method for determining the microbial inhibitory activity of serum and its application to the study of patients with leukaemia. *American Journal of Clinical Pathology*, **92**, 192–198

Tyron, V.V. and Baseman, J.B. (1987) The acquisition of

human lactoferrin by mycoplasma pneumoniae. *Microbiological Pathology*, **3**, 437–443

Van Asbeck, B.S., Marcelis, J.H., Van Kats Jaarsma, E.Y. and Verhoef, J. (1983) Synergy between the iron chelator deferoxamine and the microbial agents gentamicin, chloramphenicol, cefalothin, cefotiam and cefsulodin. *European Journal of Clinical Microbiology*, **2**, 432–438

Van Asbeck, B.S., Marks, J.J.M., Struyvenberg, A. and Verhoef, J. (1984) Functional defects in phagocytic cells in patients with iron overload. *Journal of Infection*, **8**, 232–234

Veis, J., Contiguglia, R., Kelin, M., Mishell, J., Alfrey, A. and Shapiro, J. (1986) Mucormycosis associated with desferrioxamine use in hemodialysis patients. *Kidney International*, **31**, 247

Walter, T., Arredondo, S., Arevalo, M. and Stekel, A. (1986) Effect of iron therapy on phagocytosis and bactericidal activity in neutrophils of iron deficient infants. *American Journal of Clinical Nutrition*, **58**, 877–882

Walton, E. and Gladstone, G.P. (1976) Factors affecting the susceptibility of staphylococci to killing by the cationic proteins from rabbit polymorphonuclear leucocytes: the effects of alteration of cellular energetics and various iron compounds. *British Journal of Experimental Pathology*, **57**, 560–570

Ward, C.G., Hammond, J.S. and Bullen, J.J. (1986) Effect of iron compounds on antibacterial function of human polymorphs and plasma. *Infection and Immunity*, **51**, 723–730

Waterlot, Y., Cantinieaux, B., Hariga-Muller, C. and De Maertelaere, E., Van. (1985) Impaired phagocytic activity of neutrophils in patients receiving haemodialysis: the critical role of iron overload. *British Journal of Haematology*, **291**, 501–504

Weinberg, E.D. (1978) Iron and infection. *Microbiological Reviews*, **42**, 45–66

West, S.E.H. and Sparling, P.F. (1987) Aerobactin utilisation by *Neisseria gonorrhoea* and cloning of a genomic fragment that complements *Escherichia coli* fhuB mutations. *Journal of Bacteriology*, **169**, 3414–3421

Westerhausen, M., Worsdorfer, O., Gessner, U., De Guili, R. and Senn, H.J. (1981) Immunological changes following post traumatic splenectomy. *Blut*, **43**, 345–353

Weatherall, D.J. and Clegg, J.B. (1981) In *Thalassaemia Syndromes*, 3rd edn, pp. 164–167. Oxford: Blackwell Scientific Publications.

Wilson, S.A. and Johnson, W.D. Jnr. (1980) Infections complicating surgical or functional splenectomy and gastrectomy. In *Infections in the abnormal host*, ed. M.H. Grieco. New York.

Windle, J.J., Shin, H.S. and Morrow, J.F. (1984) Induction of Interleukin 1 messenger RNA and translation in oocytes. *Journal of Immunology*, **132**, 1317–1322

Windus, D.W., Stokes, T.J., Julian, B.A. and Fenves, A.Z. (1987) Fatal Rhizopus infections in haemodialysis patients receiving deferoxamine. *Annals of Internal Medicine*, **107**, 678–680

Winterbourn, C.C. and Sutton, H.C. (1984) Hydroxyl radical production from hydrogen perioxide and enzymatically generated paraquat radicals: catalytic requirements and oxygen dependence. *Archives of Biochemistry and Biophysics*, **235**, 116–126

Yamashiro, K.M., Goldman, R.H. and Harris, D. (1971) *Pasturella pseudotuberculosis*: acute sepsis with survival. *Archives of Internal Medicine*, **128**, 605–608

Yancey, R.J., Breeding, S.A.L. and Lankford, C.E. (1979) Enterochelin (enterobactin): virulence factor for *Salmonella typhimurium*. *Infection and Immunity*, **24**, 174–180

Yetgin, S., Altay, C., Ciliv, G. and Laleli, Y. (1979) Myeloperoxidase and bactericidal function of PMN in iron deficiency. *Acta Haematologica (Basel)*, **61**, 10–14

Yinnon, A.M., Theanacho, E.N., Grady, R.N., Spira, D.T. and Herschko, C. (1989) Antimalarial effect of HBED and other phenolic and catecholic iron chelators. *Blood*, **74**, 2166–2171

3

Infections in splenectomized patients

G.M. Scott and J.D.M. Richards

Introduction

Although it is generally agreed that splenectomy renders a patient more susceptible to severe infections, this has been disputed. What is clear is that splenectomized patients occasionally present with overwhelming septicaemia, particularly caused by *Streptococcus pneumoniae* and other capsulate organisms. However, splenectomized patients form a relatively low proportion of those presenting with such infections. Arguments about the degree of enhanced susceptibility to infection can be resolved by considering the following points.

1 There is no particular reason why splenectomized patients should be more often exposed to a virulent organism than a group controlled for underlying disease. However, splenectomy may alter the pathogenesis of and affect the outcome of the infection.
2 Because the severe infection rate is low even in splenectomized patients, many patient–years of follow-up are necessary to assess the true excess risk over that in the normal population. Long-term surveys, discussed below, are often inadequate even when using a simple end-point such as death of a patient due to infection. Infections are often the terminal event in a patient with uncontrolled tumour, who may have had splenectomy earlier for palliative or diagnostic reasons. Healthy patients may easily be lost to follow up. No prospective controlled case matched study has been performed to assess the risk of infections which are not fatal.
3 A patient's underlying disease may itself affect the likelihood of severe infection and then the contribution made by the absence of the spleen cannot be easily judged. For example, Hodgkin's disease and other lymphoproliferative disorders are associated with an increased risk of severe infection in their own right. Therefore, after the immediate post-operative period, those splenectomized for trauma should, and do, appear to have a lower risk of infections than those with immunosuppressive disorders. Furthermore, straightforward splenectomy for trauma carries a lower post-operative infection risk than splenectomy following accidental trauma during abdominal surgery.
4 Factors other than severe infection are more common causes of death than overwhelming infection in patients with certain underlying diseases.
5 There are certain rare organisms, such as *Babesia* spp. and *Capnocytophaga canimorsus* which predominantly cause disease only in splenectomized subjects.

In this review, we will briefly discuss the anatomy and physiology of the spleen, the evidence that splenectomized animals are indeed more susceptible to experimental infections and the possible immunological basis for enhanced susceptibility in animals and man. Post-operative infections are considered because they appear to occur more often after splenectomy than after other similar operations. We have reviewed the literature since the excellent review by Wara (1981) on late post-splenectomy sepsis and have tried to assess risk of serious post-splenectomy sepsis from rather inadequate data. It is against this risk that decisions to do splenectomy, and the value of preventive measures such as surgical preservation, pneumococcal vaccines and antibiotic prophylaxis should be judged.

The structure and function of the spleen

The spleen may be considered as a large lymph gland interposed in the systemic circulation and has vascular and lymphoid components. The vascular component is of very special structure. The splenic artery arises from the coeliac axis and, after entering the spleen at the hilum, divides into the trabecular arteries. From the trabecular arteries, branches go into the red pulp. The arteries are surrounded by a cuff of lymphocytes and for this reason, they have been termed 'central arteries'. The cuff of lymphocytes surrounding these central arteries expands at intervals to form lymphoid follicles, the Malpighian corpuscles. When the arteries lose their lymphoid cuff, they become straight 'penicillary' arteries; becoming smaller, as arterioles, they finally terminate just short of the splenic sinuses. It is at this position that cells in the circulation may then enter either the 'closed pathway' through the splenic sinuses, or the 'open pathway' via the pulp cords. Blood cells, parasites or bacteria, entering through the pulp cords, are then subjected to a filtration process by the reticuloendothelial cells of the pulp cords. Red cells are only able to obtain re-entry into the circulation via narrow slits in the sinus walls; these have been likened to the staves of a barrel. Organisms are phagocytosed by the macrophages in their transit through the splenic pulp. Phagocytosis of capsulate organisms in the spleen is a crucial step in preventing unrestricted replication of bacteria in the circulation and so forms an important host defence mechanism.

The role of opsonins is also extremely important in relation to the phagocytosis of capsulate organisms. Opsonins act as ligands when attached to the surface of organisms and enhances the ability of the reticuloendothelial system to phagocytose. The C3b component of complement also facilitates phagocytosis. Tuftsin, a small peptide derived by enzymic cleavage of the Fc chain of IgG, is produced in the spleen and is considered to be a potent augmenter of neutrophil phagocytosis. The production of soluble factors is preserved by autoinoculation of splenic tissue after traumatic rupture.

The lymphoid component of the spleen is equally important in host defence. The anatomical structure of the spleen has been considered to be optimal for the preferential filtration of insoluble antigens from plasma and delivering them to lymphatic germinal centres (Nossal, *et al.*, 1971). The periarteriolar sheaths of lymphoid cells belong mainly to the T-subsets, whereas the germinal centres are composed essentially of B-cells. The T-cells in the periarteriolar and lymphatic sheaths are therefore ideally situated to interact with the B-cells present in the lymphoid follicles.

Splenectomy is most commonly performed either electively for haematological, malignant and immunological disorders or acutely for traumatic rupture or incidentally during abdominal surgery. It has been done for a missed acute cytomegalovirus infection and even in one case of factitious fever (Potin, Regamey and Glauser, 1983).

Hairy cell leukaemia carries a high risk of infections which correspond to a poor outcome from the underlying disease (Golomb and Hadad, 1984). In hairy cell leukaemia (Bouza, Burgaleta and Gold, 1978; Mackowiak, *et al.*, 1980) and, more controversially, in Felty's syndrome (Joyce, *et al.*, 1980; Coon, 1985), splenectomy may actually reduce the risk of infection by palliation of the condition. In the majority, however, splenectomy renders the individual at greater risk of serious infection with circulating bacterial and protozoal organisms of moderate virulence, by removal of the most important filtration and phagocytic organ in the body. Furthermore, particularly in infants, total removal of the spleen removes much of the ability to make primary antibody responses to polysaccharide antigens.

Experimental infections in splenectomized animals

Many studies in experimentally splenectomized animals indicate increased susceptibility to infectious agents. Some recent studies are summarized in Table 3.1.

Table 3.1 Effects of splenectomy in experimental infections

Reference	Species	Organism	Route*	Effects of splenectomy
		Bacteria		
Gullstrand, *et al.*, 1982	Rat	*Streptococcus pneumoniae*	iv	Fatal infection cured by penicillin given 18 but not 24 h after inoculation. Survival improved by steroids given at 24 h
Offenbartl, *et al.*, 1986	Mouse	*Streptococcus pneumoniae*	iv	Human gamma globulin in high dose reduced mortality in splenectomized mice
Schwartz, *et al.*, 1978	Rat	*Streptococcus pneumoniae*	iv	Autotransplantation of splenic tissue at splenectomy failed to protect against type 25 infection
Patel, *et al.*, 1982	Rat	*Streptococcus pneumoniae*	ip	Autotransplantation of two slices of spleen into an omental pouch reduced mortality from 44% (splenectomy alone) to 11%
Hebert, *et al.*, 1983	Mouse	*Streptococcus pneumoniae*	inhal	Mortality in splenectomized mice reduced by intra-peritoneal *Corynebacterium parvum* immediately before inhalation of pneumococci, or three days before iv pneumococci
Coil, *et al.*, 1978	Mouse	*Streptococcus pneumoniae*	inhal/iv	Pathogenicity of virulent (Type 3) bacteria enhanced by splenectomy even if given by aerosol
Lefford, *et al.*, 1978	Mouse	*Listeria monocytogenes*	lungs	Protracted pneumonitis not enhanced by splenectomy
Karanfilian, *et al.*, 1983	Mouse	*Esch. coli* endotoxin	ip	Non-splenectomized older mice were more susceptible than younger mice. Survival decreased in splenectomized young mice
Hirano, *et al.*, 1986	Rat	Experimental peritonitis	endog	Survival decreased from 48% to 17%
Butler, *et al.*, 1985	Rabbit	Dysgonic fermenter 2		Prolonged bacteraemia. No increase in risk of experimental endocarditis

Reference	Host	Parasites	Route	
Collins, et al., 1986	Aotus monkey	*Plasmodium falciparum*	iv, RBC	Increased level of parasitaemia. Model useful to examine strains from man
Wyler, et al., 1977	Rhesus monkey	*Plasmodium inui*	iv, blood	Peak parasitaemia ten-fold that in intact monkeys. Mortality greater in those splenectomized before infection. Intact but splenectomized monkeys eventually cleared parasites
Eling, 1982	Mouse	*Plasmodium berghei*	ip, RBC	Development of chronic high level parasitaemia
Oster, et al., 1980	Mouse	*Plasmodium yoelii*	ip	Splenectomized mice unable to clear infestation
		Plasmodium chabaudi adami		Chloroquine rescue of primary attack led to protection against secondary attack
Grun, et al., 1985	Mouse	*Plasmodium chabaudi adami*	iv, RBC	Fatal parasitaemia. Splenectomy after recovery led to recrudescence. Not reversed by injecting spleen cells intravenously
Dockrell, et al., 1980	Mouse	*Plasmodium yoelii*	iv, RBC	Intact animals protected by fixed parasitized red cells, but slow to clear parasitaemia if splenectomized
Waki, et al., 1985	Mouse	*Plasmodium berghei*	iv, RBC	Attenuated organism is lethal in splenectomized mice
Gysin, et al., 1980	Squirrel monkey	*Plasmodium falciparum*	iv	Enhanced susceptibility
Duffey, et al., 1985	Mouse	*Trypanosoma musculi*	ip	Anaemia and thrombocytopenia continued progressively until death
Diffley and Scott, 1984	Mouse/Rat	*Trypanosoma brucei gambiense*	iv	Fulminant first peak infestation akin to effects irradiation and cyclophosphamide
Desai, et al., 1987	Mouse	*Trypanosoma lewisi*	iv	Splenectomy did not enhance susceptibility except with concomitant C3 depletion
Benach, et al., 1978	Hamster	*Babesia microti*	iv	No increased pathogenicity
Ruebush, et al., 1979, 1981	Macaque monkey	*Babesia microti*	iv	Splenectomy 10 months after original infection and after recovery from 1–3 parasitaemic episodes, induced recurrence of parasitaemia at high levels
Hussein, 1977	Mouse	*Babesia microti* and *Babesia hylomysci*	iv	Mice that recovered lost parasitaemia by three weeks post infection. Parasitaemia did not return with splenectomy
Zaugg and Kuttler, 1987	Bison	*Babesia bigemina*	iv	Little difference in the pathogenicity between intact and splenectomized animals
Orihel and Eberhard, 1985	Monkey species	*Loa loa*	sc/insect	Microfilariae induced granulomas in the spleen and microfilaraemia recurred after splenectomy
Hof, et al., 1976	Mouse	*Toxoplasma gondii*	ip	More rapid death in splenectomized mice. Little effect of *Bordetella pertussis* (ip) or blockage of macrophages by carbon
Hayes, et al., 1975	Rat	*Fasciola hepatica*	po	No effect on infestation
Sinclair, 1970	Sheep	*Fasciola hepatica*	po	Enhanced pathogenicity

* Route of infection; iv: intravenous; ip: intraperitoneal; inhal: small particle aerosol; lungs: inoculation directly intratracheally; endog: caecal ligation and puncture; sc: subcutaneous infection or implication; insect: use of insect vector; RBC: parasitized cells; blood: citrated infected blood

Splenectomy is necessary in some animals to allow patent infection with a pathogen for another species. This is particularly so for some models of *Plasmodium* spp. parasitaemias in monkeys which are normally resistant to strains which infect humans. Similarly, some zoonoses (for example, babesiosis and *C. canimorsus* infection), are relatively avirulent for man and only cause overwhelming infection in the absence of the spleen. Important veterinary protozoal infestations such as babesiosis, anaplasmosis or theileriosis in cattle are considerably more virulent in splenectomized animals.

Infections with *S. pneumoniae* in rats or mice are clearly enhanced by splenectomy. The effects of splenic autotransplantation are controversial, depending on the technique used and the amount of tissue transplanted. In general, intraperitoneal autoinoculation of washed spleen cells at splenectomy does not protect against experimental pneumococcal infection or malaria. The route of administration of the organism is also important. Coil, Dickerman and Boulton (1978) showed that the spleen was necessary to protect mice even when *S. pneumoniae* was administered as a small particle aerosol.

Although these animal models are often used to evaluate immunotherapy or chemotherapy, it should be appreciated that they rarely mimic exactly the pathogenesis of natural infections in man.

Immunological basis for increased susceptibility to infections

Antibody levels

Several groups have studied small numbers of patients longitudinally or at point times to evaluate the effects of splenectomy on relatively simple measurements of immune status. In the early post-operative period, transient rises in circulating neutrophils and serum IgA levels have been observed, together with more persistent rises in lymphocyte and eosinophil counts (Andersen, Cohn and Sorensen, 1976). One case of profound IgA and IgE deficiency with recurrent respiratory infections post-splenectomy was reported by Skrede and coworkers (1977). This patient's identical twin who was not splenectomized had normal immunoglobulins.

Serum total IgM levels fall immediately after splenectomy (Hershman, *et al.*, 1988) in those without complications, and remain depressed at one year. Serum IgG and IgM levels may fall further with intensive chemotherapy in splenectomized Hodgkin's disease patients (Hancock, *et al.*, 1977). Lymphocyte transformation responses to antigens and mitogens fall after the operation but recover by 10 days. By one year, T-cell and B-cell counts and mitogenic responses are normal.

The protracted fall in serum total IgM levels seems to be a very consistent finding (Claret, Morales and Montaner, 1975; Chaimoff, *et al.*, 1978; Noack, Gdanietz and Muller, 1985; Schneck, *et al.*, 1984; Passl, Eibl and Egkher, 1978; Hancock, *et al.*, 1982) although Hammarstrom and Smith (1986), examining the sera from a random group of splenectomized patients, found IgM and IgG2 levels that were in the normal range. This suggests that carefully matched controls are needed to detect what are, in effect, minor abnormalities. Less impressive relative rises in serum IgA and IgG are sometimes observed.

In addition to low IgM levels, Passl, *et al.* (1976, 1978) noted that 10/22 patients had low or absent agglutinins and 16 had low or absent opsonins to *Escherichia coli*. Antibody responses to experimental challenge with dinitrophenol-Ficoll (a thymus-independent antigen) were ten-fold lower in splenectomized Hodgkin's disease patients than in those with spleens (Amlot and Hayes, 1985). If patients were immunized before splenectomy, they made normal secondary antibody responses. Similar observations have been made with pneumococcal polysaccharide vaccines (see below).

Neutrophil function

Dahl, *et al.* (1986) found abnormal polymorphonuclear function tests in 14/22 splenectomized patients who complained of recurrent infections, predominantly tonsillitis. Similarly, all of a group of splenectomized patients had neutrophils with defective capacity to reduce nitroblue tetrazolium (Falcao, Voltarelli and Bottura, 1982) but contrary results were found by Miller, *et al.* (1976), using a slightly different method and during acute infections. Splenectomy did not alter the capacity of neutrophils to phagocytose staphylococci, candida or pneumococci in malignant reticuloses (Hancock, Bruce and Richmond, 1976).

Lymphocyte populations and function

Peripheral T-lymphocyte counts tend to be higher many years after splenectomy for the staging of Hodgkin's disease, compared with matched non-splenectomized patients (Hancock, *et al.*, 1982). There is a disproportionate increase in CD8+ cells resulting in a reduced CD4:CD8 ratio (Astaldi, *et al.* 1988). The CD8+ cells are large granular lymphocytes, often remarked on in peripheral blood films, and have Natural Killer cell activity. Astaldi and coworkers suggested that the changes in T-cell populations lead to a lack of suppressor influence on B-cell function, resulting in inappropriate manufacture of IgM and a poor response to specific antigens.

In splenectomized patients. Melamed and coworkers (1982) found a decrease in circulating suppressor cell activity and *in vitro* responses to a variety of mitogens compared to matched controls. In contrast, Lanng-Nielsen, *et al.* (1983) found normal T-cell responses to phytohaemagglutinin (PHA) and enhanced responses to pokeweed mitogen (PWM) and concanavlin A (ConA). No inhibition of B-cell responses, either those dependent on T-cells or induced by PWM were seen. The changes were not related to the reason for splenectomy, to the presence of residual spleen (detected in 22/45 patients post trauma), and were present many years after the operation.

Soluble factors

Tuftsin is a tetrapeptide (thr-lys-pro-arg) manufactured in the spleen discovered by Najjar and Nishioka in 1970. It specifically stimulates neutrophil phagocytosis. There is a familial condition of tuftsin deficiency and, as expected, levels fall dramatically within days of performing splenectomy (Spirer, *et al.*, 1977; Najjar, 1978, 1979).

Splenectomized hamsters infected with Venezuelan equine encephalitis virus have a decreased plasma interferon response compared with intact animals (Jahrling, Navarro and Scherer, 1976). Reduced clearance of *Pseudomonas aeruginosa* from the blood, in a rat model of porto-caval anastomosis with splenectomy, could be reversed in part by pre-treatment with Interleukin 1 (Hamawy, *et al.*, 1986). The bases for these seemingly unrelated observations are unknown.

Changes in complement are controversial. Corry *et al.* (1979) found 10% of 58 serum specimens from splenectomized patients to have a defect in the alternative pathway of complement activation. In thalassemia, a consistently enhanced level of activation of the classical pathway was noted and was not influenced by splenectomy (Corry, *et al.*, 1981). Similarly, Nielsen and coworkers (1983) could find no evidence for deficient levels of any major complement components or of complement activation after splenectomy, even in patients who had just recovered from overwhelming infections.

In summary, many immunological disturbances have been noted in splenectomized patients. They include minor but consistent changes in immunoglobulin levels, deficient primary antibody responses to specific spleen-dependent (particularly polysaccharide) antigens, some changes in neutrophil function, decreased ability of peripheral cells to phagocytose bacteria possibly enhanced by deficiencies in important soluble products of the spleen such as tuftsin. There are also minor changes in complement in some patients and minor changes in T-cell populations.

Post-operative infections

The rate of post-operative infectious complications of splenectomy varies between 14 and 29% and depends to some extent on the presence of underlying disease. The rates are higher than after similar 'clean' intra-abdominal operations such as vagotomy (5%) (Carlstedt and Tholin, 1984). The mortality after elective splenectomy is about 1% but between 5% and 7% in all cases.

Splenectomy is a well-defined additional risk factor in post traumatic surgery deaths (Walker, *et al.*, 1985). Of 503 trauma patients who survived more than 10 days post-splenectomy, 23% developed infection, most commonly intra-abdominal sepsis. In another series, 36 out of 41 trauma patients (7% of the total), who died after day 10, were considered to have died from infection (Sekikawa and Shatney, 1983). The likelihood of sepsis increased with the severity of the trauma and therefore presumably with the surgical intervention required. Reoperation for infection after laparotomy for trauma was analysed by Blackwood and coworkers (1988). There was a much higher incidence of reoperation in the few patients who had colon trauma and required splenectomy (6/13) than in those with colon trauma (9%) or splenectomy (5%) alone.

Others have also reported a high incidence of early post-operative complications. Encke and Seufert (1986) found between 22 and 38% complications in retrospective and prospective studies; 7% of patients in both series died. Infections such as subphrenic abscess, pulmonary and pleural sepsis and failure of wound healing were the most frequent complications, and were more common in those with haematologic disease. Malmaeus and coworkers (1986) observed almost exactly the same rates of infectious complications (18%) and post-operative mortality (5%) in a similarly heterogeneous group of 167 consecutive splenectomized patients. This group noted a surprisingly low incidence in Hodgkin's disease and a high specific risk (10%) of subphrenic abscess in 52 patients with autoimmune disease. Similar rates of morbidity (24%) due mainly to pneumonia, wound infection or bleeding, and a mortality rate of 6% usually due to post-operative sepsis, were also noted by Musser and coworkers (1984) in 306 consecutive splenectomy patients. Johansson and coworkers (1990) reported a similar rate of post-operative complications (23%) but lower mortality (2/406, 0.5%) in a large retrospective series of elective splenectomies for haematological disorders. One patient died of post operative pneumonia with sepsis due to *E. coli* and *P. aeruginosa*, and one in another series due to *Staphylococcus aureus* (Rao, 1988). Occasional sepsis and mortality with these organisms will be seen in non-splenectomized individuals after abdominal surgery.

The importance of early post-operative infection with encapsulated organisms was illustrated by Malangoni and coworkers (1984). Sepsis occurred in 21/245 (9%) post-splenectomy (documented by blood culture isolation of encapsulated organisms in 9 patients), and caused death in 13 of these. Risk factors for post-operative sepsis included trauma also involving the pancreas, colon or central nervous system or fractures. In this series, of the 140 patients who survived the trauma, three went on to develop sepsis, possibly related to splenectomy at two, eight and 15 years after the operation. Two of these infections were pneumococcal but not one was fatal. Therefore in this group, the trauma and the post-operative sepsis were of far greater risk to the patients than that of delayed post-splenectomy sepsis. Documentation of serious post-operative sepsis with capsulate organisms is not unusual, suggesting that patients are at particular risk because of, and from the time of splenectomy. It is of interest to consider whether these infections are acquired in hospital or are from the patient's own flora at the time of operation. A high proportion of pneumococcal infections in hospitalized patients is considered to have been acquired in hospital (Ruben, Norden and Korica, 1984).

In a retrospective review by Cioffiro, Schein and Gliedman (1976), splenectomies necessary because of accidental trauma to the spleen during laparotomy (39/237, 16%), were more likely to be complicated by post-operative infection than those performed because of primary trauma. Inevitably, the former operations would have been prolonged and the post-operative infection risk tends to increase progressively with the length of an operation. Interestingly Langevin, Rothenberger and Goldberg (1984) tried to demonstrate the beneficial effect of spleen preservation over splenectomy during elective colonic surgery but observed no significant infections in either group!

The post-operative infection risk can probably be reduced by using a multifactorial approach. Timing the splenectomy in relation to chemotherapy, bowel preparation with antibiotics and making HLA-matched platelet concentrates available to treat haemorrhage, were specifically identified as reducing the operative mortality from 35% in a historical group to none of 20 in a prospective group (McBride and Hester, 1976).

Prophylactic antibiotics perioperatively have been recommended but there are few controlled trials to document their efficacy. Having observed a post-operative infection rate of 45% in a retrospective study, Seufert, Germann and Bottcher (1984) compared perioperative cefuroxime with no treatment in a total of 61 patients. They observed a minor reduction in sepsis and pneumonia. In a larger, though less well-controlled, study of various antibiotic regimes versus no antibiotics, Musser and coworkers (1984) noted the same rates of post-splenectomy infection (sepsis 4–6%, pneumonia 6–7%, wound infection 4–7%, urine infection 4–6%) in both groups. In a retrospective study, Walker and coworkers (1985) noted that 181/254 patients with splenic trauma had been given antibiotics from the time of admission. Sixteen different antibiotics or combinations were used for up to 10 days but there was no evidence for a reduction in infections in those who had received antibiotics.

Postoperative infections are multifactorial in origin and an unacceptably high rate in one centre cannot be reduced by using prophylactic antibiotics alone. However, if prophylactic antibiotics are to be given, then first principles should be observed: appropriate antibiotics to prevent wound and respiratory infections (particularly covering *S. pneumoniae*), no antibiotics on the days leading up to surgery, first dose to achieve circulating bactericidal antibiotic levels at the time of surgery and very few doses to be given post-operatively. For indications where prophylactic antibiotics have been shown to be better than placebo, there seems to be no value in continuing with broad-spectrum antimicrobials beyond 24 hours, even though it is tempting to do so. However, cases of overwhelming pneumococcal infections very soon after surgery have been reported (Linneman and First, 1979). Patients are likely to be exposed to new strains while in hospital and will be particularly susceptible after anaesthesia, so it is essential to continue specific prophylaxis against *S. pneumoniae* post-operatively.

Treatment of post-operative infection depends on its nature and the infecting organisms. Choice of antimicrobials should be guided by microbiological results. Empirical treatment of the septic patient must include an antibiotic regime effective against Gram negative organisms, anaerobes and *S. pneumoniae*.

Late post-splenectomy infections

General considerations

The risk of suffering from a severe bacterial infection after splenectomy can only be approximately judged from the numerous series in the literature. Many of the studies are of retrospective data often collected by question-naire. The follow-up period for each individual is highly variable. In retrospective studies, it is not satisfactory if information about some patients cannot be obtained because any infectious deaths among this group would fundamentally alter the rates (Chaikoff and McCabe, 1985). To get some idea of the true risks, recent papers have analysed the number of severe infections in terms of patient–years of exposure since operation. However, because the risk appears to decrease with time, the mean, median and range of the exposure periods should also be considered.

There is controversy about how long patients continue to be more susceptible to severe infections. The nature of most short-term studies means that the majority of infections are described in the first two years after operation, and then the incidence falls year by year. That serious infections may occur many years after splenectomy is clearly indicated by individual case reports (Evans, 1985; Sass, *et al.*, 1983), but the frequency of these late events cannot be accurately assessed. Sass and coworkers (1983) reviewed 42 cases of overwhelming sepsis in adults, 11 or more years after splenectomy. The longest interval was 42 years.

The reasons for attempting to calculate the risk of infection are to balance the view about the need for splenectomy in controversial areas to encourage the preservation of splenic tissue and to offer advice about preventing infections. Eventually it should be possible to judge whether any measures to reduce the risks have been worthwhile.

Retrospective studies often mention that splenectomized patients report an 'increase' of, or a high rate of trivial upper respiratory viral infections or tonsillitis (Dahl, *et al.*, 1986; Seifert, *et al.*, 1986). Because it is based often on hearsay, this type of data tends to be highly unreliable. The only reliable indication of infection is a positive culture. Thus positive blood and cerebrospinal fluid (CSF) cultures are used to document serious infections. However, by using positive cultures as definitive evidence for infection, mostly in patients admitted to hospital, investigators select for cases by their seriousness, and in these studies a true increase in the frequency of less severe infections in splenectomized patients cannot be detected.

It is likely that patients splenectomized for trauma are exposed to the same risk of acquiring, for example, *S. pneumoniae* as the normal population, but those splenectomized for some underlying disease may have an increased risk because of increased exposure to infections during hospital visits. Whether splenectomized patients become colonized with pneumococci many times for each overt infection is not known, but the relative rarity of documented pneumococcal infection even in this group would suggest that this is so. In healthy individuals, it is considered that the most common predisposing factor for pneumococcal pneumonia and sepsis is influenza. This is just as likely to be so for splenectomized patients and if the virus infection permits primary invasion by pneumococci in the respiratory tract, splenectomy has removed the crucial phagocytic filter which would normally constrain the replication of the bacteria in the blood-stream.

Calculated infection rates

Singer (1973) and Eraklis and Filler (1972) reviewed the literature on the rates of infection in splenectomized individuals. These papers point to wide variations in the incidence of sepsis according to underlying disease. They do not include reference to the interval between operation and infection or to the follow-up periods involved. Dickerman (1976) noted that several of the patients referred to in the earlier papers had developed infections since they had been published.

Singer calculated the expected annual rates of serious pneumococcal sepsis in normals to be 3 per 1000 for infants less than one year of age, 0.7 per 1000 for children of one to 7 years and 0.2 per 1000 for children of 5 to 14 years of age. By comparison, in all age groups, the overall rate of post-splenectomy sepsis was 7/1030 (0.7%) over an undefined period (Singer, 1973; Eraklis and Filler, 1972). In Singer's series (1973), serious infection occurred in 10/688 (1.45%) patients and 4 of these died.

Much higher rates of sepsis after splenectomy were observed where there was underlying disease, the greatest risks being in those with reticuloendothelial disorders (7/69, 10.0%), thalassaemia (14/154, 9.1%) and hereditary spherocytosis (19/850, 2.2%).

The risk also varies with the age of the patients at the time of operation. Severe infections occurred in all of five infants splenectomized before the age of six months, between six weeks and three years after the operation (King and Shumacker, 1952). Age and underlying disease

are inevitably related, children being more likely to have had splenectomy for congenital red cell abnormalities and adults for trauma or Hodgkin's disease. Furthermore the nature of the underlying condition may contribute very significantly to the risk of infection. Thus thalassaemics appear to have a much higher risk than those with hereditary spherocytosis.

In Hodgkin's disease and non-Hodgkin's lymphoma, unexpected infection in a patient in remission is by no means uncommon, though rarely fatal. In active disease, such infections may occur in the absence of granulocytopenia (Chilcote, Baehner and Hammond, 1976; Coker, et al., 1983). However, progressive disease (sometimes complicated by terminal infection) is a much more common cause of death (Notter, et al., 1980) than primary sepsis. The comprehensive studies of Coker and co-workers (1983) and Rosner and Zarrabi (1983) illustrate the complexity of infections in Hodgkin's disease, and suggest that over-whelming pneumococcal infection is relatively rare. They occurred in only 3/121 patients in remission and only one of these patients died whereas 27 bacteraemic infections occurred in 22/181 children with active disease (Donaldson, Glatstein and Vosti, 1978). Similarly, the Danish Study group (1980) noted 10 late pneumococcal infections (of which 4 were fatal) in 437 patients who had had staging laparotomy.

Splenectomy is a clear additional risk factor for severe infection during intensive chemo-therapy for Hodgkin's disease (Bishop, et al., 1981) and for bacterial and fungal sepsis after allogeneic bone marrow transplantation (Paulin, et al., 1987). Moreover, although splenectomy is associated with an additional risk of severe infections in patients with chronic leukaemia, the eventual outcome in terms of survival in comparable groups with or without splenectomy, were not different. Similarly, in matched groups of Hodgkin's disease patients allocated to splenectomy or no operation, no difference in actuarial survival between groups was seen. Disease in the spleen itself is associated with a worse prognosis (Askergren, et al., 1986).

Abrahamsen, Borge and Holte (1990) also compared infection rates in those who did and did not have splenectomy for Hodgkin's disease. Data collected by postal questionnaire administered 10 or more years after operation or diagnosis revealed infections of all types and deaths due to sepsis occurring at the same rate in both groups. However, these events were much more likely in those with stage III–IV disease who had had both radiotherapy and chemotherapy. The excellent case-control study of Mower, Hawkins and Nelson (1986), comparing splenectomized and non-splenectomized chronic leukaemics over 22 years of age, illustrated well that although the likelihood of infection was far greater if the spleen had been removed (65 vs 35%), the overall survival between the groups was not different.

Splenectomy used to be done regularly in association with renal transplantation. In one series of 323 renal transplant recipients, 181 were splectomized and four of these had late *S. pneumoniae* and one *Haemophilus influenzae* sepsis. None of the non-splenectomized patients had infections with capsulate organisms (Schroter, West and Weil, 1977). Similarly, 7 of 236 transplant recipients had sepsis between 3 and 32 months after splenectomy compared with none of 57 who were transplanted without splenectomy (Bourgault, *et al.*, 1979). Linneman and First (1979) observed pneumococcal infections less often than 10 per 1000 patient–years, and noted that these often coincided with graft failure. Cerilli and Jones (1977) and Peters and coworkers (1983), have expressed the opinion that the risk of late infections outweighs the doubtful benefits of splenectomy in transplant recipients.

Calculation of the severe risk of infection after splenectomy

In the United States of America, whereas it has been estimated that there are 0.56 cases of pneumonia per 1000 of the population per year, there are foci with much higher incidence. In San Francisco, for example, the rate of pneumococcal infection was calculated to be 2/1000/year, in Seattle 1.3/1000/year, and in the rural south-west USA to be 16/1000/year. In the latter area the rate is 46/1000/year in the over-65 age group. The rates of pneumococcal meningitis range from 0.003 to 0.05/1000/year. The increased risk of pneumococcal infection was calculated to be 5–10-fold in the post traumatic splenectomy group, 14–28-fold for congenital asplenia and 50–100-fold for Hodgkin's disease (Mufson, 1981; Austrian, 1981).

Recent reports from which it is possible to calculate late severe infection morbidity and mortality rates in splenectomized patients are summarized in Table 3.2. The rather tentative and imprecise rates extracted from these papers are roughly in the same order as those calculated by Cullingford and co-workers (1991), who carefully followed up all of 1490 patients splenectomized in Western Australia between 1971 and 1993. Limitations of this approach have been highlighted by Holdsworth, Irving and Cuschieri (1991). The mortality rates are highly variable and it is important to realize that many of those who recover from pneumococcal sepsis and meningitis are likely to have sequelae (Mouzard, *et al.*, 1979). The purist might argue that it is unreasonable to consider deaths other than due to sudden unexpected sepsis as being associated with splenectomy. It should therefore be noted that in the large series of Chaikoff and McCabe (1985), for example, 12 deaths followed peritonitis, 12 pneumonia, one encephalitis and one cellulitis, while only 2 were due to overwhelming sepsis with no apparent source of infection. However, in several series, no mortality was seen, the longest period of observation (1046 patient–years) being by Sekikawa and Shatney (1986). Similarly, Ask–Upmark (1974) saw no mortality in 100 adults followed for 8 years after splenectomy. The highest mortality rate, 21/1000 patient-years in a group of 38 children followed for a mean of 3.3 years, was observed by Mitterstiele (1979). These differences probably arise because of patients' underlying diseases and their ages at splenectomy. In general, the rate of non-fatal infection is 10–100-fold higher than the mortality rate.

Occasional patients with recurrent infections, sometimes with the same serotype of *S. pneumoniae*, are reported in many series. For example, one child had 3 separate episodes of pneumococcal sepsis at 24, 25 and 27 months after splenectomy (Chilcote, Baehner and Hammond, 1976).

Difficulties in ascribing splenectomy a role in the death of a patient are illustrated by Edwards and Digioia (1976), who felt that infection was the cause of death in only 3 of their series of 23 deaths, whereas in 9 it was contributory, and in 11 infection was only an associated factor. Infections in patients not admitted to hospital or in whom cultures are not obtained, cannot be evaluated.

Another way of assessing the relative risk of splenectomy is to analyse series of patients admitted to hospital with pneumococcal pneumonia and sepsis. Four representative studies are summarized in Table 3.3. Overall

Table 3.2 Infection rates and mortality in splenectomized individuals

Reference	Age group	Reason for splenectomy	Number of patients followed	Length of follow-up years mean or range	Morbidity		Mortality		Comments
					Severe infection episodes	Approximate rate per 1000 patient–years	Mortality due to infection	Approximate rate per 100 patient–years	
Edwards and Digioia, 1976	Adults	Malignancy	131	0.9	15	13	3	2.5	
Schwartz, *et al.*, 1982	Adults	All	193	5.6	80	73	2	1.8	36 cases died of other causes
Krivoy and Titarski, 1975	All	Haematology	104	0.3–14	NA		10	NA	
Wegelius, 1982	All	All	61	5.8	3	8.5	2	5.6	All had pneumococcal vaccination. 8 lost to follow-up
Chaikof and McCabe, 1985	Adults	All	584	7.9	NA	NA	32	7.8	Retrospective study of deaths only, 139 not traced
	Children	All	53	13.8	NA	NA	2	2.8	
Walker, 1976	Children	Haematology	791	2	NA	NA	8	5.0	Many followed up for longer, total infection deaths 17, other deaths 32

Reference	Patients	Type	No.	Follow-up					Comments
Ein, *et al.*, 1977	All	All	182	2–15	10	27	6	16.0	All infections in first 2 years
Green, *et al.*, 1986a	Adults	Trauma	144	5.1	15	20	1	1.4	
Green, *et al.*, 1986b	Children	Splenectomy	18	5.8	2	20	0	0	
		Splenorrhaphy	16	5.8	0	0	0	0	
Pederson, 1983	Children	All	384	6.2	21	8.8	6	2.5	72 patients not followed-up
Mitterstieler, *et al.*, 1979	Children	Not trauma	38	3.3	5	35	3	20.8	
Sekikawa and Shatney, 1986	All	Trauma	242	4.4	6*	5.6	0	0	*All relatively mild infections
Hays, *et al.*, 1986	Children	Hodgkin's	234	5.5	5	3.9	0	0	
Linneman and First, 1979	All	Renal transpl.	163	2.1	14	28**	NA	NA	**Functioning allografts
Constantoulakis, *et al.*, 1973	Children	Thalassaemia	72	5–15	2	2.8	1	1.4	
Chilcote, *et al.*, 1976	Children	Hodgkin's	200	NA	20	NA	10	NA	Length of follow-up not given
O'Neal and McDonald, 1981	Adults	All	256	3.8	NA		7	7.3	Controls: non-splenectomized laparotomy: fatal sepsis rate = 0/1272 patient-years
Pinna, *et al.*, 1988	Children	Thalassaemia	204	3–10	11	8.3	6	4.5	Also six cases of malaria
Cullingford, *et al.*, 1991	All	Trauma	628	6.1	8	2.1	1	0.3	
	All	Other	816	4.6	25	6.7	5	1.3	
		Total	1490	5.3	33	4.2	6	0.8	
Deodhar, *et al.*, 1993	All	Haematology	86	~5.5	NA	NA	8	16.9	Total study over 11 years

(NA: information not given.)

Table 3.3 Outcome of pneumococcal sepsis and meningitis in hospitalized patients

Reference	Patient group	Non-splenectomized		Splenectomized	
		Number	*Mortality %*	*Number*	*Mortality %*
Vachon, *et al.*, 1979	Adult ICU	96	38	4	75
Mousard, *et al.*, 1979	Paed ICU	60	50	2	100
Ruben, *et al.*, 1984	Adults	66	39	6	83
Reilly, *et al.*, 1994	All	51	12	3	67

15/288 (5%) patients of all ages with serious infections had been splenectomized, the mortality in this group being 12/15 (80%) compared to 36% in the group as a whole. Slightly better results were obtained by Selby and coworkers (1984), with only one death in 5 patients, some of whom had multiple septicaemic infections. The incidence of splenectomy in the general population is not known, so it is not possible accurately to gauge the excess serious infections in this group as a whole. In the prospective case control study of Lipsky and coworkers (1986) into the risk factors for pneumococcal sepsis, there were 63 episodes in 3074 patients, a rate of 6.3 cases per 1000 patient–years. Those risk factors identified included dementia, seizure disorders, cigarette smoking, coronary and cerebral vascular disease and institutionalization, but splenectomy had been done only in one patient and one control.

Robinette and Fraumeni (1977) studied the mortality in war veterans from Veterans Administration medical files in the USA. In 740 splenectomized ex-servicemen, the relative risks of mortality compared to those of case-matched non-splenectomized controls were 1.46 for all causes, 1.86 for ischaemic heart disease and incalculable for pneumonia. There were 6 deaths associated with pneumonia in the splenectomized cohort but none in controls.

Pimpl and coworkers (1989) compared post-mortem findings in 202 splenectomized adults with a matched group of 403 non-splenectomized controls who had had laparotomy. Splenectomy had been performed for trauma (30%), during surgery for tumour (28%) and for haematological disorders (11%). They found that pneumonia (58 vs 24%), pyelonephritis (8 vs 2%) and overwhelming sepsis (15 vs 7%) were present significantly more often in the splenectomized group. In addition, there was a higher incidence of pulmonary embolism (36 vs 10%) contributing to death in all categories of splenectomized patients, and this effect surprisingly persisted into the period more than three months after surgery. Whereas severe pneumonia was also significantly increased in all categories of splenectomized patient, sepsis had occurred significantly more often only in the group who had iatrogenic splenectomy. There was an excess mortality from sepsis in the other categories but this failed to reach statistical significance.

In summary, although there does appear to be a risk of serious sepsis after splenectomy, this risk is only slightly increased over that in the rest of the population in those splenectomized for primary trauma. It increases significantly in those with underlying malignant or other immunosuppressive disease and, for example, in thalassaemia. However, numerically many more cases of fulminant pneumococcal sepsis occur in patients who are not splenectomized, and death from causes other than late sepsis are very much more common after trauma and in malignant conditions. The effect of splenectomy *per se* may be buried in more general susceptibility to infection in severely immunosuppressed lymphoma patients.

Presentation and management of infections in splenectomized patients

In healthy subjects, the effects of acquiring *S. pneumoniae* range from healthy carriage, through minor respiratory infection and otitis media, primary peritonitis, pneumonia and meningitis. Infections with capsulate organisms are characterized by rapid onset and progress towards a fulminant course in the splenectomized patient. Linneman and First (1979) clearly differentiated between three clinical syndromes caused by *S. pneumoniae* in renal transplant recipients. Splenectomized patients presented either with severe lobar pneumonia during a rejection crisis or with sudden overwhelming fatal sepsis. One with intact spleen developed mild lobar pneumonia. Chaikoff and McCabe (1985) noted a two to three day influenza-like illness followed by the abrupt onset of clinical sepsis and massive bacteraemia from an unknown source. Bacteraemia may occur with trivial upper respiratory illness or there may be no sign of a focus of infection. In splenectomized patients, however, overwhelming sepsis with shock, altered consciousness, purpura and adrenal haemorrhage may occur irrespective of the infecting organism. This syndrome is characterized by large, diffuse, ecchymotic purpura of the peripheries (Shperber *et al.*, 1989) indistinguishable from Waterhouse-Friderichsen syndrome of non-splenectomized infants infected with *Neisseria meningitidis* and is sometimes termed overwhelming post-splenectomy infection (OPSI). In the fulminant type, signs of meningitis may be less prominent than those of sepsis because of the rapidity of progression. The cerebrospinal fluid may contain many organisms with little cellular response in the early stages: a grave prognostic sign. The peripheral neutrophil count may be high, normal or very low and is unhelpful in distinguishing bacterial from other infections.

The mortality is high and rapid death is common. In one series of 47 adults with pneumococcal sepsis more than 30 days after splenectomy for trauma, 22 died within 48 hours of their first symptom. One patient died within one hour of the first symptom and 6 of those with pneumococcal sepsis had Waterhouse-Friderichsen syndrome (Zarrabi and Rosner, 1984). Ramsay and Bouskill (1973) observed a mortality of 60% in a series of 40 infections, and Mufson (1981) a rate of 71%, compared with overall rates of 25–35% in all patients with pneumococcal pneumonia and meningitis with septicaemia.

Although microbiological specimens must be taken (particularly blood and cerebrospinal fluid cultures), it is crucial to start treatment as soon as the diagnosis is entertained. It is important to indicate to the bacteriologist that the patient is splenectomized and to identify other risk factors in the history which would point to a particular diagnosis: for example,

recent influenza predisposing to pneumococcal and meningococcal infection; dog bite for *C. canimorsus* infection: foreign travel for malaria and contact with ticks for *Babesia* spp. Blood films should be examined for parasites in the febrile patient without obvious cause, even if the patient has not been in an endemic area, because of the small risk of autochthonous infection.

The importance of clinical awareness about the risks of infection in splenectomized patients is illustrated by the following case (Report, 1984). A 19-year old man, splenectomized ten years previously for trauma, was admitted to hospital with symptoms suggesting a viral upper respiratory infection and was not treated with an antibiotic. He died 16 hours after admission from pneumococcal sepsis. The doctors were considered not negligent in diagnosing a viral infection, and it was agreed that withholding antibiotics would have been appropriate if there had been no obvious risk factors for bacterial infection. However, in the circumstances of a splenectomized patient, it was concluded that penicillin should have been started on admission to hospital.

High dose intravenous benzyl penicillin is the drug of choice for the blind treatment of sepsis in a splenectomized patient in most age groups, although in infants especially, the risk of capsulate *H. influenzae* requires the use of an antimicrobial such as cefotaxime. The vast majority of *S. pneumoniae* strains are sensitive to penicillin (minimal inhibitory concentrations (MIC) <0.1 mg/l); Occasionally a strain shows reduced sensitivity to penicillin (MIC 0.1–1.0 mg/l), but such strains would be inhibited by the large doses of penicillin currently in vogue. There have been reports of penicillin-resistant strains (MIC 2–10 mg/l), particularly causing outbreaks of infection in hospitals. In South Africa, such an outbreak occurred in children admitted with measles, and was restricted to two serotypes. In 1990, penicillin-resistant pneumococci were isolated at University College Hospital from sputum or throat swabs of three geriatric patients from North London and one child with an acute eye infection acquired in Egypt. In Spain, 50% of pneumococcal strains are resistant to penicillin but the predominant strains isolateds are included in the vaccine (Garcia-Leoni, *et al.*, 1992).

Recrudescence of pneumococcal infections

in splenectomized patients is common after stopping treatment (Selby and Toghill, 1989) and although tempting to stop early as the patient recovers, it is conventional to continue antibiotics for three weeks.

S. pneumoniae is the commonest documented organism causing serious infection in splenectomized patients yet it represents only about half of the cases (Holdsworth, Irving and Cuschieri, 1991). Surprisingly, pneumococcal infections are sometimes not seen at all. In 55 episodes of infection observed by Cormia and Campos (1973) in 35 out of 117 splenectomized patients, none was caused by the pneumococcus. Infections with *N. meningititis* (approximately 6% of the total serious infections) and *H. influenzae* are particularly likely in young splenectomized children. Other infections seen include Gram-negative bacilli (approximately 10%) (Zarrabi and Rosner, 1984) and a wide range of other organisms including *Staphylococcus aureus, Pseudomonas* spp., *H. influenzae* (Lerman, 1982; Needleman, 1973), *Streptococcus milleri* (McCulloch and Parker, 1979) and *Streptococcus agalactiae* (Hawkey and Finnegan, 1985; Small, *et al.*, 1984). Many of these are commonly seen in hospital practice and tend not to cause serious disease in healthy individuals. Some organisms are classicially not found in blood cultures during the acute illness. *Vibrio cholerae* (Thisyakorn and Reinprayoon, 1990) and *Shigella sonnei* (Christensen, Renneberg and Wallmark, 1990) are two examples of such organisms which caused sepsis in splenectomized patients.

Capnocytophaga canimorsus (formerly known as dysgonic fermenter 2: DF2) is a fastidious, slow growing Gram-negative bacillus, a commensal of the dog mouth, which rarely causes disease after dog bite in healthy subjects. It does, however, cause overwhelming sepsis in splenectomized patients (Hinrichs and Dunkelberg, 1980; Fibbe, *et al.*, 1985; McCarthy and Zumla, 1988; Krol von Straaten, Landheer and de Maat, 1990). Nine out of 26 cases reviewed by Rubin (1984) had had splenectomy. The drug treatment of choice is intravenous penicillin.

Yersinia enterocolitica occasionally is associated with ileitis or appendicitis, but septicaemia in two splenectomized patients in Italy has been reported (Rasore-Quartuo, *et al.*, 1986).

Three out of five patients identified as having clinical symptomatic primary cytomegalovirus (CMV) infection after blood transfusion and surgery were noted to have had splenectomy (Drew and Miner, 1982). It was suggested but has not been established that splenectomy might allow overt manifestations of the infection. Others have also observed that open heart or thoracic surgery is more likely to be associated with overt CMV in splenectomized patients. However, splenectomy is not an additional risk factor for herpes zoster in Hodgkin's disease patients (Redon *et al.*, 1981; Reboul, Donaldson and Kaplan, 1978).

Plasmodium falciparum infections are severe in splenectomized subjects, who should be discouraged from making trips to hyperendemic areas. *Babesia* spp. are also erythrocytic parasites, acquired through hard-tick bites (particularly *Ixodes dammini*). The organism is enzootic in deer and ticks are acquired by man in low heath or scrubland or in temperate forests. Acute babesiosis in healthy individuals is usually asymptomatic or a mild self-limited illness, though it may be associated with coincident *Borrelia burgdorferi* infection (Lyme disease). In splenectomized individuals, *Babesia* spp. may cause an overwhelming parasitaemia of red cells and is essentially unresponsive to conventional anti-protozoal agents (Healy, 1979).

These examples illustrate the unusual nature of many of the infections in splenectomized patients. While penicillin should have been started early during the illness, the treatment must be appropriately modified to cover any organism isolated from blood or CSF.

Prevention of post-splenectomy sepsis

Pneumococcal vaccines

Whereas *S. pneumoniae* accounts for approximately half of the documented cases of overwhelming infections in splenectomized patients, over 80 distinct serological variations in the capsular polysaccharide of this organism are recognized. There is limited, if any, cross protection between these serotypes. Isolated polysaccharide vaccines have been tested since the 1930s. Examination of isolates over a long period in the USA and Scandinavia, identified the most common serotypes causing disease. Vaccines containing 14, 17 and more recently,

23 of these type-specific polysaccharides have been developed into commercial vaccines (Pneumovax, Merck). Most normal subjects make a detectable antibody response to the majority but not all serotypes in the vaccine. Nevertheless, the use of a polysaccharide vaccine of this type remains controversial (Editorial, 1981). The problems may be summarized as follows:

1. It is considered that only one dose of vaccine should be given because boosting of antibody production after the second dose is poor, and because of the likelihood of severe local and systemic reactions to the large antigenic load. Even on first dose administration the vaccine causes soreness at the site of inoculation and has been reported to increase levels of isohaem-agglutinins in 0-positive subjects.

Nevertheless, Konradsen, Pedersen and Henrichsen (1980) have revaccinated children who originally received the 14-valent vaccine and had low antibody titres five years later. The 23-valent vaccine was not without local (10/20), fever (4/20) and systemic (2/20) side-effects but they were described as mild.

2. Antibodies are difficult to measure and there has been controversy about the best technique. New assays based on immunoradiometric or enzyme-linked (ELISA) techniques are more sensitive than agglutination, but reports on the affinity or quality of antibody in terms of protective efficacy have not emerged. Variable antibody responses are made by subjects to individual components of the vaccine. A serotype may rarely fail to stimulate an antibody response in an individual even after recovery from natural infection. Furthermore, because of the rarity of disease with one serotype except in an outbreak or epidemic, it has not proved possible to correlate antibody levels with protective efficacy.

3. Many serotypes are inevitably not contained in the vaccine. A vaccine containing 50 mcg of each of 23 serotypes consists of over 1 g of carbohydrate, a formidable dose to receive and to be processed immunologically. There is marked geographical variation in the prevalence of individual serotypes and there is also evidence for rapid changes in prevalence with the emergence of novel epidemic strains. Thus, there must remain a definite risk of exposure to pneumococci not represented in the vaccine, which will increase with time after the prevalence surveys, on the results of which the vaccine composition was based.

The main indication for a pneumococcal vaccine is to protect those susceptible to severe infections. Splenectomy is a relatively rare predisposing factor in most surveys, the greatest risk factors in otherwise healthy subjects being the extremes of age.

Antibody responses to pneumococcal vaccines in young children are unreliable and immunization is not recommended under two years of age. Pedersen, Hendrickse and Schiffman (1982) showed that a single dose of 14-valent vaccine may achieve a protective antibody level, assumed to be 300 ng antibody per ml, in only one half of the older children vaccinated. In a large-scale trial in the elderly, approximately the same rate of pneumococcal infections occurred in placebo and immunized individuals over a three-year follow-up period (Simberkoff, *et al.*, 1986). Infections occurred with strains carried in the vaccine as often in the immunized as in the non-immunized groups. Broome and coworkers (1980) judged the efficacy of the vaccine by analysing significant pneumococcal infections in a group of patients according to the serotypes involved and whether or not they had been vaccinated. Protection is difficult to prove in such a study but the conclusion from a relatively small number of immunized subjects, was that the vaccine had failed to protect those susceptible to infection, including some splenectomized patients. Furthermore, those over 10 years of age tended to be infected with serotypes not included in the vaccine.

There are well documented failures of protection of individuals against pneumococcal serotypes (Broome *et al.*, 1980), often to which they had made no detectable antibody response (Lanng-Nielsen, Karup-Pedersen and Ellegaard, 1982; Schlaeffer, *et al.*, 1985).

Antibody responses to pneumococcal polysaccharides are made in splenectomized patients but are variable and are further reduced if patients are receiving immunosuppressive therapy at the time of vaccination (Amman, *et al.*, 1977; Siber *et al.*, 1978). Antibody responses after splenectomy are generally in IgG2 and IgA2 but rises are much greater in post-trauma patients than in those with lymphoma, especially those who had both radiotherapy and chemotherapy (Grimfors, *et al.*, 1989). In a study of antibody responses to pneumococcal polysaccharides in Hodgkin's disease, there were no differences in responses between splenectomized and non-splenectomized patients, but if radiotherapy and chemotherapy commenced, responses were poor in both groups (Addiego, *et al.*, 1980). Donaldson and coworkers (1981) also commented on the unpredictability of responses to pneumococcal polysaccharides. Similar poor responses to *H. influenzae* capsule were observed in splenectomized Hodgkin's disease adults, again particularly those treated with chemotherapy and radiotherapy (Jakacki, *et al.*, 1990).

In contrast, Hosea and coworkers (1981) showed impaired IgM and IgG responses by ELISA to most of the serotypes tested in splenectomized patients. Certain underlying diseases contributed to even lower antibody concentrations. However, these authors pointed out the difficulties interpreting antibody responses and noted that if a two-fold increase in geometric mean titres of antibody indicated a 'satisfactory' response, then there would be no differences between patients and their controls.

Totally asplenic patients are probably unable to make primary antibody responses to polysaccharides, so it has been proposed that antibody responses to pneumococcal vaccines in these patients reflect previous natural exposure to particular serotypes. This would account for poorer responses in younger, less exposed patients and the failure of certain serotypes to induce antibodies (Caplan, *et al.*, 1983) and to protect some individuals. Antibody levels decay significantly within a period of two years after vaccination, but the relevance of this to enhanced susceptibility has not yet been clearly demonstrated (Grimfors, *et al.*, 1990).

In an attempt to unravel the response characteristics of circulating cells in different patient groups, Di Padova and coworkers (1983) studied antibody production by circulating cells and its dependence on the spleen. Circulating B-cells synthesizing antibody peaking at seven days after vaccination were not different but stimulation of B-cells synthesizing specific IgM and IgG in response to Pokeweed mitogen was deficient in splenectomized cases.

A survey of compliance with recommendations for pneumococcal vaccination and antibiotic prophylaxis in Australia (Siddins, *et al.*, 1990), revealed that whereas all of 21 patients having splenectomy for haematological disease were vaccinated prospectively, proportionately fewer in the other groups received vaccine. Only two of 18 patients who had incidental splenectomy during laparotomy were vaccinated.

No properly controlled trials of pneumococcal vaccine in splenectomized patients have been published. It is generally agreed that it is a good idea to immunize patients, preferably before splenectomy, and therefore perhaps unethical to do a placebo-controlled trial. Furthermore the data in Table 3.2 suggest that thousands of patient–years of monitoring in such a trial would be needed to prove efficacy. Recent Department of Health guidelines (1992) suggest revaccination every five years but there is little clinical experience to support such a recommendation—simply the observed fall in titre of antibodies. Case reports of failure of immunization in splenectomized patients manifest as overwhelming infections sometimes with strains not included in the vaccine (Linblad and Lindblad, 1990), suggest that other preventive steps, particularly prophylactic antibiotics must continue to be recommended.

Prophylactic antibiotics

Low dose oral phenoxymethyl penicillin (250 mg 12-hourly in adults and 125 mg 12-hourly in children) is given for the prevention of pneumococcal sepsis in splenectomized patients. Penicillin V is inconsistently absorbed and this dose schedule is ineffective in clearing sensitive organisms from the throat flora. However, *S. pneumoniae* is normally very sensitive to penicillin and we presume that its value lies in the prevention of establishment of the early stages of invasive disease. Penicillin will cover several other possible causes of bacteraemia including *C. canimorsus* and meningococci. Unfortunately, penicillin prophylaxis is not often mentioned in reports of post-splenectomy sepsis (Selby, *et al.*, 1987). Cases of vaccine failure have been clearly documented and, only recently, cases of penicillin (Deodhar, Marshall and Barnes, 1993) and ampicillin (Chadwick, Kearney and Jones, 1993) failure have been shown, the latter involving a penicillin-resistant strain of pneumococcus. (This pastient was susceptible not because of splenectomy but because of CSF rhinorrhoea.) Even if sepsis tends to occur in those not taking prophylaxis, this does not, of course, prove that the prophylaxis is actually effective.

There is little argument that this treatment should be started and continued postoperatively, but considerable debate as to how long it should continue. While most pneumococcal infections occur within the first two years after splenectomy, many occur in the next five years and there are many well-documented case reports of fatal infections occurring in otherwise healthy subjects after many years. However, these cases are very rare. If a patient is diligent about taking low-dose oral penicillin prophylaxis, then this should never be discouraged. On the other hand, it is difficult to judge the degree to which non-compliant patients should be exhorted to take prophylaxis when the risk of pneumococcal sepsis is so low. This is particularly so in those splenectomized for trauma who are completely well. Little has been written about toxicity of or hypersensitivity to low dose regimes of penicillin. Furthermore, despite penicillin, patients continue to be at risk of infections with organisms resistant to penicillin.

For patients allergic to penicillin, oral erythromycin (250 mg 12-hourly in adults) is to be recommended. Though highly active against most strains of *S. pneumoniae*, this may be less well tolerated than penicillin, and its prophylactic efficacy is unproved.

Compliance with oral antibiotics is generally poor. In the prospective study of physician compliance by Siddins, *et al.*, (1990), only 6 of 75 patients were started on long-term antibiotics. Borgna-Pignatti and coworkers (1984) assessed the compliance of 42 splenectomized thalassaemics with recommended penicillin prophylaxis. Only 3 were not taking penicillin at all, but a further 6 were taking what was considered to be inadequate intermittent therapy. Golematis and coworkers (1989) ensured that all of 98 patients splenectomized for thalassaemia were assiduously given pneumococcal vaccine preoperatively and then phenoxymethyl penicillin (625 mg po daily as a single dose). One patient who died of pneumococcal sepsis had discontinued the penicillin three months previously. The strain was not typed to determine whether it was included in the vaccine.

Patients who will not take regular penicillin prophylaxis should be urged to take this for a period of at least a month when they develop an upper respiratory tract infection. We advocate the use of amoxycillin (250 mg 8-hourly) under these circumstances because it is active against many *H. influenzae* strains and is absorbed more consistently than penicillin V. However, there is no trial work to support this recommendation. Amoxycillin is slightly less active than penicillin against *S. pneumoniae in vitro* and is more likely to cause disturbance of the gut flora with occasional diarrhoea, and overgrowth by *Candida albicans*. During outbreaks of pneumococcal infection, when a family member has established infection, or if a patient is admitted to hospital for any reason, penicillin prophylaxis should be started. Under these circumstances, we would favour giving larger doses of penicillin V (500 mg six-hourly).

General measures

Splenectomized patients should be instructed to take simple general measures to reduce the risk of acquiring an infection which may turn out to be severe. For example, influenza vaccines which are available should be offered, and patients should avoid infectious contacts as far as is reasonably possible. It is not appreciated that many viruses causing upper respiratory illness are not transmitted as well by inhalation of aerosol particles as by hand to mucosal contact. Pneumococcal infections are more common in overcrowded and poor social conditions, in mining and construction camps, in recruitment centres and in hospitals. However, a rise in incidence of pneumonia in a population often follows an epidemic of influenza or measles.

Flegg (1994) recommends other polysaccharide immunizations against meningococci (A and C) and *H. influenzae* type b. However, these infections are exceedingly uncommon and it would seem to be more worthwhile, in the first instance, to make sure that all splenectomized patients get pneumococcal vaccine and are offered antibiotic prophylaxis.

Patients should be discouraged from walking in scrub and woodland without adequate protective clothing against acquiring ticks. They should not own dogs and should take care to avoid dog bites. They should not visit areas of falciparum malaria endemicity.

Operation methods

The risks of splenectomy are obviated by not performing the operation at all. Thus computerized tomographic scanning is now advocated for the staging of Hodgkin's disease. Similarly, treatment of hairy cell leukaemia with new effective agents such as interferon-α may also reduce the need for splenectomy.

Repair of the spleen after trauma rather than removal is now a practical possibility (Roth, et al., 1982; Oakes and Charters, 1981; Bhattacharya, Ablin and Kosloske, 1989) and consideration should be given to retro-peritoneal autoinoculation of some splenic tissue, if preservation of the structural integrity of the spleen is not possible. Wetzig, Strong and Theile (1986) found that preservation of the ruptured spleen could be achieved in 25% of cases. Langevin, Rothenberger and Goldberg (1984) found no increased post-operative morbidity in cases where the spleen had been preserved following accidental trauma. After trauma to the spleen, tissue is often seeded spontaneously into the peritoneum and retro-peritoneal space. Deliberate seeding removes the normal architecture and therefore the filtration properties of the spleen, but pro-duction of soluble factors and handling of spleen dependent antigens should be preserved. However, mice reconstituted by injection of macerated filtered splenic cells into the peritoneum at the time of splenectomy, tend not to be protected against experimental *S. pneumoniae* (Schwartz, et al., 1978) or malaria (Oster, Koontz and Wyler, 1980); on the other hand implantation of large functional slices of spleen into an omental pouch, did offer some protection against *S. pneumoniae* (Patel, et al., 1982).

Splenic tissue is detectable by sulphur colloid ^{99m}Tc uptake and indirectly from peripheral blood film changes (Pearson, et al., 1978). Sass and coworkers (1983) noted that 39 of 42 patients with late post-splenectomy sepsis had no residual splenic tissue. Although immuno-globulin levels were not affected in seven patients with splenic implantation, Howell-Jolly bodies persisted, indicating inefficient filtration and phagocytosis, despite the tissue being well-vascularized (Holschneider, et al., 1983). For return of 'function' as measured by the proportion of pitted red cells in the circu-lation, radioisotope studies have suggested that 20–30 cm^3 of splenic tissue is the minimum that needs to be implanted (Corazza, et al., 1984). This is more likely to occur after trauma than after elective splenectomy.

Summary and recommendations

Splenectomy is a common operation and results in the loss of the most important phagocytic organ for filtration of the blood by the reticulo-endothelial system. The spleen is crucial for primary antibody responses to polysaccharide antigens. Surgeons should be encouraged to preserve the spleen after accidental or iatrogenic trauma.

There is justified anxiety about the risks of late post-splenectomy sepsis, but these risks are not high and may be considerably better than those from the underlying condition which prompted splenectomy and the associated risk from post-operative infections. For post-traumatic splenectomy, the incidence of over-whelming pneumococcal infection is similar to that of the general population. Relatively few patients with severe pneumococcal or other infection are actually asplenic. Although pneumococcal infections are the prominent cause of sepsis and death in splenectomized patients, about one-half of these episodes are caused by a wide variety of other organisms. Nevertheless, most efforts are directed at protecting against *S. pneumoniae*, and should include immunization and antimicrobial prophylaxis. The former does not confer complete protection and is relatively ineffective once total splenectomy has been performed and in severely immunosuppressed patients. The vaccine should be given two weeks or more before splenectomy and should be seriously considered in those for laparotomy involving a high risk of splenic trauma. Similar con-siderations apply to the use of other poly-saccharide vaccines.

There is considerable anxiety about the recommendation of long-term penicillin prophylaxis because of the emergence of resistance in pneumococci and lack of com-pliance (Read and Finch, 1994). We are not persuaded by the evidence that capsular poly-saccharide immunization is better than prophy-lactic antibiotics, nor about the recommen-dations to revaccinate with pneumococcal vaccination, which are based on the fall in circulating antibody titres rather than clinical efficacy. We recognize that infection rates are so low as to make meaningful clinical trials impractical.

Compliance with penicillin prophylaxis is poor, yet should be encouraged for the life of the patient. In those reluctant to take prophylaxis or who eventually default, advice should be given to take an antimicrobial during periods of high risk, such as following simple virus infection. Simple steps can be taken to avoid some of the other less common causes of post-splenectomy sepsis. The key to the treatment of severe infections in these patients is the immediate administration of empirical antimicrobials, intensive care support if needed and early antimicrobial change in response to microbiological results.

References

Abrahamsen, A.F., Borge, L. and Holte, H. (1990) Infection after splenectomy for Hodgkin's disease. *Acta Oncologica*, **29**, 167–170

Addiego, J.E. Jr., Ammann, A.J., Schiffman, G., Baehner, R., Higgins, G. and Hammond, D. (1980) Response to pneumococcal polysaccharide vaccine in patients with untreated Hodgkin's disease. *Lancet*, **ii**, 450-452

Amlot, P.L. and Hayes, A.E. (1985) Impaired human antibody response to the thymus-independent antigen, DNP-Ficoll, after splenectomy. Implications for post-splenectomy infections. *Lancet*, **i**, 1008–1011

Ammann, A.J., Addiego, J., Wara, D.W., Lubin, B., Smith, W.B. and Mentzer, W.C. (1977) Polyvalent pneumococcal polysaccharide immunization of patients with sickle cell anaemia and patients with splenectomy. *New England Journal of Medicine*, **297**, 897–900

Andersen, V., Cohn, J. and Sorensen, S.F. (1976) Immunological studies in children before and after splenectomy. *Acta paediatrica Scandinavica*, **65**, 409–415

Ask-Upmark, E. (1974) Infections in asplenic adults. *British Medical Journal*, **iii**, 687

Askergren, J., Bjorkholm, M., Holm, G., Johansson, B. and Mellstedt, H. (1986) Prognostic influence of early diagnostic splenectomy in Hodgkin's Disease. *Acta Medica Scandinavica*, **219**, 315–322

Astaldi, G., Airo, P. and Airo, R. (1988) Splenectomy and lymphocyte subsets. *Hematology Reviews*, **2**, 93–103. Harwood Academic Publishers

Austrian, R.R. (1981) Pneumococcus, the first hundred years. *Reviews of Infectious Diseases*, **3**, 183–189

Benach, J.L., White, D.J. and McGovern, J.P. (1978) Babesiosis in Long Island. Host-parasite relationships of rodent- and human-derived *Babesia microti* isolates in hamsters. *American Journal of Tropical Medicine and Hygiene*, **27**, 1073–1078

Bhattacharya, N., Ablin, D.S. and Kosloskie, A.M. (1989) Stapled partial splenectomy for splenic abscess in a child. *Journal of Pediatric Surgery*, **24**, 316–317

Bishop, J.F., Schimpff, S.C., Diggs, C.H. and Wiernik, P.H. (1981) Infections during intensive chemotherapy for non-Hodgkin's lymphoma. *Annals of Internal Medicine*, **95**, 549–555

Blackwood, J.M., Hurd, T., Suval, W. and Machiedo, G.W. (1988) Intra-abdominal infection following combined spleen–colon trauma. *American Surgeon*, **54**, 212–216

Borgna-Pignatti, C., De-Stefano, P., Barone, F. and Concia, E. (1984) Penicillin compliance in splenectomized thalassemics. *European Journal of Pediatrics*, **142**, 83–85

Bourgault, A.M., van Scoy, R.E., Wilkowske, C.J. and Sterioff, S. (1979) Severe infection due to *Streptococcus pneumoniae* in asplenic renal transplant patients. *Mayo Clinic Proceedings*, **54**, 123–126

Bouza, E., Burgaleta, C. and Golde, D.W. (1978) Infections in hairy cell leukemia. *Blood*, **51**, 851–859

Broome, C.V., Facklam, R.R. and Fraser, D.W. (1980) Pneumococcal disease after pneumococcal vaccination. *New England Journal of Medicine*, **303**, 549–552

Butler, T., Johnston, K.H., Gutierrez, Y., Aikawa, M. and Cardaman, R. (1985) Enhancement of experimental bacteremia and endocarditis caused by dysgonic fermenter (DF-2) bacterium after treatment with methylprednisolone and after splenectomy. *Infection and Immunity*, **47**, 294–300

Caplan, E.S., Boltansky, H., Snyder, M.J., Rooney, J., Hoyt, N.J., Schiffman, G. and Cowley, R.A. (1983) Response of traumatised splenectomized patients to immediate vaccination with polyvalent pneumococcal vaccine. *Journal of Trauma*, **23**, 801–805

Carlstedt, A. and Tholin, B. (1984) Infectious complications after splenectomy. *Acta Chirurgica Scandinavica*, **150**, 607–610

Cerilli, J. and Jones, L. (1977) A reappraisal of the role of splenectomy in children receiving renal allografts. *Surgery*, **82**, 510–513

Chadwick, P.R., Keaney, M.G. and Jones, R.A. (1993) Meningitis due to penincillin-resistant *Streptococcus pneumoniae* occurring in a patient on long-term ampicillin prophylaxis. *Journal of Infection*, **27**, 277–279

Chaikof, E.L. and McCabe, C.J. (1985) Fatal overwhelming postsplenectomy infection. *American Journal of Surgery*, **149**, 534–539

Chaimoff, C., Douer, D., Pick, I.A. and Pinkhas, J. (1978) Serum immunoglobulin changes after accidental splenectomy in adults. *American Journal of Surgery*, **136**, 332–333

Chilcote, R.R., Baehner, R.L. and Hammond, D. (1976) Septicaemia and meningitis in children splenectomized for Hodgkin's disease. *New England Journal of Medicine*, **295**, 798–800

Christensen, P., Renneberg, J. and Wallmark, E. (1990) *Shigella sonnei* sepsis after splenectomy and portacaval shunt (letter). *European Journal of Clinical Microbiology and Infectious Disease*, **9**, 148–149

Cioffiro, W., Schein, C.J. and Gliedman, M.L. (1976) Splenic injury during abdominal surgery. *Archives of Surgery*, **111**, 167–171

Claret, I., Morales, L. and Montaner, A. (1975) Immunological studies in the postsplenectomy syndrome. *Journal of Pediatric Surgery*, **10**, 59–64

Coil, J.A., Dickerman, J.D. and Boulton, E. (1978) Increased susceptibility of splenectomized mice to infection after exposure to an aerosolized suspension of type 3 *Streptococcus pneumoniae*. *Infection and Immunity*, **21**, 412–416

Coker, D.D., Morris, D.M., Coleman, J.J., Schimpff, S.C., Wiernik, P.H. and Elias, E.G. (1983) Infection among 210 patients with surgically staged Hodgkin's disease. *American Journal of Medicine*, **75**, 97–109

Collins, W.E., Skinner, J.C., Broderson, J.R., Huong, A.Y., Meha-Ffey, P.C., Stanfill, P.S. and Sutton, B.B. (1986) Infection of *Aotus azarae boliviensis* monkeys with different strains of *Plasmodium falciparum*. *Journal of Parasitology*, **72**, 525–530

Constantoulakis, M., Economopoulos, P. and Constantopoulos, A. (1973) Infections after splenectomy. *Annals of Internal Medicine*, **78**, 780–781

Coon, W.W. (1985) Felty's syndrome: when is splenectomy indicated? *American Journal of Surgery*, **149**, 272–275

Corazza, G.R., Tarozzi, C., Vaira, D., Frisoni, M. and Gasbarrini, G. (1984) Return of splenic function after splenectomy. How much tissue is needed? *British Medical Journal*, **289**, 861–864

Cormia, F.E. Jr. and Campos, L.T. (1973) Infections after splenectomy. *Annals of Internal Medicine*, **78**, 149–150

Corry, J.M., Marshall, W.C., Guthrie, L.A., Peerless, A.G. and Johnston, R.B. Jr. (1981) Deficient activity of the alternative pathway of complement in beta thalassemia major. *American Journal of Diseases of Childhood*, **135**, 529–531

Corry, J.M., Polhill, R.B. Jr., Edmonds, S.R. and Johnston, R.B. Jr. (1979) Activity of the alternative complement pathway after splenectomy: comparison to activity in sickle cell disease and hypogammaglobulinemia. *Journal of Pediatrics*, **95**, 964–969

Cullingford, G.L., Watkins, D.N., Watts, A.D.J. and Mallon, D.F. (1991) Severe late postsplenectomy infection. *British Journal of Surgery*, **78**, 716–721

Dahl, M., Hakansson, L., Kreuger, A., Olsen, L., Nilsson, U. and Venge, P. (1986) Polymorphonuclear neutrophil function and infections following splenectomy in childhood. *Scandinavian Journal of Haematology*, **37**, 137–143

Danish Hodgkin Study Group. (1980) Hodgkin's disease in Denmark. A national clinical study. *Scandinavian Journal of Haematology*, **24**, 321–334

Deodhar, H.A., Marshall, R.J. and Barnes, J.N. (1993) Increased risk of sepsis after splectomy. *British Medical Journal*, **307**, 1408–1409

Department of Health (1992) *Immunisation Against Infectious Diseases*. HMSO, London, pp. 100–103

Desai, B.B., Albright, J.W. and Albright, J.F. (1987) Cooperative action of complement component C3 and phagocytic effector cells in innate murine resistance to *Trypanosoma lewisi*. *Infection and Immunity*, **55**, 358–363

Dickerman, J.D. (1976) Bacterial infection and the asplenic host. *Journal of Trauma*, **16**, 662–668

Di Padova, F., Dürig, M., Wadström, J. and Harder, F. (1983) Role of spleen in immune response to polyvalent pneumococcal vaccine. *British Medical Journal*, **287**, 1829–1832

Diffley, P. and Scott, J.O. (1984) Immunological control of chronic *Trypanosoma brucei gambiense* in outbred rodents. *Acta Tropica (Basel)*, **41**, 335–342

Dockrell, H.M., de-Souza, J.B. and Playfair, J.H. (1980) The role of the liver in immunity to blood-stage murine malaria. *Immunology*, **41**, 421–430

Donaldson, S.S., Glatstein, E. and Vosti, K.L. (1978) Bacterial infections in pediatric Hodgkin's disease: relationship to radiotherapy, chemotherapy and splenectomy. *Cancer*, **41**, 1949–1958

Donaldson, S., Vosti, K.L., Berberich, F.R., Cox, R.S., Kaplan, H.S. and Schiffman, G. (1981). Response to pneumococcal vaccine among children with Hodgkin's disease. *Reviews of Infectious Disease*, **3**, S133–143

Drew, W.L. and Miner, R.C. (1982) Transfusion-related cytomegalovirus infection following noncardiac surgery. *Journal of the American Medical Association*, **247**, 2389–2391

Duffey, L.M., Albright, J.W. and Albright, J.F. (1985) *Trypanosoma musculi*: population dynamics of erythrocytes and leukocytes during the course of murine infections. *Experimental Parasitology*, **59**, 375–389

Editorial (1981) Indications for pneumococcal vaccine. *Lancet*, **i**, 251–253

Edwards, L.D. and Digioia, R. (1976) Infections in splenectomized patients. A study of 131 patients. *Scandinavian Journal of Infectious Diseases*, **8**, 255–261

Ein, E.H., Shandling, B., Simpson, J.S., Stephens, C.A., Bandi, S.K., Biggar, W.D. and Freedman, M.H. (1977) The morbidity and mortality of splenectomy in childhood. *Annals of Surgery*, **185**, 307–310

Eling, W.M. (1982) Chronic, patent *Plasmodium berghei* malaria in splenectomized mice. *Infection and Immunity*, **35**, 880–886

Encke, A. and Seufert, R.M. (1986) Complications following splenectomy. *Langenbecks Archiv fur Chirurgie*, **369**, 251–257

Eraklis, A.J. and Filler, R.M. (1972) Splenectomy in childhood: a review of 1413 cases. *Journal of Pediatric Surgery*, **7**, 382–388

Evans, D.I. (1985) Postsplenectomy sepsis 10 years or more after operation. *Journal of Clinical Pathology*, **38**, 309–311

Falcao, R.P., Voltarelli, J.C. and Bottura, C. (1982) The possible role of the spleen in the reduction of nitroblue tetrazolium by neutrophils. *Acta Haematologica (Basel)*, **68**, 89–95

Fibbe, W., Ligthart, G., van den Broek, P., Lampe, A. and van der Meer, J. (1985) Septicaemia with a dysgonic fermenter-2 (DF-2) bacterium in a compromised host. *Infection*, **13**, 286–287

Flegg, P.J. (1994) Long-term management after splenectomy: National guidelines please. *British Medical Journal*, **308**, 131

Garcia-Leoni, M.E., Cerceenado, E., Rodeno, P., Bernaldo de Quiros, J.C.L., Martinez-Hernandez, D. and Bouza, E. (1992) Susceptibility of *Streptococcus pneumoniae* to penicillin: a prospective microbiological and clinical study. *Clinical Infectious Diseases*, **14**, 427–435

Golomb, H.M. and Hadad, L.J. (1984). Infectious complications in 127 patients with hairy cell leukaemia. *American Journal of Hematology*, **16**, 393–401

Golematis, B., Tzardis, P., Legakis, N. and Persidou-Golemati, P. (1989) Overwhelming postsplenectomy infection in patients with thalassemia major. *Mount Sinai Journal of Medicine*, **56**, 97–98

Green, J.B., Shackford, S.R., Sise, M.J. and Fridlund, P. (1986a) Late septic complications in adults following splenectomy for trauma: a prospective analysis in 144 patients. *Journal of Trauma*, **26**, 999–1004

Green, J.B., Shackford, S.R., Sise, M.J., Powell, R.W. (1986b) Postsplenectomy sepsis in pediatric patients following splenectomy for trauma: a proposal for a multi-institutional study. *Journal of Pediatric Surgery*, **21**, 1084–1086

Grimfors, G., Bjorkholm, M., Hammarstrom, L., Askergren, J., Smith, C.I. and Holm, G. (1989) Type-specific anti-pneumococcal antibody subclass response to vaccination after splenectomy with special reference to lymphoma patients. *European Journal of Haematology*, **43**, 404–410

Grimfors, G., Soderqvist, M., Holm, G., Lefvert, A.K. and Bjorkholm, M. (1990) A longitudinal study of class and subclass antibody response to pneumococcal vaccination in splenectomized individuals with special reference to patients with Hodgkin's disease. *European Journal of Haematology*, **45**, 101–108

Grun, J.L., Long, C.A. and Weidenz, W.P. (1985) Effects of splenectomy on antibody-independent immunity to *Plasmodium chabaudi adami* malaria. *Infection and Immunity*, **48**, 853–858

Gullstrand, P., Alwmark, A. and Schalen, C. (1982) Effect of steroids on the outcome of penicillen treatment in pneumococcal sepsis in splenectomized rats. *Surgery*, **91**, 222–225

Gysin, J., Hommel, M. and Da Silva, L.P. (1980) Experimental infection of the squirrel monkey (*Saimiri sciureus*) with *Plasmodium falciparum*. *Journal of Parasitology*, **66**, 1003–1009

Hamawy, K.J., Yamazaki, K., Georgieff, M., Dinarello, C.A., Moldawer, L.L., Blackburn, G.L. and Bistrian, B.R. (1986) Improvements in host immunity by partially purified interleukin 1 in rats with portacaval anastomosis and splenectomy. *Journal of Parenteral and Enteral Nutrition*, **10**, 146–50

Hammarstrom, L. and Smith, C. I. (1986) Development of anti-polysaccharide antibodies in asplenic children. *Clinical and Experimental Immunology*, **66**, 457–462

Hancock, B.W., Bruce, L., Dunsmore, I.R., Ward, A.M. and Richmond, J. (1977) Follow-up studies on the immune status of patients with Hodgkin's disease after splenectomy and treatment, in relapse and remission. *British Journal of Cancer*, **36**, 347–354

Hancock, B.W., Bruce, L. and Richmond, J. (1976) Neutrophil function in lymphoreticular malignancy. *British Journal of Cancer*, **33**, 496–500

Hancock, B.W., Bruce, L., Whitham, M.D., Dunsmore, I.R., Ward, A.M. and Richmond, J. (1982) Immunity in Hodgkin's disease: status after five years' remission. *British Journal of Cancer*, **46**, 593–600

Hawkey, P.M. and Finnegan, O.C. (1985) Streptococcal infections following splenectomy for trauma. *Archives of Internal Medicine*, **145**, 573

Hays, D.M., Ternberg, J.L., Chen, T.T., Sullivan, M.P., Tefft, M., Fung, F., *et al.* (1986) Postsplenectomy sepsis and other complications following staging laparotomy for Hodgkin's disease in childhood. *Journal of Pediatric Surgery*, **21**, 628–632

Hayes, T.J., Bailer, J. and Mitrovic, M. (1975) Acquired immunity to *Fasciola hepatica* in splenectomised rats. *Research in Veterinary Science*, **19**, 86–87

Healy, G.R. (1979) Babesia infections in man. *Hospital Practice*, **14**, 115–116

Hebert, J.C., Gemelli, R.L., Foster, R.S. Jr., Chalmer, B.J. and Davis, J. H. (1983) Improved survival after pneumococcus in splenectomized and nonsplenectomized mice with *Corynebacterium parvum*. *Archives of Surgery*, **118**, 328–332

Hershman, M.J., Cheadle, W.G., George, C.D., Cost, K.M., Appel, S.H., Davidson, P.F. and Pork, H.C. Jr. (1988) The response of immunoglobulins to infection after thermal and nonthermal injury. *American Surgeon*, **54**, 408–411

Hinricks, J.H. and Dunkelberg, W.E. (1980) DF-2 septicaemia after splenectomy: epidemiology and immunologic response. *Southern Medical Journal*, **74**, 1638–1640

Hirano, T., Forbes, S. R., Robinson, G.T., Velky, T.S. and Greenburg, A.G. (1986) The effects of heparin and splenectomy on survival and plasma fibronectin levels in rat peritonitis. *Journal of Surgical Research*, **40**, 611–616

Hof, H., Höhne, K. and Seeliger, H.P. (1976) Macrophage function and host resistance against infection with *Toxoplasma gondii*. *Canadian Journal of Microbiology*, **22**, 1453–1457

Holdsworth, R.J., Irving, A.D. and Cuschieri, A. (1991) Postsplenectomy sepsis and its mortality: actuarial versus perceived risks. *British Journal of Surgery*, **78**, 1031–1038

Holschneider, A.M., Belohradsky, B.H., Krickz-Klimek, H. and Strasser, W. (1983) Splenectomy and reimplantation of splenic tissue in children. *Klinische Pediatrie (Stuttgart)*, **195**, 394–398

Hosea, S.W., Burch, C.G., Brown, E.J., Berg, R.A. and Frank, M.A. (1981) Impaired immune response of splenectomised patients to polyvalent pneumococcal vaccine. *Lancet*, **i**, 804–807

Hussein, H.S. (1977) The nature of immunity against *Babesia hylomysci* and *B. microti* infections in mice. *Annals of Tropical Medicine and Parasitology*, **71**, 249–253

Jahrling, P.B., Navarro, E. and Scherer, W.F. (1976) Interferon induction and sensitivity as correlates to virulence of Venezuelan encephalitis viruses for hamsters. *Archives of Virology*, **51**, 23–35

Jakacki, R., Luery, N., McVerry, P. and Lange, B. (1990) *Haemophilus influenzae* diphtheria protein conjugate immunization after therapy in splenectomized patients with Hodgkin's disease. *Annals of Internal Medicine,* **112**, 143–144

Johansson, T., Bostrom, H., Sjodah, R. and Ihse, I. (1990) Splenectomy for haematological diseases. *Acta Chirurgica Scandinavica,* **156**, 83–86

Joyce, R.A., Boggs, D.R., Chervenick, P.A. and Lalezari, P. (1980) Neutrophil kinetics in Felty's syndrome. *American Journal of Medicine,* **69**, 695–702

Karanfilian, R.G., Spillert, C.R., Machiedo, G.W., Rush, B.F. Jr. and Lazaro, E.J. (1983) Effect of age and splenectomy in murine endotoxemia. *Advances in Shock Research,* **9** 125–132

King, H. and Shumacker, H. B. (1952) Splenic studies. 1. Susceptibility to infection after splenectomy performed in infancy. *Annals of Surgery,* **136**, 239–242

Konradsen, H. B., Pedersen, F. K. and Henrichsen, J. (1990) Pneumococcal revaccination of splenectomized children. *Pediatric Infectious Disease Journal,* **9**, 258–263.

Krivoy, N. and Takarski, I. (1978) Infections after splenectomy. *New England Journal of Medicine,* **298.** 165.

Krol-van-Straaten, M.J., Landheer, J.E. and De-Maat, C.E. (1990) *Capnocytophaga canimorsus* (Formerly DE-2) infection: review of the literature. *Netherlands Journal of Medicine,* **36**, 304–309

Langevin, J.M., Rothenberger, D.A. and Goldberg, S.M. (1984) Accidental splenic injury during surgical treatment of the colon and rectum. *Surgery, Gynecology and Obstretrics,* **159**, 139–144

Lanng-Nielsen, J., Karup-Pedersen, F. and Ellegaard, J. (1982) Failure of pneumococcal vaccine in a splenectomized child. *Acta Paediatrica Scandinavica,* **71**, 331–333

Lanng-Nielsen, J., Tauris, P., Johnsen, H. E. and Ellegaard, J. (1983) The cellular immune response after splenectomy in humans. Impaired immunoglobulin synthesis *in vitro. Scandinavian Journal of Haematology,* **31**, 85–95

Lefford, M.J., Amell, L. and Warner, S. (1978) Listeria pneumonitis: induction of immunity after airborne infection with *Listeria monocytogenes. Infection and Immunity,* **22**, 746–751

Lerman, S.J. (1982) Systemic *Haemophilus influenzae* infection. A study of risk factors. *Clinics in Pediatrics (Philadelphia)* **21**, 360–364

Lindblad, B.E. and Lindblad, L.N. (1990) Fatal pneumococcal bacteremia with disseminated intravascular coagulation and Waterhouse-Friderichsen syndrome in a vaccinated splenectomized adult. *Acta Chirurgica Scandinavica,* **156**, 487–488

Linneman, C.C. Jr. and First, M.R. (1979) Risk of pneumococcal infections in renal transplant patients. *Journal of the American Medical Association,* **241**, 2619–2621

Lipsky, B.A., Boyko, E.J., Inui, T.S. and Koepsell, T.D. (1986) Risk factors for acquiring pneumococcal infection. *Archives of Internal Medicine,* **146**, 2179–2185

Mackowiak, P.A., Demian, S.E., Sutker, W.L., Murphy, F.K., Smith, J. W., Thompsett, R., *et al.* 1980)

Infections of hairy cell leukemia. Clinical evidence of a pronounced defect in cell-mediated immunity. *American Journal of Medicine,* **68**, 718–724

McBride, C.M. and Hester, J.P. (1976) The problem of splenectomy in a leukemic patient population. *Southern Medical Journal,* **69**, 715–718

McCarthy, M. and Zumla, A. (1988) DF-2 infection. *British Medical Journal,* **297**, 1355–1356

McCulloch, D.K. and Parker, A.C. (1979) Overwhelming post-splenectomy infection caused by *Streptococcus milleri. Journal of Infection,* **1**, 379–381

Malangoni, M.A., Dillon, L.D., Klamer, T.W. and Condon, R.E. (1984) Factors influencing the risk of early and late serious infection in adults after splenectomy for trauma. *Surgery,* **96**, 775–783

Malmaeus, J., Akre, T., Adami, H.O. and Hagberg, H. (1986) Early postoperative course following elective splenectomy in haematological diseases: a high complication rate in patients with myeloproliferative disorders. *British Journal of Surgery,* **73**, 720–723

Melamed, I., Zakuth, V., Tzechoval, E. and Spirer, Z. (1982) Suppressor T cell activity in splenectomized subjects. *Journal of Clinical and Laboratory Immunology,* **7**, 173–177

Miller, R.M., Garbus, J., Schwartz, A.R., Du Pont, H.L., Levine, M.M., Clyde, D.F. and Hornick, R.B. (1976) A modified leukocyte nitroblue tetrazolium test in acute bacterial infection. *American Journal of Clinical Pathology,* **66**, 905–910

Mitterstieler, G., Haas, H., Resch, R., Menardi, G. and Fischler, J. (1979) Asplenia and DIC. *Padiatrie und Padologie (Wien),* **14**, 225–232

Mouzard, A., Bompard, Y., Reinert, P. and Huault, G. (1979) Pneumococcal infections and pediatric intensive care. *Pathologie Biologie,* **27**, 537–539

Mower, W.R., Hawkins, J.A. and Nelson, E.W. (1986) Postsplenectomy infection in patients with chronic leukemia. *American Journal of Surgery,* **152**, 583–586

Mufson, M.A. (1981) Pneumococcal infections. *Journal of the American Medical Association,* **246**, 1942–1948

Musser, G., Lazar, G., Hocking, W. and Busuttil, R.W. (1984) Splenectomy for hematologic disease. The UCLA experience with 306 patients. *Annals of Surgery,* **200**, 40–45

Najjar, V.A. (1978) Molecular basis of familial and acquired phagocytosis deficiency involving the tetrapeptide, thr-lys-pro-arg, tuftsin. *Experimental Cell Biology,* **46**, 114–126

Najjar, V.A. (1979) The clinical and physiological aspects of tuftsin deficiency syndromes exhibiting defective phagocytosis. *Klinische Wochenschrift (Berlin),* **57**, 751–756

Najjar, V.A. and Nishioka, K. (1970) 'Tuftsin': a natural phagocytosis stimulating peptide. *Nature,* **228**, 672–673

Needleman, S. (1973) Infections after splenectomy. *Annals of Internal Medicine,* **78**, 149–151

Nielsen, J.L., Buskjaer, L., Lamm, L.U., Solling, J. and Ellegaard, J. (1983) Complement studies in splenectomized patients. *Scandinavian Journal of Haematology,* **30**, 194–200

Noack, L., Gdanietz, K. and Muller, G. (1985) Immunologic status of children after splenectomy. *Progress in Pediatric Surgery,* **18**, 146–149

Nossal, G.J.V. and Ada, L., (1971) *Antigens, lymphoid cells and the immune response.* Academic Press, New York

Notter, D.T., Grossman, P.L., Rosenberg, S.A. and Remington, J.S. (1980) Infections in patients with Hodgkin's disease: a clinical study of 300 consecutive adult patients. *Reviews of Infectious Diseases,* **2**, 761–800

Oakes, D.D. and Charters, A.C. (1981) Changing concepts in the management of splenic trauma. *Surgery, Gynecology and Obstetrics,* **153**, 181–185

Offenbartl, K.S., Christensen, P., Gullstrand, P. and Prellner, K. (1986) Synergism between gammaglobulin prophylaxis and penicillin treatment in experimental post-splenectomy sepsis in the rat. *International Archives of Allergy and Applied Immunology,* **79**, 45–48

O'Neal, B.J. and McDonald, J.C. (1981) The risk of sepsis in the asplenic adult. *Annals of Surgery,* **194**, 775–778

Orihel, T.C. and Eberhard, M.L. (1985) Loa loa: development and course of patency in experimentally-infected primates. *Tropical Medicine and Parasitology,* **36**, 215–224

Oster, C.N., Koontz, L.C. and Wyler, D.J. (1980) Malaria in asplenic mice: effects of splenectomy, congenital asplenia, and splenic reconstruction of the course of infection. *American Journal of Tropical Medicine and Hygiene,* **29**, 1138–1142

Passl, R., Eibl, M. and Egker, E. (1978) Immunologic examination after posttraumatic splenectomy in childhood. *Zentralblatt fur Chirurgie,* **103**, 560–566

Passl, R., Eibl, M., Egkher, E., Frisee, H., Gaudernak, T., Neugebauer, G. and Vecsei, W. (1976) Splenectomy for traumatic rupture of the spleen in childhood and its sequelae. *Wiener Klinische Wochenschrift,* **88**, 585–588

Patel, J., Williams, J.S., Naim, J.O. and Hinshaw, J.R. (1982) Protection against pneumococcal sepsis in splenectomized rats by implantation of splenic tissue into an omental pouch. *Surgery,* **91**, 638–641

Paulin, T., Ringden, O., Nilsson, B., Lonnqvist, B. and Gahrton, G. (1987) Variables predicting bacterial and fungal infections after allogeneic marrow engraftment. *Transplantation,* **43**, 393–398

Pearson, H.A., Johnston, D., Smith, K.A. and Touloukian, R.J. (1978) The born-again spleen. *New England Journal of Medicine,* **298**, 1389–1392

Pedersen, F.K., Henrichsen, J. and Schiffman, G. (1982) Antibody response to vaccination with pneumococcal capsular polysaccharides in splenectomized children. *Acta Paediatrica Scandinavica,* **71**, 451–455

Pedersen, F.K. (1983) Postsplenectomy infections in Danish children splenectomized 1969–1978. *Acta Paediatrica Scandinavica,* **72**, 589–595

Peters, T.G., Williams, J.W., Harmon, H.C. and Britt, L.G. (1983) Splenectomy and death in renal transplant patients. *Archives of Surgery,* **118**, 795–799

Pinna, A.D., Argiolu, F., Marongiu, L. and Pinna, D.C. (1988) Indications and results for splenectomy for beta thalassemia in two hundred and twenty-one pediatric patients. *Surgery, Gynecology and Obstetrics,* **167**, 109–113

Pimpl, W., Dapunt, O., Kaindl, H. and Thalhamer, J. (1989) Incidence of septic and thromboembolic-related deaths after splenectomy in adults. *British Journal of Surgery,* **76**, 517–521

Potin, M., Regamey, C. and Glauser, M. P. (1983) Factitious fevers as a cause of prolonged fevers. Five clinical cases. *Schweizerische Medizinische Wochenschrift,* **113**, 1534–1539

Ramsay, L.E. and Bouskill, K.C. (1973) Fatal pneumococcal meningitis in adults following splenectomy: two case reports and a review of the literature. *Journal of the Royal Naval Medical Service,* **59**, 102–114

Rao, G.N. (1988) Predictive factors in local sepsis after splenectomy for trauma in adults. *Journal of the Royal College of Surgeons of Edinburgh,* **33**, 68–70

Rasore-Quartino, A., Mattiello, A., Cominetti, M., Casina-Lemmi, M., Traverso, T. and Sansone, G. (1986) *Yersinia enterocolitica* sepsis in splenectomized thalassemic subjects. Description of 2 cases. *Pediatria Medica e Chirurgica (Vincenza),* **8**, 121–124

Read, R.C. and Finch, R.G. (1994) Prophylaxis after splenectomy. *Journal of Antimicrobial Chemotherapy,* **33**, 4–6

Reboul, F., Donaldson, S.S. and Kaplan, H.S. (1978) Herpes zoster and varicella infections in children with Hodgkin's disease: an analysis of contributing factors. *Cancer,* **41**, 95–99

Redon, J., Herranz, C., Montalar, J., Navarro, J.R., Blanes, A., Munarriz, B., *et al.* (1981) Infections due to herpes varicella viruses in Hodgkins disease. *Medicina clinica,* **76**, 377–380

Reilly, S., Prentice, A.G., Copplestone, J.A., Hamon, M.D. and Sarangi, J. (1994) Long-term management after splenectomy: wider criteria for vaccination. *British Medical Journal,* **308**, 131

Report (1984) Medical Defence Union, London, p. 29

Robinette, C.D. and Fraumeni, J.F. Jr. (1977) Splenectomy and subsequent mortality in veterans of the 1939–45 war. *Lancet,* **ii**, 127–129

Rosner, F. and Zarrabi, M.H. (1983) Late infections following splenectomy in Hodgkin's disease. *Cancer Investigation,* **1**, 57–65

Roth, H., Bolkenius, M., Daum, R. and Brandeis, W.E. (1982) Various aspects of pediatric surgery in surgery of the spleen. *Chirurgica (Berlin),* **53**, 687–691

Ruben, F.L., Norden, C.W. and Korica, Y. (1984) Pneumococcal bacteremia at a medical/surgical hospital for adults between 1975 and 1980. *American Journal of Medicine,* **77**, 1091–1094

Rubin, S.J. (1984) A fastidious fermentative gram–negative rod. *European Journal of Clinical Microbiology,* **3**, 253–257

Ruebush, T.K., Collins, W.E., Healy, G.R. and Warren, M. (1979) Experimental *Babesia microti* infections in non-splenectomized *Macaca mulatta. Journal of Parasitology,* **65**, 144–146

Ruebush, T.K., Collins, W.E. and Warren, M. (1981)

Experimental *Babesia microti* infections in *Macaca mulatta*: recurrent parasitemia before and after splenectomy. *American Journal of Tropical Medicine and Hygiene*, **30**, 304–307

Sass, W., Bergholz, M., Kehl, A., Seifert, J. and Hamelmann, H. (1983) Overwhelming infection after splenectomy in spite of some spleen remaining and splenosis. A case report. *Klinische Wochenschrift*, **61**, 1075–1079

Schlaeffer, F., Rosenheck, S., Baumgarten-Kleiner, A., Greiff, Z. and Alkan, M. (1985) Pneumococcal infections among immunised and splenectomised patients in Israel. *Journal of Infection*, **10**, 38–42

Schneck, H.J., von-Hundelshausen, B., Tempel, G., Oberdorfer, A. and Rastetter, J. (1984) Behaviour of immunoglobulins following traumatologically indicated splenectomy. *Fortschritte der Medizin (Leipzig)*, **102**, 263–268

Schroter, G.P., West, J.C. and Weil, R. III. (1977) Acute bacteremia in asplenic renal transplant patients. *Journal of the American Medical Association*, **237**, 2207–2208

Schwartz, A.D., Goldthorn, J.F., Winkelstein, J.A. and Swift, A.J. (1978) Lack of protective effect of auto-transplanted splenic tissue to pneumococcal challenge. *Blood*, **51**, 475–478

Schwartz, P.E., Sterioff, S., Mucha, P., Melton, L.J. and Offord, K.P. (1982) Postsplenectomy sepsis and mortality in adults. *Journal of the American Medical Association*, **248**, 2279–2283

Seifert, J., Brieler, S., Reese, F. and Hamelmann, H. (1986) Risk of infection following splenectomy. *Langenbecks Archiv Fur Chirurgie*. **369**, 269–272

Sekikawa, T. and Shatney, C.H. (1983) Septic sequelae after splenectomy for trauma in adults. *American Journal of Surgery*, **145**, 667–673

Selby, C., Hart, S., Ispahani, P. and Toghill, P.J. (1987) Bacteraemia in adults after splenectomy or splenic irradiation. *Quarterly Journal of Medicine*, **63**, 523–530

Selby, C.D. and Toghill, P.J. (1989) Meningitis after splenectomy. *Journal of the Royal Society of Medicine*, **82**, 206–209

Seufert, R.M., Germann, G. and Böttcher, W. (1984) Perioperative antibiotic prophylaxis for elective splenectomy. A randomised prospective study. *Chirurgica*, **55**, 381–384

Shperber, Y., Geller, E., Rudick, V. and Orda, R. (1989) *Purpura fulminans* associated with overwhelming sepsis and disseminated intravascular coagulation following splenectomy. *Israel Journal of Medical Science*, **25**, 657–659

Siber, G.R., Weitzman, S.A., Aisenberg, A.C., Weinstein, H.J. and Schiffman, G. (1978) Impaired antibody response to pneumococcal vaccine after treatment for Hodgkin's disease. *New England Journal of Medicine*, **299**, 442–448

Siddins, M., Downie, J., Wise, K. and O'Reilly, M. (1990) Prophylaxis against postsplenectomy pneumococcal infection. *Australia and New Zealand Journal of Surgery*, **60**, 183–187

Simberkoff, M.S., Cross, A.P., Al-Ibrahim, M., Baltch, A.L., Geiseler, P.J., Nadler, J., *et al.* (1986) Efficacy of pneumococcal vaccine in high-risk patients. *New England Journal of Medicine*, **315**, 1318–1327

Sinclair, K.B. (1970) The effect of splenectomy on the pathogenicity of *Fasciola hepatica* in the sheep. *British Veterinary Journal*, **126**, 15–29

Singer, D.B. (1973) Postsplenectomy sepsis. in H.S. Rosenberg and R.P. Bolande, eds. *Perspectives in Pediatric Pathology*, vol. 1. Chicago, Year Book Medical Publishers, 285–311

Skrede, S., Winther, F.O., Munthe, E. and Nordoy, A. (1977) Transitory IgA-deficiency and recurrent respiratory tract infectious disease after splenectomy. *Archives of Otorhinolaryngology*, **217**, 423–428

Small, C.B., Slater, L.N., Lowy, F.D., Small, R.D., Salvati, E.A., and Casey, J.I. (1984) Group B strepto-coccal arthritis in adults. *American Journal of Medicine*, **76**, 367–375

Spirer, Z., Zakuth, V., Diamant, S., Mondorf, W., Stefanescu, T., Stabinsky, Y. and Fridkin, M. (1977) Decreased tuftsin concentrations in patients who have undergone splenectomy. *British Medical Journal*, **2**, 1574–1576

Thisyakorn, U. and Reinprayoon, S. (1990) Non-01 *Vibrio cholerae* septicemia: a case report. *Southeast Asian Journal Tropical Medicine Public Health*, **21**, 149–150

Vachon, F., Carette, M.F., Gibert, C., Tremolieres, F. and Amoudry, C. (1979) Severe pneumococcal infections of adults. 100 cases collected in three years. *Pathologie Biologie*, **27**, 531–535

Waki, S., Nakazawa, S., Taverne, J., Targett, G.A. and Playfair, J.H. (1985) Immunity to an attenuated variant of *Plasmodium berghei*: role of some non-specific factors. *Parasitology*, **91**, 263–272

Walker, W. (1976) Splenectomy in childhood: a review in England and Wales, 1960–4. *British Journal of Surgery*, **63**, 36–43

Walker, W.E., Kapelanski, D.P., Weiland, A.P., Stewart, J.D. and Duke, J.H. Jr. (1985) Patterns of infection and mortality in thoracic trauma. *Annals of Surgery*, **201**, 752–757

Wara, D.W. (1981) Host defence against *Streptococcus pneumoniae*. The role of the spleen. *Reviews of Infectious Disease*, **3**, 299–301

Wegelius, R. (1982) Postsplenectomy infections. *Lancet*, **i**, 1420–1421

Wetzig, N.R., Strong, R.W. and Theile, D.E. (1986) Splenorrhaphy in the management of splenic injury. *Australia and New Zealand Journal of Surgery*, **56**, 781–784

Wyler, D.J., Miller, L.H. and Schmidt, L.H. (1977) Spleen function in quartan malaria (due to *Plamodium inui*): evidence for both protective and suppressive roles in host defence. *Journal of Infectious Diseases*, **135**, 86–93

Zarrabi, M.H. and Rosner, F. (1984) Serious infections in adults following splenectomy for trauma. *Archives of Internal Medicine*, **144**, 1421–1424

Zaugg, J.L. and Kuttler, K.L. (1987) Experimental infection of *Babesia bigemina* in American bison. *Journal of Wildlife Disease*, **23**, 99–102

4

Infections in patients with abnormal haemoglobins

L.R. Davis

Introduction

Of the clinical entities associated with the presence of abnormal haemoglobins, only those in which haemoglobin S is present modify the patient's response to infection. These, with the exception of the sickle cell trait, are grouped together as sickle cell disease. The common forms are sickle cell anaemia (homozygous haemoglobin S Disease), haemoglobin SC disease and haemoglobin S/β thalassaemia, (either β^0 or β^+). As the effects of infections are most typically seen in sickle cell anaemia the following sections will deal primarily with that condition. The last section will discuss the effect of infection on the others.

Painful crises and the role of infection

Painful crises are the most common complications of sickle cell anaemia. The exact mechanism which causes them is obscure but known precipitating factors include infection. The fever, dehydration and acidosis associated with infection contribute to starting and maintaining painful crises and the last two are particularly likely to develop in children. This has important practical implications in the management of the painful crisis. Treatment must not only aim to correct dehydration and acidosis, but also to control the fever. This may be due to the crisis itself but, may be due to the infection which precipitated the crisis. Even if examination reveals no obvious site of infection

the appropriate specimens, especially blood cultures, must still be collected. In many cases it will be necessary to start antibiotic or antimalarial therapy without awaiting the results of these investigations.

As the symptoms of painful crises overlap the general symptoms of infection, such as fever and limb pains, a test to differentiate these conditions would be of value. Studies of α-hydroxybutyrate dehydrogenase (White, et al., 1978) showed that this enzyme was raised in the steady state of sickle cell anaemia but rose even higher during painful crises and this rise could occur before the crisis was clinically apparent. Unfortunately further studies showed that it could also rise in infections in normal children (Adenuga, 1979 – unpublished).

Prevention of infection is important. Children with sickle cell anaemia should be immunized in the normal way and this should be supplemented at all ages with the appropriate immunizations when travelling overseas, and malaria prophylaxis if indicated. Regular dental examinations are important to avoid oral sepsis.

The response to bacterial infection

Two major defects in the response to infection have been recognized in sickle cell anaemia, namely, splenic hypofunction and a deficient alternative pathway of complement. Abnormalities in leucocyte function and cell mediated immunity have not been confirmed. The antibody response to infection and to immunization appears normal.

The concept of functional hyposplenism was put forward by Pearson, Spencer and Cornelius in 1969. They pointed out that even if the spleen were large it could still be non-functional as regards its ability to remove particles from the circulation. This hypofunction is mirrored in the peripheral blood by the presence of 'pitted' red cells and Howell Jolly bodies. A prognostic significance to splenic size was suggested by Rogers, Vaidya and Serjeant (1978) who showed that the greatest risk of subsequent severe infections occurred in infants in whom the spleen became palpable before one year and particularly before six months of age.

The abnormality in the alternative pathway of complement leading to defective phagocytosis of pneumococci was described by Johnston, *et al.* (1973) and of salmonellae by Hand and King (1978). Larcher, *et al.* (1982) showed that the defect in the pathway related to the functional activity of factor B. They also showed there was a separate defect in yeast opsonization and probably other defects as well since a decreased activity of the total alternative pathway could occur with normal yeast opsonization and normal functional factor B. Four patients who had had pneumococcal infections all had reduced activity of the total alternative pathway, but only two had abnormal yeast opsonization though the other two had abnormal functional activity of factor B.

Pneumococcal septicaemia and meningitis

Pneumococcal septicaemia and meningitis are two of the most serious complications of sickle cell anaemia and particularly affect children under the age of five years. There is a high mortality rate. In contrast to normal children the pneumococcus is the commonest cause of meningitis in children with sickle cell anaemia. Robinson and Watson (1966) showed it to be the cause of 13 out of 18 cases of meningitis (87%) in this condition. In the series of cases reported by Overturf, Powars and Baraff (1977) three quarters of their cases of septicaemia and meningitis occurred under the age of five years and there was a mortality of 35% for septicaemia and 10% for meningitis. In older age groups Lobel and Bove (1982) recorded deaths

at six and 20 years. Death can occur very rapidly from the onset of symptoms. Davis, Huehns and White (1981) reported two deaths within three hours of arrival at hospital. One was pneumococcal septicaemia, the other meningitis but the causal organism was not recorded. Pneumococcal infections are not an uncommon cause of admission to hospital. In two series from London reporting the causes of admission to hospital of children with sickle cell anaemia, four out of 38 (Anionwu, *et al.*, 1981) and five out of 60 (Murtaza, *et al.*, 1981) were due to pneumococci (10.5 and 7.3% respectively).

The morbidity and mortality of pneumococcal infections in early childhood emphasizes the importance of diagnosing sickle cell anaemia as early in life as possible, otherwise such an infection may be the first occasion on which the diagnosis is made. Diagnosis on cord blood is possible using standard electrophoretic techniques (Horn, *et al.*, 1986). However they pointed out that cases could be missed by relying on cord samples being collected and that it would be better to incorporate screening for sickle cell disorders into that for amino acid disorders and hypothyroidism a few days after birth, as there is a well established procedure in the United Kingdom to ensure that all neonates are tested.

Diagnosis at or around birth is of no value unless the infants are follwed up and an important function of sickle cell clinics is to encourage the patient's parents to seek medical aid if their child becomes unwell, and this applies equally well to adults. Powars, *et al.* (1981) claimed a fall in mortality in their children with sickle cell anaemia following the opening of a sickle cell centre and they attributed this to parental education.

Prevention of pneumococcal infections depends on the use of prophylactic penicillin and pneumococcal vaccine. A randomized trial of oral penicillin V versus a placebo on children under the age of three reduced the incidence of pneumococcal septicaemia by 84% in those receiving penicillin (Gaston, *et al.*, 1986). No death occurred in this group, but three died in the placebo group. Monthly intramuscular injections of long-acting benzathine penicillin were employed in a trial by John, *et al.* (1984) on children aged six months to three years. No infections were seen in those children receiving penicillin. These injections are painful and are, therefore, not suitable for long-term prophylaxis. These authors further noted that four pneumococcal infections occurred within 11 months of stopping penicillin and suggested that this might have been due to the lack of opportunity to acquire immunity to pneumococci.

Immunization with a polyvalent pneumococcal vaccine would appear to be an ideal means of preventing pneumococcal infections. Unfortunately it is ineffective in stimulating antibody production under the age of two years, cannot contain every known serotype and some of the strains are only poorly antigenic. Both the penicillin trials referred to above reported pneumococcal infections in patients who had been vaccinated. In spite of these disadvantages, pneumococcal vaccine might help to reduce the occurrence of infections if penicillin prophylaxis is stopped. Perhaps the best procedure is to start daily oral penicillin V as soon as the diagnosis is made and to vaccinate at two years of age. At present there is no firm information on how often vaccination needs repeating which is important as second vaccinations cause severe local and general reactions. It would be ideal for prophylactic penicillin to continue for life, though compliance in adults is likely to be poor. They are less likely to come to sickle cell clinics when they are well than children, who are brought by their parents and the clinic is the ideal place to issue prescriptions for penicillin. The suggestion of lifelong treatment is by analogy with the outcome of splenectomy for other haematological conditions. Evans (1985) reported two cases of pneumococcal infections occurring in adults 14 and 25 years after splenectomy for hereditary spherocytosis. He also reviewed 25 published cases of infections occurring 10 or more years after operation. Pneumococcal infections accounted for 19 (76%). The mean age at which these infections occurred was 37 years.

Osteomyelitis and Salmonella infections

A common problem in sickle cell anaemia is to distinguish between a painful crisis and osteomyelitis. The physical signs are similar and so is the distribution of the lesions. It is possible that the avascular necrosis occurring in a crisis encourages bacteria to multiply there. Usually osteomyelitis is restricted to one site whereas a painful crisis may affect several parts of the skeleton. Failure of a painful area to show signs of resolution within about 10 days would favour osteomyelitis. X-ray changes are unlikely to be helpful for about two weeks. Surgical intervention may ultimately be necessary to establish a diagnosis.

It has long been recognized that osteomyelitis is more common in patients with sickle cell anaemia than in normal persons and that many of these are due to infection with Salmonella species. The frequency of Salmonella infections probably reflects the frequency of Salmonella infections as a whole in that population. Thus, in the United Kingdom where such infections are relatively uncommon Murtaza, *et al.* (1981) only reported one admission for Salmonella osteomyelitis among a total of 60 admissions of patients with infections and sickle cell anaemia over a 20-year period. It is not clear why Salmonella infections are so common in sickle cell anaemia, though defective phagocytosis (Johnston, *et al.*, 1973) presumably plays a part and the inability of the spleen to clear organisms from the circulation.

Other bacterial infections

Haemophilius influenzae septicaemia has been considered to occur more often in children with sickle cell anaemia than in normal children. Powars, Overturf and Turner (1983) estimated it was two to four times more frequent and most of the cases were children under the age of two years. They only recorded 10 cases over a period of 18 years.

Lung complications of sickle cell anaemia are the most common cause of admission to hospital after painful crises (Anionwu, *et al.*, 1981; Murtaza, *et al.*, 1981). It remains uncertain how much of the lung pathology is due to infection and how much to infarction, especially as either may lead to the other. No particular bacterium has been consistently isolated from these cases.

The human parvovirus (B19) and aplastic crises

The causal relationship between the human parvovirus and aplastic crises was recognized by Pattison, *et al.*, 1981. Two years later it was suggested it might also be the cause of

Erythema infectiosum (Fifth disease) by Anderson, *et al.* (1983). After two more years experimental infections of volunteers with human parvovirus unified these findings and established the natural history of the disease (Anderson, *et al.*, 1985) by showing that parvovirus infection caused haematological changes in normal persons but these were less dramatic than in sickle cell anaemia.

Infection appears to occur by the nasal route. It is followed a week later by a viraemia which is accompanied by fever, malaise, myalgia and itching but no rash. The bone marrow is damaged at this point which is shown by a reticulocytopenia for about a week and a fall in the levels of haemoglobin, neutrophils, lymphocytes and platelets. In the third week recovery of the peripheral blood picture occurs, a rash appears and, more commonly in adults than children, this may be accompanied by arthralgia.

This picture is modified in sickle cell anaemia by the short half life of the mature erythrocytes and the degree of anaemia already present in the steady state. Cessation of erythropoiesis for a week allows the haemoglobin to fall as low as 2–3 g/dl and the patient may present with symptoms of acute anaemia namely pallor, dizziness and retrosternal pain. If the patient is not transfused recovery is heralded by a reticulocytosis followed by a rise in the haemoglobin level. During the period of aplasia there is a fall in the platelet level in the peripheral blood but since this is often raised in sickle cell anaemia in the steady state levels may only fall to within the normal range. A neutropenia and lymphopenia may also be detected (Anderson, *et al.*, 1982 and 1985). In the early stage of the crisis there is a virtual absence of red cell precursors from the bone marrow apart from a few pronormoblasts and a very occasional normoblast. Subsequently there is a proliferation of these cells followed by the reappearance of later forms of red cell precursors so that after a week there is erythroid hyperplasia again. Large cells resembling pronormoblasts but up to 60 microns in diameter are present during the aplastic period. Their origin and significance are uncertain. Chernoff and Josephson (1951) quoted Undritz who thought them to be the product of abnormal and incomplete mitosis of red-cell progenitors whereas Chanarin, *et al.* (1964) thought they might be megakaryocyte

precursors. In spite of the fall in lymphocytes, neutrophils and platelets in the peripheral blood there are no morphological abnormalities in the cells of these series in the bone marrow, nor do their proportions appear grossly disturbed. Studies *in vitro* by Mortimer, *et al.* (1983) showed that the parvovirus inhibited colony formation by burst-forming units and erythroid colony-forming units, but not by granulocyte macrophage progenitors.

The diagnosis of an aplastic crisis depends on showing a fall in haemoglobin level and a reticulocytopenia (<1%). It is advantageous to know the steady state values of these for each individual as levels can vary quite widely. Virus will only be detectable in the serum if obtained in the first day or two of the crisis but viral DNA is detectable for longer. IgM antibodies appear early in the crisis and IgG antibodies about a week later.

Parvovirus infection and the resulting aplastic crises are more likely to occur in children than in adults as by puberty 30% of the population have detectable antibodies to the virus. The infection will spread through a household and the detection of one case makes it important to discover whether there has been contact with other cases of sickle cell anaemia. Infection can occur without an aplastic crisis resulting (Anderson, *et al.*, 1982). Their patients had all been transfused within the previous month and although transfusion by itself would have suppressed erythroid activity in the bone marrow the expected fall in haemoglobin would have been dampened by the presence of red cells with a normal life span. Serjeant, *et al.* (1981) reported two patients with proved parvovirus infection but no evidence of aplasia. He suggested that high levels of haemoglobin F might modify the effects by increasing the lifespan of the red cells. Repeated attacks of parvovirus infection must be rare, but Anderson, *et al.* (1985) did induce infection in a volunteer who had trace amounts of IgG antibody already present. As with other infectious disorders, epidemics of parvovirus occur. Serjeant, *et al.* (1981) showed that five clusters of cases of aplastic anaemia had occurred over a 15-year period in Jamaica.

Treatment of the aplastic crisis is easily effected by blood transfusion but untreated the condition is potentially fatal. Prevention by means of a vaccine is attractive but so far the virus has not been propagated outside the body.

All the studies on the virus carried out so far have depended on obtaining the virus from the serum of infected persons. The successful use of parvovirus vaccines in domestic animals makes it probable that a human vaccine would be effective. Unfortunately, although paroviruses are widespread in animals they are virtually species specific.

Other causes of aplastic crises in sickle cell anaemia

Before the role of the human parvovirus in aplastic crises was recognized it had long been suspected that these crises had an infective origin. They tended to occur more frequently in children than in adults, affected contacts who had sickle cell anaemia, and rarely recurred. Charney and Miller (1964) described aplastic crises associated with pneumococcal, Salmonella and streptococcal infections but simultaneous infection with a parvovirus cannot be eliminated. A more interesting and recent case was described by Serjeant, *et al.* (1981) where a patient had an aplastic crisis associated with a pneumococcal infection and a parvovirus infection was excluded on serological grounds. It appears likely that the majority of aplastic crises are due to parvovirus but rarely other oganisms may produce a similar picture. No reports can be found of the bone marrow changes in such cases.

Malaria

It is generally recognized that possession of the sickle cell trait is advantageous in areas where *Plasmodium falciparum* is endemic. It is particularly of value in young children who have yet to acquire immunity. It is less certain that it is beneficial in sickle cell anaemia. Infections with *P. falciparum* certainly occur and can be severe both in themselves and by precipitating painful crises. Those who have sickle cell anaemia and have spent all their lives in non-malarial areas will not have acquired any active immunity. It is especially important that they should receive malarial prophylaxis if visiting or passing through areas in which malaria is endemic.

Infection in Haemoglobin SC disease and sickle cell/βthalassaemia

Haemoglobin SC disease is clinically milder than sickle cell anaemia. However it is subject to all the complications that occur in sickle cell anaemia and when they do occur they may be just as severe. Until recently the question of increased susceptibility to infection and of the activity or otherwise of the spleen has been controversial. However in 1982, Topley, *et al.* reported that in children with SC disease there was a significant increase in serious infections compared with a control group of normal children. The only cases of pneumococcal septicaemia were in the children with SC disease. Infections appeared more common when splenomegaly was detected at an early age as in the case of sickle cell anaemia (Topley, *et al.*, 1982). The case of fatal pneumococcal septicaemia in a patient with SC disease reported by Chilcote and Dampier (1984) was of particular interest in that evidence of asplenia was detected by increased 'pitting' of the patient's red cells. Parvovirus infection would be expected to produce a less severe aplastic crisis than those seen in sickle cell anaemia because the steady state anaemia is less and the life span of the red cells is longer. This was in fact the situation in one case in a young adult seen by the author (unpublished).

Sickle cell/β thalassaemia must be clearly distinguished into its two major varieties, that in which no adult haemoglobin is synthesized (β^0) and that in which some adult haemoglobin is produced (β^+). The β^0 variety is clinically similar to sickle cell anaemia and subject to the same degrees of severity of its complications, whereas the β^+ type is much milder and resembles haemoglobin SC disease.

The conclusions on the risks of infection in these disorders is that there is adequate evidence to recommend that patients with haemoglobin SC disease and sickle cell β^0 thalassaemia should be treated in exactly the same way as those with sickle cell anaemia as regards prophylaxis against infections. Unless screening for sickle cell disorders is carried out many patients with SC disease will go unrecognized but once diagnosed they should receive appropriate immunization against pneumococci and daily oral penicillin. In the absence of evidence to the contrary it must be assumed that patients with sickle cell β^+ thalassaemia may have some increased risk of infection and be managed accordingly.

References

Anderson, M.J., Davis, L.R., Hodgson, J., Jones, S.E., Murtaza, L., Pattison, J.R., *et al*. (1982) Occurrence of infection with a parvovirus-like agent in children with sickle cell anaemia during a two-year period. *Journal of Clinical Pathology*, **35**, 744–749

Anderson, M.J., Higgin, P.G., Davis, L.R., Willman, J.S., Jones, S.E., Kidd, I.M., *et al*. (1985) Experimental parvoviral infection in humans. *Journal of Infectious Diseases*, **152**, 257–265

Anderson, M.J., Jones, S.E., Fisher-Hoch, S.P., Lewis, E., Hall, S.M., Bartlett, C.L.R., *et al*. (1983) Human Parvovirus. The cause of Erythema infectiosum (Fifth disease)? *Lancet*, **1**, 1378

Anionwu, E., Walford, D., Brozovic, M. and Kirkwood, B. (1981) Sickle-cell disease in a British urban community. *British Medical Journal*, **282**, 283–286

Chanarin, I., Barkhan, P., Peacock, M. and Stamp, T.C.B. (1964) Acute Arrest of Haemopoiesis. *British Journal of Haematology*, **10**, 43–49

Charney, E. and Miller, G. (1964) Reticulocytopenia in Sickle Cell Disease. *American Journal of Diseases of Children*, **107**, 450–455

Chilcote, R.R. and Dampier, C. (1984) Overwhelming pneumococcal septicemia in a patient with Hb SC disease and splenic dysfunction. *Journal of Pediatrics*, **104**, 734–736

Chernoff, A.I. and Josephson, A.M. (1951) Acute erythroblastopenia in sickle-cell anemia and infectious mononucleosis. *American Journal of Diseases of Children*, **82**, 310–322

Davis, L.R., Huehns, E.R. and White, J.M. (1981) Survey of sickle-cell disease in England and Wales. *British Medical Journal*, **283**, 1519–1521

Evans, D. (1985) Postsplenectomy sepsis 10 years or more after operation. *Journal of Clinical Pathology*, **38**, 309–311

Gaston, M.H., Verter, J.I., Woods, G., Pegelow, C., Kelleher, J., Presbury, G., *et al*. (1986) Prophylaxis with oral penicillin in children with sickle cell anemia. *New England Journal of Medicine*, **314**, 1593–1599

Hand, W.L. and King, N.L. (1978) Serum opsonisation of Salmonella in sickle cell anemia. *American Journal of Medicine*, **64**, 388–395

Horn, M.E.C., Dick, M.C., Frost, B., Davis, L.R., Bellingham, A.J., Stroud, C.E., *et al*. (1986) Neonatal screening for sickle cell diseases in Camberwell: results and recommendations of a two year pilot study. *British Medical Journal* **292**, 737–740

John, A.B., Ramlal, A., Jackson, H., Maude, G.H., Sharma, A.W. and Serjeant, G.R. (1984) Prevention of pneumococal infection in children with homozygous sickle cell disease. *British Medical Journal*, **288**, 1567–1570

Johnston, R.B., Simon, L., Newman, M.S. and Strath, A.G. (1973) An abnormality of the alternate pathway of complement activation in sickle-cell disease. *New England Journal of Medicine*, **288**, 803–808

Larcher, V.F., Wyke, R.J., Davis, L.R., Stroud, C.E. and Williams, R. (1982) Defective yeast opsonisation and functional deficiency of complement in sickle cell disease. *Archives of Disease in Childhood*, **57**, 343–346

Lobel, J.S. and Bove, K.E. (1982) Clinicopathologic characteristics of septicemia in sickle cell disease. *American Journal of Diseases of Children*, **136**, 543–547

Mortimer, P.P., Humphries, R.K., Moore, J.G., Purcell, R.H. and Young, N.S. (1983) A human parvovirus-like virus inhibits haematopoietic colony formation *in vitro*. *Nature*, **302**, 426–429

Murtaza, L.N., Stroud, C.E., Davis, L.R., and Cooper, D.J. (1981) Admissions to hospital of children with sickle-cell anaemia: a study in South London. *British Medical Journal*, **282**, 1048–1051

Overturf, G.D., Powars, D. and Baraff, L.J. (1977) Bacterial meningitis and septicemia in sickle cell disease. *American Journal of Diseases of Children*, **131**, 784–787

Pattison, J.R., Jones, S.E., Hodgson, J., Davis, L.R., White, J.M., Stroud, C.E., *et al*. (1981) Parvovirus infections and hypoplastic crisis in sickle-cell anaemia. *Lancet* **1**, 664–665

Pearson, H.A., Spencer, R.P. and Cornelius, E.A. (1969) Functional asplenia in sickle-cell anemia. *New England Journal of Medicine*, **281**, 923–926

Powars, D., Weiss, J., Lee, S. and Chan, L. (1981) Pneumococcal septicemia in children with sickle cell anemia. Changing trend of survival. *Journal of the American Medical Association*, **245**, 1839–42

Powars, D., Overturf, G. and Turner, E. (1983) Is there an increased rick of *Haemophilus influenzae* septicemia in children with sickle cell anemia? *Pediatrics*, **71**, 927–931

Robinson, M.G. and Watson, R.J. (1966) Pneumococcal meningitis in sickle-cell anemia. *New England Journal of Medicine*, **274**, 1006–1008

Rogers, D.W., Vaidya, S. and Sarjeant, G.R. (1978) Early splenomegaly in homozygous sickle-cell disease: an indicator of susceptibility to infection. *Lancet*, **2**, 963–965

Serjeant, G.R., Topley, J.M., Mason, K., Serjeant, B.E., Pattison, J.R., Jones, S.E., *et al*. (1981) Outbreak of aplastic crises in sickle cell anaemia associated with parvovirus-like agent. *Lancet*, **2**, 595–597

Topley, J.M., Cupidore, L., Vaidya, S., Hayes, R.J. and Serjeant, G.R. (1982) Pneumococcal and other infections in children with sickle-cell hemoglobin C (SC) disease. *Journal of Pediatrics*, **101**, 734–736

White, J.M., Muller, M.A., Billimoria, F., Davis, L.R., and Stroud, C.E. (1978) Serum-α-hydroxybutyrate levels in sickle-cell disease and sickle cell crises. *Lancet*, **1**, 532–533

Part Two

The Bone Marrow Suppressed Patient

5

Normal flora of the bone marrow suppressed patient

P.G.R. Godwin and R.W. Lacey

Introduction

In recent years therapy for the treatment of acute leukaemias has improved survival. Necessary components of this treatment are prolonged periods of profound neutropaenia (<100 granulocytes/μl). During these episodes the patient is at risk of severe infection (Schimpff, 1980). Most of these infections are bacterial and arise from organisms that typically colonize the digestive tract. Approximately half of these are derived directly from the patient's own flora and half acquired from other sources in the hospital (Bodey and Johnston, 1971). Knowledge of the bacterial and fungal flora, and the disturbances likely to occur during therapy, may be of value in not only avoiding these episodes of infection but also helping in their diagnosis and in the selection of the most effective treatment. An aspect of this that is increasingly appreciated is the need to select agents which are not likely to result in damage to the microbiota (i.e. alteration of the bacterial community or ecosystem).

The adult human body is a community consisting of a large mass of cells of which only 10% are eukaryotic, and human in constitution (Savage, 1977), the rest are prokaryotic bacteria and a relatively small number of fungi. The majority of the bacteria (about 10^{15}) reside in the large bowel and constitute a complex flora. The oropharynx, upper respiratory tract, the outside of the body and much of the female genital tract are also extensively colonized with bacteria and some fungi. The exact composition will be discussed in this chapter.

Most different mammalian species harbour a normal flora that is characteristic for that species. The close relationship between the host and his flora is likely to have been refined over many years. It follows from that that organisms adapted to one particular host do not generally survive well in another. In particular, bacteria from food animals generally perish rapidly after ingestion by man. There are exceptions to this such as *Salmonella typhimurium*. However, in general, there is little reason to think that the theoretical flow of micro-organisms (or their genes) from animal sources to man makes a substantial contribution to the alteration of the human flora.

The normal flora is acquired soon after birth from the mother and other close attendants; if the baby is nursed for some time in hospital, then the flora may be initially atypical such as through the colonization of skin by multi-resistant coagulase-negative staphylococci. In the normal breast-fed child, there will be colonization with Bifidobacteria, later facultative anaerobes, and with the addition of solid foods, obligate anaerobes join the host flora.

The relationship between man and his microbial flora is largely commensal (i.e. the bacterial community thriving without exerting a deleterious effect on the host), but he does derive some benefits from the bacteria. This arises because the flora provides protection from colonization with organisms that may be undesirable on account of toxins or antibiotic resistance and it also produces metabolic products which are utilized by the host. This latter feature is probably not of great significance for people consuming a typical 'Western' diet.

The host/flora relationship is altered when the host is damaged by cytotoxic drugs and radiation, such that many harmless micro-organisms may now have infective potential. It is probably useful to separate two components of this disruption. First, cytotoxic drugs do alter the nature of the human cell and hence the likely relationship between microbe and the host. Second, if these new relationships in some way encourage microbial invasion of the body, cytotoxic therapy may also inhibit the elimination of these organisms. Recognizing this, attempts have been made to eliminate these organisms, predominantly Enterobacteriaceae, from patients at risk. However, alteration of a complex ecosystem, whilst easily achieved, may have unhelpful consequences even the reverse of that intended.

Normal flora of the respiratory and gastro-intestinal tracts

The bacterial flora of the bone marrow suppressed patient, before the onset of disease, is similar to that of the healthy individual.

The indigenous flora of the oral cavity is complex (Table 5.1) (Draser, Shiner and McCleod, 1969) and varies considerably with the timing of food intake. Salivary specimens reveal predominantly Streptococci (usually

Table 5.1 Salivary bacteria of the oral cavity

Salivary bacteria	Numbers (range log cfu/g) 10
Enterobacteriaceae	0–4
Enterococci	0–3
Strep. salivarius	3–6
alpha haemolytic Streps.	5–7
Neisseria	4–6
Staphylococci	0–2
Yeasts	0–2
Lactobacilli	0–3
Bacteroides	1–5
Fusobacteria	1–6
Bifidobacteria	1–4
Clostridia	0–0
Veillonella	2–6

Based on Drasar, Shiner and McCleod (1969) (4)

alpha-haemolytic on blood agar), Neisseria, Lactobacilli and some facultative Gram-negative bacilli, with small numbers of yeasts. The factors determining the composition of the oral microbiota have been studied using continuous culture models *in vitro* (McKee, *et al.*, 1985; McDermid, *et al.*, 1986). These studies have revealed the importance of pH and redox potential, which are themselves influenced by the fermentation of carbohydrate.

Salivary culture gives only a general picture of the nature and quantity of mouth organisms, many of which adhere strongly to teeth, forming dental plaque, and others such as Bacteroides and Fusobacteria inhabit gingival and dental crevices. Of particular note are Capnocytophaga species, which may cause infection in the immuno-suppressed patient (Schlaes, Dul and Lerner, 1972; Appelbaum, Ballard and Eyster, 1979). There are also minor components of the flora such as Treponemes and Actinomycetes.

Similar organisms persist into the pharynx and down the oesophagus. There is good evidence that this flora plays an important part in inhibiting the growth of potential pathogens such as *Streptococcus pyogenes* and *S. pneumoniae* and also of facultative Gram-negative organisms such as *Escherichia coli* and *Klebsiella* species. Sprunt and co-workers (1971) have demonstrated the ability of the alpha-haemolytic Streptococci to inhibit colonization with Gram-negative bacilli, and were able to demonstrate that implantation with certain bacteria enhanced resistance to further colonization. The mechanisms by which the indigenous bacteria achieve this effect will be discussed below.

The stomach, with its low pH, destroys many organisms, but alpha-haemolytic Streptococci, anaerobic cocci, *Staphylococcus epidermidis* and Candida species may be present at concentrations up to 10^3 cfu/ml (Giannella, Broitman and Zamcheck, 1972). These are present in highest numbers following the ingestion of a meal that may raise the gastric pH from 0 to 4. Mucus and lysozyme, together with IgA may also play a role in preventing adherence and consequent colonization. Over the years much attention has been focused on gastric flora due to the association of *Helicobacter pylori* with gastritis and peptic ulceration. This organism seems particularly adept at avoiding gastric protective mechanisms. It does not appear to be present in those who do not have gastritis

(Marshall and Warren, 1984). However, it is still uncertain whether we should view this organism as a primary pathogen or as a commensal in patients with gastric pathology.

Naturally, if antacids or H2-receptor or 'proton pump' blockers are given and the gastric pH rises, then the number of organisms present also increases (Stockbrugger, *et al.*, 1982), and the value of the stomach in preventing the entry of organisms to the small intestine is reduced. They may also have implications for the production of mutagens in the stomach (Stockbrugger, *et al.*, 1982). Drasar and Hill (1974) have demonstrated a direct relationship between the level of gastric pH and the numbers of bacteria in the intestine. Thus drugs used to treat epigastric discomfort may result in increased numbers of Enterobacteriaceae and other species, such as Salmonella, entering the small intestine.

Throughout the small bowel numbers of bacteria remain relatively low (10^5 cfu/ml) with counts rising towards the ileo-caecal valve. The flora of the small intestine has been studied with the use of tubes (Gorbach, *et al.*, 1967) or by taking samples during surgery for intestinal by-pass (Corrodi, *et al.*, 1978) or for trauma (Thadepelli, *et al.*, 1979). In summary, these show that the numbers of bacteria are between 0 and 10^5 cfu/ml at the proximal end, comprising Streptococci, Staphylococci, anaerobic cocci, lactobacilli and yeasts. The numbers rise to 10^9 cfu/ml at the distal end of the small bowel, with anerobes, notably Bacteroides species, becoming more dominant. The mucosal flora may, however, be quite different since biopsies were not taken in these studies to explore that possibility (Finegold, Sutter and Mathisen, 1985).

The small bowel may become abnormally colonized with bacteria as the result of increased numbers of organisms surviving in the stomach or as a consequence of abnormal anatomy, such as fistulae and diverticulae (Drasar, Shiner and McLeod, 1969). Overgrowth (i.e. the presence of large numbers of organisms not normally present) may occur in the small intestine and this can result in malabsorption (McEvoy, Dutton and James, 1983) and diarrhoea (Penny, Harendra da Silva and McNeish, 1986). In particular, after surgery, excessive growth of D-lactic acid producing bacteria can occur. The absorption of D-lactate may lead to lactic acidosis of unexpected severity, as D-lactate cannot be metabolized by the liver (Stolberg, *et al.*, 1982). Organisms such as Salmonellae produce their effects in the small gut, and whilst there is no clear evidence that they are more common in haematological conditions, their effects may be more severe (Bodey and Fainstein, 1986).

In the caecum and ascending colon the numbers of bacteria rise, with a rough parity between aerobic and anaerobic organisms. This gradually changes to an anaerobic dominance in the distal large bowel and faeces of roughly $10:1$ to $1000:1$, with a total count of 10^{11} to 10^{13} cfu/g dry weight. The dominant organisms present are Bacteroides (fragilis group), Eubacteria, Bifidobacteria, Streptococci

Table 5.2 Faecal organisms

Faecal organism	Numbers (range log cfu/g dry wt) 10	Carriage %
Actinomyces	5–11	8
Anaerobic cocci	4–13	94
Arachnia-propionibacteria	4–12	9
Bacteroides	9–13	99
Bifidobacteria	5–13	74
Clostridia	4–13	100
Eubacteria	4–13	99
Fusobacteria	5–11	98
Gram neg. facultatives	4–12	98
Other facultatives	1–12	93
Lactobacillus	3–12	78
Streptococcus	4–13	99

Based on Finegold, Sutter and Mathieson (1985) (17)

(aerobic and anaerobic), with lesser numbers of Lactobacilli, Enterobacteriaceae, Veillonellae and Clostridia (Table 5.2).

The most comprehensive studies of faecal flora conducted by Finegold and co-workers (1974, 1975 and 1977) who summarized these findings. There is a very wide range of bacterial counts between individuals, but there were striking similarities between different dietary groups (Finegold, Sutter and Mathisen, 1985). The bacterial flora once established does appear to be stable for an individual, despite changes in diet (Gorbach, *et al.*, 1967). However, there is no doubt that populations fed a typical 'Western' diet have a colonic flora different from that of people receiving other diets (Finegold, *et al.*, 1977).

It must be recognized that studies of faecal bacteria do not necessarily give satisfactory information. It is necessary to use selective media to detect minority populations of bacteria within a large mass and this may result in an incorrect count of certain species due to inhibition by the media. Furthermore, the bacteria may interact with each other during processing and on the isolation media. As has been noted in relation to the small bowel, the mucosal flora may differ substantially from that of the lumen (Savage, 1977), though studies in our department suggest that this is mainly a quantitative difference. Some bacteria may not be detected at all due to inadequate culture methods. For example, it is only recently that Spirochaetes have been successfully isolated from the colon, although they have been seen on microscopy for many years (Tompkins, *et al.*, 1986). There may be methanogens present, but few studies involving their culture have been carried out due to the complexity and their lack of medical interest.

Role of the flora of the gastro-intestinal tract

The normal microbiota has a number of effects which will be outlined. These involve resistance to colonization, food digestion and metabolism and absorption.

Colonization

Once established in the early weeks or months of life the gastro-intestinal tract flora, particu-larly that of the large bowel, is stable and is said to be in 'climax stage', resisting the establish-ment of 'foreign' strains of bacteria (Freter, 1985). This ability is commonly referred to as colonization resistance (Van der Waaij, *et al.*, 1971), although many other synonyms are used. Most investigation of this phenomenon has centred around the large bowel flora, because of its numerical preponderance, relevance to infection and accessibility of investigation.

For an organism to survive in the bowel it must either reproduce faster than it dies or is expelled (by defecation) or, alternatively, adhere to the mucosa (Freter, *et al.*, 1983). In order to reproduce at a sufficient rate, it must successfully compete with the bacteria already present for substrates and resist the toxic metabolites of the indigenous organisms. For an organism to survive in the lumen for brief periods, it only needs to attain a doubling time of 12–24 hours (Freter, 1985). Foreign strains of bacteria can often achieve this but are unable to establish themselves for prolonged periods (>10 days). This is because the bowel com-prises a stable equilibrium, with nutrients usually utilized efficiently. Thus, only organisms well adapted to these conditions become resident over the long term.

The availability of iron (Fe^{+++}) may play a part in determining the bowel flora. In neonates, who receive lactoferrin in milk, iron-requiring bacteria are inhibited to some extent, providing protection from infection (Brook, 1980). It has been noted that iron overload enhances the risk of infection (Weinberg, 1984) as does the treatment for iron over-load (Trallero, *et al.*, 1986). The avail-ability and competition for iron may be a factor determining growth of colonizing bacteria in later years, but it has not yet been fully investi-gated. If bleeding into the gut occurs over a prolonged period, this may produce changes.

In addition to nutrient competition, various physical and chemical factors such as low oxygen tension and high concentrations of short chain fatty acids may extend the lag phase for *E. coli* so that it is eliminated from the bowel before cell division can occur (Freter, *et al.*, 1983). Short chain fatty acids have also been shown to inhibit gastro-intestinal pathogens in animal models (Hudault *et al.*, 1985). Decon-jugated bile salts may adversely affect the survival of some organisms, although there is no firm evidence for the occurrence of this *in vivo*

(Savage, 1977). Bile salts may play a particular role in the small intestine (Binder, Filburn and Flock, 1974). Even organisms found higher in the digestive tract, such as Neisseria and some Bacteroides, do not find more distal conditions favourable for growth.

The role of bacteriocins within the microflora is also not clearly defined but may play a part, together with local physical conditions, in determining the oropharyngeal flora (Sanders and Sanders, 1984) and in resisting colonization with *Streptococcus pneumoniae* (Johanson, *et al.*, 1970). Stout and co-workers (1986) have produced *in vitro* evidence to suggest that some components of the pharyngeal flora – *N. meningitidis* and *Haemophilus influenzae* – may actually enhance colonization opportunities for *Legionella pneumophila* and *micdadei*.

Adhesion of bacteria to the intestinal mucosa requires a specific interaction between the bacterium and the mucosal cell surface. This specificity is determined by lectin molecules forming part of the bacterial cell surface, which only bind to certain carbohydrates on the mucosa (Beachey, 1981). Such attachment will cause competition for binding sites between extraneous and host adapted strains, the latter being likely to be successful. The host may also exhibit specific IgA mediated immunity to binding in addition to bacterial competition (Williams and Gibbons, 1982).

Studies using animal models have investigated the role of the host in determining its own flora from birth. A number of different observations have pointed to the importance of immunological tolerance in establishing a bacterial flora.

Foo and Lee (1972) injected isolates from the anaerobic flora into the host from which they were isolated (mice). The result was the production of either low levels of antibodies, or none at all. If injected into guinea-pigs, strong immune responses occurred. One reason for this phenomenon may be the presence of antigens on the bacterial cells which may be similar to host cells, thus inducing tolerance (Mattingley and Waksman, 1978). Evidence from the use of inbred mice suggests that individuals differ, facilitating the growth of only selected strains of bacteria, and this seems to be inherited. Thymus-less mice seem unable to maintain a constant aerobic flora (Van der Waaij, 1986).

The presence of an IgA coating on some strains of Enterobacteriaceae in freshly voided faeces, whilst they are absent from the anaerobic bacteria, supports the idea that there may be an immune response (Van Saene and Van der Waaij, 1979).

Removal of bacteria may occur as a result of interaction with phagocytic cells in the mucosa, or comprising the gut associated lymphoid system (which is notably undeveloped in germ-free animals). Ability to adhere may therefore be in some instances a disadvantage if an immunological response is stimulated. Encapsulated strains are more resistant to phagocytosis and in addition do not adhere as easily to epithelial cells (Beachey, 1981).

This aspect of colonization resistance will be impaired in the immune-deficient patient and therefore will limit the ability of the host to control his microbial flora.

Ill health of itself, and including leukopaenia specifically, seems to have a facilitating effect on colonization with foreign strains of bacteria, perhaps by increasing the number of receptor sites or because clearance mechanisms are impaired (Johanson, Pierce and Sanford, 1969; Johanson, *et al.*, 1972). Minah, *et al.* (1986) looked at the changes in flora at a number of sites in the mouth during myelosuppressive chemotherapy. These patients also received oral non-absorbable antibiotics. In five sites, 25–50% showed increases in Gram-negative bacilli, but this was only to 0.1% of the bacterial population. Slightly less than half of the patients showed a major shift with greater than 1% and up to 80% of the total flora being Gram-negative bacilli. The organisms present were largely of non-pathogenic species.

Metabolism

The human microbiota can metabolize most of the foodstuffs taken in by the host. In the mouth this occurs simultaneously with the initiation of digestion by oral enzymes. Further down the digestive tract partial degradation of complex polysaccharides such as cellulose, hemi-celluloses and pectin occur through bacterial enzymes, such substances not being degraded by the host. Also present in the bowel will be some unabsorbed starch, sugars and proteins originating from desquamated human cells and mucus (Cummings, 1983). To this 'cocktail' will be added host excretory material such as bile salts. In malabsorption syndromes obviously the bacterial diet will be enriched by unabsorbed material. As most host absorption occurs in the small bowel, and bacterial growth in the large bowel, little competition arises.

The large bowel fermentation process is in many ways similar to that of the ruminant stomach and contains bacteria with similar roles. In the cow, substantial quantities of short chain fatty acids are produced which satisfies the animal's major nutritional needs (McNeil, 1984). The products are the same in the human, but the nutritional need, particularly in the western world, is not great. However, the short chain fatty acids are absorbed and metabolized, and may be particularly important for mucosal cell metabolism (Roediger, 1980). Butyrate has been proposed as having an antineoplastic role in the large bowel (Kruh, 1982). Cummings (1984) considered that short chain fatty acids which are the dominant anions present in the large bowel lumen, may facilitate the uptake of water and sodium ions, resulting in the solid stool (Roediger and Rae, 1982). Bile salt metabolism may also be an important determinant of mucosal structure (Vahouny, *et al.*, 1981). Micro-organisms do, in addition, contribute important quantities of vitamins, such as vitamin K, for the benefit of the host (Rosebury 1962).

Skin flora

Over most of the body the skin is relatively dry, and the resident flora consists entirely of Gram-positive organisms – Micrococci, Staphylococci, Propionibacteria and Corynebacteria. In moist areas, such as in the toe clefts, between the buttocks and in the groins and axillae, there is colonization by a huge range of organisms, with Enterobacteriaceae often predominating. In addition, Enterococci, fungi and pseudomonads may flourish. When these sites are dried, these organisms, being susceptible to drying tend to disappear (i.e. they are transient). The precise composition of this flora depends on a number of factors: substrate competition, toxic metabolites, adherence, pH, resistance to desiccation and bacterial antagonism (Aly and Maibach, 1981). Sanders and Sanders (1984) have summarized the factors which facilitate this antagonism listing bacteriocins, hydrogen peroxide and volatile

fatty acids. Colonization of skin lesions, such as eczematous eruptions (by Staphylococci), where the patient has been shaved and under dressings (by Enterobacteriaceae) readily occurs. Probably of extreme importance for the protection of the skin against invasion by *Staph. aureus* and *Strep. pyogenes* is the synthesis of free fatty acids with inhibitory activity against these organisms. Freshly formed sebum contains neutral esterified lipid with little free fatty acids. Residents, notably coagulase-negative staphylococci, release lipases that hydrolyse such lipid to free fatty acids that may show marked antibacterial activity. Whilst it is true that some of these fatty acids may be utilized by Propionibacteria (a process likely to encourage the further generation of these acids), normal skin contains free fatty acids in sufficient amounts to destroy many potentially pathogenic Gram-positive bacteria. The fatty acids with most antibacterial activity are polyunsaturated, e.g. linolenic (C18 : 3), and it is notable that the long chain fatty acids in the body reflect their dietary intake (Lacey, *et al.*, 1963). About 30–40 years ago, there was a vogue (not then based on satisfactory clinical trial data) for treating certain skin infections with polyunsaturated fatty acids. Perhaps the time is opportune to reassess these – particularly by dietary intake. Patients who are immunosuppressed frequently develop unpleasant skin sepsis and fatty acids could be useful both therapeutically and prophylactically.

Vaginal flora

Recent quantitative studies by Masfari, Duerden and Kinghorn (1986) have shown that the normal flora consists predominantly of Lactobacilli $>10^8$ cfu/g, with coryneforms and coagulase-negative staphylococci. The flora became more anaerobic in women with abnormal conditions, for example, trichomoniasis, gonorrhoea and chlamydial infections. Organisms such as Mobiluncus and *Gardnerella vaginalis* may also be present in normal health, there being little credibility in the assignment of a primary pathogenic role to Gardnerella.

Mycoplasma hominis is carried by some 20% of women and Ureoplasma ureolyticum by 60% (Taylor-Robinson and McCormack, 1979) (and indeed they are also found in the oral cavity) but their role as components of the flora and as pathogens has not been fully defined.

The flora also changes substantially with the menstrual cycle and thus will be disrupted by drugs causing sex hormone disturbances. Post menopausally, the flora changes to contain more Enterobacteriaceae and anerobes.

Although the female genital tract is not a particularly important site in relation to infection in bone marrow suppressed patients, overgrowth can occur with yeasts in response to antibiotics, as with other patients.

Infections arising from organisms present in the normal flora or from organisms abnormally colonizing

Infections may arise from organisms which are a normal part of the host microbiota, or are present transiently or have established abnormally in the bowel or on the skin surface as a result of some disturbance to the flora (usually antibiotics) in the clinical setting. It is not always possible to distinguish between these, except where organisms are cultured that are not usually part of the normal flora, such as *Pseudomonas aeruginosa* (Buck and Cooke, 1969) and *Klebsiella pneumoniae* (Cooke, *et al.*, 1979). Colonization with potential pathogens usually occurs prior to the generation of infection and this can be anticipated by screening (Schimpff, *et al.*, 1977).

The predominant infections seen in neutropaenic patients are usually seen as septicaemias without obvious portal of entry, or respiratory tract infections, or those associated with intravenous devices. Organisms causing respiratory tract infection come from the gastro-intestinal tract, having first colonized the upper respiratory tract (Seldon, *et al.*, 1971). Aspiration of some upper respiratory and pharyngeal organisms is normal (Huxley, *et al.*, 1978), particularly during sleep, but overt infection rarely occurs because of clearance of the infecting organisms by attachment to desquamated cells, mucus and ciliated epithelium. Neutrophils in conjunction with alveolar macrophages also play an important role in removing bacteria (Pennington, Rossing, and Boerth, 1983). Presumably infection is more likely to occur when any component of the defence system is impaired, either as the result of a viral infection or chemical insults such as smoking or, important here, cytotoxic therapy.

In the small intestines organisms are able to cross the gastro-intestinal mucosa (Tancrede and Andremont, 1985) either because they have suitable pathogenic ability, e.g. Salmonellae, or because the mucosa has been damaged by cytotoxic drugs, graft versus host disease and radiotherapy (Marcus and Goldman, 1986). Particularly common too, amongst the immunodeficient, are anal fissures and other minor perianal problems with allow bacteria access to the bloodstream. Immunosuppressed patients may, in addition, respond abnormally to toxins produced by the Enterobacteriaceae, notably strains of *E. Coli*. Damage to the mucosa by enteroinvasive and enteropathogenic strains may be enhanced as a result of proliferation of indigenous bacteria or as the result of new colonization. This will result in diarrhoea but may also enhance risk of systemic infection. Immune response to these will be impaired in bone marrow suppressed patients. Antibodies to endotoxin may be important in resisting infection with Gram-negative bacteria. It has been suggested that infection characteristically occurs after prolonged neutropaenia, because of the loss of endotoxin immunity (Glauser, McCutchan and Ziegler, 1984).

From the skin, any minor lesion, even acne, which could be regarded as normal, may provide a portal of entry, particularly for Staphylococci. Immunosuppressed patients frequently have cannulae *in situ*, notably long catheters reaching to the right atrium, for the supply of cytotoxic drugs, blood, antibiotics and nutrients. Much care and attention is paid to the insertion and maintenance of these devices particularly the long catheters (Peters, *et al.*, 1984), but infection or colonization is still a common occurrence. Eykyn (1984) has reviewed the episodes of septicaemia related to intravenous catheters, finding that they are responsible for 9% of episodes of bacteraemia and 23% of all staphylococcal bacteraemia. As Hickman lines in particular are left in for many weeks, patients often require re-admission to hospital from home on account of infection (Donnelly, *et al.*, 1985). However, Weightman, *et al.*, (1986) suggest that, for Hickman lines, the organism colonizing gains access via the hub and is not related to the flora at the site of entry.

Staphylococci are responsible for over 70%

of line-related infections (Eykyn, 1984) and there are a large number of other bacteria involved, but curiously no *E. coli* in Eykyn's series. 'JK-group' diphtheroids may be a problem in immunosuppressed patients and may well be selected by the plethora of antibiotics used (Dibb and von der Lippe, 1984). However, as these organisms are often found in normal skin, their isolation from blood cultures may denote contamination. After all, their isolation from blood cultures of non-immuno-compromised patients is usually assumed to denote such contamination.

Poor dentition also provides a mechanism of access for organisms to cause local infection or infection disseminated via the bloodstream, although, there is no proof, even now, that dental procedures themselves are responsible for cardiac infections. Candida infections and herpes infections are also a noted feature of immunosuppression. Herpetic lesions may promote colonization and infection by oral bacteria.

In summary, any minor cut, blemish or local site of sepsis may result in serious infection with organisms from the host microbiota. These infections are likely to be life-threatening if the patient is severely neutropaenic with counts of below 100 neutrophils/μl (Storring, *et al.*, 1977).

Mechanisms of establishment of organisms within the host flora

Recognizing that 'foreign' organisms acquired in hospital are responsible for a large number of infections, it is worthwhile to consider how these agents gain access to the host and become established in the flora. We will consider first the disturbances of the host that facilitate colonization.

As already noted, the process of being ill, for whatever reason, seems to result in some change in the inter-relationship between host and flora, resulting in a change in its composition (Johanson, Pierce and Sandford, 1969). These alterations may be related to substrate availability (i.e. food intake and appetite), though there is little evidence for this beyond the oral cavity and stomach. Viral infection may have the effect of altering 'physical' immunity, which may facilitate colonization with new organisms. Foreign bodies such as nasogastric

and endotracheal tubes, which breach host defence mechanisms may also be a problem.

The most dramatic effects are wrought by antibiotics, which can rapidly remove sensitive bacteria within the flora even with a single oral (Mulcahy, *et al.*, 1986) or intravenous (Ambrose, *et al.*, 1985) dose. Patients with haematological malignancy are particularly likely to receive antibiotics, either because they have a genuine infection, or because pyrexia due to many causes, e.g. a transfusion reaction, is treated as a potential infection because the risks of not doing so are grave.

Antibiotics will have the effect of suppressing sensitive components of the flora, reducing its ability to resist colonization, affecting the metabolism (particularly in relation to the bowel) and also selecting resistant organisms including fungi, which may have been a minority population. Finegold, *et al.* (1985) have extensively reviewed the effects of antibiotic administration on the intestinal flora.

Once the balance of the components of the microbiota has been damaged in this way, organisms may be introduced to the host from the air, or via food and water (Buck and Cooke, 1969; Shooter, *et al.*, 1969; Remington and Schimpff, 1981; Pizzo, Purvis and Waters, 1982) or by direct transfer from other human sources. Rapidly growing, non-specializing bacteria, such as Pseudomonads and Enterobacteriaceae appear particularly able to occupy a 'microbiological vacuum'. Thus, rapid colonization throughout the gastro-intestinal tract and on the skin can result. Buck and Cooke (1969) demonstrated the ease of this occurrence in the instance of Pseudomonads by giving an oral dose to volunteers with and without concurrent antibiotics. They found that antibiotics were required for successful colonization with these extraneous organisms. Van der Waaij *et al.* (1971) found the colonizing inoculum after certain antibiotics can be very low, due largely to the destruction of the anaerobic flora. Alteration of the oropharyngeal flora will enhance colonization with *Streptococcus pneumoniae*, as noted above.

There is convincing evidence too that disturbance of the indigenous flora increases the risk of infection. This effect has been demonstrated in the axilla by the use of neomycin spray in an attempt to reduce odour. Spraying caused the selection of neomycin resistant strains of *Staphylococcus aureus* and even the development of boils. In addition, Enterobacteriaceae replaced the normal underarm flora (Shehadeh and Kligman, 1963).

Use of antibiotics can, paradoxically, increase wound infection after surgery (Day, 1975), an effect which strongly supports a protective role for the normal flora. Indeed, so striking is this effect, that Roberts (1965) has reported finding less infection in operative sites where skin flora was present than in bacteriologically sterile areas. However, not all studies have come to this conclusion!

In the gut, it is less easy to demonstrate enhanced infection rate following antibiotics, except for *Clostridium difficile* related pseudomembranous colitis, which is so closely related to the use of antibiotics (Bartlett, *et al.*, 1978).

Price and Sleigh (1970) have given the most worrying account of 'prophylactic antibiotics' actually playing a causative role in infection. In their study of a neurosurgical unit, where Klebsiella infection was widespread apparently due to the use of ampicillin and cloxacillin, prevention was achieved by stopping the use of all antibiotics.

With hazards such as these resulting from the use of antimicrobial agents, it might be imagined that there would be some reluctance in attempts to use them to modify the host microbial flora in bone marrow suppressed patients. However, this does not seem to be the case.

Prevention of infection by modification of the flora with antimicrobial agents

As a result of the high frequency of infection during neutropaenic phases in the modern treatment of haematological malignancy, many attempts have been made to modify the flora, using a variety of regimes. These regimes usually involve the administration of agents active against facultative Gram-negative organisms and may be 'non-absorbable' antibiotics such as colistin, framycetin, neomycin and gentamicin, or absorbable agents such as nalidixic acid, erythromycin and co-trimoxazole. Some antibiotic 'cocktails' also include vancomycin as an agent active against Gram-positive organisms. Nystatin or another antifungal agent, e.g. Amphotericin B, is usually added to the antibacterial drugs.

We will discuss the use of these treatments in terms of their effect on the normal flora and the host and will not consider in depth their value in the prevention of infection as this will be discussed in detail in a separate chapter. It is, however, worthwhile noting how the microbial flora changes, in a variety of directions, often unpredictably, following the prescription of prophylactic antibiotics.

The antibiotic dosages and combinations, and their success in prophylaxis, have been reviewed recently by Hann and Prentice (1984). Schimpff and coworkers (1975) used a regime of vancomycin, gentamicin and nystatin, with the aim of removing all pathogenic organisms. An additional benefit of the treatment was seen with the use of protective isolation. Levine, *et al.* (1973) showed a fall of between 87 and 99% in the numbers of bacteria in the faeces, but the oral flora and vaginal flora was altered to a lesser extent, and a high incidence of fungal infection was seen. These drugs are not palatable and this leads to poor compliance. Fracon using framycetin and colistin with nystatin tastes somewhat better (Storring *et al.*, 1977). Neocon (Watson and Jameson, 1979), neomycin replacing framycetin, is also widely used. Both are very effective at removing Enterobacteriaceae, Staphylococci and Streptococci, but leaving the anaerobic flora relatively intact (Watson and Jameson, 1979; Finegold, Mathisen and George, 1985).

Despite the improved patient acceptability, there are some drawbacks, notably diarrhoea, and neomycin has been noted to cause malabsorption with steatorrhoea and increased bile acid secretion (Paes, *et al.*, 1967). This results from the union of the basic amino-glycoside molecule with organic acid groups (Lacey, 1963). Stopping the antibiotics leads to immediate ingrowth of aerobic and facultative anaerobic Gram-negative organisms (Schimpff, 1980), which is an additional hazard where compliance is poor. Indeed, these regimes can only be shown to have any value while the neutrophil count remains below $100/\mu l$ (Schimpff, 1980).

A gentler approach to prophylaxis is that which stems from attention to 'colonization resistance' (CR) (Van der Waaij, *et al.*, 1971). This is based on the concept that retention of certain organisms of the normal flora helps to inhibit the invasion of the gut by potentially pathogenic strains of Enterobacteriaceae, etc. as discussed above. The Dutch workers have attempted to eliminate the Enterobacteriaceae with antibiotics which leave the CR largely intact. As a result of their researches they have a number of methods for detecting damage to the CR, although some are confined to animal studies. For example, increases in faecal Streptococci are considered to be a good marker for reduced CR (Van der Waaij and Berghuis de Vries, 1974). Faecal Beta-aspartyl glycine is also of value and can be measured by a variety of techniques (Welling, 1982). Beta-aspartyl glycine is not normally detectable in the faeces because it is destroyed enzymically by certain anaerobic bacteria. Armed with this tool, it is possible to look at the effect of a variety of agents for their effects on CR, before using them to examine their potential to prevent infection. Van der Waaij (1983) has reviewed a large number of agents in terms of their effects on CR. Using this method of assessing useful agents it is hoped to lessen the risks of the environment to the patient, resulting from stopping the antibiotics, reduce the cost and make the drugs easier to take.

Agents effective against aerobes alone are, for example, nalidixic acid, neomycin, trimethoprim and sulphonamides. These all eliminate a substantial number of aerobes, while leaving the anaerobic flora substantially intact and, therefore, preventing Pseudomonas colonization. However, resistance to these agents is frequent in the hospital environment. This can be circumvented by examining the aerobic flora by the use of screening cultures and switching regimes as required (Sleijfer, *et al.*, 1980).

Co-trimoxazole is used as a prophylactic agent for the prevention of *Pneumocystis carinii* pneumonia. Hughes and co-workers (1977) used this combination for this purpose and reduced the number of bacterial infections, in addition to those due to *Pneumocystis carinii*. However, most of the patients were not severely neutropaenic and this was not taken into account in the analysis of the results. Nevertheless, this provided an opportunity for cheap all-purpose prophylaxis. In small comparative studies, co-trimoxazole has been found to be as effective as oral non-absorbable antibiotices (Starke, *et al.*, 1982; Watson *et al.*, 1982) but with some marrow toxicity (Watson, *et al.*, 1982). However, in other studies, failure resulting from resistance to trimethoprim was reported almost simultaneously with these

studies (Wilson and Guiney, 1982). The European Organization for Research in the Treatment of Cancer (1984) was not able to show any benefit with prophylactic co-trimoxazole, but these patients were extremely heterogeneous, including some without neutropaenia. It was, however, observed that Gram-positive cocci were isolated less frequently from blood cultures from those patients receiving co-trimoxazole. In summary then, these drugs may not affect the anaerobic flora, but they do select for resistance, which is likely to cause problems, particularly if episodes of neutropaenia are prolonged or recurrent.

The effect on the faecal flora of newer agents such as the 4-quinolones Norfloxacin (Pecquet, Andrenant and Tanrede, 1986) and Ciprofloxacin (Brumfitt, *et al.*, 1984), and the monobactam Aztreonam (de Vries-Hosper, *et al.*, 1984) have been studied in order to assess their suitability for use as prophylactic agents. All these compounds have poor anaerobic activity. Ciprofloxacin has been used for infection prevention (Rosenberg-Arska, Dekker and Verhoef, 1985). Unfortunately, resistance, particularly in *Pseudomonas aeruginosa*, was noted during its use, which is disappointing, although it is not certain whether these resistant variants are capable of causing disease to the same extent as sensitive bacteria. In addition to these effects, the numbers of Gram-positive non-sporing bacilli were reduced in number by the 4-quinolones (Rosenberg-Arska, Dekker and Verhoef, 1985).

Antimicrobial agents may also be used to reduce the infective hazards resulting from damage to the oral mucosa. Antiseptic mouthwashes have been shown to reduce organism numbers for up to two hours (Piannotti and Pitts, 1977) and improve oral infections, such as gingivitis and periodontitis (O'Neil 1976). The use of such agents has been reviewed by Cannell (1981). Chlorhexidine and Povidone Iodine are the antiseptics generally used, the former tastes unpleasant and the latter is not always acceptable because of its colour and also has a 'metallic' taste.

Infection can sometimes result from the use of mouthwash. Stephenson, *et al.* (1984) recently reported a cluster of cases of *Pseudomonas aeruginosa* septicaemia associated with contaminated mouthwash.

In addition to producing effects on oral and large bowel bacteria, antimicrobial agents can also be used to reduce the numbers of fungi. Most fungal infections occur in patients with haematological malignancies (Bodey, 1986).

A large number of antibiotics can cause increased growth of yeasts, by suppressing their bacterial competitors in the digestive tract (Finegold, Mathison and George, 1985), in the vagina and on the skin. Orally administered antifungal drugs include the non-absorbable nystatin, miconazole and amphotericin-B, and the absorbable ketoconazole. Each of these causes reduction in fungal cell numbers and also decreases the incidence of local infection. However, no trials have detected any effect of these on the incidence of systemic infection (Brincker 1978; Brincker, 1983). This may be partly because infection of this kind is uncommon and therefore large numbers are required but also because some fungi can cause systemic infection following inhalation, e.g. Aspergillus.

Effects on the flora of agents used for the treatment of infection

Consideration of the host flora is of lesser importance in the choice of antibiotics if the patient has signs or symptoms of infection.

When a patient has, for example, a temperature exceeding 38.5 °C for two hours (or whatever criteria is taken), and is neutropaenic, with a high risk of developing Gram-negative septicaemia, early treatment is usually considered essential (as will be discussed in a later chapter). A broad-spectrum regime is usually selected in order to 'cover' as many potential pathogens as possible. This is likely to consist of an extended spectrum beta-lactam and an aminoglycoside.

This type of combination seems to be reasonably successful, though some agents such as Piperacillin and Azlocillin may well be superior to others such as Cefotaxime and Ticarcillin (Klastersky, 1984). There is little evidence that treatment with different mixtures of antibiotics has a substantial effect on long-term survival (Schimpff, 1980). However, new agents are becoming available for use, with the prospect of minimizing the mortality from bacterial infections in patients who may respond to treatment of their underlying conditions. There is currently little prospect of novel aminoglycosides becoming available in the foreseeable future.

The use of an antibiotic for the treatment of a current episode of infection is only one consideration affecting the selection of the agent, though certainly the most important. With the plethora of new agents undergoing trials and coming on to the market, it will be possible to evaluate them in terms of their subtler activities – notably for their ability to select resistant strains in the normal flora, and to cause disruption of this flora resulting in conditions such as *pseudomembranous colitis*, and their predisposition to generate fungal infections. These effects may be particularly important in second and subsequent episodes of neutropaenia.

A key feature of an antibiotic agent concerns its ability to gain access to the gastro-intestinal tract, following parenteral administration. If this occurs, it has the potential to alter the balance of organisms in the intestinal flora, including the selection of resistant organisms. Some antibiotics are particularly noted for this. Following intravenous injection, access to the gastro-intestinal tract may be gained by high biliary secretion. In the prevention of infections associated with biliary surgery, this can be seen as an advantage, although it is probable that tissue concentrations are more important in preventing post-operative sepsis (Thomas, 1982). However, in general, high biliary secretion is not an advantage because of the potential for disruption of bowel flora. Furthermore, the amount of drug gaining access to the gastro-intestinal tract through the biliary tract may be substantially in excess of the minimum inhibitory concentration (for beta-lactam agents), so that even a fraction of the possible secretion through this route may be sufficient to apply potent selection pressure in the gut.

Antibiotics may also gain access to the organisms of the gastro-intestinal tract by a number of other routes. If given orally, they may reach inhibitory concentrations before absorption, or may not be fully absorbed. In addition, they may be secreted in saliva, or directly from the intestinal mucosa (Nord, Kager and Heimdahl, 1984).

Ampicillin (Kirby and Kind, 1967) and Piperacillin (Russo, *et al.*, 1982) are actively concentrated in bile. Some 'third generation' cephalosporins are also substantially excreted in this way, which may be a reflection of their high molecular weight (Rollins and Klaasen, 1979; Wright and Line, 1980). However, the biliary excretion of ceftazidime is somewhat less than cefotaxime and ceftizoxime (Wittmann, *et al.*, 1981). Nager and Berger (1984) have made an extensive review of the biliary excretion of antibiotics.

An important additional factor influencing biliary excretion will be renal function, since if there is reduced urinary excretion serum levels will be elevated and excretion by other routes enhanced. This has been shown indirectly by finding an increased incidence of diarrhoea, secondary to antibiotic therapy, in patients with reduced renal function (Trolifors, Alestig and Norrby, 1979). Imipenem – cilastatin, in contrast to the cephalosporins is notable for poor biliary excretion (Nord, Kager and Heimdahl, 1984).

A number of antibiotics are noted for salivary secretion, such as clindamycin, erythromycin and tinidazole. Penicillin, although poorly excreted by this route, does also seem to have an effect on oral flora (Josefsson and Nord, 1982).

Many antibiotics will produce damage to the skin flora, in addition to effects in the gut. Oral trimethoprim and sulphonamides have been shown to select resistance in skin coagulase-negative staphylococci (Lacey, *et al.*, 1980).

As noted previously, integrity of the anaerobic component of the bacterial flora seems to be important in preventing colonization with resistant or potentially pathogenic strains. Unfortunately, all the agents currently used in therapy have some activity on the gastro-intestinal anaerobes, either directly or indirectly (by altering the number of facultative organisms present). Rolfe and Finegold (1981) have examined the *in vitro* activity of a wide range of currently available agents against anaerobic organisms.

The most important side-effect of antibiotic usage is *pseudomembranous colitis*, associated with *Clostridium difficile*, and most antibiotics have been noted to induce this, although it is most frequently seen with clindamycin therapy (when related to the amount used) which has no specific use in haematology patients. Broad-spectrum cephalosporins, particularly 'third generation' and extended spectrum agents, are a hazard in this respect, as *Clostridium difficile* is usually resistant to their action and their use often results in colonization with this organism (Bartlett, *et al.*, 1979). As noted above (Ambrose, *et al.*, 1985), even a single dose of antibiotic may be sufficient to select for *C. difficile*. The penicillin derivatives are, in general, more active against it, but may still sometimes cause *pseudomembranous colitis*.

The 4-aminoquinolone antibiotics have less activity against anaerobes, but are still active against the Gram-positive non-sporing bacilli and cocci (Rosenberg-Arska, Dekker and Verhoef, 1985). Aztreonam and some related drugs with a similar spectrum of activity might be very valuable therapeutic agents, since they seem to have no effect on bowel flora (Mulcahy, *et al.*, 1986). Imipenem again does not have a dramatic effect, but does increase the counts of Enterococci and Candida species (Welkon, Long and Gilligan, 1986).

The aminoglycosides too are not without effect on the flora, despite poor *in vitro* activity against anaerobes. Hazenberg, *et al.* (1985) have shown that *in vitro* gentamicin can have a concentration dependent effect on inhibiting the growth of anaerobic organisms, in addition to its effect on aerobes. These authors consider that this effect may be enhanced by binding and release of gentamicin by faeces, which may maintain concentrations, despite intermittent doses used in therapy. The implications of this study were in respect of the oral use of aminoglycosides for decontamination. In our department, Heritage, *et al.* (1988) have shown that either of the aminoglycosides, gentamicin or netilmicin, when given over 24th with metronidazole, can cause an increase in Enterobacteriaceae, Staphylococci and Enterococci in the faeces, after only three parenteral doses. The effects were remarkable a week after therapy and about 80% of patients acquired aminoglycoside resistant organisms in the gut.

Selection of resistant strains

The use of antibiotics inevitably selects for resistance in the normal flora, by eliminating sensitive strains, reducing CR and by enhancing as a result, the growth of resistant strains. The use of one antibiotic may in addition select for resistance to several. This is seen where the use of gentamicin may help selection of methicillin resistant *Staphylococcus aureus* (Speller, *et al.*, 1976; Shanson, Kensit and Duke, 1976). This has been noted too with the use of ampicillin, which may additionally select for resistance to trimethoprim (Lacey, *et al.*, 1985).

As a result of the variations in the flora due to the various mechanisms discussed, it is considered worthwhile to take screening samples from the patient, in the hope that these will be of predictive value when infection arises (Newman, *et al.*, 1981; Wingard, *et al.*, 1986). Whilst it is possible to detect specific strains of bacteria and fungi, present abnormally or in increased numbers, and while these may be the cause of the patient's infection, they may not always be involved and thus the therapy may be disappointing. However, screening cultures are of value in monitoring the level of resistance, if this has been found to be problematic, but it is difficult to justify in terms of cost efficiency, unless it results in a reduction in the use of broad-spectrum empiric therapy.

Summary

Most bacterial and fungal infections occurring in the bone marrow suppressed patient arise from organisms colonizing the patient. These may be part of his normal microbiota, or may have colonized abnormally as a result of disturbance of the flora.

The indigenous flora has a number of metabolic and nutritional roles, and is of particular relevance in preventing colonization or overgrowth with potentially pathogenic organisms.

Various strategies can be followed to reduce the risks of infection from the flora organisms, ranging from complete elimination to selective modulation.

Therapeutic and prophylactic use of antimicrobial agents may be hazardous and there is a risk of paradoxically enhancing the chances of infection, which may be with resistant organisms.

Acknowledgements

Mrs E. Ellis and Mrs S. Powis for their work in producing the manuscript.

References

Aly, R. and Maibach, H. (1981) Factors controlling skin bacterial flora. In *Skin Microbiology: relevance to clinical infection*, eds H. Malbach and R. Aly, pp. 29–39. Springer Verlag, New York

Ambrose, N.S., Johnson, M., Burdon, D.W. and Keighley, M.R.B. (1985) The influence of single dose intravenous antibiotics on faecal flora and the emergence of *Clostridium difficile*. *Journal of Antimicrobial Chemotherapy*, **15**, 319–326

Appelbaum, P.C., Ballard, J.O. and Eyster, M.E. (1979) Septicaemia due to Capnocytophaga (*Bacteroides ochraceous*) in Hodgkin's disease. *Annals of Internal Medicine*, **90**, 716–717

Bartlett, J.G., Chang, T.W., Gurwith, M., Gorbach, S.L. and Ondodonk, A.B. (1978) Antibiotic associated *pseudomembranous colitis* due to toxin producing clostridia. *New England Journal of Medicine*, **298**, 531–534

Bartlett, J.G., Wiley, S.H., Chang, T.W. and Lowe, B. (1979) Cephalosporin-associated *pseudomembranous colitis* due to *Clostridium difficile*. *Journal of the American Medical Association*, **242**, 2683–2685

Beachey, E.H. (1981) Bacterial adherence: adhesin-receptor interactions mediating the attachment of bacteria to mucosal surfaces. *Journal of Infectious Diseases*, **143**, 325–345

Binder, H.J., Fillburn, G. and Gloch, M. (1974) Bile acid inhibition of intestinal anaerobic organisms. *American Journal of Clinical Nutrition*, **28**, 119–125

Bodey, G.P. (1986) Fungal infections and fever of unknown origin in neutropaenic patients. *American Journal of Medicine*, **80**, (5C) 112–119

Bodey, G.P. and Fainstein, V. (1986) Infections of the gastro-intestinal tract in the immunocompromised patient. *Annual Review of Medicine*, **37**, 271–281

Bodey, G.P. and Johnston, D. (1971) Microbial evaluation of protected environments during patient occupancy. *Applied Microbiology*, **22**, 828–836

Brincker, H. (1978) Prophylactic treatment with miconazole in patients highly predisposed to fungal infection. A placebo-controlled double-blind study. *Acta Medica Scandinavica*, **204**, 123–128

Brincker, H. (1983) Prevention of mycosis in granulocytopaenic patients with prophylactic ketoconzole treatment. *Mykosen*, **26**, 242–247

Brumfitt, W.I., Franklin, D., Grady, J. and Hamilton-Miller, J.M.T. (1984) Changes in the pharmacokinetics of ciprofloxacin and faecal flora during the administration of a 7-day course to human volunteers. *Antimicrobial Agents and Chemotherapy*, **26**, 257–261

Brook, J.H. (1980) Lactoferrin in milk: its role in iron absorption and protection against enteric infection in the newborn infant. *Archives of Diseases of Childhood*, **55**, 417–421

Buck, A.C. and Cooke, E.M. (1969) The fate of *Pseudomonas aeruginosa* in normal persons. *Journal of Medical Microbiology*, **2**, 521–525

Cannell, J.S. (1981) The use of antimicrobials in the mouth. *Journal of International Medical Research*, **9**, 277–282

Cooke, E.M., Brayson, J.C., Edmondson, A.S. and Hall, D. (1979) An investigation into the incidence and source of Klebsiella infections in hospital patients. *Journal of Hygiene* (Cambridge), **82**, 473–480

Corrodi, P., Wideman, P.A., Sutter, V.L., Drenick, E.J., Passaro, E. and Finegold, S.M. (1978) Bacterial flora of the small bowel before and after bypass for morbid obesity. *Journal of Infectious Diseases*, **137**, 1–6

Cummings, J.H. (1983) Fermentation in the human large intestine; evidence and implications for health. *Lancet,* **i,** 1206–1209

Cummings, J.H. (1984) Colonic absorption: The importance of short chain fatty acids in Man. *Scandinavian Journal of Gastro-enterology,* (Supplement), **93,** 89–99

Day, T.K. (1975) Controlled trial of prophylactic antibiotic in minor wounds requiring suture. *Lancet,* **ii,** 1174–1176

de Vries-Hosper, H.G., Welling, G.W., Swabb, E.A. and Van der Waaij, D. (1984) Selective decontamination of the digestive tract with aztreonam: a study of 10 healthy volunteers. *Journal of Infectious Diseases,* **150,** 636–642

Dibb, W.L. and van der Lippe, E. (1984). Septicaemia in granulocytopaenic patients caused by multi-resistant diphtheroid rods. *Acta Pathologica, Microbiologica et Immunologica, Scandinavica, Section B,* **92,** 181–182

Donnelly, T.P., Cohen, J., Marcus, R.E. and Guest, J. (1985) Bacteraemia and Hickman catheters. *Lancet,* **2,** 48

Drasar, B.S. and Hill, M.J. (1974) *Human Intestinal Flora.* Academic Press. New York and London

Drasar, B.S., Shiner, M. and McCleod, G.M. (1969) Studies on the intestinal flora I. The bacterial flora of the gastro-intestinal tract in healthy and achlorhydric persons. *Gastroenterology,* **56,** 71–79

Editorial (1980). Granulocytopaenia and septicaemia. *British Medical Journal,* **281,** 1091

EORTC. International Antimicrobial Therapy Project Group (1984) Trimethoprim-Sulphamethoxazole in the prevention of infection in neutropaenic patients. *Journal of Infectious Diseases,* **150,** 372–379

Eykyn, S.J. (1984) Infection and intravenous catheters. *Journal of Antimicrobial Chemotherapy,* **14,** 203–208

Finegold, S.M., Attebery, H.R. and Sutter, V.L. (1974) Effect of diet on human faecal flora: Comparison of Japanese and American diets. *American Journal of Clinical Nutrition,* **27,** 456–469

Finegold, S.M., Flora, D.J., Attebery, H.R. and Sutter, V.L. (1975) Faecal bacteriology of colonic cancer and control patients. *Cancer Research,* **35,** 3407–3417

Finegold, S.M., Mathiesen, G.E. and George, W.L. (1985) Changes in human intestinal flora related to the administration of antimicrobial agents. In *Human intestinal microflora in health and disease,* ed. D.J. Hentges, pp. 355–446. Academic Press, New York

Finegold, S.M., Sutter, V.L. and Mathieson, G.E. (1985) Normal indigenous intestinal flora. In *Human Intestinal Microflora in Health and Disease,* ed. D.J. Hentges, pp. 3–31. Academic Press, New York

Finegold, S.M., Sutter, V.L., Sugihara, P.T., Elder, M.A., Lehman, S.M. and Phillips, R.C. (1977) Faecal bacteriology in Seventh Day Adventist populations and control subjects. *American Journal of Clinical Nutrition,* **30,** 1781–1792

Foo, M. and Lee, A. (1972) Immunological response of the autochthonous intestinal flora. *Infection and Immunity,* **6,** 525–532

Freter, R. (1985). Mechanisms that control the microflora of the large intestine. In *Human Intestinal Flora in Health*

and Disease, ed. D.J. Hentges, pp. 33–54. Academic Press, New York

Freter, R., Brickner, H., Botley, M., Cleven, D. and Aranki, H. (1983) Mechanisms which control bacterial propulations in continuous flow culture models of mouse large intestinal flora. *Infection and Immunity,* **39,** 676–685

Freter, R., Brickner, H., Fekete, J. and Vickerman, M.M. (1983) Survival and implantation of *Escherichia coli* in the intestinal tract. *Infection and Immunity,* **39,** 686–703

Giannella, R.A., Broitman, S.A. and Zamcheck, N. (1972) Gastric acid barrier to ingested micro-organisms in man: Studies *in vivo* and *in vitro. Gut,* **13,** 251–256

Glauser, M.P., McCutchan, J.A. and Ziegler, E. (1984) Immuno-prophylaxis and immuno-therapy of Gram-negative infections in the immuno-compromised host. *Clinics in Haematology,* **13,** 549–555; **22,** 249–256

Gorbach, S.L., Nahas, L., Lerner, P.I. and Weinstein, L. (1967) Studies of the intestinal microflora I: Effects on diet, age and periodic sampling on numbers of faecal micro-organisms in man. *Gastroenterology,* **53,** 845–855

Hann, I.M. and Prentice, H.G. (1984). Infection prophylaxis in the patient with bone marrow failure. *Clinics in Haematology,* **13,** 523–547

Hazenberg, M.P., Pennock-Schroder, A.M. and van der Merwe, J.P. (1985) Binding to and antibacterial effect of Aztreonam, temocillin, gentamicin and tobramycin on human faeces. *Journal of Hygiene* (Cambridge), **95,** 255–263

Heritage, J., Dyke, G.W., Johnston, D. and Lacey, R.W. (1988) Selection of resistance to gentamicin and netilmicin in the faecal flora following prophylaxis for colorectal surgery. *Journal of Antimicrobial Chemotherapy,* **22,** 249–256

Hudault, S., Bewa, H., Bridonneau, C. and Raibaud, P. (1985) Efficiency of various bacterial suspensions derived from the cecal floras of conventional chickens in reducing the population level of *Salmonella typhimurium* in gnotobiotic mice and chicken intestines. *Canadian Journal of Microbiology,* **31,** 832–838

Hughes, W.T., Kuhn, S., Chaudhury, S., Feldman, S., Verzosa, M., Aur, R.J.A., Pratt, C. and George, S.L. (1977) Successful chemoprophylaxis for *Pneumocystis carinii* pneumonitis. *New England Journal of Medicine,* **297,** 1419–1426

Huxley, E.J., Viroslav, J., Gray, W.R. and Pierce, A.K. (1978) Pharyngeal aspiration in normal adults and patients with depressed consciousness. *American Journal of Medicine,* **64,** 564–568

Johanson, W.G. Jr., Blackstock, R., Pierce, A.K. and Sanford, J.P. (1970) The role of bacterial antagonism in pneumococcal colonization of the human pharynx. *Journal of Laboratory Clinical Medicine,* **75,** 946–952

Johanson, W.G., Pierce, A.K. and Sanford, J.P. (1969) Changing pharyngeal bacterial flora of hospitalized patients. *New England Journal of Medicine,* **281,** 1137–1140

Johanson, W.G., Pierce, A.K., Sanford, J.P. and Thomas,

G.D. (1972) Nosocomial respiratory infections with Gram-negative bacilli. The significance of colonization of the respiratory tract. *Annals of Internal Medicine, 77,* 701–706

Josefsson, K. and Nord, C.E. (1982) Effects of phenonymethyl penicillin and erythromycin in high oral doses on the salivary microflora. *Journal of Antimicrobial Chemotherapy,* **10**, 325–333

Klastersky, J. (1984) New Antibacterial agents: the role of new penicillins and Cephalosporins in the management of infection in granulocytopaenic patients. *Clinics in Haematology,* **13**,(3), 587–598

Kirby, W.M.M. and Kind, A.C. (1967) Clinical pharmacology of ampicillin and netacillin. *Annals of the New York Academy of Science,* **145**, 291

Kruh, J. (1982). Effects of sodium butyrate, a new pharmacological agent, on cells in culture *Molecular and Cellular Biochemistry,* **42**, 65–82

Lacey, R.W. (1963) Binding of neomycin and analogues by fatty acids *in vitro. Journal of Clinical Pathology,* **21**, 564–566

Lacey, R.W. and Lord, V.L. (1981). Sensitivity of Staphylococci to fatty acids: novel inactivation of Linolenic Acid by serum. *Journal of Medical Microbiology,* **14**, 41–49

Lacey, R.W., Lord, V.L., Howson, G.L., Luxton, D.E.A. and Trotter, I.S. (1983) Double-blind study to compare the selection of antibiotic resistance by amoxycillin or cephradine in the commensal flora. *The Lancet,* i, 529–532

Levine, A.S., Siegel, S.E., Schreiber, A.D., Hauser, J., Preisler, H. and Goldstein, I.M. (1973) Protected environment and prophylactic antibiotics. A prospective controlled study of their utility in the therapy of acute leukaemia. *New England Journal of Medicine,* **288**, 477–483

Marcus, R.E. and Goldman, J.M. (1986) Management of infection in the neutropaenic patient. *British Medical Journal,* **293**, 406–408

Marshall, B.J. and Warren, J.R. (1984) Unidentified curved bacilli in the stomach of patients with gastritis and peptic ulceration. *Lancet,* i, 1311–1315

Masfari, A.N., Duerden, B.I. and Kinghorn, G.R. (1986) Quantitative studies of vaginal bacteria. *Genito-urinary Medicine,* **62**, 256–263

Mattingley, T.A. and Waksman, B.H. (1978) Immunlogic suppression after oral administration of antigen I. Specific suppressor cells formed in fat Peyer's patches after oral administration of sheep erythrocytes and their systemic migration. *Journal of Immunology,* **121**, 1878–1883

McDermid, A.S., McKee, A.S., Ellwood, D.C. and Marsh, P.D. (1983) Effect of lowering pH on the composition and metabolism of a community of nine oral bacteria grown in a chemostat. *Journal of general microbiology,* **132**, 1205–1214

McEvoy, A., Dutton, J. and James, O.F.W. (1983) Bacterial contamination of the small bowel is an important cause of malabsorption in the elderly. *British Medical Journal,* **287**, 789–793

McNeil, N.I. (1984) The contribution of the large intestine to energy supplies in man. *American Journal of Clinical Nutrition,* **39**, 338–342

McKee, A.S., McDermid, A.S., Ellwood, D.C. and Marsh, P.D. (1985) The establishment of reproducible complex communities of oral bacteria in the chemostat using defined inocula. *Journal of Applied Bacteriology,* **59**, 263–275

Minah, G.E., Rednor, J.L., Peterson, D.E., Overholser, C.D., Depaola, L.G. and Suzuki, J.D. (1986) Oral succession of Gram-negative bacilli in suppressed cancer patients. *Journal of Clinical Microbiology,* **24**, 210–213

Mulcahy, F.M., Lacey, C.J., Barr, K.W. and Lacey, R.W. (1986) Resistance in *Escherichia coli* after single dose ampicillin to treat gonorrhoea. *Genito-urinary Medicine,* **62**, 166–169

Nagar, H. and Berger, S.A. (1984) The excretion of antibiotics by the biliary tract. *Surgery, Gynaecology and Obstetrics,* **158**, 601–607

Newman, K.A., Schimpff, S.L., Young, V.M. and Wiernick, P.H. (1981) Lessons learned from surveillance cultures in patients with ante non-lymphoblastic leukaemia. Usefulness for epidemiologic, preventative and therapeutic research. *American Journal of Medicine,* **70**, 423–431

Nord, C.E., Kager, L. and Heimdahl, A. (1984) Impact of antimicrobial agents on the gastro-intestinal microflora and the risk of infections. *American Journal of Medicine,* **76**, (suppl. 5A), 99–107

O'Neill, T.L. (1976) The use of chlorhexidine mouthwash in the control of gingival inflammation. *British Dental Journal,* **141**, 276–280

Paes, I.C., Searl, P., Rubert, M.W. and Faloon, W.W. (1967) Intestinal lactase deficiency and saccharide malabsorption during oral neomycin administration. *Gastroenterology,* **53**, 49–58

Pecquet, S., Andremont, T. and Tancrede, C. (1986) Selective antimicrobial modulation of the intestinal tract by norfloxacin in human volunteers and gnotobiotic mice associated with a human faecal flora. *Antimicrobial Agents and Chemotherapy,* **29**, 1047–1052

Pennington, J.E., Rossing, T.H. and Boerth, L.W. (1983) The effect of human alveolar macrophages on the bactericidal capacity of neutrophils. *Journal of Infectious Diseases,* **148**, 101–109

Penny, M.E., Harendra da Silva, D.G. and McNeish, A. (1986) Bacterial contamination of the small intestine of infants with enteropathogenic *Escherichia coli* and other enteric infections: a factor in the aetiology of diarrhoea. *British Medical Journal,* **292**, 1223–1226

Peters, J.L., Belsham, P.A., Taylor, B.A. and Watt-Smith, S. (1984) Long-term venous access. *British Journal of Hospital Medicine,* **32**, 230–242

Piannotti, R. and Pitts, G. (1977) Effects of an antiseptic mouthrinse on crevicular anaerobes. *Journal of Dental Research,* **56**, A560

Pizzo, P.A., Purvis, D.S. and Waters, C. (1982) Microbiological evaluation of food items for patients undergoing gastro-intestinal decontamination and protected isolation. *Journal of the American Dietetics Association,* **81**, 272–279

Price, D.J.E. and Sleigh, J.D. (1970) Control of infection due to *Klebsiella aerogenes* in a neurosurgical unit by withdrawal of all antibiotics. *Lancet,* **ii**, 1213–1215

Remington, T.S. and Schimpff, S.C. (1981) Please don't eat salads. *New England Journal of Medicine,* **304**, 433–435

Roberts, D.R. (1965) Significance of clean wound cultures. *American Surgeon,* **31**, 153–155

Roediger, W.E.W. (1980) Role of anaerobic bacteria in the metabolic welfare of the colonic mucosa in man. *Gut,* **21**, 793–798

Roediger, W.E.W. and Rae, D.A. (1982) Trophic effect of short chain fatty acids on mucosal handling of ions by the defunctioned colon. *British Journal of Surgery,* **69**, 23–25

Rolfe, R.D. and Finegold, S.M. (1981) Comparative *in vitro* activity of new Beta-lactam antibiotics against anaerobic bacteria. *Antimicrobial Agents and Chemotherapy,* **20**, 600–609

Rollins, D.E. and Klasser, C.D. (1979) Biliary excretion of drugs in man. *Clinical Pharmacokinetics,* **4**, 368–369

Rosebury, T. (1962) *Micro-organisms indigenous to man.* New York, McGraw-Hill

Rosenburg-Arska, M., Dekker, A.W. and Verhoef, J. (1985) Ciprofloxacin for selective decontamination of the alimentary tract in patients with acute leukaemia, during remission induction treatment. The effect on faecal flora. *Journal of Infectious Diseases,* **152**, 104–107

Russo, J., Thompson, M.I.B., Russo, M.E., Swann, B.H., Matsen, J.M., Moody, F.G. and Rikkers, L.F. (1982) Piperacillin distribution in bile, gallbladder wall, abdominal skeletal muscle, and adipose tissue, in surgical patients. *Antimicrobial Agents and Chemotherapy,* **22**, 488–492

Savage, D.C. (1977) Microbial ecology of the gastrointestinal tract. *Annal Review of Microbiology,* **31**, 107–133

Sanders, W.C. and Sanders, S.C. (1984) Modification of normal flora by antibiotics: effects on individuals and the environment. In *New dimensions in Antimicrobial Chemotherapy,* eds R.K. Root and M.E. Sane, pp. 217–241. Churchill Livingstone, New York

Schimpff, S.C. (1980) Infection prevention during profound granulocytopaenia. *Annals of Internal Medicine,* **93**, 358–361

Schimpff, S.C., Greene, W.H., Young, V.M., Fortner, C.L., Jepsen, L., Cusack, N., Black, J.M. and Wiernick, P.H. (1975) Infection prevention in acute lymphocytic leukaemia; laminar air flow room reverse isolation with oral, non-absorbable antibiotic prophylaxis. *Annals of Internal Medicine,* **82**, 351–358

Schimpff, S.C., Young, V.M., Green, W.H., Verneulen, C.D., Moody, M.R. and Wiernik, P.H. (1977) Origin of infection in ante non-lymphocystic leukaemia: significance of hospital acquisition of potential pathogens. *Annals of Internal Medicine,* **77**, 707–714

Schlaes, D.M., Dul, M.J. and Lerner, P.I. (1982) Capnocytophaga bacteraemia in the compromised host. *American Journal of Clinical Pathology,* **77**, 358–361

Seldon, R., Lee, S., Wang, W.L.L., Bennett, J.V. and Eickhoff, T.C. (1971) Nosocomial Klebsiella infections: intestinal as a reservoir. *Annals of Internal Medicine,* **74**, 657–664

Shanson, D.C., Kensit, T.G. and Duke, R. (1976) Outbreak of hospital infection with a strain of *S. aureus* resistant to gentamicin and methicillin. *Lancet,* **ii**, 1347–1348

Shehadeh, N.H., and Kligman, A.M. (1963) The effect of topical antibacterial agents on the bacterial flora of the axilla. *Journal of Investigative Dermatology,* **40**, 61–71

Shooter, R.A., Cooke, E.M., Gayer, H., Kumar, P., Patel, N., Parker, M.T., Thom, B.T. and France, D.R. (1969) Food and medicaments as possible sources of hospital strains of *Pseudomonas aeruginosa. Lancet,* **i**, 1227–1229

Sleijfer, D.T., Mulder, N.H., de Vries-Hosper, H.G. *et al.* (1980) Infection prevention in granulocytopaenic patients by selective decontamination of the digestive tract. *European Journal of Cancer,* **16**, 859–869

Snydman, D.R., Gorbea, H.F., Roper, B.R., Meyka, J.A., Murray, S.A. and Perry, L.K. (1982) Predictive volume of surveillance skin cultures in total-parental-nutrition-related infection. *Lancet,* **ii**, 1385–1388

Speller, D.C.E., Raghurath, D., Stephens, M., Viant, A.C., Reeves, D.S., Wilkinson, P.J., Broughall, T.M. and Holt, H.A. (1976) Epidemic infection by a gentamicin-resistant *S. aureus* in three hospitals. *Lancet,* **i**, 464–466

Sprunt, K., Leidy, G.A. and Redman, W. (1971) Prevention of bacterial overgrowth. *Journal of Infectious Diseases,* **123**, 1–10

Starke, I.D., Catovsky, D., Johnson, S.A., Donnelly, P., Darrell, J., Goldman, T.M. and Galton, D.A.G. (1982) Co-trimoxazole alone for prevention of bacterial infection in patients with acute leukaemia. *Lancet,* **i**, 5–6

Stephenson, T.R., Heard, S.R., Richards, M.A. and Tabaqchali, S. (1984) Outbreak of septicaemia due to contaminated mouthwash. *British Medical Journal,* **289**, 1584

Stockbrugger, R.W., Cotton, P.B., Eugenides, N., Bartholomew, B.A., Hill, M.J. and Walters, C.C. (1982) Intragastric nitrites, nitrosamines and bacterial overgrowth during cimetidine treatment. *Gut,* **23**, 1048–1054

Stolberg, L., Rolfe, R., Gitlin, N., Mann, L., Linder, J. and Finegold, S. (1982) D-lactic acidosis due to abnormal gut flora. *New England Journal of Medicine,* **306**, 1344–1348

Storring, R.A., Jameson, B., McElwain, T.J., Wiltshaw, E., Spiers, A.S.D. and Gaya, H. (1977) Oral non-absorbed antibiotics prevent infection in acute non-lymphoblastic leukaemia. *Lancet,* **ii**, 837–840

Stout, J.E., Best, M.G., Yu, V.L. and Riks, J.D. (1986) A note on symbiosis of *L. pneumophila* and *T. micdadei* with human respiratory flora. *Journal of Applied Bacteriology,* **60**, 297–299

Tancrede, C. and Andremont, A. (1985). Bacterial translocation and Gram-negative bacteraemia in patients with haematological malignancies. *Journal of Infectious Diseases,* 151, 99–103

Taylor-Robinson, D. and McCormack, W.M. (1979). Mycoplasmas in human genito-urinary infection. In *The Mycoplasmas,* eds J.G. Tully and R.F. Whitcomb, vol. 22 pp. 307–366. New York, Academic Press

Thadepelli, H., Lou, M.A., Bach, V.T., Matsui, T.K. and Mandal, A.K. (1979) Microflora of the human small intestine. *American Journal of Surgery,* 138, 845–850

Thomas, M. (1982) Antibiotics in bile. *Journal of Antimicrobial Chemotherapy,* 12, 419–422

Tompkins, D.S., Foulkes, S.J., Godwin, P.G. and West, A.P. (1986) Isolation and characterization of intestinal spirochaetes. *Journal of Clinical Pathology,* 39, 535–541

Trallero, E.P., Cilla, G.C., Lopez-Lopategui, C. and Arratibel, C. (1986) Fatal septicaemia caused by *Yersinia enterocolitica* in *Thalassaemia major. Paediatric infectious diseases,* 5, 483–485

Trollfors, B., Alestig, K. and Norrby, R. (1979) Local and gastro-intestinal reactions to intravenously administered cefoxitin and cefuroxime. *Scandinavian Journal of Infectious Diseases,* 11, 315–316

Vahouny, G.V., Cassidy, M.M., Lightfoot, F., Grau, L. and Kritchivsky, D. (1981) Ultrastructural modifications of internal and colonic mucosa induced by free and bound bile acids. *Cancer Research,* 41, 3764–3765

Van der Waaij, D. (1983) *Antibiotic choice: the importance of colonization resistance.* Research Studies Press (John Wiley) Chichester

Van der Waaij, D. (1986) The apparent role of the mucous membrane and the gut associated lymphoid tissue in the selection of the normal flora of the digestive tract. *Clinical Immunology Newsletter,* 7, 4–7

Van der Waaij, D. and Berghuis de Vries, J.M. (1974) Selective elimination of Enterobacteriaceae species from the digestive tract in mice and monkeys. *Journal of Hygiene* (Cambridge) 72, 205–211

Van der Waaij, D., Berghuis de Vries, J.M. and Lekkerkerk van der Wees, J.E.C. (1971) Colonization resistance of the digestive tract in conventional and antibiotic treated mice. *Journal of Hygiene* (Cambridge), 69, 405–411

Van Saene, H.K.F. and Van der Waaij, D. (1979) A novel technique for detecting IgA coated, potentially pathogenic micro-organisms in the human intestine. *Journal of Immunological Methods,* 30, 87–96

Watson, J.G. and Jameson, B. (1979) Antibiotic prophylaxis for patients in protective isolation. *Lancet,* i, 1183

Watson, J.G., Powles, R.L., Lawson, D.N., Morgenstern, G.R., Jameson, B., McElwain, T.J., Judson, I., Lumley, H. and Kay, H.E.M. (1982) Co-trimoxazole versus non-absorbable antibiotics in acute leukaemia. *Lancet,* i, 6–9

Weightman, N.C., Simpson, E.M. and Speller, D.C.E. (1986) Source of infection in Hickman catheters. *Journal of Clinical Pathology,* 39, 1046

Weinberg, E.D. (1984). Iron withdrawal: a defence against infection and neoplasia. *American Journal of Physiology,* 64, 65–102

Welling, G.W. (1982) Comparison of methods for the determination of -aspartylglycine in faecal supernatants of leukemic patients treated with antimicrobial agents. *Journal of Chromatography,* 232, 55–62

Welkon, C.J., Long, S.S. and Gilligan, P.H. (1986) Effect of imipenen-Cilastatin therapy on faecal flora. *Antimicrobial Agents and Chemotherapy,* 29, 741–743

Williams, R.C. and Gibbons, R.J. (1982) Inhibition of bacterial adherence by secretory immunoglobulin A: a mechanism of antigen disposal. *Science,* 177, 679–697

Wilson, T.M. and Guiney, D.G. (1982) Failure of oral trimethoprim-sulphaemethoxazole prophylaxis in acute leukaemia. *New England Journal of Medicine,* 306, 16–20

Wingard, T.R., Dick, J., Charachie, P. and Saral, R. (1986) Antibiotic resistant bacteria in surveillance stool cultures of patients with prolonged neutropaenia. *Antimicrobial Agents and Chemotherapy,* 30, 435–439

Wittmann, D.H., Schhasan, H.H., Kohler, F. and Seibert, W. (1981) Pharmacokinetic studies of ceftazidime in serum, bone, bile, tissue, fluid and peritoneal fluid. *Journal of Antimicrobial Chemotherapy,* 8, (suppl. B), 293–297

Wright, W.E., Line, V.D. (1980) Biliary excretion of cephalosporins in rats: influence of molecular weight. *Antimicrobial Agents and Chemotherapy,* 17, 842–846

6

The effects of antileukaemic cytoreductive therapy on host defences

E.J. Bow and A.R. Ronald

Introduction

The successful management of patients with acute leukaemia is frequently obstructed by severe, potentially life-threatening infections. The increased incidence of infection in these patients is attributable to a multiplicity of serious defects in the host defence system. Host defence against invading micro-organisms is a complicated series of cooperative interactions between the cellular and humoral components of the system. The system can be described by its four basic components: the epithelial/mucosal barrier; humoral immunity characterized by serum and mucosal immunoglobulins and the components of complement; cellular immunity characterized by the interactions of thymus-derived lymphocytes and macrophages; and the neutrophilic phagocyte. One or more of these components are severely damaged in patients with acute leukaemia. This may be secondary to a pure primary defect imposed by the leukaemic process itself or secondary to secondary defects imposed by the myelotoxic, immunotoxic and mucosal toxic effects of the multi-modal treatment regimens for leukaemia. The wide spectrum of infectious agents observed in these patients all too often reflects host defence defects of a combined primary and secondary nature. It is the purpose of this chapter to discuss how these mechanisms become defective and the role that these defects play in the pathogenesis of infection in patients undergoing remission induction therapy for acute leukaemia with regimens containing anthracyclines and cytosine arabinoside.

The myelotoxic effects of remission induction therapy

Remission induction therapy for acute leukaemia consists of regimens containing one or more highly myelotoxic agents. These regimens result in a predictable reduction of the numbers of circulating peripheral blood neutrophils. This reduction is inversely related to the risk of acquired infection (Bodey, et al., 1966; Pizzo, 1984). Although the lower limit for the absolute neutrophil count for adult caucasians is 1.5×10^9/l (Zacharski, Elvebach, Linman, 1971; Bain and England, 1975), the risk of infection is only slightly increased in the range of $0.5–1.5 \times 10^9$/l (Bow, et al., 1985; Bow, et al., 1987). Severe neutropaenia occurs when the number of circulating neutrophils falls below 0.5×10^9/l, and this is association with a substantially higher risk of infection (Bodey, et al., 1966; Wade, et al., 1983; Bow, et al., 1987; Whimbey, et al., 1987). Circulating neutrophil counts of less than 0.1×10^9/l sustained longer than a week are virtually always associated with fever and infection. Furthermore, the risk of life-threatening bacteraemias is markedly increased compared to lesser degrees of neutropaenia (Wade, et al., 1983; Bow, et al., 1987).

Neutrophil count

The absolute number of circulating neutrophils is calculated as the proportion of circulating leukocytes that are segmented (polymorphonuclear) neutrophils. This is usually based upon a differential count of 100 leukocytes on a Romanowsky stained peripheral blood smear. The accuracy of the neutrophil count depends upon the number of leukocytes counted on the blood smear (Rumke, 1979). As the total leukocyte count falls as a result of cytotoxic therapy, the error associated with the differential count rises substantially. In patients undergoing induction chemotherapy for acute leukaemia, it is common to have total leukocyte counts of $0.3-0.7 \times 10^9/l$ and differential counts based upon only 25 to 50 leukocytes on the peripheral blood smear. In this situation, perhaps only 2 or 3 segmented neutrophils may be observed. The range of error for the differential leukocyte count based upon these small numbers is so high that the reliability of the absolute neutrophil count is substantially reduced. For this reason, requests for frequent differential counts as a means of monitoring the patient's risk of infection are often discouraged (Shapiro and Greenfield, 1987). Although an absolute neutrophil count of $0.010 \times 10^9/l$ is less than a count of $0.075 \times 10^9/l$, the most clinically relevant information with respect to infection risk is that the count falls in the category of less than $0.1 \times 10^9/l$. Accordingly, it is suggested that the risk of infection be based not upon the results of the absolute neutrophil count but rather the category (less than $0.1 \times 10^9/l$, $0.1-0.499 \times 10^9/l$, $0.5-0.999 \times 10^9/l$ and $>1.0 \times 10^9/l$) in which the count falls.

It is important for clinicians who are managing patients undergoing remission induction therapy for acute leukaemia to know the degree and duration of neutropaenia associated with induction regimen. This allows the clinician to anticipate the resources needed for patient support (such as blood product support or allocation of isolation facilities) and to plan infection prevention and management strategies. The myelotoxicity of antileukaemic therapy is often reported as time to the nadir or to the recovery of the peripheral leukocyte or neutrophil counts. It is difficult to glean the risk of infection from this kind of data. It would be more useful to know the expected duration of time a patient might spend at particular degrees of neutropaenia. There is so much variability in the reporting of this information that data for specific antileukaemic regimens is hard to find and even harder to compare.

Induction chemotherapy

The cornerstone of therapy for acute non-lymphocytic leukaemia has been the use of regimens containing an antimetabolite, cytosine arabinoside (ARA-C) and an anthracycline, adriamycin or daunorubicin (ADR or DNR). Although there are few controlled trials comparing the efficacy of the anthracyclines, DNR is generally preferred because of fewer non-haematologic toxicities (Yates, *et al.*, 1982). The combination of ARA-C and DNR is highly myelotoxic and results in a rapid drop in the number of circulating leukocytes and neutrophils within 7 to 10 days of beginning therapy. Circulating neutrophil counts of less than $1.0 \times 10^9/l$ persist on the average for 30 days. Table 6.1 shows the degree and duration of neutropaenia for adult patients undergoing remission induction therapy with ARA-C and DNR from our own institution (the University of Manitoba) (E.J. Bow, 1987, personal communication), the University of Maryland Cancer Center (Wade, *et al.*, 1983) and from the European Organization for Research and Treatment of Cancer (Gnotobiotic Project Group) (Kurrle, *et al.*, 1986). These data

Table 6.1 Degree and duration (mean number of days) of neutropaenia for patients with acute leukaemia undergoing remission induction with cytosine arabinoside and daunorubicin

Neutrophil count ($\times 10^9/l$)	Duration of neutropaenia (mean days)			
	<0.1	0.1–0.499	0.5–0.999	<1.0
University of Manitoba, 1987 (n = 55)	15.8	8.4	4.4	28.6
Wade, *et al.*, 1983 (n = 64)	20.1	7.6	4.7	27.7
Kurrle, *et al.*, 1986 (n = 140)	17.9	11.5	6.1	35.5

demonstrates that patients are at high risk of infection for an average of just over three and a-half weeks when the circulating neutrophil counts of less than $0.5 \times 10^9/l$. Furthermore, persistent life-threatening neutropaenia (less than $0.1 \times 10^9/l$) lasts for an average of two and a-half weeks. Overall, lesser degrees of neutropaenia (peripheral neutrophil counts of 0.1–0.499 and 0.5–0.999 $\times 10^9/l$) last approximately 7–10 days and 5–7 days respectively. This time is usually distributed prior to and following the period of persistent life-threatening neutropaenia.

The rate at which the bone marrow recovers following the nadir varies dependent upon the degree of stem cell and marrow damage attributable to either the chemotherapeutic regimen or the underlying disease itself. Vaughan, Karp and Burke (1980) showed in serial studies of 19 patients with acute leukaemia receiving timed-sequential regimen of high dose ARA-C (45 mg/kg continuous infusion days 1–3 and 8–11) and DNR (1.0 mg/kg IV day 1–3) that by day 13 from the start of therapy only stromal elements could be observed within patients' bone marrow and that this persisted until day 20–24. Peripheral blood leukocytes appeared 7–10 days following reappearance of normal cells in the bone marrow. Peripheral T lymphocytes, B-lymphocytes and monocytes and neutrophils recovered at days 18–22, days 23–27 and days 28–32 respectively. Although the regimen used in this study utilized higher doses than are customarily used in remission induction therapy, the marrow recovery pattern is similar to that observed with standard dosing regimens where ARA-C is used in doses of 100–200 mg/M^2 as a continuous infusion over 5 to 7 days.

These recovery times are substantially longer than those observed for patients receiving pulse dose cyto-reductive therapy for solid tissue malignancies (deJongh, *et al.*, 1983; Schreml, Lohrmann and Anger, 1985; Minah, *et al.*, 1986; Bunn, *et al.*, 1987). In these circumstances the period of severe neutropaenia (less than $0.5 \times 10^9/l$) usually averages less than 7–10 days.

Encouraging response rates have been reported for relapsed patients receiving doses of ARA-C that are substantially higher (high dose ARA-C, HDARA-C) than the standard 100–200 mg/M^2 doses (Hines, *et al.*, 1984; Herzig, *et al.*, 1985; Wells, *et al.*, 1985; Arlin, *et al.*,

1987; Barnett, *et al.*, 1987; Ganesan, *et al.*, 1987; Hiddemann, *et al.*, 1987).

Although the dosing schedules have varied among different institutions, doses of 2–3 grams/M^2 infused over 1–3 hours every 12 hours for periods of 2–6 days have been used most frequently. The degree and duration of neutropaenia for HDARA-C containing regimens have been similar to that reported for anthracycline/standard dose ARA-C regimens (Slevin, *et al.*, 1982; Herzig, *et al.*, 1985; Barnett, *et al.*, 1987; Preisler, *et al.*, 1987). The median time until the circulating neutrophil count rises above $0.5 \times 10^9/l$ is 25–30 days with a range of 19–50 days. This period can be extended as long as 60–90 days for heavily pretreated patients where there may be more prolonged direct effects of cytotoxic therapy on the marrow stem cell pool or the marrow microenvironment (Schreml, Lohrmann and Anger, 1985).

Non-myelotoxic effects of remission induction therapy upon integumental surfaces

The integumental barrier is one of the major host defence mechanisms that becomes damaged during therapy for acute leukaemia. The most important integumental barriers in this regard are the skin and the epithelial mucosal surfaces lining the upper and lower gastrointestinal tract. The source of the majority of the infections observed in neutropaenic patients with acute leukaemia is the pool of micro-organisms colonizing these surfaces (Schimpff, *et al.*, 1972). The increased use of indwelling central venous catheters for venous access in leukaemic patients has been paralleled by an increased incidence of infections due to Gram-positive micro-organisms such as *Staphylococcus epidermidis* (Wade, *et al.*, 1982; Winston, *et al.*, 1983). However, the pathogenetic role of the indwelling central venous access catheters in infection has been relatively minor in comparison to the role played by cytotoxic therapy induced intestinal mucosal damage in the presence of severe neutropaenia (Wade, *et al.*, 1982). Gram-positive infections appear to occur more frequently in association with the use of prophylactic antibacterial regimens which suppress aerobic Gram-negative bacilli (Bow, *et al.*, 1985; Bow, *et al.*, 1987).

Clinical syndrome of gut toxicity

Gastrointestinal mucosal toxicity is common among patients receiving ARA-C containing regimens. Figure 6.1 illustrates the natural history of the clinical syndrome associated with progressive cytotoxic therapy associated mucosal damage. This is characterized initially by the appearance of nausea and vomiting within 3 to 4 days of beginning therapy in 80–90% of patients (Slavin, Dias and Saral, 1978; Johnson, Smith and DesForges, 1985). The normal colonic mucosal surface is replaced by very atypical undifferentiated cells and the glandular lumena are plagued by necrotic and degenerated cells. Progressive cellular necrosis occurs resulting in depopulation of the mucosal surface over the next 5 to 10 days. This is associated with loss of water, electrolytes and protein across the gut wall resulting in abdominal pain, watery diarrhoea, hypokalaemia and hypoalbuminaemia (Slavin, Dias and Saral, 1978). The spectrum of clinical manifestations extends from only mild symptoms to abdominal catastrophes simulating

acute appendicitis, a perforated viscus or ischaemic bowel. This syndrome of abdominal pain, distension and severe diarrhoea has been reported in 5–25% of patients receiving standard dose ARA-C/anthracycline regimens (Peterson, *et al.*, 1980; Rai, *et al.*, 1981; Slevin, *et al.*, 1982; Yates, *et al.*, 1982) and in up to three-quarters of patients receiving various HDARA-C regimens (Herzig, *et al.*, 1985; Arlin, *et al.*, 1987; Barnett, *et al.*, 1987; Hiddemann, *et al.*, 1987). Furthermore, older patients (>60 years) may suffer these symptoms more frequently (Yates, *et al.*, 1982). Unfortunately, the true incidence of nausea/vomiting and diarrhoea as markers for gut mucosal toxicity among leukaemic patients receiving induction or re-induction therapy is unclear due to the inconsistency in defining and reporting these toxicities in the literature. Table 6.2 illustrates the incidence of nausea/vomiting and of diarrhoea among patients receiving HDARA-C containing regimens for relapsed or progressive acute leukaemia. Nausea and vomiting was reported in 72–93% of the patients. The addition of an anthracycline, m-AMSA or mitoxantrone to the HDARA-C did not appear greatly to influence the incidence of this. Although diarrhoea was observed in

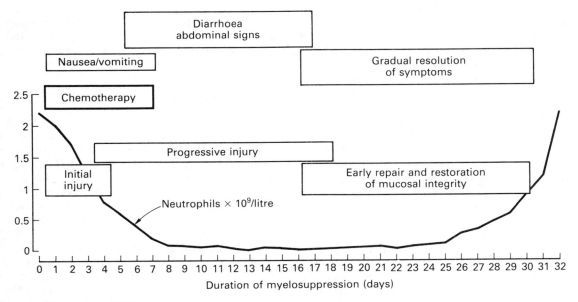

from: Slavin *et al.*, 1978

Figure 6.1 Natural history of the clinical syndrome associated with the gastrointestinal mucosal toxicity induced by cytosine arabinoside containing cytoreductive remission induction regimens for acute leukaemia

Table 6.2 Gastrointestinal toxicity associated among patients with relapsed acute leukaemia receiving regimens containing high dose cytosine arabinoside (HDARA-C)

Reference	HDARA-C dose	Other agents dose	Mucositis n, (%)	Nausea/ n, (%)	Diarrhoea n, (%)
Hines, *et al.*, 1984 (n = 40)	$3\,g/M^2$ q12h 6d	m-AMSA[a] 75–100 mg/M^2 d7–9	20 (50%)	37 (93%)	NR*
Herzig, *et al.*, 1985 (n = 34)	$3\,g/M^2$ q12h 6d	—	NR	30 (88%)	13 (39%)
Herzig, *et al.*, 1985 (n = 44)	$3\,g/M^2$ q12h 6d	DNR/ADR[b] 20 mg/M^2 30 mg/M^2 d7–9	NR	38 (86%)	15 (34%)
Arlin, *et al.*, 1987 (n = 47)	$3\,g/M^2$ q12h 5d	m-AMSA[a] d1–3	18 (38%)	34 (72%)	23 (49%)
Hiddemann, *et al.*, 1987 (n = 43)	$3\,g/M^2$ q12h 4d	MTO[c] d2–6	30 (70%)	39 (91%)	35 (81%)

[a] 4'-(9 acridinylamino) methane sulfon-m-ansidine, amsacrine
[b] Daunorubicin/Adriamycin
[c] Mitoxanthrone
* Not reported

34–81% of patients, there was no consistent definition of severity (number of watery stools per day), duration of symptoms, when in the cycle the symptoms developed and the presence of guaic-positivity reflecting GI bleeding. Furthermore, data were lacking about other symptoms related to gastrointestinal toxicity during the induction cycle such as abdominal distension and pain.

The symptoms of abdominal pain, distension, diarrhoea and nausea/vomiting are associated with the pathologic changes in the intestinal mucosa and thus contribute significantly to the morbidity of these regimens. It would be desirable to report intestinal mucosal toxicity in a manner similar to that for myelotoxicity. The clinician should know the expected incidence of these symptoms with respect to patient age, their duration, severity and when they occur in the cycle. This would aid physicians in planning of supportive strategies such as electrolyte replacement and parenteral nutrition.

The denuded intestinal epithelium provides a surface that may be easily colonized by potentially pathogenic bacteria and fungi. Bacterial proliferation in this environment leads to further mucosal damage, necrosis, vascular thrombosis and ulceration (Slavin, Dias and Saral, 1978). In the absence of a neutrophilic response, these areas provide the major unobstructed portals of entry for the colonizing microflora. Figure 6.2 illustrates the typical gross appearance of the ulcerated lesions that are characteristically distributed over the colonic mucosal surface. Figure 6.3 represents a PAS-stained section through one of these ulcers and shows the mucosal invasion by budding yeasts and pseudohyphae characteristic of invasive Candidiasis. This patient died of disseminated *Candida albicans* infection. Further studies are needed to identify cytoreductive regimens that minimize the gastrointestinal mucosal toxicity and to identify more effective ways of suppressing gastrointestinal colonization by potentially pathogenic micro-organisms.

Oral toxicity

A high proportion of patients undergoing cytoreductive therapy for acute leukaemia experience painful, often debilitating, inflammatory lesions within the oral cavity (Lockhart and Sonis, 1979; Yates, *et al.*, 1982; Dreizen, *et al.*, 1986; Arlin, *et al.*, 1997; Hiddemann, *et al.*, 1987). The tissues of the periodontium, gingival surfaces and oral mucosa are affected. Investigators at the M.D. Anderson Hospital and Tumor Institute reported chemotherapy related oral mucositis, infection or haemorrhage in about half of the cases of acute leukaemia studied between 1966 and 1986 (Dreizen, *et al.*, 1986). Anthracycline/ARA-C containing regimens exert their effects on the developing basal epithelial cells of the oral

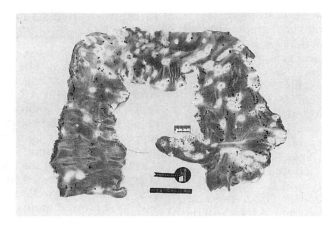

Figure 6.2 Photograph of colon at post-mortem examination of a 62-year-old man who died day 18 of primary induction therapy for acute non-lymphocytic leukaemia. The mucosal surface was characterized by multiple necrotic ulcers diffusely distributed over the entire length of the colon

mucosa resulting in decreased cell renewal in a manner which parallels the effect on the marrow stem cell (Lockhart and Sonis, 1979) and the intestinal mucosal surface (Slavin, Dias and Saral, 1978). Mucosal atrophy, cytolysis and denudation of the mucosal surface causes the typical painful foci of local ulceration within 4 to 7 days following the administration of

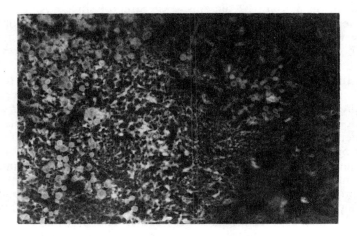

Figure 6.3 Pas-stained photomicrograph (× 100) of a section through one of the colonic ulcers depicted in Figure 6.2. The base of the ulcer and submucosa is infiltrated by budding yeasts and pseudohyphae. The cause of death was disseminated infection due to *Candida albicans*

cytotoxic agent. This usually spontaneously resolves between day 14 to 21 (Bottomley, *et al.*, 1977; Guggenheimer, *et al.*, 1977; Lockhart and Sonis, 1979).

The natural history of oral mucositis is influenced by the cytotoxic therapy induced neutropaenia which itself plays a permissive role in allowing the clinical expression of acute upon chronic periodontal infection (Overholser, *et al.*, 1982). This process usually reaches its maximum intensity at the time of the neutrophil nadir, approximately day 14 (Bodey, 1971; Lockhart and Sonis, 1979). This period between day 7 and 14 represents the time when polymicrobic infections become superimposed upon the chemotherapy induced mucositis thus extending the morbidity into the 3rd and 4th week (McGraw and Belch, 1985). In retrospective review, fungi accounted for 61% of the oral infections among acute leukaemics in one study (Dreizen, *et al.*, 1986). In another report, oropharyngeal candidiasis developed in 60% of patients undergoing induction chemotherapy (DeGregorio, Lee and Ries, 1982). In this series, oropharyngeal candidiasis appeared more frequently among patients who had chemotherapy induced mucositis. *Herpes simplex* virus infections of the oral cavity reported in 50–90% of seropositive patients undergoing remission induction therapy or bone marrow transplantation have a median onset between 7 and 11 days (Montgomery, Redding and LeMaistre, 1986). Acute exacerbations of pre-existing, asymptomatic, chronic periodontitis occurred in 59% of 22 patients aged 23 to 67 years undergoing remission induction therapy for acute non-lymphocytic leukaemia (Overholser, *et al.*, 1982). These infections occurred when the neutrophil count was less than 0.1×10^9/l. The severity and duration of chemotherapy induced mucositis correlates with pre-existing levels of dental plaque and periodontal disease (Linquist, Hickey and Drane, 1978). There is evidence accumulating that much of the extra infectious morbidity superimposed upon the chemotherapy induced mucositis can be significantly reduced by the prophylactic use of antiviral agents such as acyclovir (Gold and Corey, 1987), antiseptics such as chlorhexidine (McGraw and Belch, 1985) or antifungal agents such as ketoconazole (Estey, *et al.*, 1984). Further work is required to determine the optimal duration of therapy and most appropriate patient population for whom these strategies may be best applied.

Immunosuppressive effects

The remission-induction regimens commonly used for acute leukaemia have important immunosuppressive effects in addition to the myelosuppressive effects discussed earlier. Anthracyclines and ARA-C have a profound suppressive effect upon the numbers of circulating T- and B-lymphocytes which parallel the suppressive effects upon the function of cell mediated and humoral immune mechanisms. At the clinical level the consequences of these effects are a heightened susceptibility to pathogens normally controlled by these mechanisms and a depressed potential for immunologic control of the leukaemic process. The effects of anthracyclines and ARA-C on immune responsiveness appears to be dependent upon the schedule of administration. This has been reviewed in detail previously (Leventhal, Cohen and Triem, 1974).

T-cell function

T-lymphocyte function may be moderately depressed in patients with acute leukaemia. This is suggested from studies evaluating cutaneous, delayed-type, hypersensitivity reactions and *in vitro* lymphocyte responsiveness to mitogens such as phytohaemagglutinin or Streptolysin 'O'. Among patients responding to induction and consolidation therapy a decrease in immune responsiveness can be detected beginning 2 to 5 months after beginning therapy (Hersh, *et al.*, 1974). Immunologic competence appears to recover at approximately six months (Hersh, *et al.*, 1974). Immune function has been observed to become depressed as early as one month prior to a relapse (Hersh, *et al.*, 1974). Immunocompetence in patients undergoing chemotherapy for acute leukaemia has been studied by administering a battery of intradermal skin tests serially over the course of therapy and recovery (Dupuy, *et al.*, 1971; Hersh, *et al.*, 1974). Hersh, *et al.* (1974) demonstrated a gradual decline in responsiveness to skin recall antigens that corresponded to the period on remission induction and consolidation therapy (Figure 6.4). Responsiveness increased to base-

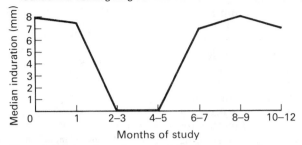

Delayed-type hypersensitivity reactions
to five skin test recall antigens in patients with acute
leukaemia undergoing remission induction chemotherapy

Figure 6.4 Delayed-type hypersensitivity responses to five
recall antigens in patients achieving remission following
remission induction therapy for acute leukaemia (Modified
from Hersh, *et al.*, 1974)

line pre-therapy levels after 6 months. Dupuy, *et al.* (1971) correlated a decrease in the intensity of cutaneous delayed hypersensitivity reactions associated with induction of marrow aplasia and an increase with the achievement of remission status (Figure 6.5). These studies showed not only that remission skin test results were similar to pre-treatment results, but that the magnitude of the cutaneous reactivity was substantially less than that observed among matched controls. This illustrates that the underlying disease itself has a significant suppressive effect on this aspect of host defence.

B-cell function

Modern therapy for acute leukaemia has a more profound qualitative and quantitative effect upon B-cell function than T-cell function (Leventhal, Cohen and Triem, 1974). Immunoglobulins have been reported to be quantitatively normal in leukaemic patients prior to therapy (McKelvey and Carbone, 1965; Kiran and Gross, 1969). Induction therapy results in a fall in immunoglobulin G over a 5-week period after which it returns to normal. Schiffer, *et al.* (1976) showed that 50–66% of patients developed major blood group antibody or lymphocytotoxic antibody while undergoing acute leukaemia induction therapy with DAT (Daunorubicin/ARA-C/thioguanine). This was contrasted with the expected 95% sero-conversion rate among normal controls immunized with group A or group B red blood cells reported by Fairley (Fairley and Akers, 1962). Dupuy, *et al.* (1971) immunized patients undergoing remission induction for acute leukaemia with polio vaccine containing the three strains of killed poliovirus. Half of the patients failed to respond to any of the 3 strains compared to 92% of the controls. In contrast 83% of patients achieving remission had a

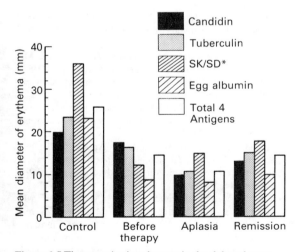

Figure 6.5 The quantitative changes in the delayed-type hypersensitivity responses to cutaneous recall antigens in patients with acute leukaemia undergoing remission induction therapy. The impact of the underlying disease on these responses is illustrated by the decrease in intensity of response to the four antigens tested (candidin, tuberculin, streptokinase/streptodornase, egg albumin) compared to control subjects. Further the impact of the induction therapy is illustrated by decrease in intensity of response from before therapy to the time of marrow aplasia. Immune responsiveness increases again with the achievement of remission (Modified from Dupuy, *et al.*, 1971)

response to one or more strains of poliovirus in the vaccine. Further, the titres of antibody developed in response to primary and secondary antigenic stimulation were also diminished (Dupuy, *et al.*, 1971; Schiffer, *et al.*, 1976).

These studies demonstrate that antileukaemic therapy is associated with at least a moderate effect on both T and B cell function. It has been difficult, however, to separate the effects of therapy from the immunosuppressive effects of the leukaemic process. There does not appear to be a prognostically useful parameter of T or B-cell function that predicts specific infection risk analogous to the predictive value of the circulating neutrophil count for pyogenic bacterial or fungal infection in patients with acute leukaemia.

References

Arlin, Z.A., Ahmed, T., Mittelman, A., Feldman, E., Mehta, R., Weinstein, P., Rieber, E., Sullivan, P. and Baskind, P. (1987) A new regimen of amsacrine with high-dose cytarabine is safe and effective therapy for acute leukemia. *Journal of Clinical Oncology*, **5**, 371–375

Bain, B.J. and England, J.M. (1975) Normal haematological values: sex differences in neutrophil count. *British Medical Journal*, **1**, 306–309

Barnett, M.J., Rohatiner, A.Z.S., Ganesan, T.S., Richards, M.A., Miller, A. and Lister, T.A. (1987) A phase II study of high-dose cytosine arabinoside in the treatment of acute leukaemia in adults. *Cancer Chemotherapy and Pharmacology*, **19**, 169–171

Bodey, G.P., Buckley, M., Sathe, Y.S. and Freireich, E.J. (1966) Quantitative relationships between circulating leukocytes and infection in patients with acute leukemia. *Annals of Internal Medicine*, **64**, 328–340

Bodey, G.P. (1971) Oral manifestations of the myeloproliferative diseases. *Postgraduate Medicine*, **49**, 115–121

Bottomley, W.K., Perlin, E. and Ross, G.R. (1977) Antineoplastic agents and their oral manifestations. *Oral Surgery*, **44**, 527–534

Bow, E.J., Rayner, E., Scott, B.A. and Louie, T.J. (1987) Selective gut decontamination with nalidixic acid or trimethoprim-sulfamethoxazole for infection prophylaxis in neutropenic cancer patients: relationship of efficacy to antimicrobial spectrum. *Antimicrobial Agents and Chemotherapy*, **31**, 551–557

Bow, E.J., Louie, T.J., Rayner, E. and Pitsanuk, J. (1985) Norfloxacin (N) versus trimethoprim/sulfamethoxazole (T/S) for infection prophylaxis in patients (PTS) with acute leukemia (AL). [abs. 150]. *In Proceedings of the 25th Interscience Conference on Antimicrobial Agents and Chemotherapy*. Washington, D.C.: American Society for Microbiology

Bunn, P.A., Lichter, A.S., Makuch, R.W., Cohen, M.H.,

Veach, S.R., Matthews, M.J. *et al.* (1987) Chemotherapy alone or chemotherapy with chest radiation therapy in limited stage small cell lung cancer: a prospective, randomized trial. *Annals of Internal Medicine*, **106**, 655–662

DeGregorio, M.W., Lee, W.M.F. and Ries, C.A. (1982) Candida infections in patients with acute leukemia: ineffectiveness of nystatin prophylaxis and relationship between oropharyngeal and systemic candidiasis. *Cancer*, **50**, 2780–2784

deJongh, C.A., Wade, J.C., Finley, R.S., Joshi, J.H., Aisner, J., Wiernik, P.H. and Schimpff, S.C. (1983) Trimethoprim/sulfamethoxazole versus placebo: a double-blind comparison of infection prophylaxis in patients with small cell carcinoma of the lung. *Journal of Clinical Oncology*, **1**, 302–306

Dreizen, S., McCredie, K.B., Bodey, G.P. and Keating, M.J. (1986) Quantitative analysis of the oral complications of antileukemia chemotherapy. *Oral Surgery, Oral Medicine and Oral Pathology*, **62**, 650–653

Dupuy, J.M., Kourilsky, F.M., Fradelizzi, D., Feingold, N., Jacquillat, C.I., Bernard, J. and Dausset, J. (1971) Depression of immunologic reactivity of patients with acute leukemia. *Cancer*, **27**, 323–331

Estey, E., Maksymiuk, A., Smith, T., Fainstein, V., Keating, M., McCredie, K.B. *et al.* (1984) Infection prophylaxis in acute leukemia: comparative effectiveness of sulfamethoxazole and trimethoprim, ketoconazole, and a combination of the two. *Archives of Internal Medicine*, **144**, 1562–1568

Fairley, G.H. and Akers, R.J. (1962) Antibodies to blood group A and B substances in reticuloses. *British Journal of Haematology*, **8**, 375–391

Ganesan, T.S., Barnett, M.J., Amos, R.J., Piall, E.M., Aherne, G.W., Man, A. and Lister, T.A. (1987) Cytosine arabinoside in the management of recurrent leukaemia. *Hematological Oncology*, **5**, 65–69

Gold, D. and Corey, L. (1987) Acyclovir prophylaxis for herpes simplex virus infection. *Antimicrobial Agents and Chemotherapy*, **31**, 361–367

Guggenheimer, J., Verbin, R.S., Appel, B.N. and Schmutz, J. (1977) Clinicopathologic effects of cancer chemotherapeutic agents on human buccal mucosa. *Oral Surgery*, **44**, 58–63

Hersh, E.M., Gutterman, J.U., Mauligit, G.M., McCreadie, K.B., Burgess, M.A., Matthews, A. and Freireich, E.J. (1974) Serial studies of immunocompetence of patients undergoing chemotherapy for acute leukemia. *The Journal of Clinical Investigation*, **54**, 401–408

Herzig, R.H., Lazarus, H.M., Wolff, S.N., Phillips, G.L. and Herzig, G.P. (1985) High-dose cytosine arabinoside therapy with and without anthracycline antibiotics for remission reinduction of acute nonlymphocytic leukemia. *Journal of Clinical Oncology*, **3**, 992–997

Hiddemann, W., Kreutzmann, H., Straif, K., Ludwig, R., Mertelsmann, R., Donhuijsen-Ant, R., Lengfelder, E., Arlin, Z. and Buchner, T. (1987) High-dose cytosine arabinoside and mitoxantrone: a highly effective regimen in refractory acute myeloid leukemia. *Blood*, **69**, 744–749

Hines, J.D., Oken, M.M., Mazza, J.J., Keller, A.M., Strecter, R.R. and Glick, J.H. (1984) High-dose cytosine arabinoside and m-Amsa is effective therapy in relapsed acute nonlymphocytic leukemia. *Journal of Clinical Oncology*, **2**, 545–549

Johnson, H., Smith, T.J. and Desforges, J. (1985) Cytosine-arabinoside-induced colitis and peritonitis: nonoperative management. *Journal of Clinical Oncology*, **3**, 607–612

Kiran, O. and Gross, S. (1969) The G immunoglobulins in acute leukemia in children: hematologic and immunologic relationships. *Blood*, **33**, 198

Kurrle, E., Dekker, A.W., Gaus, W., Haralambie, E., Krieger, D., Rozenberg-Arska, M., deVries-Haspers, H.G., Van der Waaij, D. and Wendt, F. (1986) Prevention of infection in acute leukemia: a prospective randomized study on the efficacy of two different drug regimens for antimicrobial prophylaxis. *Infection*, **14**, 226–232

Leventhal, B.G., Cohen, P. and Triem, S.C. (1974) Effect of chemotherapy on the immune response in acute leukemia. *Israel Journal of Medical Science*, **10**, 866–887

Lindquist, S.F., Hickey, A.J. and Drane, J.B. (1978) Effect of oral hygiene on stomatitis in patients receiving cancer chemotherapy. *Journal of Prosthetic Dentistry*, **40**, 312–314

Lockhart, P.B. and Sonis, S.T. (1979) Relationship of oral complications to peripheral blood leukocyte and platelet counts in patients receiving cancer chemotherapy. *Oral Surgery*, **48**, 21–28

McGraw, W.T. and Belch, A. (1985) Oral complications of acute leukemia: prophylactic impact of a chlorhexidine mouth rinse regimen. *Oral Surgery, Oral Medicine and Oral Pathology*, **60**, 275–280

McKelvey, E. and Carbone, P.P. (1965) Serum immuno-globulin concentrations in acute leukemia during intensive chemotherapy. *Cancer*, **18**, 1295

Minah, G.E., Rednor, J.L., Peterson, D.E., Overholser, C.D., Depaola, L.G. and Suzuki, J.B. (1986) Oral succession of gram-negative bacilli in myelosuppressed cancer patients. *Journal of Clinical Microbiology*, **24**, 210–213

Montgomery, M.T., Redding, S.W. and LeMaistre, C.F. (1986) The incidence of oral herpes simplex virus infection in patients undergoing cancer chemotherapy. *Oral Surgery, Oral Medicine and Oral Pathology*, **61**, 238–242

Overholser, C.D., Peterson, D.E., Williams, L.T. and Schimpff, S.C. (1982) Periodontal infection in patients with acute nonlymphocytic leukemia, prevalence of acute exacerbations. *Archives of Internal Medicine*, **142**, 551–554

Peterson, B.A., Bloomfield, C.D., Bosl, G.J., Gibbs, G. and Malloy, M. (1980) Intensive five-drug combination chemotherapy for adult acute non-lymphocytic leukemia. *Cancer*, **46**, 663–668

Pizzo, P.A. (1984) Granulocytopenia and cancer therapy – past problems, current solutions, future challenges. *Cancer*, **54**, 2649–2661

Preisler, H.D., Rustum, Y., Henderson, E.S., Bjornsson, S., Creaven, P.J., Higby, D.J., *et al.* (1979) Treatment of acute nonlymphocytic leukemia: use of anthracycline-cytosine arabinoside induction therapy and comparison of two maintenance regimens. *Blood*, **53**, 455–464

Preisler, H.D., Raza, A., Early, A., Kirshner, J., Brecher, M., Freeman, A., *et al.* (1987) Intensive remission consolidation therapy in the treatment of acute non-lymphocytic leukemia. *Journal of Clinical Oncology*, **5**, 722–730

Rai, K.R., Holland, J.F., Glidewell, O.J., Weinberg, V., Brunner, K., Obrecht, J.P., *et al.* (1981) Treatment of acute myelocytic leukemia: a study by cancer and leukemia group B. *Blood*, **58**, 1203–1212

Rumke, C.L. (1979) The statistically expected variability in differential leukocyte counting. In *Differential Leukocyte Counting* (edited by J.A. Koepke), pp. 39–45. Skokie, Illinois: College of American Pathologists

Schiffer, C.A., Lightenfeld, J.L., Wiernik, P.H., Mardiney, M.R. and Joseph, J.M. (1976) Antibody response in patients with acute non-lymphocytic leukemia. *Cancer*, **37**, 2177–2182

Schimpff, S.C., Young, V.M., Greene, W.H., Vermeulen, G.D., Moody, M.R. and Wiernik, P.H. (1972) Origin of infection in acute nonlymphocytic leukemia, significance of hospital acquisition of potential pathogens. *Annals of Internal Medicine*, **77**, 707–714

Schreml, W., Lohrmann, H-P. and Anger, B. (1985) Stem cell defects after cytoreductive therapy in man. *Experimental Hematology*, **13**, 31–42

Shapiro, M.F. and Greenfield, S. (1987) The complete blood count and leukocyte differential count. *Annals of Internal Medicine*, **106**, 65–74

Slavin, R.E., Dias, M.A. and Saral, R. (1978) Cytosine arabinoside induced toxic alterations in sequential chemotherapeutic protocols. *Cancer*, **42**, 1747–1759

Slevin, M.L., Rohatiner, A.Z.S., Dhaliwal, H.W., Henry, G.P., Bell, R. and Lister, T.A. (1982) A comparison of two schedules of cytosine arabinoside used in combination with adriamycin and 6-thioguanine in the treatment of acute myelogenous leukemia. *Medical and Pediatric Oncology*, **1**, 185–192

Vaughan, W.P., Karp, J.E. and Burke, P.J. (1980) Long chemotherapy-free remissions after single-cycle time-sequential chemotherapy for acute myelocytic leukemia. *Cancer*, **45**, 859–865

Wade, J.C., Schimpff, S.C., Newman, K.A. and Wiernik, P.H. (1982) Staphylococcus epidermidis: an increasing cause of infection in patients with granulocytopenia. *Annals of Internal Medicine*, **97**, 503–508

Wade, J.C., deJongh, C.A., Newman, K.A., Crowley, J., Wiernik, P.H. and Schimpff, S.C. (1983) Selective antimicrobial modulation as prophylaxis against infection during granulocytopenia: trimethoprim-sulfamethoxazole vs. nalidixic acid. *The Journal of Infectious Diseases*, **147**, 624–634

Wells, R.J., Feusner, J., Devney, R., Woods, W.G., Provisor, A.J., Cairo, M.S., *et al.* (1985) Sequential high-dose cytosine arabinoside – asparaginase treatment in advanced childhood leukemia. *Journal of Clinical Oncology*, **3**, 998–1004

Whimbey, E., Kiehn, T.E., Brannon, P., Blevins, A. and

Armstrong, D. (1987) Bacteremia and fungemia in patients with neoplastic diseases. *The American Journal of Medicine*, **82**, 723–730

Winston, D.J., Dudnick, D.V., Chapin, M., *et al.* (1983) Coagulase-negative staphylococcal bacteremia in patients receiving immunosuppressive therapy. *Archives of Internal Medicine*, **143**, 32–36

Yates, J., Glidewell, O., Wiernik, P., Cooper, M.R., Steinberg, D., Dosik, H., *et al.* (1982) Cytosine arabinoside with daunorubicin or adriamycin for therapy of acute myelocytic leukemia: a CALGB study. *Blood*, **60**, 454–462

Zacharski, L.R., Elvebach, L.R. and Linman, L.W. (1971) Leukocyte counts in healthy adults. *American Journal of Clinical Pathology*, **56**, 148–150

7

Pulmonary infection in the immunosuppressed patient

A.C. Newland and J.A. Wedzicha

The survival of patients with haematological malignancies has improved with more effective use of chemotherapy and better support therapy, including the use of combinations of antibiotics for the infective problems. These are an almost inevitable consequence of the neutropenia that is associated with the treatment and often the disease.

Pulmonary infections are second only in importance to septicaemia as the major cause of morbidity and mortality in neutropenia, although they themselves often rapidly progress to disseminated infection (Tobias, Wrigley and O'Grady, 1978; Slevin, et al., 1981). This has been especially documented in adult acute leukaemia where the use of intensive chemotherapy protocols and bone marrow transplantation are associated with profound and occasionally prolonged periods of neutropenia (Stevens, et al., 1991; Preisler, et al., 1991; Schiller, et al., 1992; Vogler, 1992).

The risk of infection increases as the neutrophil count falls below 0.5×10^9/l and is particularly severe when the count is less than 0.1×10^9/l (Bodey, et al., 1966a). The majority of patients receiving intensive cytotoxic chemotherapy will develop neutropenia at some stage during their treatment and most will become infected. Studies correlating the development of fever with subsequent documentation of infection have shown that approximately 20–30% of these episodes are due to bacteraemias, 20% to clinically documented infections, 20% to non-bacteraemic microbiologically documented infections and the remaining 30–40%

are possible or doubtful infections (de Pauw, Verhagan and Novakova, 1987).

The range of pulmonary disease includes both gram negative and gram positive pneumonias and opportunistic infections particularly with fungi, *Pneumocystis carinii* and cytomegalovirus. These may be complicated by the presence of leukaemic infiltration, pulmonary haemorrahge and oedema and quite frequently several of these processes may be present at the same time (Bodey, et al., 1966b). Between 25–50% of adults will die of infection at some stage during the treatment for acute non-lymphocytic leukaemia (Levine, et al., 1974) and this is usually associated with neutropenia. The reported mortality rate when there are associated pulmonary complications may reach 70% in some patient groups (Singer, et al., 1979) with survival depending on early, aggressive investigation and treatment as death may occur within a few days of the appearance of an abnormality on a chest radiograph (Wardman, et al., 1984).

Although the presence of neutropenia is an important factor in increasing the susceptibility to infection other factors need to be taken into consideration. Following chemotherapy both cell and humorally mediated immunity may be depressed for several months, despite the return to normal of the blood count. This is highlighted in the treatment of childhood lymphoblastic leukaemia where neutropenia is less profound, pneumonia occurring in less than 5% of children during the initial induction chemotherapy (Chessels and Leiper, 1980) but with a peak instance at 40 to 80 days after diagnosis, during maintenance chemotherapy, when the child is generally haematologically normal (Siegel, *et al.*, 1980). The changes in the immune mechanism and the disruption to the body's defence is even more profound and long lasting following bone marrow transplantation (Burakoff, Lipton and Nathan, 1983; Deeg, Storb and Thomas, 1984).

Pneumonia

The large area of mucous membrane in the lung has multiple protective mechanisms. It is coated by mucous which contains IgA at the level of the bronchi and IgG in the alveoli. There are in addition the presence of alveolar macrophages and T-cells (Green, *et al.*, 1977). As a further protection, 50% of the body's neutrophils marginate in the lungs at any one time. Therefore any disruption of this protective mechanism will encourage colonization and subsequent infection. The presence of leukaemic infiltration, pulmonary haemorrhage or oedema which may disrupt the protective integument will enhance the risk.

The clinical picture is of fever, shortness of breath and unproductive cough, although in many cases pyrexia alone may be present. The severely neutropenic patient is unable to form a local reaction and limit the infection and in up to 70% bacteraemia develops early. The impaired inflammatory response also leads to a reduction in the normal physical signs. Chest auscultation may be normal and a chest X-ray is always indicated in the febrile neutropenic patient and may demonstrate a pulmonary infiltrate in a clinically 'silent' patient.

The primary haematological disease may be responsible for the lung appearances, however, when the changes are diffuse and follow a prolonged period of neutropenia, opportunistic infection is more likely (Tenholder and Hooper, 1980). Although in this setting pulmonary haemorrhage can occur and may be extensive (Blank, Castellino and Shah, 1975) and difficult to diagnose (Golde, *et al.*, 1975).

Although there might be a variation in the prevalent pathogens from hospital to hospital a significant change from gram negative to gram positive bacteria, as the most frequently isolated causative organism, has been recently recognized (Wade, *et al.*, 1982; Kelsey, *et al.*,

1992). This change in infection pattern has been largely due to a combination of gut decontamination measures and the use of long-term indwelling, tunnelled catheters (Hickman, *et al.*, 1979) which become colonized by skin commensals, such as the coagulase negative staphylococci. Morbidity and mortality resulting from infection with gram positive organisms has increased concomitantly (Klastersky, 1986).

Escherichia coli, Klebsiella species, Pseudomonas species and *Staphylococcus aureus* are still among the primary pathogens to be considered but the 'non-pathogens', including *Staphylococcus epidermidis*, the coryneforms and the viridans streptococci, need to be increasingly considered (Wade, *et al.*, 1982; Cohen, *et al.*, 1993; Winston, *et al.*, 1983; Whimbey, *et al.*, 1987). In addition polymicrobial infections may be found in up to 20% of the patients.

Fungal infections have become an increasing problem in the immune compromised host and in some series have been identified in as many as 25% of patients (Sickles, *et al.*, 1973). However, the true magnitude is difficult to determine because of under reporting. In general, experience suggests that the disseminated mycoses, particularly candida, aspergillus and cryptococcus, are increasingly considered and/or diagnosed in tertiary care centres (Stevens, 1987). This change in incidence is due to the increasing use of combination broad spectrum antibacterial agents, the use of central catheters and the increasingly aggressive chemotherapeutic regimes for malignancy.

The role of herpes viruses has also been underestimated. Herpes simplex occurs in 80% of seropositive patients following bone marrow transplantation, due to reactivation of latent virus, and usually manifests as oral ulceration but can progress to H simplex pneumonia. Varicella zoster infection due also to reactivation of latent virus is particularly common in Hodgkin's disease and in the late post bone marrow transplant period. This often disseminates and has a high mortality rate.

Interstitial pneumonia due to cytomegalovirus is a major problem for allogeneic bone marrow transplant recipients and is exacerbated by the use of total body irradiation and the presence of graft versus host disease (Meyers, Flournoy and Wade, 1983). The incidence of infection varies from 10–50% but up to two-thirds progress to interstitial pneumonitis which has a mortality rate of between 50 and 90% (Watson, 1983; Ljungman, *et al.*, 1992). The infection is usually due to reactivation of latent virus but may be transmitted by blood products, particularly granulocyte transfusions (Clift, *et al.*, 1978). Measles pneumonia is the commonest cause of death in remission in children treated for acute lymphoblastic leukaemia and may develop without the classic rash. Parents, patients and teachers should be warned always to report the viral contact as early as possible.

Pneumocystis carinii pneumonia (PCP) has in the past been a problem in children with acute lymphoblastic leukaemia, occurring during maintenance therapy (Wolff, *et al.*, 1977), the risk directly relating to the degree of immunosuppression (Rapson, *et al.*, 1980). The discovery, however, that co-trimoxazole when used as prophylaxis against bacterial infection appeared to protect almost completely from PCP has all but eliminated this as a problem in this group.

Tuberculosis is an unusual but recognized complication of lymphoma, especially Hodgkin's disease, but is also a risk to all patients on steroids or other immunosuppressive therapy. Elderly patients are especially at risk as they may have suffered tuberculosis in the past and have old healed tuberculosis foci that may harbour viable *Mycobacterium tuberculosis*. The pulmonary infiltrates on the chest X-ray may be variable with either upper lobe cavitation, lobar consolidation or miliary infiltrate (Matthay and Greene, 1980) and such patients should receive prophylactic therapy while receiving chemotherapy.

Nocardia asteroides, a gram positive acid fast bacillus, is an important pulmonary pathogen in the immune suppressed patients. Infection in the lungs may present as lobar pneumonia, single or multiple nodules and miliary abscesses. Response to treatment is poor and less than 30% of patients with disseminated infection recover (Bodey, 1975).

Diagnostic approaches

Faced with the febrile neutropenic patient with an abnormal chest X-ray, the necessity for the early initiation of empirical broad spectrum antibiotic therapy is well established (Schimpff, *et al.*, 1971). A combination of bactericidal antibiotics are usually used in order to provide a broad spectrum antibacterial activity and to exploit possible synergy between antibiotics (Klastersky and Zinner, 1982). If there is no response, further investigation will be needed to differentiate between the various etiological factors.

Chest radiographs are usually normal in neutropenic patients who have no chest symptoms, but can be helpful in patients at risk from aspergillosis. Chest computerized tomography may detect otherwise unrecognized pulmonary infiltrates in patients with recurrent or persistent fever who have normal chest radiographs (Feusner, *et al.*, 1988; Barloon, *et al.*, 1991).

The most important factor in directing therapy is identification of the infecting organism. Blood cultures should always be taken in the febrile patient prior to commencement of antibiotic therapy. However, they are helpful in less than 50% (Sickles, *et al.*, 1973; Bodey, *et al.*, 1978). As many of the organisms responsible for the infections arise from endogenous microbial flora or are hospital acquired, some centres practice routine surveillance cultures during periods of neutropenia. However, the predictive power of these is low and they are not cost-effective (Kramer, *et al.*, 1982). If sputum is produced, which is unusual in the neutropenic setting, culture and sensitivity tests are frequently unreliable. It is common to isolate gram negative organisms such as Klebsiella sp. or Pseudomonas sp. but this often occurs because the sputum is collected after the patient has commenced an empiric antibiotic regimen in practice antibiotics tend to be started at the time the blood cultures are taken and sputum collection often occurs later. The isolates found in sputum usually represent the change in colonization in the upper respiratory tract flora due to the antibiotics and may occur within hours of commencing treatment. They should rarely be used alone as an indication to alter therapy.

In the patient who fails to respond to the first choice antibiotic regimen the choice is, therefore, to alter treatment empirically or follow an 'invasive' diagnostic approach. A combination of approaches is often used as, despite intensive therapy, many patients remain febrile while still neutropenic and early diagnostic information, even if negative, may allow rational decisions to be made. In one series, however, a prospective study of immunosuppressed patients with pulmonary infiltrates only one-third demonstrated a causative agent despite extensive investigation (Singer, *et al.*, 1979).

Bronchoscopy and bronchoalveolar lavage

In the febrile neutropenic patient who has not responded to initial empirical therapy, those with pulmonary infiltrates represent a diagnostic and therapeutic problem, since prolonged fever of unknown origin is encountered regularly (Whimbey, *et al.*, 1987). Under these circumstances invasive procedures, such as tracheal aspirates, bronchoalveolar lavage and biopsies may be warranted. In view of the frequently coexisting haemorrhagic diathesis, protection with platelet concentrates is mandatory during invasive investigation. Among these procedures fibreoptic bronchoscopy together with bronchoalveolar lavage should be the first line investigation in view of the ease of performance and safety (Stover, *et al.*, 1984).

During bronchoalveolar lavage the bronchoscopy is wedged in a segmental bronchus in an area of lung which shows shadowing on the radiograph. Warmed, sterile saline is then passed down the bronchoscope into the segment of the lung during inspiration and aspirated during expiration. This technique allows sampling of the cells and secretions from the lower respiratory tract and the lavage fluid is sent as soon as possible for bacteriological, viral, fungal and cytological examination (Hunninghake, *et al.*, 1979). This procedure is well tolerated by patients and has few complications compared with lung biopsy procedures.

Bronchoalveolar lavage can be safely used in thrombocytopenic patients and in those undergoing assisted ventilation, without any risk of causing a pneumothorax. A fall in the arterial oxygen saturation has been shown during the procedure but can be prevented by administration of nasal supplemental oxygen during the procedure (Hendy, Bateman and Stableforth, 1984). In the immunosuppressed patient with pulmonary infiltration, bronchoalveolar lavage has an overall diagnostic yield of 66–93%, using a combination of cytological and microbiological techniques. It provides a high

diagnostic yield for each major group of pathogens with minimal complications (Young, Hopkin and Cuthbertson, 1984; Abramson, *et al.*, 1987). It has enabled the diagnosis of infections with *Pneumocystis carinii*, Cytomegalovirus, *Legionella pneumophila*, fungi and mycobacteria (Hopkin, *et al.*, 1983; Stover, *et al.*, 1984; Milburn, Prentice and DuBois, 1987).

The technique is also helpful for diagnosis of pulmonary haemorrhage when the alveolar macrophages isolated from the lavage fluid will be laden with haemosiderin (Drew, Finlay and Golde, 1977). However bronchoalveolar lavage is less useful for diagnosing malignancy or drug induced toxicity (Stover, *et al.*, 1984).

Results are obtained rapidly which is important for the immediate management of these patients, allowing the early institution of appropriate treatment. Drugs that may be toxic or suppressive to the bone marrow and kidneys can be added with greater confidence once the necessity for these compounds has been established.

Sputum induction with nebulized saline has been suggested as an alternative aid to diagnosis in some patients and may replace bronchoalveolar lavage in patients in whom infection with the human immunodeficiency virus is suspected (de Blic, *et al.*, 1987).

Transbronchial lung biopsy

Transbronchial lung biopsy through a fibreoptic bronchoscope has also been widely used to investigate pulmonary infiltrates in immunosuppressed patients (Stableforth, *et al.*, 1978). During this procedure a small sample of lung is obtained, approximately 1.5 mm in diameter, but this technique is associated with a higher risk of complications, especially pulmonary haemorrhage and pneumothorax.

In a series of immunosuppressed patients who also underwent transbronchial lung biopsy, 19% developed pneumothoraces and 26% haemorrhage, which was especially common in patients with renal failure, probably due to impaired platelet function associated with uraemia (Cunningham, *et al.*, 1977). Transbronchial biopsy is contraindicated in patients with thrombocytopenia or other coagulation abnormalities.

Bronchial brushings can also be obtained

during the procedure by using a sheathed brush, which is passed through the bronchoscopy and aids isolation of organisms. The diagnostic yield of transbronchial lung biopsy on its own (48%), is less than for bronchoalveolar lavage (Poe, *et al.*, 1979), but when the procedure is combined with bronchial brushings and lavage, bronchoscopy had a sensitivity of 77% for all diagnoses. However, for all pulmonary infection the sensitivity of the procedure was higher at 90% (Williams, *et al.*, 1985).

Transtracheal aspiration

Transtracheal aspiration has been used for some time to obtain samples for analysis in immunocompromised patients when no sputum is available. The procedure needs to be performed with care in the thrombocytopenic patient and may lead to mediastinitis. In a study of pyrexial patients with neutropenia and respiratory symptoms, whose underlying diagnosis was acute leukaemia or myeloma, a positive bacterial isolate was obtained in 56% of cases (Slevin, *et al.*, 1981). Although 2 cases of aspergillus infection were identified, it is not claimed that this technique is designed to identify opportunist infections. Some of the patients in this study, however, were already on antibiotics. In this group coliforms were found in 10 of the 16 patients compared with one of 16 not having antibiotics. This highlights the problems seen in routine sputum analysis with an associated rapid secondary colonization by coliforms following empirical antibiotic therapy. Similar misleading results may also be obtained, if candida are identified, as fungi may colonize the trachea and main bronchi without invading the lung parenchyma (Matthay, *et al.*, 1980).

Percutaneous lung biopsy

Trephine drill biopsy (Steel and Winstanley, 1969) has been used to obtain samples, but the incidence of haemorrhage and pneumothorax is high, making the procedure inappropriate in patients with haematological abnormalities (Cunningham, *et al.*, 1977; Tenholder and Hooper, 1980; Palmer, Davidson and Lusk, 1980). Percutaneous fine needle biopsy with fluoroscopic guidance (Flower and Verney,

1979) is very useful for obtaining material for cytological and microbiological examination in localized disease but in patients with diffuse pulmonary infiltrates the sample recovered may be small and inadequate for examination.

Open lung biopsy

Open lung biopsy under general anaesthetic gives a specific diagnosis in patients with pulmonary infiltration of 50–80% in the various series (Wilson, Cockerill and Rosenow, 1985). During biopsy the surgeon can inspect the lung and take the sample from the most appropriate area, avoiding the lingula and the tips of the middle-lobe, where non-specific changes can be present. There is a higher incidence of complications and procedure-related mortality than with other techniques. Pulmonary infection may be recurrent in these patients and repeated surgical procedures to obtain biopsies are obviously inappropriate. Children, however, may be intolerant of other procedures and an open biopsy under anaesthetic may be indicated, although in adults bronchoscopy with bronchoalveolar lavage and the addition of transbronchial biopsy, if appropriate, should be the first line of investigation. Open lung biopsy should be only considered if other methods fail and the result will affect treatment and survival.

Rapid diagnostic techniques

The investigatory techniques discussed usually still rely on culture to identify an organism and often this delay can lead to complications in the unresponsive, neutropenic patient. Therefore, several newer techniques have been developed to aid the process of diagnosis, including lysis-centrifugation blood cultures for bacteria and yeasts, shell-vial cultures for viruses, immuno-fluorescent and enzyme-linked immunosorbent assays for antigen detection, and the polymerase chain reaction (Peter, 1991).

Diagnosis of CMV pneumonitis depends upon demonstration of the virus or the immune response. The latter may be suppressed for several months following the bone marrow transplant and, therefore, serodiagnosis of CMV is not ideal. Direct visualization of CMV inclusions in Giemsa-stained lung biopsy provides a rapid and specific diagnosis but requires open lung biopsy to obtain the material with its higher morbidity and mortality. Immuno-fluorescent techniques have been developed using cells obtained at bronchoalveolar lavage. Developed by Griffiths, *et al.* (1984) these demonstrate the presence of CMV in the cells by utilizing a panel of fluorescein labelled monoclonal antibodies directed against early antigens in CMV development. This test which detects early antigen fluorescent foci (DEAFF) will be positive in 80% of patients, allowing confirmation of the diagnosis within 24 hours of the procedure.

The diagnosis of invasive aspergillosis raises similar problems to that of CMV and is also associated with high mortality if treatment is delayed. Definitive diagnosis rests on the histo-logical demonstration or culture of an organism from open lung or transbronchial biopsy speci-mens. More recently the demonstration of aspergillus antigen in serum, urine and bronchoalveolar lavage fluid has provided an alternative approach to diagnosis. A large, recent study has proved its value, using an enzyme linked immunoabsorbent assay to monitor 121 patients who were profoundly neutropenic after leukaemic therapy. The technique was shown to have a 95% chance of identifying aspergillus infection before it became clinically apparent (Rogers, *et al.*, 1990) allowing specific aggressive therapy. This technique may also be adapted for identi-fication of other infections, e.g. Candida species (Walsh, Hathorn and Sobel, 1991).

Summary

Despite the range of investigations available, infection (particularly pulmonary) remains the major cause of mortality in the immuno-suppressed host (Levine, *et al.*, 1974) and continuing improvement in the therapeutic approach is necessary. Rapid diagnosis is of little help if there is no effective therapy and until very recently this has been the case in a number of the opportunist infections seen (Hirsch and Schooley, 1983). In general, how-ever, the early infections are bacterial; oppor-tunist infections occur in only 13% of initial episodes (Tenholder and Hooper, 1980). A failure to commence early therapy may be fatal due to irreversible endotoxaemic shock which may occur within hours, treatment is usually started with a combination of bactericidal antibiotics. A popular and widely used combi-nation would consist of a ureidopenicillin and aminoglycoside (Norrby, *et al.*, 1987) but because of the well recognized nephro and oto-toxicity of the aminoglycosides, the efficacy of double beta lactam combinations have also been explored (Young, 1985) and more recently monotherapy (Hathorn, Rubin and Pizzo, 1987). Early monotherapy studies using carboxypenicillins (Bodey, *et al.*, 1971) and the ureidopenicillins (Wade, *et al.*, 1981) were discouraging because of the poor response rates and the development of resistance. The introduction of newer agents such as Ceftazidime and Ciprofloxacin have provided an important alternative to the penicillin/aminoglycoside combinations (Pizzo, *et al.*, 1986; Kelsey, *et al.*, 1992). The more recent increase in incidence of gram positive infections has also lead some investigators to suggest that glycopeptides should be added routinely to these agents, thus removing the advantages of monotherapy (de Pauw, 1990).

If the initial approach is associated with a lack of response and if culture data are not available from the blood with diffuse changes present on the chest X-ray then it is reasonable to proceed to early bronchoalveolar lavage before broadening the empirical treatment to include amphotericin B, co-trimoxazole or anti-viral agents. In the patient who continues to be un-responsive with continuing pulmonary changes, open lung biopsy could be considered. However the majority of patients are not fit enough to withstand the procedure and most physicians would require hard evidence from clinical trials that this approach is likely to affect the outcome.

References

Abramson, M.J., Stone, C.A., Holmes, P.W. and Tai, E.H. (1987) The role of bronchoalveolar lavage in the diagnosis of suspected opportunistic pneumonia. *Aust. NZ. J. Med.*, **17**, 407–412

Barloon, T.J., Galvin, J.R., Mori, M., Stanford, W. and Gingrich, R.D. (1991) High resolution ultrafast chest CT in the clinical management of febrile bone marrow transplant patients with normal or non-specific chest roentgenograms. *Chest*, **99**, 928–933

Blank, N., Castellino, R.A. and Shah, V. (1973) Radio-graphic aspects of pulmonary infection in patients with altered immunity. *Radiol. Clinc. North Am.*, **II**, 175–190

Bodey, G.P. (1975) Infection in cancer patients. *Cancer Treatment Rev.*, **2**, 89–128

Bodey, G.P., Buckley, M., Sathe, Y.S. and Freireich, E.J.

(1966a) Quantitative relationship between circulating leucocytes and infection in patients with acute leukaemia. *Annals of Internal Medicine*, **64**, 328–340

Bodey, G.P., Powell, R.D., Hersh, E.M., Yetevian, A. and Freireich, E.J. (1966b) Pulmonary complications of acute leukaemia. *Cancer*, **19**, 781–793

Bodey, G.P., Rodriguez, V., Chang, H-Y. and Narboni, G. (1978) Fever and infection in leukaemic patients. *Cancer*, **41**, 1610–1622

Bodey, G.P., Whitecar, J.P., Middleman, E. and Rodriquez, V. (1971) Carbenicillin therapy for Pseudomonas infections. *Journal of American Medical Association*, **290**, 62–66

Burakoff, S.J., Lipton, J.M. and Nathan, D.G. (1983) Recapitulation of the immune response and haemopoietic system in bone marrow transplantation. In: *Clinics in Haematology* (ed.) D.G. Nathan, 695–720, W.B. Saunders Co. Ltd., London, Philadelphia, Toronto

Chessells, J.M. and Leiper, A.D. (1980) Infection during remission induction in childhood leukaemia. *Arch. Dis. Child*, **55**, 118–123

Clift, R.A., Sanders, J.E. and Thomas, E.D. (1978) Granulocyte transfusions for the prevention of infection in patients receiving bone marrow transplants. *N. Engl. J. Med.*, **198**, 1052–1057

Cohen, J., Donnelly, J.P., Worsley, A.M., Catovsky, D., Goldman, J.M. and Galton, D.A.G. (1983) Septicaemia caused by viridans streptococci in neutropenic patients with leukaemia. *Lancet*, **ii**, 1452–1454

Cunningham, J.H., Zavala, D.C., Corry, R.J. and Keim, C.W. (1977) Trephine air drill, bronchial brush and fibreoptic transbronchial lung biopsies in immunosuppressed patients. *Am. Rev. Respir. Dis.*, **115**, 213–220

deBlic, J., McKelvie, P., LeBourgeois, M., Blanche, S., Benoist, M.R. and Scheinmann, P. (1987) Value of bronchoalveolar lavage in the management of severe acute pneumonia and interstitial pneumonitis in the immunocompromised child. *Thorax*, **42**, 759–765

Deeg, J.H., Storb, R. and Thomas, E.D. (1984) Bone marrow transplantation; a review of delayed complications. *British Journal of Haematology*, **57**, 185–208

de Pauw, B.E., Verhagan, S. and Novakova, I. (1987) Antibiotic therapy in cancer patients with fever and septicaemia. *N. Engl. J. Med.*, **316**, 410–412

de Pauw, B.E. (1990) Treatment of infection in neutropenia. *Current Opinion in Infectious Disease*, **3**, 197–202

Drew, S.L., Finley, J.N. and Golde, D.W. (1977) Diagnostic lavage and occult pulmonary haemorrhage in thrombocytopenic, immunosuppressed patients. *Am. Rev. Respir. Dis.*, **116**, 215–221

Feusner, J., Cohen, R., O'Leary, M. and Beach, B. (1988) Use of routine chest radiography in the evaluation of fever in neutropenic oncology patients. *Journal of Clinical Oncology*, **6**, 1699–1702

Flower, C.D.R. and Verney, G.I. (1979) Percutaneous needle biopsy of thoracic lesions – an evaluation of 300 biopsies. *Clinc. Radiol*, **30**, 215–218

Golde, D.W., Drew, W.L., Klein, H.Z., Finley, T.N. and Cline, M.J. (1975) Occult pulmonary haemorrhage in acute leukaemia. *Brit. Med. J.*, **ii**, 166–168

Green, G.M., Jakab, G.J., Low, R.B. and Davis, G.S. (1977) Defense mechanisms of the respiratory membrane. *Am. Rev. Respir. Dis.*, **115**, 479–514

Griffiths, P.D., Panjwani, D.D., Stirk, P.R., Ball, M.G., Ganczakowski, M., Blacklock, H.A. and Prentice, H.G. (1984) Rapid diagnosis of cytomegalovirus infection in immunocompromised patients by detection of early antigen fluorescent foci. *Lancet*, **ii**, 1242–1245

Hathorn, J.W., Rubin, M. and Pizzo, P. (1987) Empirical antibiotic therapy in the febrile neutropenic cancer patients. *Antimicrobial Agents and Chemotherapy*, **31**, 971–977

Hendy, M.S., Bateman, J.R.M. and Stableforth, D.E. (1984) The influence of transbronchial lung biopsy and bronchoalveolar lavage on arterial blood gas changes occurring in patients with diffuse interstitial lung disease. *Br. J. Dis. Chest*, **78**, 363–368

Hickman, R.O., Buckner, C.D., Clift, R.A., Sanders, J.E., Stewart, P. and Thomas, E.D. (1979) A modified right atrial catheter for access to the venous system in marrow transplant recipients. *Surg. Gynaecol. Obstet.*, **148**, 871–875

Hirsch, M.S. and Schooley, R.T. (1983) Treatment of herpes virus infections. *New Engl. J. Med.*, **309**, 1034–1039

Hopkin, J.M. Turney, J.H., Young, J.A., Aden, D. and Michael, J. (1983) Rapid diagnosis of obscure pneumonia in immunosuppressed renal patients by cytology of alveolar lavage fluid. *Lancet*, **ii**, 299–301

Hunninghake, G.W., Gadek, J.E., Kawanami, O., Ferrans, V.J. and Crystal, R.G. (1979) Inflammatory and immune processes in the human lung in health and disease – evaluation by bronchoalveolar lavage. *Am. J. Pathol.*, **97**, 149–206

Kelsey, S.M., Weinhardt, B., Collins, P.W. and Newland, A.C. (1992) Teicoplanin plus ciprofloxacin versus gentamicin plus piperacillin in the treatment of febrile neutropenic patients. *Eng. J. Clin. Microbiol. Infect. Dis.*, **11**, 509–514

Klastersky, J., Zinner, S.H. (1982) Synergistic combinations of antibiotics in gram negative bacillary infections. *Reviews in Infectious Diseases*, **4**, 294–301

Klastersky, J. (1986) Concept of empiric therapy with antibiotic combinations. *Am. J. Med.*, **80**, 2–12

Kramer, B.S., Pizzo, P.A., Robichaud, K.J., Witebsky, F.G. and Wesley, R. (1982) Role of serial microbiologic surveillance and clinical evaluation in the management of cancer patients with fever and granulocytopenia. *American Journal of Medicine*, **72**, 561–568

Levine, A.S., Schimpff, S.C., Graw, R.G. and Young, R.C. (1974) Haematological malignancies and other marrow failure states: progress in the management of complicating infections. *Seminars in Haematology*, vol. II, no. 2, 141–202

Ljungman, P., Engelhard, D., Link, H., Biran, P., Brandt, L., Brunet, S., Cordonnies, C., Debussches, L., De Laurenzi, A., Kolb, H.J., Messina, C., Newland, A.C. and Prentice, H.G. (1992) Treatment of interstitial pneumonitis due to cytomegalovirus with Ganciclovir and intravenous immune globulin:

experience of the EBMTG. *Clinical Infectious Diseases*, **14**, 831–835

Matthay, R.A., Greene, W.H. (1980) Pulmonary infections in the immunocompromised patient. *Med. Clin. North Am.*, **64**, 529–551

Meyers, J.D., Flournoy, N. and Wade, J.C. (1983) Biology of interstitial pneumonia after marrow transplantation. *In*: Gale, R.P. *ed.*: Recent advances in bone marrow transplantation: *Proceedings of the UCLA Symposia Conference*, New York: Alan R. Liss: 405–423

Milburn, H.L., Prentice, H.G. and Du Bois, R.M. (1987) Role of bronchoalveolar lavage in the evaluation of interstitial pneumonia in recipients of bone marrow transplant. *Thorax*, **42**, 766–772

Norrby, S.R., Vandercam, B., Louie, T., Runde, V., Norberg, B. and Amika, M. (1987) Imipenem/cilastatin versus amikacin plus pipericillin in the treatment of infections in neutropenic patients. *Scand. J. Inf., Dis.*, **52**, 65–78

Palmer, D.L., Davidson, M. and Lusk, R. (1980) Needle aspiration of the lung in complex pneumonias. *Chest*, **78**, 16–21

Peter, J.B. (1991) The polymerase chain reaction: amplifying our options. *Review of Infectious Disease*, **13**, 166–171

Pizzo, P.A., Hathorn, J.W., Hiemenz, J., Brown, M., Commess, T. and Cotton, D. (1986) A randomized trial comparing ceftazidime alone with combination antibiotic therapy in cancer patients with fever and neutropenia. *New Engl. J. Med.*, **315**, 552–558

Poe, R.H., Utell, M.J., Israel, R.H., Hall, W.J. and Eshleman, J.D. (1979) Sensitivity and specificity of the non-specific transbronchial lung biopsy. *Am. Rev. Respir. Dis.*, **119**, 25–31

Preisler, H.S., Lasson, R.A., Raza, A., Browman, G., Goldberg, J., Vogler, R., Day, R., Gottlieb, A., Vardiman, J.W., Bennett, J., Kukla, C. and Grunwald, H. (1991) The treatment of patients with newly diagnosed poor prognosis acute myelogenous leukaemia. *Brit. J. Haematol.*, **79**, 390–397

Rapson, N.T., Cornbleet, M.A., Chessells, J.M., Bennett, A.J. and Hardistry, R.M. (1980) Immunosuppression and serious infection in children with acute lymphoblastic leukaemia: a comparison of three chemotherapy regimes. *Brit. J. Haematol.*, **45**, 41–52

Rogers, T.R., Haynes, K.A. and Barnes, R.A. (1990) Value of antigen detection in predicting invasive pulmonary aspergillosis. *Lancet*, **ii**, 1210–1213

Schiller, G., Gajewski, J., Nimes, S., Territo, M., Ho, W. and Champlin, R. (1992) A randomised study of intermediate versus conventional dose cytarabine induction for acute myelogenous leukaemia. *Brit. J. Haematol.*, **81**, 170–177

Schimpff, S., Satterlee, W., Young, V.M. and Serpeck, A. (1971) Empirical therapy with combination and gentamicin for febrile neutropenic patients with cancer and granulocytopenia. *New Engl. J. Med.*, **284**, 1061–1065

Sickles, E.A., Young, V.M., Greene, W.H. and Wiernik,

P.H. (1973) Pneumonia in acute leukaemia. *Annals of Internal Medicine*, **79**, 528–534

Siegel, S.E, Nesbit, M.E., Baehner, R., Sather, H. and Hammond, D. (1980) Pneumonia during therapy for childhood acute lymphoblastic leukaemia. *Am. J. Dis. Child*, **134**, 28–34

Singer, C., Armstrong, D., Rosen, P.P., Walzer, P.D. and Bessie, Y. (1979) Diffuse pulmonary infiltrates in immunosuppressed patients. *Am. J. of Med.*, **66**, 110–120

Slevin, M., Rohatiner, A., Malpas, J.S. and Lister, A. (1981) Pneumonia during treatment of acute leukaemia. *Brit. Med. J.*, **282**, 473

Slevin, M.L., Bell, L.R., Catto-Smith, A.G., Ford, J.M., Malpas, J.S. and Lister, T.A. (1981) The role of transtracheal aspiration in the diagnosis of respiratory infection in neutropenic patients with acute leukaemia. *Leuk. Res.*, **5**, 165–168

Stableforth, D.E., Knight, R.K., Collins, J.V., Heard, B.E. and Clarke, S.W. (1978) Transbronchial lung biopsy through the fibreoptic bronchoscope. *Br. J. Dis. Chest*, **72**, 108–114

Steel, S.J. and Winstanley, D.P. (1969) Trephine biopsy of the lung and pleura. *Thorax*, **24**, 576–584

Stevens, D.A. (1987) Problems in antifungal therapy. *Infection*, **15**, 87–92

Stevens, R.F., Hann, I.F., Wheatley, K. and Gray, R. (1991) Intensive chemotherapy with or without additional bone marrow transplantation in pediatric AML. *Leukaemia*, **6**, 55–58

Stover, D.E., Zaman, M.B., Hajdu, S.I., Lange, M., Gold, J. and Armstrong, D. (1984) Bronchoalveolar lavage in the diagnosis of diffuse pulmonary infiltrates in the immunosuppressed host. *Ann. Intern. Med.*, **101**, 1–7

Tenholder, M.F. and Hooper, R.G. (1980) Pulmonary infiltrates in leukaemia. *Chest*, **78**, 3, 468–473

Tobias, J.S., Wrigley, P.F.M. and O'Grady, F. (1978) Bacterial infection and acute myeloblastic leukaemia: an analysis of two hundred patients undergoing intensive remission induction therapy. *Europ. J. Cancer*, **14**, 383–391

Vogler, W.R. (1992) Strategies in the treatment of acute myelogenous leukaemia. *Leukaemia Research*, **16**, 1141–1153

Wade, J.C., Schimpff, S.C., Newman, K.A., Fortner, C.L., Standiford, H.C. and Wiernik, P.H. (1981) Piperacillin or ticarcillin plus amikacin, a double blind prospective comparison of empiric antibiotic therapy for febrile granulocytopenic cancer patients. *Am. J. Med.*, **71**, 983–990

Wade, J.C., Schimpff, S.C., Newman, K.A. and Wiernix, P.H. (1982) Staphylococcus epidermidis: an increasing cause of infection in patients with granulocytopenia. *Ann. Intern. Med.*, **97**, 503–508

Wardman, A.G., Milligan, D.W., Child, J.A., Delamore, I.W. and Cooke, N.J. (1984) Pulmonary infiltrates and adult acute leukaemia – empirical treatment and survival related to the extent of pulmonary radiological disease. *Thorax*, **39**, 568–571

Watson, J.G. (1983) Problems of infection after bone marrow transplantation. *J. Clin. Path.*, **36**, 683–692

Walsh, T.J., Hathorn, J.W. and Sobel, J.D. (1991) Detection of circulating candidal enolase by immunoassay in patients with cancer and invasive candidiasis. *N. Eng. J. Med*, **324**, 1026–1031

Whimbey, E., Kiehn, T.E., Brannon, P., Blavins, A. and Armstrong, D. (1987) Bacteremia and fungemia in patients with neoplastic disease. *Am. J. Med.*, **82**, 723–730

Williams, D., Yungbluth, M., Adams, G. and Glassroth, U. (1985) The role of fibreoptic bronchoscopy in the evaluation of immunocompromised hosts with diffuse pulmonary infiltrates. *Am. Rev. Respir. Dis.*, **131**, 880–885

Wilson, W.R., Cockerill, F.R. and Rosenow, E.C. (1985) Pulmonary disease in the immunocompromised host. *Mayo Clinic Proc.*, **60**, 610–631

Winston, D.J., Dudnick, D.V., Chapin, M., Ho, W.G.,

Gale, R.P. and Martin, W.J. (1983) Coagulase-negative staphylococcal bacteraemia in patients receiving immunosuppressive therapy. *Archive Internal Medicine*, **143**, 32–36

Wolff, L.F., Bartlett, M.S., Baehner, R.L., Grosfeld, J.L. and Smith, J.W. (1977) The causes of interstitial pneumonia in immunocompromised children: an aggressive systemic approach to diagnosis. *Pediatrics*, **60**, 41–45

Young, L.S. (1985) Double B-Lactam therapy in the immunocompromised host. *Journal of Antimicrobial Chemotherapy*, **16**, 4–7

Young, J.A., Hopkin, J.M. and Cuthbertson, W.P. (1984) Pulmonary infiltration in immunocompromised patients: diagnosis by cytological examination of bronchoalveolar lavage fluid. *J. Clin. Path.*, **37**, 390–397

8

Invasive mycoses in neutropenic patients

J.P. Burnie

Introduction

Invasive mycoses in neutropenic patients pose three main problems for the clinician. They are difficult to diagnose, difficult to prevent and difficult to treat even when on the drug which is the gold standard for that particular fungus. Mortality on therapy varies from 75% for systemic candidiasis to 90% for invasive aspergillosis. These facts have led to a considerable endeavour in recent years to rectify this situation. This chapter will summarize the current state for the most important of the fungi as well as comment on the rarer pathogens where appropriate.

Systemic candidiasis

Systemic candidiasis (candidosis) is the term for invasive infection due to one of the yeasts of the Candida group. Clinically this includes *Candida albicans*, *Candida parapsilosis*, *Candida tropicalis*, *Candida krusei*, and *Torulopsis glabrata*. The development of this disease is due to autoinfection by yeast colonizing the patient's bowel or intravenous catheters. Yeast cells are capable of passing through the intestinal wall by 'persorption'. This was shown when a normal healthy volunteer orally ingested 10^{12} blastospores which resulted in positive blood cultures and urine samples (Krause, *et al.*, 1969). *C. albicans* causes infection in neutropenic patients by first setting up a localized oral lesion in the mouth. Yeasts

are then swallowed by the patient. Normally these would not be a problem as they would be destroyed by gastric acid and prevented from causing infection by the competing bacterial flora. The intactness of the patient's mucosa also prevents the uptake of whole yeast cells. In the neutropenic host, the bacterial flora has been diminished by the prior administration of antibiotics and the mucosa has been compromised by cytotoxic agents. The consequence of this is that the clinical manifestations of the disease include oral thrush, oesophageal candidiasis, intestinal candidiasis and finally disseminated candidiasis.

The second way *C. albicans* can produce a systemic infection is by colonizing indwelling and central venous line catheters, particularly in patients on total parenteral nutrition. Catheters develop thrombi which act as a source of infection. *Candida parapsilosis* is particularly predisposed to do this and may lead to the patient developing endocarditis.

Clinical manifestations

Oral candidiasis

There are focal lesions on the dorsum of the tongue, on the buccal mucosa and gingiva and on the oropharynx. These are white with an adherent pseudomembrane of desquamated epithelial cells, yeasts and necrotic tissue. On removal they leave a raw painful bleeding ulcer.

Oesophageal candidiasis

The most common symptom of this condition is pain on swallowing which may be so severe that it prevents the patient eating. Oral candidiasis is found in about 50% of patients. Barium swallow shows a wide range of findings none of which are specific. The classic picture is a shaggy appearing mucosal surface due to mucosal ulceration. This technique is neither sensitive nor specific but is of value in following the response to therapy. These superficial candidal lesions have been found at autopsy examination in about 10% of patients with lymphoma, 15% of patients with acute leukaemia and in 2% of patients with a carcinoma (Myerowitz, *et al.*, 1975). Rarely *C. albicans* may form a more widespread disease in the gastrointestinal tract where there are abscesses extending the whole length.

Disseminated candidiasis

There is no typical clinical picture of systemic candidiasis. Patients tend to be considered at risk if they are pyrexial, neutropenic and unresponsive at 48 hours to broad spectrum antibiotics such as a third generation cephalosporin and an aminoglycoside. In about 10% of cases a typical exanthem is seen and the yeast can be isolated from this. Some patients develop chorioretinitis which can be progressive leading to blindness. It is often associated with previous intravenous line colonization and a similar syndrome has been described in heroin addicts. Terminally the patient may develop candidal meningitis. This may mimic a cerebrovascular accident and produce a frank neurological deficit. The patient tends to be very confused and the deficit fluctuates in a way impossible for a stroke. Recent years have seen the description of hepatosplenic candidiasis. This appears on recovery from neutropenia and the patient becomes progressively jaundiced. Diagnostic imaging shows lesions measuring > 5–10 mm in the liver, spleen and occasionally the lung and kidney. Blood cultures are typically negative. Biopsy confirms the presence of yeasts histopathologically but they may fail to grow on culture.

Diagnosis

The lack of a classic presentation of disseminated candidiasis has heightened interest in the development of diagnostic tests. The gold standard is blood culture. In the United Kingdom about 50% of cases proved to have disseminated candidiasis at necropsy are blood culture positive during life. The lysis centrifugation (Isolator, Dupont, DE) system yields better results with both a reduction in the time for recovery of Candida and an increase in the frequency of isolation (Guerra-Romero, *et al.*, 1987).

The profusion of the literature on the serodiagnosis of systemic candidiasis reflects the difficulty in defining an antigen–antibody system which characterizes the disease. *C. albicans* is immunologically not a homogeneous yeast. Hasenclever and Mitchell (1961) demonstrated serotype A and serotype B strains and this has been further subdivided by immunoblot fingerprinting to demonstrate at least 17 different serotypes (Lee, *et al.*, 1986). *C. albicans* exists in both a yeast and a mycelial phase *in vivo*. Most of the antigens involved in serological tests are derived from the yeast phase, whereas the mycelial form is more typical of deep-seated infections (Munoz, *et al.*, 1980). Thus, the identification of mycelial specific antigens might form the basis of a serological test which would reliably differentiate between invasive disease and colonization. Current knowledge is that, although there may be mycelial-specific antigens, these are valueless diagnostically. Diagnosis can be made by detecting antibody, antigen, a metabolite or circulating DNA. These will be discussed in turn.

Candida antibody detection

The traditional tests for the serodiagnosis of candidal infections have been antibody detection by whole cell agglutination and counterimmunoelectrophoresis (CIE). The results with whole cell agglutination reflect the serum IgM whilst the results with CIE are thought mainly to measure serum IgG. These tests have been disappointing as up to 50% of neutropenic patients with serious candidal infections are falsely negative (Preisler, *et al.*, 1971). False positive results have also occurred in a variety of other fungal infections as well as patients with minor *Candida* infections. This positivity has varied from 3% to 60% (Wheat, 1984).

Immunoblotting has been applied to the sera of patients with systemic candidiasis. Matthews, *et al.*, (1984) described a 47 kDa antigen to which the production of antibody correlated with survival from disease. Other workers have defined similar antigens whose molecular weight have varied from 44,000–52,000 kDa (Greenfield and Jones, 1981; Strockbine, *et al.*, 1984; Au-Young, *et al.*, 1985). Neutropenic patients differed from non-neutropenic patients in that they produced mainly an IgM response, failing to convert to IgG. Non-neutropenic patients produced both classes of antibody. The difference between the 47 kDa and 48 kDa antigens of *C. albicans* will be discussed separately.

Candida antigen detection

In 1983 Gentry *et al.*, described the first latex agglutination test for detecting circulating *Candida* antigen. The original latex agglutination test found that 30 out of 33 patients with disseminated candidiasis had an antigen titre of one in four or greater. A titre of one in eight was virtually diagnostic of invasive disease. The antiserum was raised against heat-killed candidal blastospores but measured a heat labile antigen. It was marketed as the CandTec System. Burnie and Williams (1985) evaluated the test in 30 cases of systemic candidiasis. They demonstrated that in 20 of these the antigen titres reached one in four and in 10 it reached a titre of one in eight. In only one of the 81 colonized patients was there an antigen titre of greater than one in four and this came from a patient with a colonized intravenous catheter. No positive results (titres greater than one in two) were obtained in 400 control sera once rheumatoid factor had been excluded.

Bailey, *et al.* (1985) compared the CandTec test with another latex test in which particles were coated with rabbit antiserum raised against heat-killed *Candida albicans* blastospores. Both tests produced disappointingly low titres and antigen was only detected late in the disease. Sera were pre-treated with a protease and heated so as to dissociate antigen–antibody complexes.

Kahn and Jones (1986) compared the Cand-Tec test with a latex test for mannan in which particles were coated with antibody against *Candida mannan*. In 23 episodes of cases with invasive candidiasis in leukaemic patients, antigenaemia was detected in 18 cases (78%) by the test detecting mannan and 11 (48%) by Cand-Tec. Fung, Dontar and Tilton (1986) examined 83 serum samples from 24 patients infected with *Candida albicans*. Six of these had invasive disease. They reported the CandTec test to have a sensitivity of 71% and a specificity of 98% at a titre of >8. Ness, *et al.*, 1979 evaluated the test during 217 admissions of 200 patients involving intensive chemotherapy or bone marrow transplantation. Eleven patients developed systemic candidiasis and 6 gave positive antigen results. Of the 60 patients who died 41 underwent autopsy examination and 29 had detectable antigen. The latex test was positive in 30 (20.5%) of the survivors and 10 (53%) of the unautopsied patients. The false positive results were associated with a raised serum creatinine concentration, a finding which was contested (Price and Gentry, 1990).

Burnie (1985) developed a latex test for detected candidal antigens. Antibody was raised against an extract of *Candida albicans* strain NCPG 3153 and coated onto latex particles. Colonized patients gave a lower maximum antigen titres than systematically infected cases. The only exceptions were patients where an intravenous line was colonized or the patient had a candida urinary tract infection. In both these types of patients antifungal therapy was occasionally necessary. The systemically infected patients were sub-divided into those who had neutropenia and those with normal white counts. The 126 non-neutropenic patients gave higher maximum antigen titres than the 74 neutropenic patients. The distribution of maximum antigen detected in the latter was as follows: no antigen (5 cases), titre of 2 (10 cases), titre of 4 (17 cases), 8 (15 cases), 10 (14 cases), 20 (7 cases), 40 (4 cases) and 80 (2 cases). The individuals with the very high maximum antigen titres died (Burnie, 1991).

These results refer to maximum antigen titres detected and contrast with those when the original diagnosis was first suggested. For example only three out of six patients with neutropenia had an antigen titre of eight when they presented clinically. Nevertheless, two patients reached this titre once amphotericin B treatment had been started. The titre changed with therapy. After an initial rise when therapy started it would fall rapidly back to undetectable levels if the patients survived but remained persistently positive if the patient died. The test detected infection due to *Candida parapsilosis* well, produced some cross-reaction with *Candida tropicalis*, *Candida krusei* and *Candida guilliermondii*. It missed infection due to *Torulopsis glabrata* (Matthews and Burnie, 1988a; Matthews, *et al.*, 1990).

These tests have recently been outdated by tests aimed at either the 47 kDa or 48 kDa antigen of *Candida albicans*.

47 kDa or 48 kDa?

Stockbine, *et al.* (1984) identified an immunodominant cytoplasmic antigen of 48 kDa. Antibody production was strongly associated with deep candidiasis amongst patients with neoplastic diseases. This 48 kDa was subsequently found to be *Candida enolase* (Mason, *et al.*, 1988; Franklyn, *et al.*, 1990). Studies of experimental disseminated candidiasis in mice and rabbits demonstrated that 48 kDa antigen detected by ELISA was expressed in the absence of fungaemia, correlated with deep tissue infection, distinguished superficial from deep involvement and declined in response to antifungal therapy. A monoclonal was prepared against this antigen and this was assessed in high risk cancer patients as a prospective clinical trial between four medical oncology centres over a two-year period (Walsh, *et al.*, 1991, 1992). Antigen was detected by double sandwich liposomal immunoassay for *Candida enolase* in serial collected sera. One hundred and seventy cancer patients were entered in the study and 684 serum samples assayed. Among the 24 cases who were subsequently shown to have invasive candidiasis the enolase test performed with a sensitivity of 54%. Multiple serum sampling improved the detection of antigenaemia which was found in 11 out of the 13 cases of deep proved tissue infection and in 7 of the 11 cases of fungaemia.

This 48 kDa antigen has to be distinguished from the 47 kDa antigen. Both antigens were defined by immunoblotting sera from patients with systemic candidiasis but only antibody against the 47 kDa antigen was claimed to protect from invasive disease. The 47 kDa antigen has been identified as an immuno-

dominant breakdown product of a 90 kDa heat shock protein (hsp 90). Monoclonals against the enolase antigen cross-react on the immunoblot with antigenic bands at 120–135 kDa and at 35–38 kDa (Strockbine, *et al.*, 1984). In contrast antibodies both polyclonal and monoclonal against a synthetic peptide LKVIRKNIVKKMIE reacted with the band at 47 kDa and a band at 92 kDa (Matthews and Burnie 1989; Matthews, *et al.*, 1991). A dot immunobinding assay based on an affinity purified antibody against this antigen was capable of detecting circulating antigen in the sera of patients. The rate of detection of systemic candidiasis in neutropenic patients was 77% compared with 55% when a total antibody probe was used (Matthews and Burnie, 1988b). The identity of the 47 kDa was established by cloning into lambda gt 11 and screening with rabbit hyperimmune serum and sera from patients with AIDS. The importance of the antigen in disseminated candidiasis was shown by the fact that patients who seroconverted to the 47 kDa antigen also seroconverted to a fusion protein made when the antigen was expressed in *E. coli* Y1089. The 47 kDa antigen is expressed at 23, 30 and 37 °C. At 30° and 37° the higher molecular weight antigen of apparent molecular weight 92 kDa is also expressed. Antigen is conserved with all the isolates of *Candida albicans* so far examined and is present in both the yeast and mycelial form. The 47 kDa antigen has also been directly isolated from a patient by Neill, *et al.*, 1987 and shown to be immunodominant in an animal model (Ferriera, *et al.*, 1990).

Detection of *Candida* metabolites

The cyclopentol D-arabinitol is the most extensively studied metabolite of *Candida albicans* (Wong, *et al.*, 1982). Serum concentrations of D-arabinitol detected by gas liquid chromatography have been used as a diagnostic test. Currently, however, this has become unfashionable as the GLC assay is expensive and difficult to do.

Amplification of *Candidal* DNA by the polymerase chain reaction

This has been suggested as a possible way of improving the diagnosis of disseminated candidiasis. Amplification of the gene C14 demethylase as a fungus specific gene has been recently utilized by Buckman, *et al*. (1990). The test seems capable of detecting *Candida* when it grows in a body fluid. The detection of *Candida* DNA in either serum or blood has proved difficult. The gene detecting *Candida* hsp 90 has been detected in a case of *Candidal meningitis* (personal observation).

Treatment of disseminated candidiasis

Chemoprophylaxis

In 1982 Hann, *et al*., reported that ketoconazole greatly reduced the likelihood of fungal infection in immunocompromised patients. Their study evaluated 37 patients receiving 400 mg ketoconazole orally and 35 patients receiving 40 mg oral amphotericin B plus 1.2 million international units of nystatin per day. A fungal infection occurred in 70% of patients receiving amphotericin B plus nystatin and in only 30% of patients receiving ketoconazole. During an outbreak of systemic candidiasis on an intensive care unit Burnie, *et al*. (1985) demonstrated that ketoconazole helped break the spread of infection but cases occurred whilst the patients were receiving full chemoprophylaxis. These results underlined the importance of adequate gut absorption as the patients who developed systemic disease had all undergone oesophago-gastrectomies.

Recent years have seen the introduction of fluconazole as a prophylactic agent against fungal infection in neutropenic patients. It has the advantage that it can be given orally and intravenously. It penetrates the CSF readily. It has been used in combination with teicoplanin to prevent both Gram positive and candidal infections in a randomized study in neutropenic children (Schaison, *et al*., 1990). Fluconazole prophylaxis is also associated with an increase in the incidence of *Torulopsis glabrata* a fungus which tends to be intrinsically resistant to the compound. Resistant isolates of *Candida albicans* have also been reported with a minimum inhibitory concentration of 32 to 252 times higher than standard strains. These isolates also failed to respond to fluconazole in *in vivo* models (Galgiani, 1990). Fluconazole has the advantages that it is non-toxic and is well tolerated by patients. Its exact role in antifungal prophylaxis remains to be demarcated. It must be remembered that at the levels

currently given to patients it will have no clinical effect against *Aspergilli*.

Treatment of systemic candidiasis

The most effective antibiotic in the treatment of systemic candidiasis is amphotericin B. It is given systematically by the intravenous route and may remain attached to receptor sites in tissues for months after the last dose is given. It does not penetrate the cerebrospinal fluid and urine well. Nephrotoxicity is a major hazard and the patients may develop hypokalaemia, hypercalcaemia and metabolic acidosis. These defects are reversible in the initial phase of treatment but becomes progressive with further amphotericin B. They are not dose-related nor do serum levels of amphotericin B reflect clinical efficacy.

Other complications include nausea, vomiting, fevers, headaches, general aching and anorexia upon initial infusion of the drug. Anaemia is often seen in these patients and this is due to suppressed red cell production. Thrombocytopenia is rare but associated with decreased platelet production. All of these complications appear to be reversible despite prolonged administration of the drug. Neurological complications are rare but include peripheral neuropathies, hearing loss and convulsions. Intrathecal administration may result in arachnoiditis and a methyl ester of amphotericin B has been associated with dementia (Ellis, *et al*., 1982). The combination of amphotericin B and leucocyte transfusions has produced an acute respiratory deterioration which contributed to the death of five leukaemic patients (Wright, *et al*., 1981).

The dose of amphotericin B recommended varies but a typical dose would be 0.6 mg/kg per day. This is administered by slow intravenous infusion over a period of six hours after an initial test dose of 1 mg in 250 ml dextrose. The total dose of amphotericin B given over several days should be at least 200 mg. The amount of further amphotericin B required depends on the improvement in the clinical state of the patient, the resolution of pyrexia and the disappearance of circulating antigen. Problems with the toxicity of amphotericin B have led to the development of several liposomal formulations.

Vestar prepared a formulation with distearoyl phosphatidyl glycerol, cholesterol and soya lecithin. This formulation was found to be therapeutic in mice with either candidiasis (Gondal, *et al.*, 1987) or cryptococcosis. Vestar did not pursue clinical trials in the United States but named the formulation AmBisome and launched it for compassionate use in Europe. Further results have tended to confirm that the level of nephrotoxicity was reduced (Meunier, *et al.*, 1990). The most extensive reported experience is from University College Hospital. Here AmBisome was used to treat 40 neutro-penic patients with either proved or suspected fungal infection. All patients had failed con-ventional amphotericin B. The entry criteria for the study were: (1) progression of clinical signs and symptoms after at least 250 mgs of conventional amphotericin B or 2) progression of radiological abnormalities after 250 mgs of amphotericin B or 3) deterioration of renal function with a rising creatinine above 125 μmols/l. Nine of the 40 patients had a proven fungal infection, 6 had pulmonary aspergillosis, 3 had oesophagitis and stomatitis with *Candida* species isolated from throat swabs. 31 patients had a suspected fungal infection. Of the 9 proven cases commenced on AmBisome 7 had a complete remission whilst 2 died. Of the 31 suspected cases 11 showed a complete resolution on their clinical signs and symptoms, 4 showed no clinical resolution of their clinical condition and 12 patients died either from suspected fungal or progressive haematological disease. Chopra, *et al.* (1992) felt that this study was encouraging and AmBisome should be assessed further.

Bristol-Myers Squibb have also produced a liposomal preparation named ABLC. The drug was well tolerated in normal volunteers but the area under the curve was only a fifth of that of Fungizone. (Kan, *et al.*, 1991). Clinical trials are now being pursued by the manufacturer at a dose up to 5 mg/kg daily.

The latest formulation of Amphotericin B has been a colloidal dispersion similar to Fungizone but with cholesteryl sulphate instead of desoxy-cholate. This was originally marketed by Liposome Technology under the name ABCD but has subsequently been licensed by Zeneca as Amphocil. Initial studies have been encouraging.

The second antifungal of value in the management of systemic candidiasis is flu-cytosine. It is a synthetic drug which is well absorbed orally and can be given intravenously.

It penetrates the CSF and urine well. It can be toxic especially when given in combination with amphotericin B. Gastrointestinal toxicity is common and fatalities from bone marrow sup-pression have been reported. For these reasons it is important to measure the serum flucytosine levels during therapy and keep the dose such that the serum concentration is well below 100 μg/ml. Horne, *et al.* (1985) recommend a dose of 100 mg/kg per day in four divided doses for days 1–2 which is reduced to 50 mg/kg after this. This is because the renal excretion of flu-cytosine may decline with the concomitant administration of amphotericin B. In the treatment of systemic candidiasis the combi-nation of amphotericin B plus flucytosine is controversial. Haematologists tend to be reluctant to use flucytosine because of its poten-tial suppression effects on the bone marrow. They feel that the patient is most likely to recover from infection when no longer neutro-penic so that any compound which might prolong this is contra-indicated.

Flucytosine is of great value when the primary site of infection is either in the brain or in the urinary tract. A dose of 50 mg/kg per day for three days in a patient with normal renal function prevents the development of toxicity and is effective at treating candidal urinary tract infections. It is difficult to judge the dose with fluctuating renal failure but this becomes easier if the patient is on dialysis. Most of the antibiotic is removed by dialysis so that a dose of 10 mg/kg can be given after each dialysis and this produces adequate levels of circulating flucytosine.

The third group of antifungal compounds is the imidazole and triazole derivatives. There are three compounds of interest in the treat-ment of systemic candidiasis. The first is keto-conazole which can only be given orally. The major reported problem is hepato-toxicity which is an idiosyncratic reaction occurring in about one in 10,000 patients (Lake-Bakaarg, *et al.*, 1987). Ketoconazole has successfully treated heroin addicts for disseminated candidiasis (Dupont and Drouhet, 1985). The second compound is fluconazole. The role of fluconazole as a front-line antifungal in dis-seminated candidiasis is at present contentious. Its major advantages are that it can be given as both an oral and intravenous preparation and its lack of nephrotoxicity. The third compound is Itraconazole. This has a much higher activity against invasive aspergillosis and is discussed in detail under that disease.

Personal comments on therapy

The drug of choice in disseminated candidiasis is still amphotericin B. Fluconazole should be confined to those cases where either there is pre-existing nephrotoxicity or there is evidence of fungal meningitis. I have seen two patients where the systemic infection was successfully treated with either amphotericin B or liposomal amphotericin B and where a complicating choroidoretinitis progressed despite this. In both of these, successful therapy was achieved by adding in fluconazole at 800 mgs per day. The dose of amphotericin B is 0.6 mgs/kg/day. This should be started after a test dose at the full dose. There is no logic in introducing it in a step wise fashion. 5-flucytosine can be added at a low dose of 50 mg/kg/day in patients where there is either definite renal involvement or evidence of candidal meningitis. I am reluctant to give the higher doses described in the literature due to problems with drug induced thrombocytopaenia even when the levels were within the normal range. In an adult the minimum total dose of amphotericin B is 200 mgs given over about 10 days. In the case of an uncomplicated candidal septicaemia this should be adequate. In complicated cases where there is a local source of infection such as candidal endocarditis the therapy should be continued for a minimum of six weeks.

The new liposomal formulations pose an exciting advance in the field. I have successfully treated a patient with hepatic candidiasis who failed to repond to both fluconazole and then prolonged amphotericin B therapy with AmBisome.

Torulopsis glabrata tends to be intrinsically resistant to fluconazole and so should be treated with amphotericin B. *T. glabrata* septicaemias can be fatal but the overall mortality is considerably lower than with *C. albicans*. In the case of *C. parapsilosis* the source of infection is often a colonized intravenous line and the infection can be resolved by the removal of this line. There may be no need for antifungal therapy. It must be remembered however that *Candida parapsilosis* tends to infect heart valves and I have seen two patients develop *C. parapsilosis* endocarditis following infected intravenous lines.

Cryptococcus

Introduction

Cryptococcus neoformans is a yeast found in the soil on fruits and vegetables and in abundance in pigeon faeces. The yeasts enter through the respiratory tract in most cases. In rare cases skin lesions occur through traumatic direct contact.

Clinical features

Pulmonary cryptococcosis in non-immunocompromised patients may be asymptomatic. Haemoptysis is rare and on chest X-ray there may be nodular shadows with a cryptococcoma. In patients infected with the human immunodeficiency virus (HIV) it may produce mediastinal lymphadenopathy or pneumonia. It may then disseminate to the central nervous syndrome. The onset of CNS symptoms may be insidious or very abrupt. They may resemble a non-specific meningoencephalitis or a brain tumour. There may be violent headaches due to increased intracranial pressure and this is often an early and important symptom. Patients are often afebrile or have a mildly elevated temperature peaking at 39 °C. Papilloedema occurs in about one-third of cases and cranial nerve palsies in about one-fifth. Hydrocephalus may be a complication. Pleocytosis in the CSF may vary from a predominance of neutrophils to a predominance of mononuclear cells. In HIV infected patients the cell count is lower and there are no or few CNS symptoms.

Skin and mucosal involvement can occur. The skin is affected in about 10% of cases and the lesions may be solitary or multiple. The mucosa is affected in about 3% of cases.

Diagnosis

In the case of heavy infection in neutropenic patients the cryptococci can be seen in the CSF by an Indian ink smear. A drop of the sediment of 5 ml CSF is mixed on a slide with an equal volume of Indian ink and a cover slip is set in place. The specimen is examined for budding yeasts which have a doubly refractile cell wall within a distinctly outlined capsule. In HIV positive patients the number of *Cryptococci* seen is typically higher.

In biopsy specimens, when stained by mucicarmine, the cell wall and capsule appear red and there may be radiating spines around the cell wall. The cells are free in tissues or enclosed in giant cells and macrophages. Budding may be seen in active lesions with the buds attached to the parent cells by a narrow neck. There are no true hyphae.

In 1963, Bloomfield, *et al.* described a rapid latex agglutination test for the detection of cryptococcal polysaccharide antigen. The test is highly accurate with up to 100% of infected patients detected in some series. The test has prognostic value in predicting likely treatment failures and can be applied to both serum and CSF (Diamond, *et al.*, 1974). The antigen detected by the latex system is the capsular polysaccharide.

Anti-cryptococcal antibodies can also be measured by latex agglutination. These occur in normal subjects so are of limited value diagnostically. Their appearance carries a good prognosis. Infection due to *Trichosporon beigelii* can give a false positive cryptococcal latex test (MacManus and Jones, 1985). In HIV positive patients the titres of cryptococcal antigen in both CSF and serum are enormously elevated exceeding one in 100,000 and even reaching one in 2,000,000 (Eng, *et al.*, 1986).

Treatment

In the non-immunosuppressed patient the treatment of pulmonary cryptococcosis is difficult. This is because of the frequency of harmless respiratory isolates of *C. neoformans*, the discovery of cryptococcus at surgical resection which has received no treatment and caused no illness and because the beneficial effect of amphotericin B may be minimal. In many cases the diagnosis is made at thorocotomy and this procedure may be curative. About 10% of these patients may go on to develop disseminated cryptococcosis and meningitis (Campbell, 1966). In the case of immunosuppressed patients the situation is simpler in that they all need treatment. The classic regime for neutropenic patients is a combination or amphotericin B 0.3–0.5 mg/kg per day and 5-flucytosine 150 mg/kg per day. This should be continued for a period of at least 6 weeks (Bennett, *et al.*, 1979).

In HIV positive patients flucytosine is often associated with leukopenia or gastrointestinal adverse effects. Doses must be reduced to <100 mg/d if the drug can be taken at all (Chuck, *et al.*, 1989). An alternative approach

is a prolonged course of amphotericin B at 0.6 mg/kg/day.

The desire for effective oral therapy has led to trials with fluconazole. This penetrates the CSF well at doses of 400 or 800 mg/day and is becoming established as standard treatment (Esposito, *et al.*, 1989). The role of this compound in neutropenic patients with invasive cryptococcus needs to be evaluated. Itraconazole has also been shown to be successful (Denning, *et al.*, 1989).

Invasive aspergillosis

Introduction

Aspergillus species are ubiquitous and are found in the dust, soil and air samples. They cause three different sorts of disease namely invasive aspergillosis, allergic bronchopulmonary aspergillosis and a discrete fungal ball – aspergilloma. Recent papers have shown an increase in the incidence of invasive aspergillosis. This is thought to mirror both an increase in the number of patients with predisposing conditions and also the severity of their treatment. The incidence varies considerably but in some series as many as 15–40% of patients who die of acute leukaemia have evidence of aspergillosis (Meyer, *et al.*, 1975). The primary organ involved is the lung in more than 90% of cases.

Clinical features

The classic clinical presentation is that of unremitting fever usually higher than 39 °C in a neutropenic patient. Dyspnoea and a non-productive cough are often absent during the early stage of the disease. The reported frequency of repeated pleuritic chest pain and pleural rub varies from 15–61% (Young, *et al.*, 1970; Meyer, *et al.*, 1975). The non-specific clinical presentation and the lung involvement suggest that an abnormal chest X-ray and a positive sputum culture would be helpful in diagnosis. Unfortunately chest X-rays may show no abnormality at the time the first symptoms develop and in one study 10% of patients who had necropsy confirmed disease had had a normal chest X-ray the previous week (Fisher, *et al.*, 1981). Aspergilli have a predilection for arterial vessels so that they may mimic an embolus. They also may present as a discrete mass.

The value of sputum culture is limited; 50% of patients with pulmonary disease produce no sputum (Fisher, *et al.*, 1981) and two-thirds of those who do produce sputum are culture-negative. Positive cultures can occur in the absence of clinical disease (Armstrong, 1989) and this may reflect the aspiration of spores or possible aspergillus fragments which may contaminate respiratory secretions. Tregar, *et al.*, 1985 reviewed 89 patients with positive sputum cultures. In nine cases there were two or more positive sputum cultures. This included a group of eight patients who subsequently had histological proved invasive aspergillosis. Cultures from infected patients had a heavier growth of and contained mixed aspergillus species less often than did cultures from uninfected patients. Tregar, *et al.*, 1985 concluded that the culture of respiratory specimens was still of some value.

Some investigators have used the result of nasal swabs to make predictions about subsequent pulmonary infection with *Aspergilli* especially *Aspergillus flavus* (Aisner, *et al.*, 1977). This method has not become a widely accepted practice (Armstrong, 1989).

The definitive diagnosis of invasive aspergillosis is the demonstration of both cultural and histological presence of fungus on lung biopsy. This may be difficult to achieve as the patient may be both thrombocytopenic and hypoxic. One solution to this is bronchoscopy which is safe and well tolerated. Unfortunately, Albelda, *et al.*, 1984 found that it established or suggested the diagnosis in only 50% of leukaemic patients. False-negative results were particularly likely to appear early in the disease when it is localized and still treatable. Blood cultures are occasionally of value in endocarditis but are negative in disseminated aspergillosis. A positive culture is normally due to contamination.

The failure of conventional diagnostic techniques has led to numerous attempts to produce a serodiagnostic test. These can be divided into earlier tests where antibody was measured and more recent studies measuring antigen. A key study by Young and Bennett (1971) measured antibody by double-diffusion, complement fixation, immunoelectrophoresis and direct fluorescence. It failed to show any antibody in 15 patients with widespread invasive disease.

This conflicted with the results of Coleman and Kaufman, 1972 who found precipitins in 82% of proved cases of invasive aspergillosis and in 83% of suspected cases.

Antibody production in invasive aspergillosis has been examined by immunoblotting serial serum samples against an extract of *Aspergillus fumigatus* NCPF 2109 (Matthews, *et al.*, 1985; Burnie and Matthews, 1991). This demonstrated the immunodominance of antigenic bands at 88, 84, 51 and 40 kDa. Monoclonal antibodies raised against the hsp 90 complex of *C. albicans* and the water mould *Achlya ambisexualis* identified these four antigenic bands as homologous proteins. Aspergillus hsp 90 was also extracted from the sera of two patients with invasive aspergillosis by affinity chromatography. Its expression has been shown in an aspergilloma surgically removed from a patient. An immunodominant antigen with an apparent molecular weight of 58 kDa (52–62 kDa) has also been confirmed in 38 patients with invasive aspergillosis (Fratamico, *et al.*, 1991).

Antibody in invasive aspergillosisis is only present in about 52% of cases (Burnie and Matthews, 1991). It is prognostic rather than diagnostic in that patients who survive invariably mount an antibody response, although patients may die with some antibody. The prolonged course of invasive aspergillosis in contrast to invasive candidiasis means that it is still worth measuring. Antibody against the lower molecular weight *Aspergillus* bands does not occur outside patients who have on-going *Aspergillus* infection.

Antigen detection in invasive aspergillosis is a research tool. Early work has detected galactomannan. It has been demonstrated in the sera of animals experimentally infected and in man both by radio-immune assay and enzyme immunoassay (Weiner, *et al.*, 1983; Sabetta, *et al.*, 1985). Rogers, *et al.*, 1990 developed two ELISAs to detect serum and urinary aspergillus antigen. The presence of antigen correctly predicted invasive pulmonary aspergillosis in 16 patients. In two other cases antigen appeared only after the clinical diagnosis and in one case antigen was undetectable. Two ELISAs were used, the first employed a human high titre aspergillus serum. The nature of the aspergillus antigen detected was obscure although the antigen reacted on immunoblot with *Aspergillus* antigens of apparent molecular weights

29, 18 and 11 kDa. The second test employed a rat IgM monoclonal antibody specific to galactomannan.

The test with the human antibody was positive in four out of 174 urines (20%) and in 61 out of 482 sera (13%). The monoclonal based ELISA was positive in 74 out of 170 urines (44%) and in 63 out of 135 sera (18%). The differences in these results suggest that at least two sorts of *Aspergillus* antigen circulate during disease. The first of these is heat stable galacto-mannan and the second a heat labile cyto-plasmic antigen.

Burnie (1991) developed a reverse passive latex agglutination test and dot-blot assay for the diagnosis of invasive aspergillosis. At a latex titre cut-off of >1 in 8, the test had a sensitivity of 29.4% specificity of 94.3%. This was in sera taken early in the infection when the diagnosis was first suggested. The sensitivity rose to 55.1% when sera with the maximum level of antigen were assayed. The dot-blot immuno-assay was more sensitive and 33.3% of cases were positive in the initial sera. This increased to 61.5% when the serum with the maximum antigen level was taken. The effect of heating the sera was inconsistent suggesting at least two separate antigen complexes. The direct isolation of hsp 90 from the sera of patients with invasive aspergillosis proves that this is the cytoplasmic antigen detected by Burnie (1991), and in experimentally infected rats by Yu *et al.* (1990). Phillips and Radigan (1989) developed a rabbit model of invasive aspergillosis. They showed by immuno-affinity chromatography followed by immunoblotting that an antigen of 80 kDa circulated during infection.

These test systems are of low sensitivity and limited value. An alternative approach would involve the polymerase chain reaction and several groups are examining this. My own experience of PCR in invasive aspergillosis is that it can be used to confirm *Aspergillus* in a biopsy from which it has grown but as yet cannot detect aspergillus DNA in the blood of patients with invasive aspergillosis.

Treatment

In invasive aspergillosis as previously stated, chest X-rays are unreliable, sputum unhelpful or misleading and sero-diagnosis insensitive. Treatment thus has to be started on the basis of clinical suspicion. Treatment was recently reviewed by Denning and Stevens (1990). They appraised 2,121 cases reported in 497 articles in the literature and analysed 440 courses of treat-ment in 379 patients. They concluded that the overall mortality from pulmonary aspergillosis in bone marrow transplants exceeded 94% regardless of therapy. Amphotericin B at 1 mg/kg per day with flucytosine was stated as lowering the mortality in neutropenic patients with pulmonary aspergillosis who did not receive a bone marrow transplant. The latter comment is somewhat controversial as the animal data assessing flucytosine is difficult to interpret and does not clearly support the idea that flucytosine should routinely be used in *Aspergillus* infection. I would advocate Amphotericin B 1 mg/kg on its own for this disease. It is customary to give at least 1 gm of compound until the clinical signs of the disease have resolved.

The alternative approach is itraconazole. It has the disadvantage that currently only an oral preparation is available. Its value is in early infection when the diagnosis has not been con-clusively proved but there are changes in the chest X-ray coincident with a deteriorating pulmonary function. At this stage in their disease the patient can still tolerate oral therapy so can start itraconazole. Denning, *et al.* (1989b) reported their experience of treating 15 patients with invasive aspergillosis with up to 400 mg of itraconazole orally per day. Four out of the five patients with invasive pulmonary disease, two out of the two with skeletal disease, one out of the two with pleural disease and one out of one with pericardial, sinus, mastoid or hepatosplenic aspergillosis and onychomycosis responded.

These results support the idea that itra-conazole is an important anti-*Aspergillus* drug. Its major limitation lies in the lack of an intra-venous formulation. The new liposomal amphotericin B compounds are also active, but there is currently too little data available to assess their value in invasive disease.

Mucormycosis

Introduction

Mucormycosis refers to clinically similar mycoses caused by the members of the order *Mucorales* and its families. The most common genera of fungi leading to infection are Absidia,

Mucor and Rhizopus. They are classified together because on histopathological examination they all produce broad, non-septate hyphae.

The fungi enter the body either via the rhinopharynx, the lungs, the gut or more readily through the skin. They almost invariably develop infection deep in the tissues and invade blood vessels leading to thrombosis. They may metastasize to the lung, brain, liver, kidney or other sites.

Predisposing factors include leukaemia, lymphoma, carcinoma, diabetes mellitus, renal failure and a persistent enteritis in children.

Clinical manifestations

Rhinocerebral mucormycosis

This is associated with uncontrolled diabetes mellitus and can be its presenting feature. It may run a fulminant course of ten days or less but chronic presentations over weeks or months have been described. The typical history is 1–7 days of unilateral headache, eye irritation, swelling and epistaxis. The patient becomes progressively lethargic and then comatosed. There is orbital cellulitis and proptosis in about two-thirds of cases and black necrotic lesions can be found on the hard palate or on the nasal mucosa. There is progressive involvement of the cranial nerves and subsequent thrombosis of the internal carotid artery leading to hemiplegia in about one-third of cases. Coma has been reported in about two-thirds and this carries a poor prognosis (Ferry *et al.*, 1961).

Pulmonary mucormycosis

The lung may be involved on its own or this may form part of a disseminated picture. There is often fever, haemoptysis and chest X-ray changes include consolidation, cavitation, solitary nodules and the presence of a fungal ball. Sputum examination is frequently negative and the diagnosis can only be confirmed by bronchoscopy or transbronchial biopsy.

Disseminated mucormycosis

This frequently arises in the lung and spreads to the central nervous system where it causes infarcts and abscesses. Skin lesions are rare but have been described in infection due to *Rhizomucor pusillus* where they resembled ecthyma gangrenosum (Krammer, *et al.*, 1975). Mucormycosis involving the gastrointestinal tract has also been described.

Diagnosis

The definitive diagnosis is made by the biopsy of a deep site where they are broad, irregular, non-septate, branching hyphae with no spores. There may be evidence of blood vessel invasion.

Treatment

In the case of rhinocerebral mucormycosis in diabetes mellitus the underlying ketoacidosis must be corrected. Where appropriate surgical removal of infected tissue is performed and this is combined with intravenous amphotericin B therapy. Amphotericin B is the only drug with demonstrated clinical efficacy and the fungi are resistant to flucytosine and the imidazole compounds. Amphotericin B is given at a high dose of at least 1 mg/kg per day. The total dose should be between 2–3 g but depends on the response of the lesions to therapy as well as the nephrotoxicity of the amphotericin B administered. The value of the liposomal amphotericin B compounds is unknown.

Pseudallescheriasis

This disease is caused by the fungus *Pseudallescheria boydii*. It has caused cases of endocarditis, prostatitis, meningitis and mycetoma. In immunocompromised hosts, the commonest infection is that involving the lung where it causes a necrotizing pneumonia. It can then disseminate to other organs within the body.

It is a non-fastidious fungus and grows well on Sabouraud's medium. The colonies are initially white with abundant aerial mycelia but become a brown to grey colour with maturation. Treatment of disseminated infection is difficult and has involved surgical resections of the lung lesions, and the use of miconazole and ketoconazole. Isolates of *P. boydii* are consistently resistant to both amphotericin B and flucytosine, *in vitro* as well as *in vivo* (Lutwick, *et al.*, 1976). Ketoconazole has been used to treat the infection successfully (Galgiani, *et al.*, 1986).

Normally pathogenic fungi which cause disease in immunocompromised hosts

The fungi which cause Histoplasmosis, Blasto-mycosis, Coccidioidomycosis and Paracocci-dioidomycosis in non-immunocompromised hosts can also cause infection in neutropenic patients. It is beyond the scope of this chapter to deal with these in detail but their existence should be remembered when dealing with patients from the appropriate country.

Conclusion: The role of empiric amphotericin B

The early diagnosis of invasive fungal infection in a neutropenic patient still remains unreliable. Amphotericin B is the drug of choice in the majority of these patients so that it is logical to suggest that it might be used empirically in pyrexial neutropenic patients. Pizzo, *et al.* (1982) showed with an amphotericin B dose of 0.5 mg/kg/day that empiric antifungal therapy did reduce the development of invasive fungal infection in high risk patients with no apparent source of fever. This trend was confirmed in subsequent randomized trials performed both by the EORTC (EORTC, 1989) and at the National Cancer Institute, Bethesda (Walsh, *et al.*, 1991b).

Problems with the diagnosis of invasive fungal infections in neutropenic patients will continue to dominate the literature. The roles of the newer antifungal triazole compounds and of liposomal and lipid complexes of ampho-tericin B will be the subject of further clinical investigation.

References

Aisner, J., Schimpff, S.C. and Wiernick, P.H. (1987) Treatment of invasive aspergillosis: relation of early diagnosis and treatment to response. *Ann. Intern. Med.,* **86**, 539–543

Albelda, S.M., Talbot, G.H., Gerson, S.L., Miller, W.T. and Cassieleth, P.H. (1984) Role of fibreoptic broncho-scopy in the diagnosis of invasive aspergillosis in patients with acute leukaemia. *Am. J. Med.,* **76**, 1027–1034

Armstrong, D. (1989) Problems in management of opportunistic fungal diseases. *Rev. Inf. Dis.,* **11**, suppl. 7, S1591–1599

Au-Young, J.K., Troy, F.A. and Goldstein, E. (1985) Serologic analysis of antigen specific reactivity in patients with systemic candidiasis. *Diag. Microbiol. Inf. Dis.,* **3**, 419–432

Bailey, J.W., Sada, E., Brass, C. and Bennett, J.E. (1985) Diagnosis of systemic candidiasis by latex agglutination for serum antigen. *J. Clin. Microbiol.,* **21**, 749–752

Bennett, J.E., Dismukes, W.E., Duma, R., *et al.* (1979) A comparison of amphotericin B alone and combined with flucytosine in the treatment of cryptococcal meningitis. *NE J. Med.,* **30**, 126–131

Bloomfield, M., Gordon, M.A. and Elmendorf, D.F. (1963) Detection of *Cryptococcus neoformans* antigen in body fluids by latex particle agglutination. *Proc. Soc. Exp. Biol. Med.,* **114**, 64–67

Buckman, T.G., Russier, M., Merz, W.C. and Charache, P. (1990) Detection of surgical pathogens by *in vitro* DNA amplification. Part I. Rapid identification of *Candida albicans* by *in vitro* amplification of a fungus specific gene. *Surgery,* **108**, 338–346

Burnie, J.P. (1985) A reverse passive agglutination test for the diagnosis of candidosis. *J. Immunol. Meths.,* **82**, 267–280

Burnie, J.P., Odds, F.C., Lee, W., Webster, C. and Williams, J.D. (1985) Outbreak of systemic *Candida albicans* in intensive care unit caused by cross-infection. *Brit. Med. J.* **290**, 746–748

Burnie, J.P. (1991) Antigen detection in invasive aspergillosis. *J. Immunol. Meths.* **143**, 187–195

Burnie, J.P and Williams, J.D. (1985) Evaluation of the Ramco latex agglutination test in the early diagnosis of systemic candidiasis. *Eur. J. Clin. Microbiol.* 98–101

Burnie, J.P. and Matthews, R.C. (1991) HSP 88 and *Aspergillus fumigatus. J. Clin. Microbiol.,* **29**, 2099–2106

Campbell, G.D. (1981) Primary pulmonary cryptococcosis. *Am. Rev. Resp. Dis.,* **94**, 236–243

Chopra, R., Fielding, A. and Goldstone, A.H. Ambisome: UCH experience (personal communication)

Chuck, S.L. and Sande, M.A. (1989) Infections with *Cryptococcus neoformans* in the acquired immuno-deficiency syndrome. *N. Engl. J. Med.,* **321**, 794–799

Coleman, R.M. and Kaufman, L. (1972) Use of immuno-diffusion test in the serodiagnosis of aspergillosis. *Appl. Microbiol.,* **23**, 301–308

Denning, D.W., Tucker, R.M., Hanson, L.H., Hamilton, J.R. and Stevens, D.A. (1989a) Itraconazole therapy for cryptococcal meningitis and cryptococcosis. *Arch. Intern. Med.,* **149**, 2301–2308

Denning, D.W., Tucker, R.W., Hanson, L.H. and Stevens, D.A. (1989b) Treatment of invasive aspergillosis with itraconazole. *Am. J. Med.,* **86**, 791–800

Denning, D.W. and Stevens, D.A. (1990) Antifungal and surgical treatment of invasive aspergillosis: Review of 2,121 published cases. *Rev. Infect. Dis.,* **12**, 1147–1201

Diamond, R.D. and Bennett, J.E. (1974) Prognostic factors in cryptococcal meningitis. A study of 111 cases. *Annals Int. Med.,* **80**, 176–181

Dupont, B. and Drouhet, E. (1985) Cutaneous, ocular and osteoarticular candidiasis in heroin addicts: New clinical and therapeutic aspects in 38 patients. *J. Infect. Dis.,* **152**, 577–591

Eng, R.H.K., Bisburg, E., Smith, S.M. and Kapila, R. (1986) Cryptococcal infections in patients with the acquired immune deficiency syndrome. *Am. J. Med.*, **81**, 19–23

EORTC International Antimicrobial Therapy Cooperative Group. (1989) Empiric antifungal therapy in febrile granulocytopenic patients. *Am. J. Med.*, **86**, 668–672

Esposito, K., Foppa, C.U. and Antonio, S. (1989) Fluconazole for cryptococcal meningitis. (letter) *Ann. Intern. Med.*, **110**, 170

Franklyn, K.M., Warmington, J.P., Ott, A.K. and Ashman, R.D. (1990) An immunodominant antigen of *Candida albicans* shows homology to the enzyme enolase. *Immun. Cell Biol.*, **68**, 173–178

Fratamico, P.M. and Buckley, H.R. (1991) Identification and characterisation of immunodominant 58 kilodalton antigen of *Aspergillus fumigatus* recognized by sera of patients with invasive aspergillosis. *Infect. Immun.*, **59**, 309–315

Fung, J.C., Donta, S.T. and Tilton, R.C. (1986) *Candida* detection system (CandTec) to differentiate between *Candida albicans* colonization and disease. *J. Clin. Microbiol.*, **24**, 542–547

Galgiani, J.N., Stevens, D.A., Graybill, J.R., Stevens, D.L., Tillinghost, A.J. and Levine, H.B. (1986) *Pseudallescheria boydii* infections treated with ketoconazole. *Chest*, **86**, 219–224

Galgiani, J.N. (1990) Susceptibility of *Candida albicans* and other yeasts to fluconazole; relation between *in vitro* and *in vivo* studies. *Rev. Infect. Dis.*, **12**, (suppl. 13) S272–S275

Gondal, J.A., Swartz, R.P. and Rahman, A. (1989) Therapeutic evaluation of free and liposome-encapsulated amphotericin B in the treatment of systemic candidosis in mice. *A.A.C.*, **33**, 1544–1548

Greenfield, R.A. and Jones, J.M. (1981) Purification and characterization of a major cytoplasmic antigen of *Candida albicans. Infect. Immun.*, **30**, 78–89

Guerra-Romero, L., Edson, R.S., Cockerill, F.R., Hostmeicer, C.D. and Roberts, G.D. (1987) Comparison of Dupont Isolator and Roche Septi-Chek for detection of fungaemia. *J. Clin. Microbiol.*, **25**, 1623–1625

Hann, I.M., Prentice, H.G., Corringham, R., Keaney, M., Noone, P., Fox, J., Szawatkowski, M., Blacklock, H.A., Shannon, M., Gasgoine, E., Bosen, E. and Hoffbrand, A.V. (1982) Ketaconazole versus nystatin plus amphotericin B for fungal prophylaxis in severely immuno-compromised patients. *Lancet,* **i**, 826–829

Hasenclever, H.F. and Mitchell, W.O. (1961) Antigenic studies of *Candida*. I. Observation of two antigenic groups in *Candida albicans. J. Bact.*, **82**, 570–573

Horne, R., Wong, B. and Kiehn, T.E. (1985) Fungemia in a cancer hospital: changing frequency, earlier onset, and results of therapy. *Rev. Infect. Dis.*, **7**, (5), 646–655

Kahn, E.W. and Jones, J.M. (1986) Latex agglutination tests for the detection of *Candida* antigens in sera of patients with invasive candidiasis. *J. Immunol. Meths.*, **153**, 579–585

Kan, V.L., Bennett, J.E. and Amantec, M.A. (1991) Comparative safety, tolerance and pharmacokinetics of amphotericin B lipid complex and amphotericin B desoxychocolate in healthy male volunteers. *J. Infect. Dis.*, **164**, 418–421

Krammer, V.S., Hernandez, A.D., Reddick, R.L., *et al.* (1975) Cutaneous infarction. Manifestation of disseminated mucor-mycosis. *Arch. Derm.*, **113**, 1075

Krause, W., Matheis, H. and Wulf, K. (1969) Fungaemia and funguria after oral administration of *Candida albicans. Lancet*, **i**, 598–599

Lake-Bakaarg, G., Scheuer, P.J. and Sherlock, S. (1987) Hepatic reaction associated with ketaconazole in the UK. *Brit. Med. J.*, **29**, 419–422

Lee, W., Burnie, J.P. and Matthews, R.C. (1986) Fingerprinting *Candida albicans. J. Immunol. Meths.*, **93**, 177–182

Lutwick, L., Galgiani, J., Jojnson, R. and Stevens, D. (1976) Disseminated fungal infections due to *Pseudallescheria boydii. In vitro* drug sensitivity studies. *Am. J. Med.*, **61**, 632–640

MacManus, D.J. and Jones, J.M. (1085) Detection of *Trichosporon beigelii* antigen cross-reactive with *Cryptococcus neoformans* capsular polysaccharide in serum from a patient with disseminated *Trichosporon* infection. *J. Clin. Microbiol.*, **21**, 681–685

Mason, A.B., Brandt, M.E. and Buckley, H.R. (1988) Enolase activity associated with *Candida albicans* cytoplasmic antigen. *Yeast*, **5**, S231–S240

Matthews, R.C., Burnie, J.P. and Tabaqchali, S. (1984) Immunoblot analysis of the serological response in systemic candidosis. *Lancet*, **ii**, 1415–1418

Matthews, R.C., Burnie, J.P., Fox, A. and Tabaqchali, S. (1985) Immunoblot analysis of serological responses in invasive aspergillosis. *J. Clin. Path.*, **38**, 1300–1303

Matthews, R.C., Burnie, J.P. and Tabaqchali, S. (1987) Isolation of immunodominant antigens from sera of patients with systemic candidosis and characterization of serological response to *Candida albicans. J. Clin. Microbiol.*, **25**, (2), 230–237

Matthews, R.C. and Burnie, J.P. (1988a) A prospective assessment of a reverse passive latex agglutination test in the serodiagnosis of systemic infection. *Serodiag. Immun.*, **2**, 95–103

Matthews, R.C. and Burnie, J.P. (1988b) Diagnosis of systemic candidiasis by a dot immunobinding assay for the immunodominant 47 kDa antigen. **26**, 459–463

Matthews, R.C. and Burnie, J.P. (1989) Cloning of a DNA sequence encoding a major fragment of the 47 kilo-dalton stress protein homologue of *Candida albicans. FEMS Microbiol. Letts.*, **60**, 25–30

Matthews, R.C., Lee, W., Donohoe, M.S., Damani, N.N. and Burnie, J.P. (1990) *Torulopsis glabrata* fungaemia; clinical features and antibody responses. *Serodiag. Immun.*, **4**, 209–216

Matthews, R.C., Burnie, J.P. and Lee, W. (1991) The application of epitope mapping to the development of a new serological test for systemic candidosis. *J. Immunol. Methods*, **143**, 73–79

Meunier-Carpentier, F., Gorin, N., Kuse, E.R., Prentice,

H.G., Rinden, O., Thra, S. and Viriani, M. (1990) Safety of Ambisome; results from a multicenter study. *Abstract 260 Thirteenth ICAAC.*

Meyer, R.D., Young, L.S., Armstrong, D. and Yu, B. (1975) Aspergillosis complicating neoplastic disease. *Am. J. Med.,* **54**, 6–15

Munoz, M., Estes, G., Kilpatrick, M., Di Salvo, A. and Virella, G. (1980) Purification of cytoplasmic antigens from the mycelial phase of *Candida albicans*: possible advantages of its use in *Candida* serology. *Mycopathologia,* **72**, 47–53

Myerowitz, R.L., Layman, H., Pertursson, S. and Yee, R.B. (1979) Diagnostic value of *Candida* precipitins determined by counterimmunoelectrophoresis in patients with acute leukaemia. A protective study. *Am. J. Clin. Pathol.,* **72**, 963–967

Neale, T.J., Muir, J.C. and Drake, B. (1987) The immuno-chemical characterisation of circulating immune complex constituents in *Candida albicans* osteomyelitis by isoelectric focusing, immunoblot and immunoprint. *Aut. NZ J. Med.,* **17**, 201–209

Ness, M.J., Vaughan, W.P. and Woods, G.L. (1989) *Candida* antigen latex test for detection of invasive candidiasis in immunocompromised patients. *J. Infect. Dis.,* **159**, 495–502

Pizzo, P.A., Robichaud, K.L., Gill, F.A. and Witebsky, F.G. (1982) Empiric antibiotic and antifungal therapy for cancer patients with prolonged fever and granulocytopenia. *Am. J. Med.,* **72**, 101–111

Philips, P. and Radigan, G. (1989) Antigenemia in a rabbit model of invasive aspergillosis. *J. Infect. Dis.,* **159**, 1147–1150

Price, M.F. and Gentry, L.O. (1990) *Candida* antigen latex test. *J. Infect. Dis.* **161**, 807–808

Preisler, H.D., Hasenclever, H.L. and Henderson, E.S. (1971) Anti-*Candida* antibodies in patients with acute leukaemia. *Am. J. Med.,* **51**, 352–261

Rogers, T.R., Haynes, K.A. and Barnes, R.A. (1990) Value of antigen detection in predicting invasive pulmonary aspergillosis. *Lancet,* **336**, i, 1210–1213

Sabetta, J.R., Miniter, P. and Andriole, V.T. (1988) The diagnosis of invasive aspergillosis by an enzyme-linked immunosorbent assay for circulating antigen. *J. Infect. Dis.,* **152**, 946–953

Schaison, G., Baruchel, A. and Arlet, G. (1990) Prevention of Gram positive and *Candida albicans* infections using teicoplanin and fluconazole: a randomized study in neutropenic children. *Brit. J. Haematol.,* **76**, suppl. 12, 24–26

Strockbine, N.A., Largen, M.T., Zweibel, S.M. and Buckley, H.R. (1984) Identification and molecular weight characterization of antigens from *Candida albicans* that are recognized by human sera. *Infect. Immun.,* **43**, 715–721

Tregar, T.R., Visscher, P.W., Bartlett, M.S. and Smith, J.W. (1975) Diagnosis of pulmonary infection caused by *Aspergillus*: usefulness of respiratory cultures. *J. Infect. Dis.,* **152**, 572–576

Walsh, T.J., Hathorn, J.W. and Sobel, J.D. (1991a) Detection of circulating *Candida* enolase by immunoassay in patients with cancer and invasive candidiasis. *N. Engl. J. Med.,* **324**, 1026–1031

Walsh, T.J., Lee, J., Lecciones, J., Rubin, M., Butler, K., Francis, P., Weinberger, M., Roilides, E., Marshall, D., Gress, J. and Pizza, P.A. (1991b) Empiric therapy with amphotericin B in febrile granulocytopenic patients. *R. I. D.* **13**, 496–503

Walsh, T.J., Lee, J.W. and Pizzo, P.A. (1992) Immuno-diagnosis of invasive candidiasis in patients with neoplastic diseases. *New Stratergies in Fungal Disease,* eds J.E. Bennett, R.J. Hay and P.K. Peterson. Churchill Livingstone, 227–242

Weiner, M.H., Talbot, G.H., Gerson, S.L., Filice, G. and Caseileth, P.A. (1983) Antigen-detection in the diagnosis of invasive aspergillosis. *Ann. Intern. Med.,* **99**, 777–781

Wheat, L.J. (1984) *The role of the serologic diagnostic laboratory and the diagnosis of fungal disease.,* Ch. 3, 43–68

Wong, B., Bernard, E.M., Gold, J.W.M., Fong, D., Silber, A. and Armstrong, D. (1982) Increased arabinitol levels in experimental candidiasis in rats; arabinotol appearance rate, arabinitol/creatine ratios, and severely infectious. *J. Infect. Dis.,* **146**, 346–352

Wright, D.J., Robichard, K.J., Pizzo, P.A. and Deisseroth, A.B. (1981) Lethal pulmonary reactions associated with the combined use of amphotericin B and leucocyte transfusions. *N. Engl. J. Med.,* **304**, 1185–1189

Young, R.C., Bennett, J.E., Vogel, C.I., *et al.* (1970) Aspergillosis. The spectrum of the disease in 98 patients. *Medicine* (Baltimore), **49**, 147

Young, R.C. and Bennett, J.E. (1971) Invasive aspergillosis. *Am. Rev. Resp. Dis.,* **104L**, 710–716

Yu, B., Niki, Y. and Armstrong, D. (1990) Use of immunoblotting to detect *Aspergillus fumigatus* antigen in sera and urines of rats with experimental invasive aspergillosis. *J. Clin. Microbiol.,* **28**, 1575–1579

9

Planned progressive therapy: Logical sequence of management of infection in the neutropenic patient

Harold Gaya and Lynda E. Fenelon

Empiric antibiotic therapy for seriously ill patients must be selected with the knowledge that even the most effective antibiotics cannot produce a successful response in every patient. It is likely that modification of the initial regimen will be required in some patients. Therefore, initial regimens should include antibiotics that do not complicate future therapeutic decisions because of a propensity to cause bacterial resistance, superinfection or other complications.

Planned progressive therapy is a logical and disciplined strategy for selection of empiric antibiotic therapy in the febrile, neutropenic patient. Initial therapy is selected to achieve an optimal therapeutic response; however, the need to modify therapy for continuing fever or future febrile episodes is an equally important consideration. By avoiding regimens associated with a high rate of antibacterial resistance, superinfection, or toxicity, planned progressive therapy preserves future therapeutic options for febrile, neutropenic patients.

Why is there a need for planned progressive therapy? First, oncologists are prescribing more aggressive chemotherapeutic regimens in order to improve tumour response. Thus, patients are experiencing more prolonged periods of profound neutropenia (<100 cells/μl). In addition, patients receive multiple cycles of chemotherapy and develop repeated episodes of infection. It is therefore essential to preserve bacterial sensitivity to antibiotics.

Second, some newer antibiotics (e.g. third-generation cephalosporins, imipenem) tend to induce multiple antibiotic resistance during therapy with the result that repeated febrile episodes in the neutropenic patient are becoming increasingly difficult to treat. Nosocomial outbreaks of multi-antibiotic-resistant Gram-negative infections during unrestricted antibiotic use have also been reported (Brun-Buisson, *et al.*, 1987).

Concern over the consequences of inappropriate antibiotic therapy in febrile, neutropenic patients and the recognized need to preserve future therapeutic options have led several groups of physicians to suggest a sequential approach to empiric therapy (Barnes and Rogers, 1987; Hoffken, *et al.*, 1987). In this monograph, results from comparative studies of standard ureidopenicillin plus aminoglycoside therapy and newer antimicrobial regimens in high-risk cancer patients are reviewed. Based on these data, the rationale for recommending a logical sequence of antibiotic therapy, planned progressive therapy, is presented.

Considerations in the selection of antibiotic therapy

In patients with cancer, the most common cause of treatment-related mortality is infection. Neutropenic patients ($<1,000$ cells/μl) with Gram-negative bacteraemia, especially due to *Pseudomonas aeruginosa*, are at greatest risk for morbidity and mortality (Klastersky, 1983;

Pizzo, *et al.*, 1984; Gaya, 1986). Such patients include those with haematologic malignancies and solid tumours and those patients with severely compromised host defences due to aplastic anaemia, bone marrow transplant, radiation therapy or immunosuppressive therapy (Pizzo, *et al.*, 1984, 1985).

The primary objective of antibiotic therapy in high-risk patients is to decrease mortality from infectious complications (Pizzo, *et al.*, 1985). Mortality rates during the 1960s were as high as 50% among febrile, neutropenic patients with documented Gram-negative bacteraemia, and most deaths occurred during the first 48 to 72 hours (Schimpff, *et al.*, 1971; Bryant, *et al.*, 1971). Without effective treatment, over 50% of neutropenic patients infected with *P. aeruginosa* died within 48 hours of the onset of fever (Bodey and Rodriguez, 1973).

Fortunately, mortality has dramatically declined with the early use of effective empiric antibiotic regimens. The combination of an antipseudomonal penicillin plus an aminoglycoside provides excellent antibacterial activity against the most common potentially fatal pathogens including *P. aeruginosa*, *Escherichia coli*, *Klebsiella pneumoniae*, *Staphylococcus aureus* and streptococci. The value of this type of synergistic combination of antibiotics in achieving optimal response is well documented (Klastersky and Zinner, 1982).

Empiric antibiotic regimens were initially designed to provide broad coverage that included *S. aureus* and the Gram-negative pathogens *P. aeruginosa*, *E. coli* and *K. pneumoniae* (Klastersky, 1983; Pizzo, 1985). These organisms plus *Candida* sp. accounted for 70% of the episodes of septicaemia diagnosed at a major cancer centre (Whimbey, *et al.*, 1987). The changing prevalence of pathogens in neutropenic patients has necessitated changes in empiric antibiotic regimens. While Gram-negative pathogens are the most rapidly fatal causes of infection, Gram-positive pathogens including streptococci, *Staphylococcus epidermidis*, corynebacteria and *Listeria* are also recognized as causal agents in the seriously ill, neutropenic patient (Pizzo *et al.*, 1985; Whimbey, *et al.*, 1987). In a recent survey of bacterial pathogens isolated from febrile, granulocytopenic patients, Gram-positive organisms were identified in 46% of patients, and Gram-negatives in 54%. The common Gram-negative pathogens represented only

Table 9.1 Bacterial pathogens isolated from febrile, neutropenic patients (Adapted from J.W. Hathorn, P.A. Pizzo: Is there a role for monotherapy with β-lactam antibiotics in the initial empirical management of febrile neutropenic cancer patients? *J. Antimicrob. Chemother.* 1986, **17** (suppl. A), 41–54, with permission)

Pathogen	No.	%
Gram-negative	140	54
Enterobacter sp.	13	5
Escherichia coli	42	16
Klebsiella sp.	31	12
Proteus sp.	5	2
Pseudomonas aeruginosa	34	13
Other	15	6
Gram-positive	118	46
Enterococci	7	3
Staphylococcus aureus	41	16
Staphylococcus epidermidis	29	11
Other *Streptococcus* sp.	32	12
Other	9	3

41% of the organisms isolated (Hathorn and Pizzo, 1986; Table 9.1).

Three factors are important in the choice of empiric antibiotic therapy in the seriously ill patient (Hathorn and Pizzo, 1986). The first factor is efficacy. Broad-spectrum coverage of the most likely pathogens is essential, preferably with a synergistic combination of antibiotics. The regimen must provide effective treatment of rapidly fatal Gram-negative and Gram-positive pathogens including *P. aeruginosa*. Even though the occurrence of *P. aeruginosa* in neutropenic patients has declined, the potentially fatal outcome from *P. aeruginosa* bacteraemia necessitates optimal coverage. Second, the risk of adverse drug reactions should be minimal. Third, the risk of causing infections that are more difficult to treat should be minimized by selecting antibiotics with a low potential for induction of bacterial resistance and superinfections.

Antimicrobial therapy in the seriously ill patient

Selection of an antimicrobial regimen that provides optimal coverage of the likely pathogens is crucial when treating seriously ill, febrile, neutropenic patients for suspected infections. Which antibiotic regimen is most appropriate for empiric therapy has been a matter of debate

Table 9.2 Antibacterial agents for treating infections in febrile, neutropenic patients

Established agents	New agents
Penicillins	Cephalosporins
Azlocillin	Cefoperazone
Carbenicillin	Cefsulodin
Mezlocillin	Ceftazidime
Piperacillin	Ceftizoxime
Ticarcillin	Moxalactam
Aminoglycosides	Carbapenem
Amikacin	Imipenem
Gentamicin	
Netilmicin	Monobactam
Tobramycin	Aztreonam
	Quinolones
	Ciprofloxacin
	Enoxacin
	Norfloxacin

(Table 9.2). *In vitro* antibacterial activity and the use of synergistic antibiotic combinations are important considerations in selecting an antibiotic regimen.

In vitro activity

Ureidopenicillin-aminoglycoside combination: The ureidopenicillins, azlocillin, mezlocillin and piperacillin, are broad-spectrum penicillins with an expanded spectrum of activity (Winston, *et al.*, 1986). Compared with carbenicillin and ticarcillin, the ureido-penicillins have increased activity against enterobacteria including *P. aeruginosa*, *Klebsiella*, *Serratia* and *Acinetobacter* and Gram-positive pathogens such as streptococci (including enterococci), and *Listeria* (Moody, *et al.*, 1984). Piperacillin is the most active against anaerobic organisms, although all three ureido-penicillins inhibit anaerobic bacteria including *Bacteroides fragilis*. In general, mezlocillin and piperacillin are more active than azlocillin against enterobacteria, and piperacillin is the most active against *Pseudomonas* sp.

Newer antibiotics: Among the newer anti-biotics, aztreonam, a monobactam, has good activity against most Gram-negative bacteria including *P. aeruginosa*. However, it has no activity against Gram-positive or anaerobic bacteria (Winston, *et al.*, 1986). Imipenem, a carbapenem, is active against most Gram-

positive, Gram-negative and anaerobic bacteria. It is inactive against methicillin-resistant *S. aureus* and *Pseudomonas* sp. other than *P. aeruginosa*. Unfortunately, its broad spectrum of activity may pose a problem by promoting colonization and superinfection with Gram-negative bacteria which develop multi-antibiotic resistance (Hathorn and Pizzo, 1986).

New third-generation cephalosporins have a broader spectrum of activity than older agents in this class. Cefoperazone, cefsulodin and ceftazidime are the only members of this group with adequate activity against *Pseudomonas* sp., but empiric therapy with cefsulodin is limited by its lack of activity against other Gram-negative bacteria (Hathorn and Pizzo, 1986). Ceftazidime has no activity against anaerobic bacteria and is similar to other third-generation cephalosporins in that it has inadequate activity against important Gram-positive pathogens such as methicillin-resistant *S. aureus*, *S. epidermidis*, enterococci and *Listeria* sp. (Pizzo, *et al.*, 1985; Hathorn and Pizzo, 1986; Young, 1986).

Synergy and antagonism

Synergy is the supra-additive effect achieved with a combination of two or more antibiotics, compared with the effect of each individual antibotic (Klastersky and Zinner, 1982; Young, 1982). Synergistic effects may occur because (1) each antibiotic acts at a different target site in the organism; (2) one drug inhibits beta-lactamase, thus protecting the second drug; or (3) one drug increases membrane permeability, allowing the second drug easier access to its target site (Klastersky and Zinner, 1982; Gutmann, *et al.*, 1986). The best example of the first mechanism is the combination of a penicillin and an aminoglycoside.

Antibiotic synergy implies a greater bacterial cell kill with an antibiotic combination than with either drug alone and is determined in the laboratory using one or more *in vitro* techniques that measure antibacterial activity (Young, 1982). Typically, a four-fold or greater decrease in the minimum inhibitory concentrations (MIC) and minimum bactericidal concen-trations (MBC) is observed with significantly synergistic combinations. The ureidopenicillin-aminoglycoside combination is synergistic against most enterobacteria, *S. aureus*, and enterococci (Drusano, *et al.*, 1984). Piperacillin plus amikacin was the most synergistic combination against *P. aeruginosa* (Kurtz, *et al.*, 1981).

Measurement of serum bactericidal activity (SBA) is one of the most effective methods of correlating clinical response with antibiotic synergy. Several investigators have correlated *in vitro* tests of synergy with clinical response in granulocytopenic patients with serious infections (Anderson, *et al.*, 1978; de Jongh, *et al.*, 1986a; Klastersky, *et al.*, 1975). In two respective studies, 71 of 76 (93%) granulocytopenic patients with Gram-negative bacteraemia had a favourable response when the peak SBA was 1 : 16 or higher, while only 8 of 21 patients (38%) responded when the SBA was less than 1 : 16 (Figure 9.1; de Jongh *et al.*, 1986b; Sculier and Klastersky, 1984). In studies of cancer patients with Gram-negative bacteraemia, an improved outcome was clearly shown when *in vitro* synergy was demonstrated. In contrast, clinical response was significantly lower when *in vitro* synergy was absent (Table 9.3). Klastersky, *et al.* (1972, 1975) compared the results of *in vitro* tests of

synergy with clinical outcome in cancer patients treated with empiric therapy consisting of ticarcillin plus tobramycin, ticarcillin plus caphalothin, or cephalothin plus tobramycin. Combinations that demonstrated *in vitro* synergy were significantly ($P < 0.05$) more effective than nonsynergistic combinations.

In a retrospective study, the correlation between clinical response and antimicrobial synergy was evaluated in patients with Gram-negative bacteraemia (Anderson, *et al.*, 1978). Overall, the clinical response was significantly ($P < 0.05$) higher in patients when a synergistic combination was used (80%) than when a non-synergistic combination was used (64%). *In vitro* synergy was significantly ($P < 0.05$ to 0.005) correlated with clinical response in patients with rapidly fatal disease, neutropenia ($< 2,000$ cells/μl), and shock. Similar results were observed in another study by the same group (Lau, *et al.*, 1977). It was concluded that an improved clinical response could be obtained in patients with the poorest prognosis through the use of synergistic antibiotic combinations.

In one report, the correlation between *in*

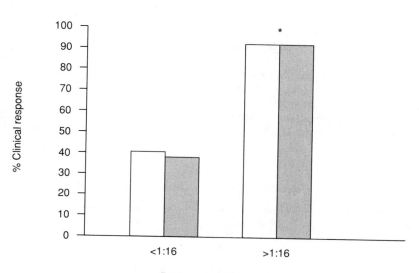

*P < 0.001

☐ de Jongh *et al.*, 1986b

▨ Sculier and Klastersky, 1986

Figure 9.1 Correlation between clinical response and serum bactericidal activity in patients with Gram-negative bacteraemia treated with empiric antibiotic therapy

Table 9.3 Correlation between clinical response and *in vitro* synergy of antibiotics in cancer patients with Gram-negative bacillary bacteraemia

Reference	% response (no. of patients)		
	Synergy	No synergy	P value
Anderson, *et al.* (1978)	79 (23/29)	33 (8/24)	<0.001
de Jongh, *et al.* (1986a)	59 (20/34)	44 (11/25)	0.005[a]
Klastersky, *et al.* (1972)	85 (17/20)	41 (7/17)	<0.01
Klastersky, *et al.* (1977)	75 (18/24)	41 (9/22)	<0.01
Lau, *et al.* (1977)	82 (18/22)	44 (7/16)	<0.05
Total	74 (96/129)	40 (42/104)	<0.001

[a] Significant difference only for patients with profound neutropenia (<100 cells/μl).

vitro synergy of antibiotic combinations and outcome was evaluated (de Jongh, *et al.*, 1986a). The response of 41 patients with Gram-negative bacteraemia and profound neutropenia (<100 cells/μl) to empiric therapy with broad-spectrum antibiotic combinations was evaluated. In 31 evaluable patients, a favourable outcome was observed in 8 of 18 patients in whom synergy was present, compared with one of 13 patients in whom synergy was absent ($P = 0.005$). Synergy was important even when the pathogen was susceptible to both antibiotics: 7 of 11 patients in whom synergy was present responded, compared with none of 6 patients treated with nonsynergist combinations.

Antagonism occurs with some antibiotic combinations. Antagonism may arise from induction of beta-lactamase production by one drug (e.g. cefoxitin), which increases enzymatic hydrolysis of a second beta-lactam. Therefore, caution should be exercised when choosing a double beta-lactam combination. Antagonism may also be caused by changes in membrane permeability induced by one drug (e.g., imipenem) of a combination (Nayler, 1987). Evidence from *in vitro* and *in vivo* studies shows that indifferent or even antagonistic effects may be produced by some combinations (Gutmann, *et al.*, 1986; Winston, *et al.*, 1986; Table 9.4). Ureidopenicillin-cephalosporin combinations may produce antagonistic effects, especially with respect to Gram-negative pathogens (Kuck, *et al.*, 1981; Zinner *et al.*, 1981). Other studies have shown antagonism of the bactericidal effects, both *in vitro* and *in vivo*, with combinations of imipenem or cefoxitin plus aztreonam (Brorson and Larsson, 1984) and combinations of aztreonam with beta-lactam antibiotics (Stutman, *et al.*, 1984; Wu, *et al.*, 1984). Clearly, antimicrobial antagonism is a concern when choosing combination therapy

Table 9.4 *In vitro* antagonism between beta-lactam antibiotics (From Gutmann, *et al.*, 1986; Winston, *et al.*, 1986)

Antagonistic antibiotic	Target	Bacterial species
Cefoxitin	Aziocillin	Enterobacteriaceae
	Aztreonam	*Enterobacter*
	Mezlocillin	Enterobacteriaceae
Imipenem	Aziocillin	*Pseudomonas*
	Aztreonam	*Pseudomonas*
	Cefoperazone	*Serratia*
	Piperacillin	*Pseudomonas*
Aztreonam	Chloramphenicol	*Klebsiella*
	Moxalactam	*Pseudomonas, Enterobacter*
Cefamandole	Mezlocillin	*Enterobacter*
	Piperacillin	*Serratia, Proteus*

Table 9.5 Beta-lactamase induction potency of different antibiotics in *Enterobacter cloacae*[a]

Low	Medium	High
Cefsulodin	Carbenicillin	Cefamandole
Piperacillin	Cefotaxime	Cefoxitin
	Cefuroxime	Ceftazidime
		Clavulanic acid
		Imipenem
		Moxalactam

[a] Arvilommi, 1983; Minami, *et al.*, 1980.

for the febrile, neutropenic patient, and agents that are not high inducers or beta-lactamases should be selected (Table 9.5).

Clinical experience with antibiotic therapy

Important factors in the design of trials of empiric therapy

When reviewing the results of studies of antibiotic combinations for empiric therapy in febrile, granulocytopenic patients, it is necessary to keep in mind the criteria for an acceptable study design. Many comparative clinical trials of antibiotic therapy have been reported in the literature. However, the number of studies that meet the criteria of a well-designed trial is small when important characteristics of study design, execution and data analysis are considered (Young, 1986; Hathorn and Pizzo, 1986; Pizzo, *et al.*, 1985).

A large number of patients must be enrolled in a clinical trial of empiric antibiotic therapy in order to detect a statistically significant difference in clinical response (Gaya, 1983). For this reason, many of the larger antibiotic studies have been carried out by multicentre collaborative groups such as the European Organization for Research and Treatment of Cancer (EORTC) International Antimicrobial Therapy Cooperative Group.

For example, in a preliminary report of a trial comparing two drug regimens as empiric therapy for febrile, granulocytopenic patients, the statistical basis for determining sample size was presented (Wade, *et al.*, 1987). To attain a 5% level of significance, assuming a 70% response in the control group and at least 20% response with the trial drug, the investigators required enough patients to provide 465 febrile episodes (or 246 documented infections).

Randomization of a prospective study using double-binding is essential to minimize bias, but this is not always practical. Although it may not be possible to have a true placebo control, the use of an appropriate comparative regimen with a proved record of efficacy is important in order to provide a meaningful comparison.

Heterogeneity of patient characteristics, underlying disease, and host immune status limits the ability to gather large numbers of similar patients and introduces confounding factors when these patients are grouped together. For example, a large number of antibiotic studies have been conducted in febrile, neutropenic cancer patients; treatment of these patients probably represents the most severe test of an antibacterial regimen. However, the type of malignancy can influence the response to treatment. Remission rates associated with the neoplastic disorder, antineoplastic treatment or surgery and age group are among the factors that vary among types of cancer and can influence the response to antimicrobial therapy. The degree and duration of neutropenia are major factors that influence recovery from an infectious episode: a marked decrease in response is seen when the neutrophil count remains less than 100 cells/μl. Patient characteristics should be specified in the study report, and analyses should be stratified when appropriate. The site and source of infection and the organisms isolated can have a significant impact on the response to treatment; detailed descriptions of this information should be available.

Criteria for entering patients into a trial and evaluating response must be clear and concise to allow for accurate analysis of response. Several classifications of infection have been used by investigators, including microbiologically documented infection with or without bacteraemia, clinically documented infection, possible infection and doubtful infection on retrospective review (EORTC International Antimicrobial Therapy Project Group, 1978).

The criteria by which patients are judged evaluable may differ considerably among studies. In Europe, the definition of a favourable response is generally based on the response to the initial antibiotic regimen. In contrast, a few centres in the United States define the overall response rate as a combination of favourable response to initial therapy together with a response following modification of the initial regimen. Thus, a considerable difference in response rates may be noted (Pizzo, *et al.*, 1986).

Based on these criteria, the following discussion of clinical trials of empiric antibiotic therapy is limited to prospective, randomized studies with large numbers of patients. Only patients with microbiologically or clinically documented infections are considered with respect to response rates. *Favourable response* refers only to episodes in which there was no modification of the original empiric regimen. When possible, response rates in bacteraemic patients, patients with persistently profound granulocytopenia (<100 cells/μl throughout therapy) and patients with pseudomonal infections are considered separately, because they represent particularly difficult therapeutic situations.

Ureidopenicillin plus aminoglycoside

Before the introduction of the ureidopenicillins (azlocillin, mezlocillin and piperacillin), the combination of an antipseudomonal penicillin (carbenicillin or ticarcillin) plus an aminoglycoside was considered optimal therapy in the febrile, neutropenic patient (EORTC Group, 1978, 1983a). Because of their expanded spectrum of activity against gram-negative bacilli, streptococci and anaerobic bacteria, ureidopenicillins have replaced carbenicillin and ticarcillin in empiric regimens (Table 9.6; Pizzo, *et al.*, 1985).

The first large, well-designed clinical trials of ureidopenicillins studied the piperacillin-amikacin combination. In 1981, 92 febrile, granulocytopenic patients were randomly assigned to treatment with piperacillin plus amikacin or ticarcillin plus amikacin (Wade, *et al.*, 1981). The overall response in patients with documented infection was 58% in the piperacillin group and 56% in the ticarcillin group. However, 17 patients in the ticarcillin group were colonized with resistant Gram-negative bacilli during therapy, compared with only three patients in the piperacillin group.

The following year, a comparison of piperacillin plus amikacin and carbenicillin plus amikacin was reported in 244 febrile, granulocytopenic patients (Winston, *et al.*, 1982). In patients with documented infections, a response occurred in 38 of 53 (72%) patients treated with the piperacillin regimen and 48 of 66 (73%) patients treated with the carbenicillin

Table 9.6 Prospective, randomized clinical trials of ureidopenicillin-aminoglycoside combinations versus antipseudomonal penicillins plus aminoglycosides in febrile, granulocytopenic patients[a]

Reference	Number of evaluable episodes (patients)	Therapy (episodes)	Favourable responses/ documented infections (%)[b]	Favourable responses/ bacteraemia (%)[c]
Klastersky, *et al.* (1986)	(582)	Azlocillin + amikacin (197) versus	82/120 (68)	33/50 (66)[d]
		cefotaxime + amikacin (162) versus	59/99 (60)	18/43 (42)
		ticarcillin + amikacin (223)	80/152 (53)	25/60 (42)
Lawson, *et al.* (1984)	358 (225)	Mezlocillin + tobramycin (75) versus	23/43 (53)	13/22 (59)
		ticarcillin + tobramycin (135) versus	36/54 (67)	14/20 (70)
		ticarcillin + tobramycin + cephalothin (148)	44/64 (69)	8/11 (47)
Wade, *et al.* (1981)	121 (92)	Pipercillin + amikacin (59) versus	22/38 (58)	5/15 (33)
		ticarcillin + amikacin (62)	19/34 (56)	6/11 (55)
Winston *et al.* (1982)	297 (244)	Piperacillin + amikacin (143) versus	38/53 (72)	16/25 (64)
		carbenicillin + amikacin (154)	48/66 (73)	20/36 (56)

[a] Neutropenia defined as $<1,000$ cells/μl in all studies
[b] Microbiologically and clinically documented ('possible' infections or 'fever of unknown origin' categories excluded)
[c] Includes Gram-negative and Gram-positive bacteraemias
[d] Significantly improved response compared with other treatment groups ($P<0.05$).

regimen. The response in patients with bacteraemia was also similar: 16 of 25 (64%) patients receiving piperacillin and 20 of 36 (56%) patients receiving carbenicillin responded. However, in patients with Gram-negative infections, only 27 of 36 (75%) who received carbenicillin responded versus 20 of 22 (91%) who received piperacillin. Of those with Gram-negative bacteraemia, 11 of 12 (92%) treated with piperacillin versus only 11 of 19 (58%) treated with carbenicillin had a favourable response. Hypokalemia occurred significantly ($P = 0.001$) more often in carbenicillin-treated patients than in piperacillin-treated patients.

The most comprehensive study was the third EORTC trial (Klastersky, *et al.*, 1986). This was a prospective, randomized study designed to compare the efficacy and toxicity of three combination antibiotic regimens – (1) azlocillin plus amikacin; (2) cefotaxime plus amikacin; and (3) ticarcillin plus amikacin – in 582 febrile, granulocytopenic cancer patients. The overall response rate and the response rate for documented infections were similar in the three treatment groups: azlocillin plus amikacin – 70% and 68%, cefotaxime plus amikacin – 65% and 60%, and ticarcillin plus amikacin – 59% and 53%, respectively. But for bacteraemic patients, the response rate with azlocillin plus amikacin (66%) was significantly ($P < 0.05$) higher than with the other two regimens. In addition, the response in patients with Gram-negative bacteraemia was greater ($P = 0.080$) with azlocillin plus amikacin (66%) than with cefotaxime plus amikacin (37%).

In a subset of 23 patients with *P. aeruginosa* bacteraemia, a response was observed in 7 of 10 patients receiving azlocillin plus amikacin, 5 of 8 receiving ticarcillin plus amikacin, but none of 5 patients receiving cefotaxime plus amikacin. A significantly ($P = 0.001$) better response was observed when the Gram-negative pathogen was susceptible to both antibiotics, and a poor response was correlated with profound, persistent granulocytopenia (<100 cells/μl). In summary, the combination of a ureidopenicillin and an aminoglycoside was more efficacious than the other combinations, especially for patients with gram-negative bacteraemia.

In a large trial, tobramycin combined with mezlocillin, ticarcillin, or the triple drug combination was evaluated for the treatment of febrile episodes in 225 granulocytopenic cancer patients (Lawson, *et al.*, 1984). In 161 patients with documented infections, there was no significant difference in response rates among the three therapies. Only 59 patients had bacteraemia, and the response ranged from 47% to 70%. However, this response rate included patients in whom the antibiotic regimen was modified during therapy.

Other antibiotic combinations

The efficacy of other antibiotic combinations in febrile, granulocytopenic patients has been evaluated in five prospective, randomized, comparative trials (Table 9.7). Third-generation cephalosporins plus an aminoglycoside or double beta-lactam combinations were evaluated in over 1,200 patients with a suspected infection. The overall response in patients with documented infections averaged 71%, which is similar to the response observed with ureidopenicillinaminoglycoside combinations. No particular regimen was superior in efficacy to the standard ureidopenicillin-aminoglycoside regimen. In addition, an increased frequency of superinfections and toxicity was observed in patients treated with cephalosporins and double beta-lactam regimens.

One study compared an aminoglycoside combined with either a cephalosporin or a penicillin. Moxalactam plus amikacin was compared with ciarcillin plus amikacin in 122 cancer patients with 191 febrile episodes (de Jongh, *et al.*, 1982). The response for all documented infections was greater than 80% with each regimen, but in patients with bacteraemia, only 11 of 18 (61%) in the moxalactam group and 7 of 14 (50%) in the ticarcillin group responded.

The other four studies compared a double beta-lactam combination with a beta-lactam plus aminoglycoside combination. A favourable response in documented infections was observed in 202 of 294 (69%) patients treated with a double beta-lactam combination compared with 83 of 125 (66%) patients treated with a beta-lactam plus aminoglycoside combination. Consistent with other studies in febrile, granulocytopenic patients, the response was correlated with the sensitivity of isolated pathogens to the antibiotics and the degree and duration of granolocytopenia. In general, there were no significant differences in response

Table 9.7 Prospective, randomized clinical trials of antibiotic combinations in febrile, granulocytopenic patients[a]

Reference	Number of evaluable episodes (patients)	Therapy (episodes)	Favourable responses/ documented infections (%)[b]	Favourable responses/ bacteraemia (%)[c]
de Jongh, *et al.* (1982)	191 (122)	Moxalactam + amikacin (98) versus	45/54 (83)	11/18 (61)
		ticarcillin + amikacin (93)	45/56 (80)	7/14 (50)
Fainstein, *et al.* (1984)	445 (219)	Moxalactam + ticarcillin (217) versus	73/113 (65)	29/34 (85)
		moxalactam + tobramycin (228)	76/118 (64)	27/36 (75)
Feld, *et al.* (1985)	220 (195)	Moxalactam + ticarcillin (117) versus	38/64 (59)	10/20 (50)
		ticarcillin + tobramycin (103)	38/69 (55)	10/24 (42)
Joshi, *et al.* (1984)	198 (–)[d]	Piperacillin + ceftazidime (99) versus	46/56 (82)	10/15 (67)
		ceftazidime + tobramycin (99)	46/61 (75)	11/20 (55)
Winston, *et al.* (1984b)	272 (219)	Moxalactam + piperacillin (136) versus	45/61 (74)	17/23 (74)
		moxalactam + amikacin (136)	41/50 (82)	13/18 (72)

[a] Neutropenia defined as <1,000 cells/μl
[b] Includes microbiologically and clinically documented infections
[c] Includes Gram-negative and Gram-positive bacteraemias
[d] Data not supplied.

between antibiotic combinations when type of pathogen or source of infection was considered.

Unfortunately, the significance of these favourable results is limited by concerns about the study design. None of these studies used the standard ureidopenicillin-aminoglycoside regimen for comparison, and only two studies used a penicillin-aminoglycoside regimen for comparison (de Jongh, *et al.*, 1982; Feld, *et al.*, 1985). Thus, it is not possible to make a direct comparison of the results. It is noteworthy that bacterial resistance and superinfection occurred with an unexpectedly high frequency during therapy with moxalactam and ceftazidime regimens (see Resistance and Superinfection, below).

The results of therapy in a subgroup of patients with gram-negative bacteraemia were recently reported from the fourth EORTC trial (EORTC Group, 1987). Febrile, granulocytopenic patients received either azlocillin plus amikacin, or ceftazidime combined with either a short course (three days) or a full course of amikacin. The overally response and response in profoundly neutropenic patients in the ceftazidime plus full course amikacin group were significantly ($P < .05$) better than in the other two groups. Ceftazidime plus short course amikacin resulted in a poor response in patients with *Pseudomonas* or *E. coli* bacteraemia, and

the poor response was not due to the development of bacterial resistance. These results emphasize the importance of the aminoglycoside to the empiric regimen. The poor response with azlocillin was due to a high incidence of azlocillin-resistant gram-negative organisms.

Efficacy of monotherapy

In numerous published reports, third-generation cephalosporins, imipenem, aztreonam and quinolone antibiotics have been used as empiric therapy in the febrile, granulocytopenic patient, but only ten studies used a prospective, randomized study design (Tables 9.8 and 9.9). Most compared single drug therapy with combination antibiotic regimens. There is considerable variation in the study methodology and data reporting of trials of monotherapy; thus, a summary of overall results is not possible. In addition, few studies compared monotherapy with the standard ureidopenicillin-aminoglycoside combination regimen. Therefore, response rates for monotherapy and combination therapy cannot be directly compared. However, some observations can be drawn from the results.

Most antibiotics are inadequate for empiric monotherapy in the febrile, neutropenic

Table 9.8 Prospective, randomized clinical trials comparing ceftazidime with combination therapy in febrile, neutropenic patients

Reference	Number of evaluable episodes/ patients	Therapy (episodes)	Number of documented infections[a]	Response without modification (%)
dePauw, *et al.* (1983)	–[b]/87	Ceftazidime (42)	18	15 (83)[c]
		versus		
		cefotaxime + gentamicin (45)	14	8 (57)
Donnelly, *et al.* (1985)	65/50	Ceftazidime (33)	28	15 (54)
		versus		
		piperacillin + netilmicin + cefotaxime (32)	25	16 (64)
Fainstein, *et al.* (1984)	172/–[b]	Ceftazidime	51	30 (59)[c]
		versus		
		ceftazidime + tobramycin	52	37 (71)
Granowetter, *et al.* (1984)	107/–[b]	Ceftazidime (48)	19	10 (53)
		versus		
		cephalothin + carbenicillin + gentamicin (59)	26	14 (54)
Pizzo, *et al.* (1986)	550/–[b]	Ceftazidime (282)	92	45 (49)
		versus		
		cephalothin + carbenicillin + gentamicin (268)	64	41 (64)
Ramphal, *et al.* (1983)	–/44	Ceftazidime (21)	–[b]	9 (43)
		versus		
		cephalothin + carbenicillin + gentamicin (23)	–[b]	13 (56)

[a] Includes clinically and microbiologically documented infections
[b] Data not available
[c] Includes patients in whom the initial regimen may have been modified during the course of therapy.

patient. Cefotaxime, cefsulodin, cefoperazone, and moxalactam do not provide a sufficient antibacterial spectrum for *Pseudomonas* sp., Enterobacteriacea, and Gram-positive pathogens to make them useful as monotherapy (Hathorn and Pizzo, 1986). Cefotaxime was significantly ($P < .05$) less effective than ceftazidime for empiric therapy even when

Table 9.9 Prospective, comparative trials comparing imipenem with other antibiotics in febrile, neutropenic patients

Reference	Number of evaluable episodes/ patients	Therapy (episodes)	Number of documented infections[a]	Favourable responses[b] (%)
Falloon, *et al.* (1987)	126/–[c]	Imipenem (61)	21	6 (29)
		versus		
		ceftazidime (65)	24	5 (21)
Mortimer, *et al.* (1985)	–[c]/61	Imipenem (31)	9	(58)[d]
		versus		
		cefoperazone + mezlocillin (30)	16	(40)[d]
Norrby, *et al.* (1987)	61/44	Imipenem (31)	8	–[c]
		versus		
		piperacillin + amikacin (30)	4	–[c]
Vandercam, *et al.* (1984)	–[c]/74	Imipenem (36)	29	26 (90)
		versus		
		piperacillin + amikacin (38)	33	25 (76)

[a] Includes clinically and microbiologically documented infections
[b] Includes response with and without modification
[c] Data not available
[d] Response rate for all febrile episodes.

combined with gentamicin (de Pauw, *et al.*, 1983).

Cefoperazone was effective in 50% to 67% of patients with documented infections; however, treatment was modified if a Gram-positive pathogen was isolated during therapy, and patients were excluded from analysis if they were treated for less than 48 hours (Piccart, *et al.*, 1984).

Ceftazidime was evaluated as monotherapy for febrile, neutropenic patients in six controlled trials (Table 9.8). The number of patients studied was too small for statistical analysis, but in most cases, the favourable response rate was lower for ceftazidime than for the comparative combination antibiotic regimen. Ceftazidime's value as monotherapy may be limited by problems with resistance, superinfection, or breakthrough infections from Gram-positive pathogens. In one study, multiple antibiotic resistance secondary to ceftazidime usage improved when the initial empiric regimen was changed to piperacillin and netilmicin (Swann, *et al.*, 1988).

Only four prospective, randomized trials have been reported in which imipenem was compared with another antibiotic regimen in febrile, neutropenic patients (Table 9.9). Incomplete data were available for the number of episodes of bacteremia and types of organisms responsible for the infection, and response was reported for less than 70 episodes of documented infection in the imipenem group. Conclusions about the comparative efficacy of imipenem in the febrile, neutropenic patient must await the results of additional trials.

Safety

Ureidopenicillin-aminoglycoside combination: The ureidopenicillins possess the well-documented safety profile of the penicillins; the most important adverse effect clinically is hypersensitivity reactions. Occasionally aminoglycoside-induced nephrotoxicity and rarely ototoxicity occur, but these are usually mild and transient effects. However, aminoglycoside serum concentrations and renal function should be monitored.

Newer antibiotics: Toxicities with newer antibiotics and with new combinations (e.g. double beta-lactam combinations) are not well defined. Relatively few side-effects have been reported with aztreonam, imipenem, and the quinolones, but these agents have fairly recently been introduced into clinical practice, and thus have been evaluated in relatively few patients. An accurate assessment of their toxicity profile will require more extensive clinical use.

Cephalosporins may produce a number of hematologic abnormalities. They inhibit platelet aggregation, and their combination may produce synergistic bleeding abnormalities (Sattler, *et al.*, 1986). The incidence of hypoprothrombinaemia ranged from 4% to 68% in one report, and cancer patients represented a high-risk group (Sattler, *et al.*, 1986). Neutropenia was observed during therapy in 4 of 41 patients treated with ceftazidime for serious infections, but these abnormalities resolved after antibiotic therapy was stopped (Eron, *et al.*, 1983).

Cephalosporin-aminoglycoside combinations may produce synergistic nephrotoxicity. Klastersky, *et al.* (1975) reported that a cephalothin-tobramycin regimen was associated with a significantly ($P < 0.05$) higher frequency of nephrotoxicity than the ticarcillin-tobramycin regimen (21% vs 6%). However, nephrotoxicity is seen much less commonly with second- and third-generation cephalosporins.

A similar finding was reported in the first EORTC trial (EORTC Group, 1978). During therapy with cephalothin plus gentamicin, there was a 26% incidence of nephrotoxicity in older patients with an elevated baseline serum creatinine. Thus, a ureidopenicillin-aminoglycoside regimen may be preferred, especially in patients at risk for nephrotoxicty.

Quinolones as a group cause central nervous system effects (dizziness, headache, restlessness and tremors), and crystalluria rarely may occur with ciprofloxacin therapy, particularly in the presence of an alkaline urine (Arcieri, *et al.*, 1987). As with other oral agents, gastrointestinal disturbances (nausea, vomiting and diarrhoea) may occur. Clinically important drug interactions between ciprofloxacin and theophylline, and ciprofloxacin and antacids or cimetidine may also affect therapy (Rubinstein and Segev, 1987).

Quinolones are limited to use in the adult population. In animal studies, quinolones inhibit normal joint formation and produce cartilage damage in juvenile weight-bearing joints (Schlüter, 1987). Consequently, ciprofloxacin is contraindicated in patients less than

16 years of age. A recent report cited a case of arthropathy that occurred in a 16-year-old patient during and after therapy with cipro-floxacin, but the true risk of arthropathy in humans during ciprofloxacin therapy remains to be determined (Alfaham, *et al.*, 1987).

Imipenem has been associated with gastro-intestinal disturbances in 7.4% and allergic reactions in 2.7% of patients. Nausea and vomiting are associated with rapid rates of infusion in some patients. Allergic reactions to imipenem may occur in patients with a history of penicillin allergy, and grand mal seizures and convulsions have been reported (Clissold, *et al.*, 1987).

Clinical consequences of induced resistance

The choice of therapy in the seriously ill patient is also influenced by considerations of resis-tance to antibiotics. The usefulness of currently available antibiotics will be preserved only by judicious use of those agents known to cause multiple antibiotic resistance. Antibiotics capable of inducing multiple resistance (e.g., imipenem, ceftazidime, quinolones) pose a serious therapeutic problem.

The primary mechanism of concern for resis-tance is a change in enzyme production by bacteria, which leads to hydrolysis or trapping of beta-lactam antibiotics (Sanders and Sanders, 1985). Several antibiotics have been identified as potent inducers of beta-lactamase both *in vitro* and *in vivo* (see Table 9.5). Recently, the changes in bacterial cell membrane permeability were identified as an additional mechanism of resistance for gram-negative pathogens (Büscher, *et al.*, 1987a, b; Gutmann, *et al.*, 1985; Quinn, *et al.*, 1986; Stratton and Tausk, 1987).

Thus, stable derepression of chromosomal type I beta-lactamase production together with associated changes in outer membrane per-meability can lead to resistance to virtually all beta-lactam antibiotics, aminoglycosides, quinolones and other antibiotics currently available. This phenomenon is inherent in *Pseudomonas*, *Serratia* and *Enterobacter* sp. (Sanders and Sanders, 1985).

Development of resistance to most of the newer antimicrobial agents during therapy has been documented in a number of case reports (Table 9.10). Bacterial resistance and treatment

failures are frequently reported during therapy with third-generation cephalosporins. Follath, *et al.* (1987) reported on the frequency of resistant isolates during therapy with third-generation cephalosporins. Over a five-year period, 18 of approximately 150 patients with initially sensitive Gram-negative isolates became resistant to therapy. Cross-resistance to all other cephalosporins and penicillins was invariably present. Resistance developed most commonly in *Enterobacter cloacae* (14), but *Serratia marcescens* (4), *Klebsiella oxytoca* (3), *P. aeruginosa* (2) and *Citrobacter freundii* (2) were also involved. Recurrent infection occur-red in 12 of the 18 patients, and 7 patients died from the infection caused by antibiotic-resistant bacteria. The authors concluded that develop-ment of resistant bacteria during treatment with third-generation cephalosporins is relatively frequent and may have serious clinical conse-quences in patients with impaired host-defence mechanisms.

Multiresistant Gram-negative pathogens are increasingly being reported in neutropenic patients and patients with cystic fibrosis (Gaya, unpublished data; Swann, *et al.*, 1988). In one institution where ceftazidime was used as second-line therapy, multi-antibiotic resistant bacteria were isolated from febrile, neutropenic patients (Swann, *et al.*, 1988). Over half of the isolates were resistant to piperacillin and over 30% were resistant to gentamicin and ceftazidime. The increased incidence of resis-tance was thought to be caused by increased use of ceftazidime, and the problem resolved when the use of ceftazidime as empiric therapy was discontinued. All subsequent gram-negative isolates were sensitive to piperacillin or netilmicin, and 69% were sensitive to both antibiotics. Caution was suggested with wide-spread use of ceftazidime.

Emergence of bacterial resistance during therapy with imipenem has been reported in *Proteus* sp., *S. epidermidis*, group D strepto-cocci and *Pseudomonas* sp. (Clissold, *et al.*, 1987). Acquired resistance most frequently develops with *Pseudomonas*. In one series of adult patients, 75 of 424 (18%) *P. aeruginosa* isolates acquired resistance to imipenem during therapy (Clissold, *et al.*, 1987). Other reports have noted a similar rate of imipenem resistance that has developed during therapy (Pedersen, *et al.*, 1985; Salata, *et al.*, 1985; Winston, *et al.*, 1984a).

Table 9.10 Summary of reports of bacterial resistance during therapy with ceftazidime, ciprofloxacin, and imipenem

Reference	Number of patients	Diagnosis	Duration of therapy (days)	Resistant pathogen	MIC Before	MIC After	Outcome
Ceftazidime Bragman, *et al.* (1986)	27	Bacteraemia	5 to 20	*P. aeruginosa*	<8	>50	9 failures 5 resistant 4 deaths 7 superinfections
Eron, *et al.* (1983)	41	Serious infections	3 to 57	*Enterobacter cloacae* (1), *Enterobacter agglomerans* (1), *P. aeruginosa* (1)	–[a]	–[a]	4 failures 3 resistant 7 superinfections
Ramphal, *et al.* (1983)	21	Fever neutropenia	2 to 38	*Clostridium* sp (1), enterococci (3)	–[a]	–[a]	5 deaths 8 superinfections
Ciprofloxacin Chapman, *et al.* (1985)	5	Bacteraemia, respiratory tract infection, osteomyelitis	5 to 21	*P. aeruginosa* (3), *K. pneumoniae* (1), *E. cloacae* (1)	0.03–0.5	1–8	4 deteriorated
Lode, *et al.* (1987)	12	Respiratory tract infection	7 to 51	*P. aeruginosa*	0.25–0.5	2–8	1 failure 7 resistant
Roberts, *et al.* (1985)	37	Cystic fibrosis	–[a]	*P. aeruginosa*	–[a]	–[a]	14 resistant
Imipenem Pedersen, *et al.* (1985)	10	Cystic fibrosis	14	*P. aeruginosa*	5[b]	25	10 resistant
Salata, *et al.* (1985)	10	Pneumonia	10	*P. aeruginosa*	1.9[b]	23[c]	2 failures 6 resistant
Winston, *et al.* (1984a)	17	Bacteraemia, pneumonia, other	14	*P. aeruginosa*	1–2	>8	3 failures 6 resistant

[a] Data not available
[b] Mean MIC for ten isolates of *P. aeruginosa*
[c] Mean MIC for six resistant isolates of *P. aeruginosa*.

The development of multi-antibiotic resistance during quinolone therapy is described in a number of reports. A high frequency of bacterial resistance has been reported with ciprofloxacin. In one report, ciprofloxacin-resistant *P. aeruginosa* were isolated in 14 of 37 (38%) cystic fibrosis patients during treatment (Roberts, *et al.*, 1985). In a separate report, 7 of 12 clinical isolates of *P. aeruginosa* persisted in patients with serious infections despite treatment with ciprofloxacin, and there was an eight-fold increase in the MIC for ciprofloxacin during therapy (Lode, *et al.*, 1987). A similar eight-fold or greater increase in ciprofloxacin's MIC for *P. aeruginosa* was reported during therapy in five patients in whom treatment failed (Chapman, *et al.*, 1985).

Superinfection

The incidence of superinfection during antimicrobial therapy has been correlated with the duration of both antibiotic therapy and neutropenia (EORTC Group, 1978). Data from animal studies indicate that superinfection occurs more frequently with single drug therapy, and the results of clinical studies confirm these findings.

Ceftazidime has excellent bactericidal activity against most Gram-negative bacilli including *P. aeruginosa*, but it has relatively little activity against Gram-positive pathogens. In two recent studies, modification of the empiric regimen to include an agent with Gram-positive coverage was needed more frequently during the first 72 hours in patients treated with ceftazidime than with comparative agents (Donnelly, *et al.*, 1985; Pizzo, *et al.*, 1986). Modification of the original therapy was needed in 49% of ceftazidime-treated patients and 34% of combination therapy patients within 72 hours; the most frequent cause was isolation of Gram-positive bacteria (Pizzo, *et al.*, 1986). Twenty-one episodes of breakthrough bacteraemia occurred; 11 were in patients receiving ceftazidime alone, and 9 of the 11 were due to Gram-positive pathogens (Pizzo, *et al.*, 1986). Three of five episodes of Gram-negative bacteraemia were fatal pseudomonal infections (two episodes in patients receiving combination therapy and one in the mono-therapy group). Two of the fatal cases involved a *Pseudomonas* isolate that was resistant to both ceftazidime and the combined regimen.

In three additional studies, superinfections with Gram-positive organisms were observed during ceftazidime therapy (Fainstein, *et al.*, 1983; Granowetter, *et al.*, 1984; Ramphal, *et al.*, 1983). Superinfections due to *Clostridium* sp. (4) and enterococci (3) were reported in 5 of 21 patients treated with ceftazidime (Ramphal, *et al.*, 1983). Four of five patients died from the superinfection. These results suggest that an antibiotic with better activity against Gram-positive pathogens must be combined with ceftazidime when treating febrile, neutropenic patients.

Of 71 febrile, neutropenic patients treated with imipenem as initial empiric therapy, eight developed superinfection during therapy (Bodey, *et al.*, 1986). Two patients developed fungal superinfection (*Candida* septicaemia and *Aspergillus* pneumonia), and two patients had pseudomonal superinfection – one imipenem-sensitive and one imipenem-resistant: The pathogen could not be isolated in the remaining four patients.

There are few published reports in which aztreonam was used as empiric therapy in seriously ill, neutropenic patients. Addition of an antibiotic with Gram-positive activity will be required when aztreonam is used for empiric therapy in these patients because aztreonam is not a broad-spectrum antibiotic.

Additional considerations for persistent infections

After 48 to 72 hours of treatment, the initial empiric antibiotic regimen should be reassessed according to the response to therapy and the results of pretreatment cultures (Pizzo, *et al.*, 1984). If an organism is isolated from the infected site and the patient is not responding to therapy, the antibiotic regimen should be modified to provide the most appropriate therapy. Many infectious disease specialists recommend tailoring the new regimen to provide specific coverage of the causative organism in an effort to avoid superinfection. However, maintaining broader coverage may protect against the development of a secondary infection, particularly in the granulocytopenic patient.

Vancomycin therapy

When a granulocytopenic patient fails to defervesce during empiric treatment, the possibilities of inadequate coverage, superinfection, or development of resistance must be explored. The addition of vancomycin may be required in the granulocytopenic patient who remains febrile after 48 to 72 hours of empiric treatment. The incidence of Gram-positive infections has increased among these patients, possibly because of quinolone prophylaxis and routine use of indwelling central venous catheters, which predispose to local infection with common Gram-positive skin organisms (Pizzo, *et al.*, 1985; Karp, *et al.*, 1986). *S. epidermidis*, *S. aureus* and streptococci are among the most frequent Gram-positive organisms causing bacteraemia. These organisms are often resistant to cephalosporins and penicillins, and vancomycin is the most effective treatment (Pizzo, *et al.*, 1984; Lowder, *et al.*, 1982; Pearson, *et al.*, 1977; Christensen, *et al.*, 1982; Lowy and Hammer, 1983).

Antifungal therapy

The granulocytopenic patient who remains febrile in the absence of a documented pathogen after three or more days of broad-spectrum antimicrobial therapy appears to be at high risk for the development of systemic fungal infections (Holleran, *et al.*, 1985; Whimbey, *et al.*,

1987). The frequency of systemic fungal infection in cancer patients has increased dramatically in recent years due to increased use of broad-spectrum antibiotics, more aggressive antineoplastic therapy, invasive procedures, and parenteral nutrition (Myerowitz, *et al.*, 1977; Meunier-Carpentier, 1984; Horn, *et al.*, 1985). Unfortunately, it is often difficult to document a disseminated fungal infection. In one series, blood cultures were positive for fungal organisms in only 12% to 34% of patients with acute leukaemia in whom a fungal infection was documented by another method (Holleran, *et al.*, 1985). Because of the difficulty with diagnosis and high mortality associated with untreated fungemia in granulocytopenic patients, empiric antifungal therapy using amphotericin B is recommended by several authors (Solomkin, *et al.*, 1982; Fainstein, *et al.*, 1987; Holleran, *et al.*, 1985; Pizzo, *et al.*, 1982; Horn, *et al.*, 1985). Once initiated, antifungal therapy should be continued throughout the granulocytopenic period (Holleran, *et al.*, 1985). Despite its drawbacks, amphotericin B is the only effective antifungal agent for empiric therapy in neutropenic patients.

Granulocyte transfusions

Granulocyte transfusions are used as an adjunct to appropriate antibiotic treatment in patients with persistently profound granulocytopenia; however, the efficacy of this treatment for all granulocytopenic patients is not well established (Wade, *et al.*, 1981; Lawson *et al.*, 1984; Gaya, 1983; Schimpff, 1977; Morse, *et al.*, 1966; Vogler and Winton, 1977; Alavi, *et al.*, 1977). The EORTC Group (1983b) administered granulocyte transfusions with empiric antibiotic therapy at the onset of fever in neutropenic patients. The overall response in the granulocyte transfusion group (69%) was not significantly different from that of the control group (78%), which suggests that empiric use of granulocyte transfusions is not beneficial. However, results from two other studies showed an increased response with granulocyte transfusions when administered to profoundly neutropenic patients with a documented infection (Klastersky, 1979; Vogler and Winton, 1977). Both groups found a significant ($P < 0.05$) improvement in response and prolonged survival when granulocyte transfusions

were administered to a subgroup of patients with documented infections. This topic is more fully discussed in Chapter 13.

The paediatric patient

Paediatric patients require special consideration when empiric antimicrobial therapy is begun; there are fewer therapeutic options available for use in this patient group. Some antimicrobial agents are not approved for use in paediatric patients while others may have adverse effects that preclude their use in children (e.g. quinolones; Schlüter, 1987). Therefore, a ureidopenicillin-aminoglycoside combination as initial empiric therapy in the pediatric patient would seem to be logical.

Rational treatment of the seriously ill patient

The febrile, granulocytopenic patient is at high risk for infectious complications, and Gramnegative bacteraemia in these patients is frequently fatal. They require early institution of empiric antimicrobial therapy with a synergistic combination which is rapidly bactericidal. The concept of Planned Progressive Therapy is based on the premise that seriously ill patients need the most efficacious therapy at the onset of infection. This therapy should provide broadspectrum coverage of the most likely pathogens based on local susceptibility patterns. Further, the initial regimen should not prejudice treatment of future infections through the development of multiple antibiotic resistance, superinfection or toxicity. It should be designed to take into account the different infections seen after repeated courses of antibiotic therapy and allow for the orderly introduction of anti-Grampositive and antifungal therapy.

A logical, stepwise approach to therapy in the febrile (Figure 9.2) granulocytopenic patient is presented in the treatment algorithm. Therapy should be initiated with a ureidopenicillin, such as piperacillin, plus an aminoglycoside. Within 48 to 72 hours, when initial culture results become available, appropriate modifications may be implemented. In the absence of a microbiologically documented infection but with clear evidence of a clinical response, therapy should be continued until the patient has been afebrile for five days. If the patient remains

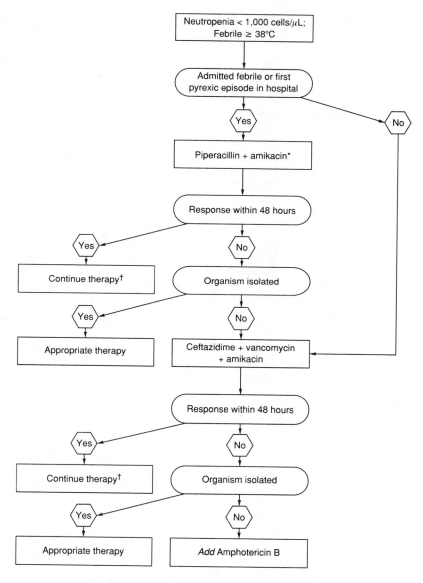

*If aminoglycoside is contraindicated, use piperacillin + ciprofloxacin.
†Until patient is afebrile for five days.

Figure 9.2 Treatment algorithm for the febrile, granulocytopenic patient requiring empiric antibiotic therapy

febrile or has recurrent fever, vancomycin is added to the treatment regimen; this is particularly indicated in the patient at risk for Gram-positive infections from the use of indwelling venous catheters. Because vancomycin covers all likely Gram-positive pathogens, a third-generation cephalosporin may be substituted at this stage to cover ureidopenicillin-resistant Gram-negative pathogens. The aminoglycoside is retained for synergy. On day 4, the patient's condition should be re-evaluated. If a response has not been observed and there is no documented source of infection, antifungal therapy with amphotericin B should be started and continued until resolution of neutropenia. In all instances, therapy should be guided by the clinical situation and local sensitivity and resistance patterns.

When faced with a suspected infection in the febrile, neutropenic patients, the clinician needs an antibiotic regimen with proved efficacy and a low potential for induction of resistance of superinfection during therapy. All drugs carry the risk of adverse reactions, and while it is tempting to use the newer antimicrobial agents (either as monotherapy or in combination) in an effort to avoid toxicity, there is no guarantee that this objective will be achieved.

In the absence of resistance problems, the efficacy of a ureidopenicillin-aminoglycoside combination in the febrile, neutropenic patient is well documented. Its use for initial therapy allows us to reserve alternative antimicrobials as a therapeutic option for future or persistent episodes of fever. It permits a planned and progressive response to a clinical situation which is infinitely variable and constantly changing.

The authors thank the copyright holders for the permission to publish this article from *Therapeutic Conferences*, *Planned Progressive Therapy*, by kind permission of Advanced Therapeutics Communications International, Secaucus, New Jersey.

References

Alavi, J.B., Root, R.K., Djerassi, I., *et al.* (1977) A randomized clinical trial of granulocyte transfusions for infection in acute leukemia. *N. Engl. J. Med.,* **296**, 706–711

Alfaham, M., Holt, M.E. and Goodchild, M.C. (1987) Arthropathy in a patient with cystic fibrosis taking ciprofloxacin. *Br. Med. J., 296*, 699

Anderson, E.T., Young, L.S. and Hewitt, W.L. (1978) Antimicrobial synergism in the therapy of gram-negative rod bacteremia. *Chemotherapy, 24*, 45–54

Arcieri, G., Griffith, E., Gruenwaldt, G., *et al.* (1987) Ciprofloxacin: An update on clinical experience. *Am. J. Med., 82* (suppl. 5a), 381–386

Arvilommi, H. (1983) Induction of beta-lactamase in clinical bacterial isolates by beta-lactam antibiotics. *13th International Congress of Chemotherapy*, Vienna

Barnes, R.A. and Rogers, T.R. (1987) An evaluation of empirical antibiotic therapy in febrile neutropenic patients. *Br. J. Haematol., 66*, 137–140

Bodey, G.P. and Rodriguez, V. (1973) Advances in the management of *Pseudomonas aeruginosa* infections in cancer patients. *Eur. J. Cancer, 9*, 435–441

Bodey, G.P., Alvarez, M.E., Jones, P.G., *et al.* (1986) Imipenem-cilastatin as initial therapy for febrile cancer patients. *Antimicrob. Agents Chemother., 30*, 211–214

Bragman, S., Sage, R., Booth, L., *et al.* (1986) Ceftazidime in the treatment of serious *Pseudomonas aeruginosa* sepsis. *Scand. J. Infect. Dis., 18*, 425–429

Brorson, J.E. and Larsson, P. (1984) Cefoxitin and imipenem (N-formimidoyl thienamycin) can be antagonistic to aztreonam (letter). *J. Antimicrob. Chemother., 14*, 667–668

Brun-Buisson, C., Legrand, P., Philippon, A., *et al.* (1987) Transferable enzymatic resistance to third-generation cephalosporins during nosocomial outbreak of multi-resistant *Klebsiella pneumoniae. Lancet, 2*, 302–306

Bryant, R.E., Hood, A.F., Hood, C.E., *et al.* (1971) Factors affecting mortality of gram-negative rod bacteremia. *Arch. Intern. Med., 127*, 120–128

Büscher, K.H., Cullmann, W., Dick, W., *et al.* (1987a) Imipenem resistance in *Pseudomonas aeruginosa* is due to diminished expression of outer membrane proteins. *J. Infect. Dis., 156*, 681–684

Büscher, K.H., Cullmann, W., Dick, W. *et al.* (1987b) Imipenem resistance in *Pseudomonas aeruginosa* resulting from diminished expression of an outer membrane protein. *Antimicrob. Agents Chemother., 31*, 703–708

Chapman, S.T., Speller, D.C.E. and Reeves, D.S. (1985) Resistance to ciprofloxacin (letter). *Lancet, 2*, 39

Christensen, G.D., Bisno, A.L., Parisi, J.T., *et al.* (1982) Nosocomial septicemia due to multiply antibiotic-resistant *Staphylococcus epidermidis. Ann. Intern. Med., 96*, 1–10

Clissold, S.P., Todd, P.A., Campoli-Richards, D.M. (1987) Imipenem/cilastatin: A review of its antibacterial activity, pharmacokinetic properties and therapeutic efficacy. *Drugs, 33*, 183–241

de Jongh, C.A., Wade, J.C., Schimpff, S.C., *et al.* (1982) Empiric antibiotic therapy for suspected infection in granolocytopenic cancer patients: A comparison between the combination of moxalactam plus amikacin and ticarcillin plus amikacin. *Am. J. Med., 73*, 89–96

de Jongh, C.A., Joshi, J.H., Newman, K.A., *et al.* (1986a) Antibiotic synergism and response in gram-negative bacteremia in granulocytopenic cancer patients. *Am. J. Med., 80* (suppl. 5c), 96–100

de Jongh, C.A., Joshi, J.H., Thompson, B.W., *et al.* (1986b) A double beta-lactam combination versus an aminoglycoside-containing regimen as empiric antibiotic therapy for febrile granulocytopenic cancer patients. *Am. J. Med., 80*(suppl. 5C), 101–111

dePauw, B.E., Kauw, F., Muytjens, H., *et al.* (1983) Randomized study of ceftazidime versus gentamicin plus cefotaxime for infections in severe granulocytopenic patients. *J. Antimicrob. Chemother., 12*(suppl. A), 93–99

Donnelly, J.P., Marcus, R.E., Goldman, J.M., *et al.* (1985) Ceftazidime as first-line therapy for fever in acute leukaemia. *J. Infect., 2*, 205–215

Drusano, G.L., Schimpff, S.C. and Hewitt, W.L. (1984) The acylampicillins: Mezlocillin, piperacillin, and azlocillin. *Rev. Infect. Dis. 6*, 13–32

EORTC (1978) International Antimicrobial Therapy Project Group: Three antibiotic regimens in the treatment of infection in febrile granulocytopenic patients with cancer. *J. Infect. Dis.,* **137**, 14–29

EORTC (1983a) International Antimicrobial Therapy Project Group: Combination of amikacin and carbenicillin with or without cefazolin as empirical treatment of febrile neutropenic patients. *J. Clin. Oncol.,* **1**, 597–603

EORTC (1983b) International Antimicrobial Therapy Project Group: Early granulocyte transfusions in high risk febrile neutropenic patients. *Schweiz Med. Wochenschr.* **113**(suppl14), 46–48

EORTC (1987) International Antimicrobial Therapy Cooperative Group: Ceftazidime combined with a short or long course of amikacin for empirical therapy of gram-negative bacteremia in cancer patients with granulocytopenia. *N. Eng. J. Med.* **317**, 1692–1698

Eron, L.J., Park, C.H., Hixon, D.L., *et al.* (1983) Ceftazidime in patients with *Pseudomonas* infections. *J. Antimicrob. Chemother.,* **12**(suppl.A), 161–169

Fainstein, V., Bodey, G.P., Elting, L., *et al.* (1983) A randomized study of ceftazidime compared to ceftazidime and tobramycin for the treatment of infections in cancer patients. *J. Antimicrob. Chemother.,* **12**(suppl.A), 101–110

Fainstein, V., Bodey, G.P., Bolivar, R., *et al.* (1984) Moxalactam plus ticarcillin or tobramycin for treatment of febrile episodes in neutropenic cancer patients. *Arch. Intern. Med.,* **144**, 1766–1770

Fainstein, V., Bodey, G.P., Elting, L., *et al.* (1987) Amphotericin B or ketoconazole therapy of fungal infections in neutropenic cancer patients. *Antimicrob. Agents Chemother.,* **31**, 11–15

Falloon, J., Rubin, M., Hathorn, J., *et al.* (1987) Is a carbapenem as effective as a 3rd generation cephalosporin when used as monotherapy in the empiric treatment of the febrile neutropenic patient? Program and abstracts of the 27th Interscience Conference on Antimicrobial Agents and Chemotherapy. Washington, DC., *American Society for Microbiology*, p. 315

Feld, R., Louie, T.J., Mandell, L., *et al.* (1985) A multicenter comparative trial of tobramycin and ticarcillin vs moxalactam and ticarcillin in febrile neutropenic patients. *Arch. Intern. Med.,* **145**, 1083–1088

Follath, F., Costa, E., Thommen, A., *et al.* (1987) Clinical consequences of development of resistance to third generation cephalosporins. *Eur. J. Clin. Microbiol.,* **6**, 446–450

Gaya, H., Klastersky, J. and Schimpff, S.C. (1975) Protocol for an international trial of initial therapy regimens in neutropenic patients with malignant disease. *Eur. J. Cancer,* **11**(suppl.), 51–54

Gaya, H. (1983) Rational basis for the choice of regimens for empirical therapy of sepsis in granulocytopenic patients: A report of the EORTC International Antimicrobial Therapy Project Group. *Schweiz. Med. Wochenschr.,* **113**(suppl.14), 49–57

Gaya, H. (1986) Combination therapy and monotherapy in the treatment of severe infection in the immunocompromised host. *Am. J. Med.,* **80**(suppl.6B), 149–155

Granowetter, L., Wells, H. and Lange, B. (1984) Ceftazidime versus cephalothin, carbenicillin and gentamicin as the initial therapy of the febrile neutropenic pediatric cancer patient (abstract). *Pediatr. Res.,* **18**(suppl.4 part 2), 276A

Gutmann, L., Williamson, R., Moreau, N., *et al.* (1985) Cross-resistance to nalidixic acid, trimethoprim, and chloramphenicol associated with alterations in outer membrane proteins of *Klebsiella, Enterobacter,* and *Serratia. J. Infect. Dis.,* **151**, 501–507

Gutmann, L., Williamson, R., Kitzis, M.D., *et al.* (1986) Synergism and antagonism in double beta-lactam antibiotic combinations. *Am. J. Med.,* **80**(suppl. 5C), 21–29

Hathorn, J.W. and Pizzo, P.A. (1986) Is there a role for monotherapy with β-lactam antibiotics in the initial empirical management of febrile neutropenic cancer patients? *J. Antimicrob. Chemother.,* 17(suppl. A), 41–54

Höffken, G., Link, H., Maschmeyer, G., *et al.* (1987) Empiric antimicrobial therapy in neutropenic patients: Preliminary results of a prospective randomized trial (abstract). Program and abstracts of the 27th Interscience Conference on Antimicrobial Agents and Chemotherapy. Washington, DC, *American Society for Microbiology,* p. 322

Holleran, W.M., Wilbur, J.R. and DeGregorio, M.W. (1985) Empiric amphotericin B therapy in patients with acute leukemia. *Rev. Infect. Dis.,* **7**, 619–624

Horn, R., Wong, B., Kiehn, T.E., *et al.* (1985) Fungemia in a cancer hospital: Changing frequency, earlier onset, and results of therapy. *Rev. Infect. Dis.,* **7**, 646–655

Joshi, J., Ruxer, R., Newman, K., *et al.* (1984) Double β-lactam versus an aminoglycoside + β-lactam combination as empiric therapy for granulocytopenic cancer patients (abstract). Program and abstracts of the 24th Interscience Conference on Antimicrobial Agents and Chemotherapy. Washington, DC, *American Society for Microbiology,* p. 158

Karp, J.E., Dick, J.D., Angelopulos, C., *et al.* (1986) Empiric use of vancomycin during prolonged treatment-induced granulocytopenia: Randomized, double-blind, placebo-controlled clinical trial in patients with acute leukemia. *Am. J. Med.,* **81**, 237–242

Klastersky, J., Cappel, R. and Daneau, D. (1972) Clinical significance of *in vitro* synergism between antibiotics in gram-negative infections. *Antimicrob. Agents Chemother.,* **2**, 470–475

Klastersky, J., Hensgens, C. and Debusscher, L. (1975) Empiric therapy for cancer patients: Comparative study of ticarcillin-tobramycin, ticarcillin-cephalothin, and cephalothin-tobramycin. *Antimicrob. Agents Chemother.,* **7**, 640–645

Klastersky, J., Meunier-Carpentier, F. and Prevost, J.M. (1977) Significance of antimicrobial synergism for the outcome of gram negative sepsis. *Am. J. Med. Sci.,* **273**, 157–167

Klastersky, J. (1979) Granulocyte transfusions as a therapy and a prophylaxis of infections in neutropenic patients. *Eur. J. Cancer,* **15**, 15–22

Klastersky, J. and Zinner, S.H. (1982) Synergistic

combinations of antibiotics in gram-negative bacillary infections. *Rev. Infect. Dis.,* **4**, 294–301

Klastersky, J. (1983) Empiric treatment of infections in neutropenic patients with cancer. *Rev. Infect. Dis.,* **5**(suppl.), S21–S31

Klastersky, J., Glauser, M.P., Schimpff, S.C., *et al.* (1986) Prospective randomized comparison of three antibiotic regimens for empirical therapy of suspected bacteremic infection in febrile granulocytopenic patients. *Antimicrob. Agents Chemother.,* **29**, 263–270

Kuck, N.A., Testa, R.T. and Forbes, M. (1981) *In vitro* and *in vivo* antibacterial effects of combinations of beta-lactam antibiotics. *Antimicrob. Agents Chemother.,* **19**, 634–638

Kurtz, T.O., Winston, D.J., Bruckner, D.A., *et al.* (1981) Comparative *in vitro* synergistic activity of new beta-lactam antimicrobial agents and amikacin against *Pseudomonas aeruginosa* and *Serratia marcescens Antimicrob. Agents Chemother.,* **20**, 239–243

Lau, W.K., Young, L.S., Black, R.E., *et al.* (1977) Comparative efficacy and toxicity of amikacin/carbenicillin versus gentamicin/carbenicillin in leukopenic patients: A randomized prospective trial. *Am. J. Med.,* **62**, 959–966

Lawson, R.D., Gentry, L.O., Bodey, G.P., *et al.* (1984) A randomized study of tobramycin plus ticarcillin, tobramycin plus cephalothin and ticarcillin, or tobramycin plus mezlocillin in the treatment of infection in neutropenic patients with malignancies. *Am. J. Med. Sci.,* **287**, 16–23

Lode,, H., Wiley, R., Höffken, G., *et al.* (1987) Prospective randomized controlled study of ciprofloxacin versus imipenem-cilastatin in severe clinical infections. *Antimicrob. Agents Chemother.,* **31**, 1491–1496

Lowder, J.N., Lazarus, H.M. and Herzig, R.H. (1982) Bacteremias and fungemias in oncologic patients with central venous catheters: Changing-spectrum of infection. *Arch. Intern. Med.,* **142**, 456–459

Lowy, F.D. and Hammer, S.M. (1983) *Staphylococcus epidermidis* infections. *Ann. Intern. Med.,* **99**, 834–839

Meunier-Carpentier, F. (1984) Chemoprophylaxis of fungal infections. *Am. J. Med.,* **76**, 652–656

Minami, S., Yotsuji, A., Inoue, M., *et al.* (1980) Induction of beta-lactamase by various beta-lactam antibiotics in *Enterobacter cloacae. Antimicrob. Agents Chemother.,* **18**, 382–385

Moody, J.A., Peterson, L.R. and Gerding, D.N. (1984) *In vitro* activities of ureidopenicillins alone and in combination with amikacin and three cephalosporin antibiotics. *Antimicrob. Agents Chemother.,* **26**, 256–259

Morse, E.E., Freireich, E.J., Carbone, P.P., *et al.* (1966) The transfusion of leukocytes from donors with chronic myelocytic leukemia to patients with leukopenia. *Transfusion,* **6**, 183–192

Mortimer, J., Miller, S., Black, D., *et al.* (1987) Cefoperazone and mezlocillin versus impenemcilastatin in febrile granulocytopenic cancer patients: A randomized trial. Program and abstracts of the 27th Interscience Conference on Antimicrobial Agents and Chemotherapy. Washington, DC, *American Society for Microbiology,* p. 315

Myerowitz, R.L., Pazin, G.J. and Allen, C.M. (1977) Disseminated candidasis: Changes in incidence, underlying diseases, and pathology. *Am. J. Clin. Pathol.,* **68**, 29–38

Nayler, J.H.C. (1987) Resistance to β-lactams in gram-negative bacteria: Relative contributions of β-lactamase and permeability limitations. *J. Antimicrob. Chemother.,* **19**, 713–732

Norrby, S.R., Norberg, B., Lundberg, S., *et al.* (1987) Imipenem/cilastatin versus amikacin plus piperacillin for treatment of febrile episodes in patients with marked neutropenia. Clinical Evaluation of Imipenem/Cilastatin: *Monotherapy of Hospital Infections.* Istanbul, Turkey, July 21

Pearson, T.A., Braine, H.G. and Rathbun, H.K. (1977) *Corynebacterium* sepsis in oncology patients: Predisposing factors, diagnosis, and treatment. *JAMA,* **238**, 1737–1740

Pedersen, S.S., Pressler, T., Hoiby, N., *et al.* (1985) Imipenem/cilastatin treatment of multiresistant *Pseudomonas aeruginosa* lung infection in cystic fibrosis. *J. Antimicrob. Chemother.,* **16**, 629–635

Piccart, M., Klastersky, J., Meunier, F., *et al.* (1984) Imipenem/cilastatin treatment of multiresistant *Pseudomonas aeruginosa* lung infection in cystic fibrosis. *J. Antimicrob. Chemother.,* **16**, 629–635

Pizzo, P.A., Robichaud, K.J., Gill, F.A., *et al.* (1982) Empiric antibiotic and antifungal therapy for cancer patients with prolonged fever and granulocytopenia. *Am. J. Med.,* **72**, 101–111

Pizzo, P.A., Commers, J., Cotton, D., *et al.* (1984) Approaching the controversies in antibacterial management of cancer patients. *Am. J. Med.,* **76**, 436–449

Pizzo, P.A. (1985) Empiric therapy and prevention of infection in the immunocompromised host, in G.L. Mandell, R.G.J. Douglas, J.E. Bennett (eds) *Principles and Practice of Infectious Diseases,* ed. 2. New York, John Wiley, pp. 1680–1688

Pizzo, P.A., Thaler, M., Hathorn, J., *et al.* (1985) New beta-lactam antibiotics in granulocytopenic patients: New options and new questions. *Am. J. Med.,* **79**(suppl. 2A), 75–82

Pizzo, P.A., Hathorn, J.W., Hiemenz, J., *et al.* (1986) A randomized trial comparing ceftazidime alone with combination antibiotic therapy in cancer patients with fever and neutropenia. *N. Engl. J. Med.,* **315**, 552–558

Quinn, J.P., Dudek, E.J., DiVincenzo, C.A., *et al.* (1986) Emergence of resistance to imipenem during therapy for *Pseudomonas aeruginosa* infections. *J. Infect. Dis.,* **154**, 289–294

Ramphal, R., Kramer, B.S., Rand, K.H., *et al.* (1983) Early results of a comparative trial of ceftazidime versus cephalothin, carbenicillin and gentamicin in the treatment of febrile granulocytopenic patients. *J. Antimicrob. Chemother.* **12**(suppl. A), 81–88

Roberts, C.M., Batten, J. and Hodson, M.E. (1985)

Ciprofloxacin-resistant *Pseudomonas* (letter to the editor). *Lancet,* **1**, 1442

Rubinstein, E. and Segey, S. (1987) Drug interactions of ciprofloxacin with other non-antibiotic agents. *Am. J. Med.,* **82**(suppl. 4A), 119–123

Salata, R.A., Gebhart, R.L., Palmer, D.L., *et al.* (1985) Pneumonia treated with imipenem/cilastatin. *Am. J. Med.,* **78**(suppl. 6A), 104–109

Sanders, C.C. and Sanders, W.E. (1985) Microbial resistance to newer generation β-lactam antibiotics: Clinical and laboratory implications. *J. Infect. Dis.,* **151**, 399–406

Sattler, F.R., Weitekamp, M.R. and Ballard, J.O. (1986) Potential for bleeding with the new betalactam antibiotics. *Ann. Intern. Med.,* **105**, 924–931

Schimpff, S.C., Satterlee, W., Young, V.M., *et al.* (1971) Empiric therapy with carbenicillin and gentamicin for febrile patients with cancer and granulocytopenia. *N. Engl. J. Med.,* **284**, 1061–1065

Schimpff, S.C. (1977) Therapy of infection in patients with granolocytopenia. *Med. Clin. North Am.,* **61**, 1101–1118

Schlüter, G. (1987) Ciprofloxacin: Review of potential toxicologic effects. *Am. J. Med.,* **82**(suppl. 4A), 91–93

Sculier, J.P. and Klastersky, J. (1984) Significance of serum bactericidal activity in gram-negative bacillary bacteremia in patients with and without granulo-cytopenia. *Am. J. Med.,* **76**, 429–435

Solomkin, J.S., Flohr, A.M. and Simmons, R.L. (1982) Indications for therapy for fungemia in post-operative patients. *Arch. Surg.,* **117**, 1272–1275

Stratton, C.W. and Tausk, F. (1987) Synergistic resistance mechanisms in *Pseudomonas aeruginosa. J. Antimicrob. Chemother.,* **19**, 413–416

Stutman, H.R., Welch, D.F., Scribner, R.K., *et al.* (1984) *In vitro* antimicrobial activity of aztreonam alone and in combination against bacterial isolates from pediatric patients. *Antimicrob. Agents Chemother.,* **25**, 212–215

Swann, R.A., Mitchell, C.J. and Wood, J.K. (1988) Successful reduction in the incidence of multiresistance in gram-negative rod bacteraemias in neutropenic patients by withdrawal of ceftazidime. *Sixth Mediterranean Congress of Chemotherapy.* Italy, May

Vandercam, B., Michaux, J.L., Agaliotis, D., *et al.* (1987) Imipenem/cilastatin versus piperacillin plus amikacin as empiric therapy of febrile episodes in neutropenic patients with hematologic malignancies. Clinical Evaluation of Imipenem/Cilastatin: Monotherapy of Hospital Infections. Istanbul, Turkey, July 21

Vogler, W.R. and Winton, E.F. (1977) A controlled study of the efficacy of granulocyte transfusions in patients with neutropenia. *Am. J. Med.,* **63**, 983–990

Wade, J.C., Schimpff, S.C., Newman, K.A., *et al.* (1981) Piperacillin or ticarcillin plus amikacin: A double-blind prospective comparison of empiric antibiotic therapy for febrile granulocytopenic cancer patients. *Am. J. Med.* **71**, 983–990

Wade, J., Bustamante, C., Devlin, A., *et al.* (1987) Imipenem vs. piperacillin plus amikacin, empiric therapy for febrile neutropenic patients: A double-blind trial. Program and abstracts of the 27th Interscience Conference on Antimicrobial Agents and Chemotherapy. Washington, DC, *American Society for Microbiology,* p. 315

Whimbey, E., Kiehn, T.E., Brannon, P., *et al.* (1987) Bacteremia and fungemia in patients with neoplastic disease. *Am. J. Med.,* **82**, 723–730

Winston, D.J., Ho, W.G., Young, L.S., *et al.* (1982) Piperacillin plus amikacin therapy *v* carbenicillin plus amikacin therapy in febrile, granolocytopenic patients. *Arch. Intern. Med.,* **142**, 1663–1667

Winston, D.J., McGrattan, M.A. and Busuttil, R.W. (1984a) Imipenem therapy of *Pseudomonas aeruginosa* and other serious bacterial infections. *Antimicrob. Agents Chemother.,* **26**, 673–677

Winston, D.J., Barnes, R.C., Ho, W.G., *et al.* (1984b) Moxalactam plus piperacillin versus moxalactam plus amikacin in febrile granulocytopenic patients. *Am. J. Med.,* **77**, 442–450

Winston, D.J., Ho, W.G., Champlin, R.E., *et al.* (1986) Ureidopenicillins, aztreonam, and thienamycin: Efficacy as single-drug therapy of severe infections and potential as components of combined therapy. *J. Antimicrob. Chemother.,* **17**(suppl. A), 55–66

Wu, D.H., Baltch, A.L., Smith, R.P., *et al.* (1984) Effect of aztreonam in combination with azlocillin or piperacillin on *Pseudomonas aeruginosa. Antimicrob. Agents Chemother.,* **26**, 519–521

Young, L.S. (1982) Combination or single drug therapy for gram-negative sepsis, in J.S. Remington and M.S. Swartz (eds) (1982) *Current Clinical Topics in Infectious Diseases,* vol. 3. New York, McGraw-Hill, pp. 177–205

Young, L.S. (1986) Problems of studying infections in the compromised host. *Rev. Infect. Dis.,* **8**(suppl. 3), S341–S349

Zinner, S.H., Klastersky, J., Gaya, H., *et al.* (1981) *In vitro* and *in vivo* studies of three antibiotic combinations against gram-negative bacteria and *Staphylococcus aureus. Antimicrob. Agents Chemother.,* **20**, 463–469

10

Virus infections in the immuno-compromised host

S.A. Schey, C. Aitken and A.G. Dalgleish

Introduction

The immunocompromised patient is becoming an ever increasing proportion of the hospital workload. Immunosuppression may be a result of primary disease (such as AIDS) or subsequent to iatrogenic chemotherapy, radiotherapy or specific immunosuppressive regimens. Although there are similarities between these different groups of patients there are also important differences which strongly suggest that in addition to immunosuppression other factors are required to produce clinical manifestations of a viral mediated disease. This is illustrated by the different clinical presentation of Cytomegalovirus (CMV) in AIDS and bone marrow transplant patients. In the former, pneumonitis is uncommon and the main morbidity is CMV induced retinitis, yet in the bone marrow recipient, CMV pneumonitis is the biggest threat to survival. This implies a selective imbalance between the virus and the immune system resulting in a particular dysfunction as opposed to suppression. For example clinical CMV associated pneumonitis requires an active cytotoxic lymphocyte response to occur and this is why it is rare in AIDS patients. Immune dysfunction may represent selective defects of the humoral or cellular components or both. For example patients with hypogammaglobulinaemia develop selective problems such as chronic enterovirus (ECHO) meningitis, whereas cell mediated immunity deficits may allow an uncontained measles infection resulting in giant cell pneumonia or disseminated herpes infections.

In this chapter we will confine ourselves to problems of viral infections in bone marrow transplant recipients. There are two important situations to be considered. First, where there is an infection with a new virus and, second, the failure of the immune system to prevent reactivation of a latent virus such as CMV, HSV, etc. In this respect if a patient has not been exposed to CMV every effort should be made to avoid exposure to the virus when immunosuppressed. Therefore where possible only CMV seronegative blood products and bone marrow should be given to seronegative patients. Unfortunately, this is not always possible as between 40–80% of most populations have been exposed to CMV by late adolescence. Furthermore screening costs of blood donors is prohibitive in some centres and in an emergency situation it may not be possible to provide seronegative blood in large quantities.

Ubiquitous viruses, such as measles, are more likely to be a problem in younger patients with immune dysfunction as they have had only limited exposure and, therefore, less opportunity to develop immunity. When immune dysfunction is established live virus vaccines are contraindicated but may be used prior to the induction of immunosuppression by, for example, the administration of cancer chemotherapy prior to bone marrow transplantation.

Management of these patients requires rapid and accurate diagnosis. The problem of diagnosing virus infections in the immuno-compromised patient is compounded by the non-specific nature of symptoms such as fever, the absence of localizing signs and often, the failure of these patients to mount a white cell response. Serology is also unhelpful because these patients are unable to mount an appro-priate immune response.

Because of these problems better methods have been developed to identify early infection, particularly as delay in initiating treatment is usually associated with a poorer prognosis. Virus may be identified by electron microscopy, rapid culture methods, immunofluorescence and nucleic acid probe techniques. Specific, effective treatment is unavailable for many virus infections, and in such cases prophylactic measures should be taken whenever possible. Hence for patients known, or suspected, of being exposed to common childhood viral infections, e.g. measles, mumps or varicella zoster, the administration of hyperimmune immunoglobulin is recommended. For a number of common viruses, such as entero-viruses, adenoviruses, parainfluenza and influenza viruses, hyperimmune globulin is not available and no therapy is possible (perhaps with the possible exception of amantadine). Where possible, exposure to these viruses should be vigorously avoided. Many viruses are latent, the virus lying dormant in a non-infectious state at specific sites in the body, and becoming reactivated during periods of immunosuppression. Attempts to eradicate these viruses in the latent state are ineffective, identification of those patients at risk of reacti-vation is important, so that prophylaxis or early treatment can be instituted if required.

Table 10.1 Virus infections in immunocompromised patients

Virus	Syndrome	Cause of reduced immunity
CMV Primary or recurrent	Pneumonitis Disseminated Gastroenteritis	Transplants
	Retinitis	AIDS
HSV	Reactivation Disseminated	Tumours Chemotherapy AIDS
	Persistent local	Transplants
Varicella zoster Primary or recurrent	Disseminated infection Pneumonitis	Transplants Tumours Chemotherapy AIDS
Measles	Disseminated infection Pneumonitis Subacute encephalitis	Transplants Chemotherapy AIDS
Adenovirus	Pneumonia Cystitis Gastroenteritis	Transplants AIDS
Polyomavirus	Cystitis Progressive multifocal Leukoencephalopathy AIDS tumours	Transplants AIDS Tumours
EBV	Fatal mononucleosis Lymphomas	Transplants AIDS
Others Hepatitis viruses Rotavirus Enteroviruses Papillomaviruses		

Killed vaccines have been used successfully in immunocompromised hosts. Thus, annual influenza vaccines reduce the incidence of influenza in populations such as the elderly, and hepatitis B vaccine should be given to patients at risk that includes health care workers. Anti CMV and varicella zoster vaccines are currently under evaluation and their efficacy is being assessed.

The following section will address specific viral problems (Table 10.1).

The herpes virus family

This family compromises a heterologous group of viruses united by a common basic structure. This is an internal double stranded DNA core coding for 80–100 proteins enclosed in a protein capsid. The capsid is surrounded by a lipo-protein envelope derived from the host cell membrane containing both host and viral antigens. Although there are over 60 viruses in this family only five have man as a natural host and are capable of causing clinical problems. These are herpes zoster (the cause of chicken-pox and shingles), herpes simplex (the virus associated with labial, genital and ophthalmic infections), cytomegalovirus (the cause of an infectious mononucleosis syndrome, ophthalmic, gastrointestinal infections and pneumonitis), Epstein–Barr virus (the virus causing infectious mononucleosis and malignances in rare circumstances) and human herpes-6-virus (roseola infantum).

Herpes simplex

Two types of HSV have been identified, types I and II, and the primary infection with these tends to affect different areas of the body. Thus type I is an infection largely of the mouth, face, oesophagus and brain whilst type II infections tend to involve the genital area, rectum, skin of the lower body and meninges. Type II infections tend to be more common as a cause of abnormal ulceration (in patients with AIDS) than type I.

The major clinical features are a vesicular rash which may ulcerate and can involve the oesophagus and rectum. The virus may persist in a latent phase without replication with no detectable immune response. In addition HSV can cause hepatitis, encephalitis and

pneumonia. Although pre-existing antibody may protect against reinfection, the herpes simplex virus tends to set up latent infection so that 90% of all HSV infections in a group of patients with acquired immunosuppression are due to reactivation. The incidence of infection has been shown to be high in leukaemia patients undergoing intensive chemotherapy (60%) and higher still for bone marrow recipients (70–80%), the median time to recurrence being 17–18 days post treatment, i.e. herpes simplex infections tend to occur with greatest frequency early in the neutropenic period. The experience of most groups is that the majority of these infections are type I (approximately 90%) whilst type II is seen in the remaining 10%. The mucocutaneous lesions are clinically distinct between the two viruses. Whereas both types of virus can cause significant morbidity, they are not a major cause of mortality. However, most centres report an overall mortality from HSV infection of <5% in all bone marrow transplant recipients usually due to pneumonia. More recently, an association of HSV infection with mucositis has been more widely recognized. Baglin, *et al.* (1989) reported an increased incidence of isolation of herpes simplex from the mouth in those pyrexial neutropenic patients whose temperature did not settle with antibiotics, compared to those whose temperature did settle on an antibiotic combination.

Diagnosis

E.M. may give a rapid result, otherwise scrapings may show a classical cytopathic effect in 48 hours. Serological titres can confirm the diagnosis retrospectively, but a failure to do so does not exclude the diagnosis.

Management

The nucleoside analogue, acyclovir, or rather its phosphorylated derivative is an extremely effective treatment for herpes simplex infections, it has virtually replaced all its predecessors such as vidarabine and idoxuridine, and is the drug of choice. Due to its selective phosphorylation in infected cells it is a highly specific antiviral agent with few side-effects. Concern over the development of resistance was raised when three cases of H. simplex pneumonia were associated with resistant strains (Ljungman, *et al.*, 1990). Acyclovir resistance in H. Simplex is most commonly associated with thymidine kinase mutants, although polymerase mutants and mutants with altered binding affinities have also been identified. On the whole, thymidine kinase deficient variants appear to be less virulent and their appearance seems to be related to repeat exposure to acyclovir as opposed to its use in prophylaxis, hence the incidence of resistance rises post bone marrow transplantation from 2% after the first episode to 11% after a second episode, nevertheless resistance does not pose a problem at present although it may do so in the future.

Varicella zoster

VZV produces the clinical symptoms of chickenpox and 'shingles', the latter being a reactivation of the dormant virus. VZV infection will occur in 46–50% of bone marrow transplant patients at a median onset of five months post transplantation although some cases may present 3–4 years after transplantation (Locksley, *et al.*, 1985). In the majority of these patients infection is due to reactivation of latent virus which results in local dermatome involvement in 85% and a generalized rash and disseminated disease in the remaining 15%. Herpes zoster will occur in up to 15% of patients with Hodgkin's disease and a slightly smaller proportion (10%) of patients with non-Hodgkin's lymphoma; 30% of these patients progress to disseminated disease with lung, heart, CNS and gastrointestinal tract involvement (Saral, *et al.*, 1984). Varicella poses a particular problem because of dissemination, usually to the lungs, in up to 25% of cases. Mortality due to life-threatening organ involvement is greatest in those presenting with generalized rash or those who disseminate after presenting with initial localized involvement. It is important to note that shingles may involve a single dermatome, overlapping dermatomes or non-contiguous dermatomes and may be complicated by pneumonitis, hepatitis and encephalitis. In those with progressive disease, pulmonary involvement and meningo-encephalitis are reported (in up to 5%) as a cause of death.

Diagnosis

This is often made on clinical grounds. Isolation of virus or virus particles from vesicle fluid in virus culture and identification by direct immunofluorescence or electron microscopy, where available, allows confirmation of the diagnosis. Serology may also be helpful in identifying those at risk of a primary infection; an IgM response may be mounted in both chicken pox and shingles although this may not be reliable in the immunocompromised patient.

Management

Acyclovir is currently the drug of choice, it must be administered intravenously at approximately twice the dose of that required to treat herpes simplex infections. Using such a regimen, acyclovir has been shown to be efficacious in enhancing clinical and virological clearance of lesions in placebo controlled trials. Other agents have been tested *in vitro*. These include the new nucleoside group, oxetanocins which seem to have quite a broad spectrum of activity against most members of the herpes family (Takashi, *et al.*, 1991), and also a series of 6-alkylaminopurine arabinosides whose activity seems to be limited to VZV (Koszalka, *et al.*, 1991). However these drugs are really only at the experimental stage but may offer scope for the future providing any problems with toxicity are reduced. Because of the potential for dissemination in the immunocompromised host, prophylaxis is essential when exposure of these patients to a known case of varicella-zoster has occurred. Zoster immune globulin, ZIG is prepared from the sera of blood donors with a high titre of antibody to VZV, it should be administered to those susceptible preferably within 72 hours. Unfortunately ZIG does not reliably prevent infection, its administration is an attempt to prevent the serious disseminated form of the infection.

Successful immunization with a live attenuated varicella strain has also been achieved (Takahashi, *et al.*, 1974). The vaccine has been shown to confer significant protection to immunocompromised children (i.e. the group most at risk); breakthrough infections can occur in 10–15% vaccinees as antibody levels wane but these are usually mild. Although the vaccine virus can establish latency and has the potential for reactivation as shingles this seems to be less frequent than with the wild strain. The vaccine is not yet licensed in UK or USA but is undergoing extensive clinical trials.

Cytomegalovirus

CMV infection is a serious complication occurring in the early (after 4–16 weeks) post-transplant period and accounting for 15–20% of deaths in this time. Infection is most quickly confirmed by detecting virus antigen or nucleic acid. Important points concerning pathogenesis of CMV have become clear. These include:

1 Infection rates are lower in seronegative compared to seropositive recipients, indicating the importance of viral reactivation
2 Approximately 50% of adult patients develop evidence for active CMV infection
3 Allograft recipients are at a greater risk for development of pneumonitis compared to Autograft recipients
4 Presence of graft versus host disease (GVHD) is associated with an increased incidence of CMV
5 Age of recipient
6 Degree of HLA match between donor and recipient

Wingard, *et al.* (1990) confirmed that the incidence of CMV disease is less than that of active infection, the major determinant being type of transplant – 10% allograft but only 2% autograft recipients were affected.

One of the most serious and dreaded complications is the development of pneumonitis it predominately affects the allograft recipient and may be compounded by the risk factors outlined above. Interestingly the use of cyclosporin as prophylaxis for GVHD seems to be protective (Meyers, *et al.*, 1990).

Many patients with CMV infection remain asymptomatic so that simply demonstrating a rise in virus titre or isolating the virus from saliva or urine are not indications for treatment. The clinical manifestations of this infection, however, are manifold and appear to be influenced by the setting in which infection occurs. Thus, pneumonitis occurs in up to 10% of patients post bone marrow transplantation, with enteritis being seen in only 1% of patients and retinitis only rarely (<0.2% in reported series). In the setting of CMV infection occurring in AIDS patients however, retinitis is the commonest clinical manifestation, followed by enteritis. Whilst CMV pneumonitis can occur it is usually as a co-pathogen and commonly resolves with treatment of the other pathogen. Post bone marrow transplantation pneumonitis still carries an 80–90% mortality in most centres. Interestingly, some centres are now reporting a fall in the incidence of CMV pneumonitis post transplant and it has been suggested that this is secondary to the reduced incidence of GvHD that is seen with the more widespread and judicious use of cyclosporin A as GvHD prophylaxis.

Diagnosis

Serological tests for CMV are not sensitive or reliable enough to confirm CMV disease. Even during a primary infection IgM may or may not be produced and the length of time it persists can vary greatly.

Because of the above problems and the inherent delay in serological diagnosis, efforts have been concentrated on the rapid detection of the virus in patient specimens to confirm the diagnosis. The standard technique of observing a cytopathic effect in cell culture is time consuming, taking up to 21 days before a negative result can be claimed. The advent of monoclonal antibodies, however, has allowed the rapid identification of viral antigens in biopsy samples (e.g. bronchoalveolar lavage centrifugation) or in cell culture, or in detection of early antigen fluorescent foci (DEAFF test) (Stirk and Griffiths, 1987). Meyers, *et al.* (1990) have found that viraemia is a positive predictor for the development of pneumonitis and is superior to the detection of virus shedding in urine or saliva. The implication being that regular surveillance cultures will identify those most at risk of developing pneumonitis, thus allowing time to institute treatment with ganciclovir. This approach was also used by Schmidt, *et al.* (1991) who investigated the outcome of bone marrow transplant patients who underwent a diagnostic bronchoalveolar lavage on day 35. If CMV was isolated the patients were randomized to receive ganciclovir or not (Schmidt, *et al.*, 1991). A significant improvement in mortality was seen in the treated group compared to the untreated.

Management

Until recently the therapeutic strategies available for the treatment of these infections have been disappointing, but the use of new agents has resulted in encouraging results and greater optimism for the future (Miescher and Jaffe, 1990). Whilst the use of ganciclovir, as a single agent, has met with limited success in the treatment of pneumonitis when given together with high dose intravenous immunoglobulin the combination is reported to cause 50–70% resolution of infection although controlled trials of this combination are still awaited (Reed, *et al.*, 1988); (Wingard, 1990).

The mechanism of action of the combination has not been fully elucidated, but it is thought (Grundy, 1987) that the immunoglobulins may block T-cell mediated destruction of lung tissue, while ganciclovir reduces the viral load. Even if these results are confirmed problems still remain because up to 30% of cases will fail to respond.

CMV gastroenteritis can also occur, this may present as a gastritis, gastric ulcerations, duodenitis, oesophagitis, pyloric perforation or haemorrhagic colitis. Endoscopy is usally required to make the diagnosis and the lesions usually respond to ganciclovir alone, although they may relapse.

The toxicity profile of ganciclovir is considerable, particularly post bone marrow transplantation where the myelo-suppressive complications, particularly neutropenia, may compromise the use of this drug in adequate doses for prolonged periods, although this is usually reversible on discontinuing the drug.

CMV prophylaxis needs to weigh the advantages of treatment against its side-effects, and thus the use of CMV negative blood products or an in-line leucocyte depletion filter, which removes up to 98% of leucocytes, are advocated for seronegative recipients receiving a bone marrow from a seronegative donor. Such products are not, however, always readily available and if this is the case, or a seronegative recipient is receiving marrow from a seropositive donor. Another option is the administration of intravenous immune globulin. A schedule of repeated doses for up to a year reduced the incidence of interstitial pneumonia although the reduction due to CMV was less impressive. In the same study a significant reduction in the incidence of acute GVHD was also observed (Sullivan, *et al.*, 1990). The use of acyclovir in high dose ($500\,mgs/m^2$ intravenously 8-hourly) throughout the transplant period has also been shown to be an effective prophylaxis in the CMV seropositive recipient group. Not only was the incidence of infection and active disease reduced but also the overall mortality (Meyers, *et al.*, 1988). It should be noted in this context that acyclovir given to some AIDS patients with H2V infection has been associated with progression of CMV retinitis to blindness and should be used with caution in this setting.

A more economical approach to prophylaxis has been in the development of a vaccine. The final results of a 10-year study by Plotkin *et al.* have recently shown that the Towne strain of CMV as a live attenuated vaccine reduces the severity of CMV disease (not infection) in the recipient negative donor positive group of renal transplant patients (Plotkin, *et al.*, 1991). However, there is still the worry about its oncogenic potential and possible teratogenesis in pregnant women – a subunit vaccine would be a safer and more acceptable alternative. Until the immunogenic epitopes of CMV are full elucidated the development of a subunit vaccine will be slow.

Foscarnet also has activity against CMV but it is a toxic agent and must be given intravenously, its major side-effects are renal and electrolyte dysfunction. The combination of ganciclovir and foscarnet may well be synergistic as suggested by a recent case report of CMV retinitis in an HIV patient which failed to respond to either agent alone. The combination prevented further deterioration, and the retinitis remained quiescent (Nelson, *et al.*, 1991).

The most important determinant of survival from CMV infection, however, is the development of a cytotoxic cellular response by the NK or T-lymphocytes. A novel approach to the treatment and prophylaxis of CMV infections which is currently in a pre-clinical stage is to boost cellular immunity of the recipient by administering isolated subpopulations of anti-CMV lymphocytes whose cellular responses have been amplified by the use of cytokines. More recently an anti-CMV vaccine has been developed which in clinical trials of CMV negative patients post renal transplantation has been shown to be effective in reducing the incidence of primary CMV infection. Further developments in this field are awaited.

Epstein–Barr virus (EBV)

The role of EBV as a pathogen in immuno-compromised hosts remains to be elucidated. Although EBV can be isolated from a high proportion of immunocompromised patients it is only rarely associated with any clinical syndrome. These include fever, hepatitis, cytopenia and lymphomas. Interestingly there is increased evidence for an association between B cell lymphomas in CNS and EBV in AIDS patients and perhaps other immunocom-promised groups (Anonymous, 1991). Most infections probably represent recrudescence of a latent virus because up to 90% of adult patients can be shown to have protective neutralizing antibodies. Hence, although the virus is associated with white cells and may be transmitted by transfusion, primary infections are less common perhaps because antibody present in the sera transfused with the leuco-cytes may be protective.

Diagnosis

Diagnosis is dependent on detecting rising titres of anti-EBV IgM antibody or the presence of heterophile antibody. More recently antibody to specific viral epitopes, such as the capsid and early antigen, has enabled a more specific diagnosis. Cell culture can show active EBV replication using DNA hybridization. An oligo-clonal lymphoproliferative disorder is associ-ated with EBV infection post renal trans-plantation. These tumours do not exhibit any consistent chromosomal abnormalities and are sensitive to T-cell control, perhaps via the same lipid membrane protein that acts as the receptor for the Epstein–Barr virus on the B-cell. The Epstein–Barr nuclear antigen is expressed by the Burkitt lymphoma cells in 90% of the African variety and a somewhat smaller pro-portion (20%) of the non-endemic 'American' form of the disease. Furthermore, the tumour cells are monoclonal and express a consistent chromosomal abnormality involving reciprocal translocation from chromosome 8 to, most usually, chromosome 14 t(8–14). Less com-monly, chromosome 2 or 22 t(2:8), t(8:22) is involved. This abnormality is not seen in patients with infectious mononucleosis and the tumour is not sensitive to T-cell control.

In addition to the lymphoma and suscepti-bility to viral infections seen in generalized immunodeficiency states, there are a number of families reported possessing a selective defect in resistance to the EB virus that is transmitted genetically in an X-linked recessive manner. In the proband of patients with this X-linked lymphoproliferative syndrome (Purtillo, *et al.*, 1974), primary infection with the EB virus results in secondary hypogammaglobulinaemia bilirubinaemia, chronic lymphoproliferative disease or an acute fatal infectious mono-nucleosis syndrome. Only in a few patients does Burkitt's lymphoma develop. These patients appear to be unable to mount an anti-EBNA antibody response and do not produce NK cells in response to interferon. The immunological abnormality, however, remains unresolved.

Treatment

Acyclovir does not appear to affect the clinical course or outcome of EB virus disease although it may reduce oropharyngeal shedding of the virus. No other specific treatment of the virus has been found effective and treatment should therefore be directed to the lymphoma (Sullivan, *et al.*, 1984). There is no effective prophylactic therapy. Spontaneous resolution of the lymphoma has been reported with cessation of immunosuppression if this can be done safely.

Human herpes 6 virus (HHV-6)

HHV-6 was first isolated in 1986 by Salaluddin, *et al.* It is a double-stranded DNA virus, distinct from other members of the herpes family which has an associated seroprevalence of between 20 and 100% in normal populations. Disease associations include *Roseola infantum*, post viral fatigue syndrome and possibly lympho-proliferative conditions. A recent report by Carrigan, *et al.* (1991) have implicated HHV-6 in 2 bone-marrow transplant patients who developed fatal pneumonitis. In both instances its close relative, CMV, was excluded and it is postulated that the disease process occurred secondary to reactivation of HHV-6, previous exposure shown by seropositivity. In vitro studies have shown HHV-6 is susceptible to ganciclovir (Reed, *et al.*, 1988).

Hepatitis B virus (HBV)

Haematological patients used to be at great risk from acquiring HBV via blood products and in some parts of the world they still are. An acute HBV infection may lead to complete recovery, asymptomatic antigenaemia or chronic hepatitis. In all cases the virus genome persists in the liver. Reactivation can occur irrespective of patients' HBsAg status and can be diagnosed by the presence of hepatitis B e antigen (HBeAg), HBsAg, HBV-DNA or HBV-DNA polymerase in the serum. Again, the role of the immune response in the pathogenesis of disease is underscored by the fact that immunosuppressed patients may not suffer from destructive hepatitis but successful reconstitution, i.e. after a marrow transplant, may lead to an exacerbation which may be fulminant. There is no effective antiviral agent currently available but alpha interferon is showing promising results.

Measles

Vaccinated immunocompromised children do not get measles, therefore the at risk population are young native unvaccinated children.

The major clinical features are giant cell pneumonia seen in children with malignancy, where it is the biggest single cause of treatment-related mortality, and subacute measles encephalitis (SME). The latter occurs usually within six months of initial illness and may be rapidly progressive; it does not occur in normal hosts. Subacute sclerosing panencephalitis (SSPE) can occur in the immunocompetent, it is a fatal slowly progressive degeneration of the brain, and usually occurs after an interval of 6–8 years. It is thought that the virus replicates slowly in the CNS, probably in a mutant form.

The typical rash of measles may be absent in the immunocompromised host due to the lack of cell mediated immunity. Therefore diagnosis is by isolation from mucous washing, urine or lymphocytes. Unfortunately, the diagnosis of measles is occasionally first suspected only at autopsy. No specific treatment exists although gammaglobulin is often given if the patient is known, or suspected of being exposed to the virus before symptoms develop. The measles vaccine is a live virus and should not be given to those already immunocompromised.

Adenoviruses

These cause fever, diarrhoea and pneumonia and occasionally death. Fatal pneumonia is associated with types 1, 5 and 7 (Shields, *et al.*, 1985). Haematuria is associated with urine isolates of types 31–34. Hepatitis has also been described.

Diagnosis

Diagnosis is by EM and isolation with typing defined by serological and restriction endonuclease mapping techniques. There is no consistently effective treatment and the only vaccine that is currently available contains a few serotypes only.

Polyomaviruses

Isolates BK and JC are ubiquitous and may be associated with unrelated ureteric stenosis and progressive multifocal leucoencephalopathy (PML). This latter complication is associated with the JC virus which, although commonly isolated in immunosuppressed patients, rarely leads to clinical signs of PML. BK is associated with haemorrhagic cystitis following bone marrow transplantation. Diagnosis is by culture on human embryo fibroblasts and PML is confirmed by CT scan and brain biopsy in suspected cases. No effective treatment or prophylaxis is available.

Papillomaviruses

Warts are a feature of patients with a cell mediated defect and as such are common (18–30%) in patients with leukaemia and Hodgkin's disease. Mucosal infections and cervical neoplasia are at least nine times higher in transplant patients than normal patients. Diagnosis requires cytological examination of smears and biopsies, by direct DNA-DNA hybridization and by polymerase chain reaction (PCR).

Other viruses

Less commonly severe gastrointestinal and respiratory infections may be caused by other viruses usually only associated with mild illnesses in the immunocompetent. Respiratory syncytial virus, the causative agent in bronchiolitis, may be life threatening in the immunocompromised setting and has been reported as the cause in three severe cases of pneumonia in BMT recipients (Martin, *et al.*, 1988). It should always be considered as a potential pathogen especially during the winter months. Similarly enteroviruses have resulted in disseminated fulminant infections (Briggs, *et al.*, 1990).

Conclusion

The main viruses affecting haematological patients which can be treated are HSV, VZV and CMV. Fortunately, acyclovir is non-toxic and prophylactic therapy can be given. The main problem is CMV pneumonitis which is often fatal. The problem is whether or not to give prophylactic therapy. As the disease takes over a month to declare itself, prophylaxis requires a non-toxic drug. Ganciclovir is the only agent with major anti-CMV activity but at the expense of marked bone marrow. Clearly there is a need for a non-toxic anti-CMV agent which could be given to all patients prophylactically. The role of CMV immunoglobulin is also not clear. These and other questions remain to be conclusively answered in order to cope adequately with these major clinical problems. The main solution in all these patients is to try to redress the underlying immune deficiency as soon as possible, a situation which is not always easily obtained.

Newer methods of detection which are both more rapid and sensitive are being developed. The polymerase chain reaction (PCR) previously regarded as a research tool, is rapidly being included in the routine diagnostic armamentarium offered by most virology laboratories. Although it promises to overshadow previous techniques in terms of speed and sensitivity, the test does lack a certain 'robustness', necessary for use as a routine diagnostic test. Quantification of virus in clinical specimens by PCR is also being developed (Fox, *et al.*, 1992). This is necessary as PCR does not distinguish between active or latent infections, and therefore to be of use prognostically it is important to be able to assess viral load, and monitor any changes.

References

Anonymous (1991) Epstein-Barr virus and AIDS-associated lymphomas [editorial]. *Lancet*, **338**, 979–981

Baglin, T.P., Gray, J.J., Marcus, R.E. and Wreghitt, T.G. (1989) Antibiotic resistant fever associated with herpes simplexvirus infection in nuetropenic patients with haematological malignancy. *Journal of Clinical Pathology*, **42**, 1255–1258

Biggs, D.D., Toorkey, B.C., Carrigan, D.R., Hanson, G.A., Ash, R.C. (1990) Disseminated echovirus infection complicating bone marrow transplantation. *American Journal of Medicine*, **88**, 421–425

Carrigan, D.R., Drobyski, W.R., Russler, S.K., Tapper, M.A., Knox, K.K. and Ash, R.C. (1991) Interstitial pneumonitis associated with human herpesvirus-6 infection after marrow transplantation. *Lancet*, **338**, 147–149

Fox, J.C., Griffiths, P.D. and Emery, V.C. (1992) Quantification of human cytomegalovirus DNA using the polymerase chain reaction. *Journal of General Virology*, **73**(9), 2405–2408

Grundy, J.E., Shanley, J.D. and Griffiths, P.D. (1987) Is cytomegalovirus interstitial pneumonitis in transplant recipients an immunopathological condition? *Lancet*, **2**, 996–999

Holland, H.K., Wingard, J.R. and Saral, R. (1990) Herpes virus and enteric viral infections in bone marrow transplantation: clinical presentations, pathogenesis and therapeutic strategies. *Cancer Investigation*, **8**, 509–521

Koszalka, G.W., Averett, D.R., Fyfe, J.A., Roberts, G.B., Spector, T., Biron, K. and Krenitsky, T.A. (1991) 6-N-substituted derivatives of adenine arabinoside as selective inhibitors of varicella-zoster virus. *Antimicrobials Agents and Chemotherapy*, **35**, 1437–1443

Levin, M.J. (1990) Current approaches to the prevention and treatment of cytomegalovirus disease after bone marrow transplantation: an overview. *Seminars in Hematology*, **27**(Suppl 1), 1–4

Ljungman, P., Ellis, M., Hackman, R.C., Shepp, D.H. and Meyers, J.D. (1990) Acyclovir-resistant herpes simplex virus causing pneumonia after marrow transplantation. *Journal of Infectious Diseases*, **162**, 244–248

Locksley, R.M., Flournoy, N., Sullivan, K.M. and Meyers, J.D. (1985) Infection with varicella-zoster virus after marrow transplantation. *Journal of Infectious Diseases*, **152**, 1172–1181

Martin, M.A., Bock, M.J., Pfaller, M.A. and Wenzel, R.P. (1988) Respiratory syncytial virus infections in adult bone marrow transplant recipients. *Lancet*, **1**, 1396–1397

Meyers, J.D., Reed, E.C., Shepp, D.H., Thornquist, M., Dandliker, P.S., Vicary, C.A., Flournoy, N., Kirk, L.E., Kersey, J.H., Thomas, E.D., *et al.* (1988) Acyclovir for prevention of cytomegalovirus infection and disease after allogeneic marrow transplantation. *New England Journal of Medicine*, **318**, 70–75

Meyers, J.D., Ljungman, P. and Fisher, L.D. (1990) Cytomegalovirus excretion as a predictor of cytomegalovirus disease after marrow transplantation: importance of cytomegalovirus viraemia. *Journal of Infectious Diseases*, **162**, 373–380

Nelson, M.R., Barter, G., Hawkins, D. and Gazzard, B.G. (1991) Simultaneous treatment of cytomegalovirus retinitis with ganciclovir and foscarnet. *Lancet*, **338**, 250

Plotkin, S.A., Starr, S.E., Friedman, H.M., Brayman, K., Harris, S., Jackson, S., Tustin, N.B., Grossman, R., Dafoe, D. and Barker, C. (1991) Effect of Towne live virus vaccine on cytomegalovirus disease after renal transplant. A controlled trial. *Annals of Internal Medicine*, **114**, 525–531

Purtilo, D.T., Cassel, C. and Yang, J.P. (1974) Fatal infectious mononucleosis in familial lymphohistiocytosis. *New England Journal of Medicine*, **291**, 736

Reed, E.C., Bowden, R.A., Dandliker, P.S., Lilleby, K.E. and Meyers, J.D. (1988) Treatment of cytomegalovirus pneumonia with ganciclovir and intravenous cytogalovirus immunoglobulin in patients with bone marrow transplants. *Annals of Internal Medicine*, **109**, 783–788

Sakuma, T., Saijo, M., Suzutani, T., Yoshida, I., Saito, S., Kitagawa, M., Hasegawa, S. and Azuma, M. (1991) Antiviral activity of oxetanocins against varicella-zoster virus. *Antimicrobial Agents and Chemotherapy*, **35**, 1512–1514

Saral, R., Burns, W.H. and Prentice, H.G. (1984) Herpes virus infections: clinical manifestations and therapeutic strategies in immunocompromised patients. *Clinics in Haematology*, **13**, 645–660

Schmidt, G.M., Horak, D.A., Niland, J.C., Duncan, S.R., Forman, S.J. and Zaia, J.A. (1991) A randomized, controlled trial of prophylactic ganciclovir for cytomegalovirus pulmonary infection in recipients of allogenic bone marrow transplants; The City of Hope-Stanford-Syntex CMV Study Group. *New England Journal of Medicine*, **324**, 1005–1011

Shields, A.F., Hackman, R.C., Fife, K.H., Corey, L. and Meyers, J.D. (1985) Adenovirus infections in patients undergoing bone-marrow transplantation. *New England Journal of Medicine*, **312**, 529–533

Stirk, P.R. and Griffiths, P.D. (1987) Use of monoclonal antibodies for the diagnosis of cytomegalovirus infection by the detection of early antigen fluorescent foci (DEAFF) in cell culture. *Journal of Medical Virology*, **21**, 329–337

Sullivan, J.L., Medveczky, P., Forman, S.J., Bakerm S.M., Monroe, J.E. and Mulder, C. (1984) Epstein-Barr-virus induced lymphoproliferation. Implications for antiviral chemotherapy. *New England Journal of Medicine*, **311**, 1163–1167

Sullivan, K.M., Kopecky, K.J., Jocom, J., Fisher, L., Buckner, C.D., Meyers, J.D., Counts, G.W., Bowden, R.A., Peterson, F.B., Witherspoon, R.P., *et al.* (1990) Immunomodulatory and antimicrobial efficacy of intravenous immunoglobulin in bone marrow transplantation. *New England Journal of Medicine*, **323**, 705–712

Takahashi, M., Otsuka, T., Okuno, Y., Asano, Y. and Yazaki, T. (1974) Live vaccine used to prevent the spread of varicella in children in hospital. *Lancet*, **2**, 1288–1290

Wingard, J.R. (1990) Advances in the management of infectious complications after bone marrow transplantation. *Bone Marrow Transplantation*, **6**, 371–383

Wingard, J.R., Piantadosi, S., Burns, W.H., Zahurak, M.L., Santos, G.W. and Saral, R. (1990) Cytomegalovirus infections in bone marrow transplant recipients given intensive cytoreductive therapy. *Reviews of Infectious Diseases*, **12**(Suppl 7), S793–804

11

Oral and peri-anal infections in the immunocompromised host

Stephen M. Kelsey and C. Daniel Overholser

Introduction

The numerous advances in the treatment of patients with haematological malignancy have led to an increased awareness of the infective complications of these diseases and their treatment. Infections of the oropharynx and peri-anal regions are important causes of morbidity in immunosuppressed patients, particularly those receiving chemotherapy or undergoing bone marrow transplantation (BMT). Long periods of neutropenia in these patients predispose the mouth and ano-rectal regions to local infection by a wide variety of agents. In addition, the breakdown of intact mucosa at these sites provides a portal of entry into the bloodstream for colonizing or commensal, but potentially pathogenic, organisms. Oropharyngeal infections may occur in around 40% of patients receiving chemotherapy for haematological malignancy (Sonis, Sonis and Lieberman, 1978; Peterson and Overholser, 1981a; Dreizen, et al., 1986; Barrett, 1987) and in up to 60% of patients undergoing BMT (Barrett, 1986). Peri-anal infections have been documented in 3–14% cases (Schimpff, et al., 1972a; Howard, 1983).

There are a number of reasons why these sites are particularly prone to infective complications. Periodontal disease (gingivitis and periodontitis) is the inflammatory response to a mixed bacterial infection that occurs on the surface of the teeth next to the gingiva. Periodontal disease pre-exists in a large proportion of patients presenting for treatment, largely due to poor oral hygiene. The effects of periodontal disease are exacerbated by chemotherapy (Overholser, 1986). In addition, chemotherapeutic agents are toxic to the rapidly proliferating cells of the gastro-intestinal mucosa (Bottomley, Perlin and Ross, 1977). The resulting mucositis, together with neutropenia, removes the barrier to local tissue infection and bloodstream invasion by colonizing organisms. Mucosal damage may be even more severe following total body irradiation (TBI), often used as part of conditioning regimens prior to BMT (Meyers, 1986). A broad range of potentially pathogenic organisms can be isolated from the mouth and ano-rectum of patients receiving chemotherapy (Schimpff, et al., 1972). It has been estimated that approximately half of these organisms colonize the patient during hospitalization and therapy, whereas the other half are present at initial diagnosis. Up to 86% of infections occurring in neutropenic patients after chemotherapy can be documented to have arisen from endogenous flora (Pizzo, 1981). In addition, infections of the oropharynx and ano-rectal regions, together with those of the lower respiratory tract, are more likely to be associated with bloodstream invasion than infection at other sites.

Oral infections in immunosuppressed patients can be broadly divided into dental infections (periodontal, pulp and periapical disease) and those of the mucosa and surrounding tissues. Bacteria are the commonest infecting agents causing, or exacerbating, the former. The immunosuppressed patient, however, is also susceptible to viral and fungal infection. Peri-anal disease and its management will be discussed separately.

Bacterial infections

Bacterial infection of the oropharynx occurs in approximately 12% of patients following chemotherapy, thus accounting for one-third of oral infections during the neutropenic period (Dreizen, *et al.*, 1986). Infection predominantly involves the periodontal and pulpal regions of the teeth and gums. Local and systemic invasion may also occur.

Periodontal disease

It has been estimated that 83% to 98% of adults in the general population are affected by periodontal disease, the incidence increasing with age (Goldman and Cohen, 1973). Colonization of dental plaque by bacteria, and the resultant inflammatory response, causes toxin production and metabolism of local nutrients. This leads to gingival ulceration. Such ulceration creates a portal of entry for organisms directly into surrounding soft tissues and bloodstream, particularly during periods of neutropenia (Overholser, 1986). Severity and duration of oral infective problems after chemotherapy have been shown to correlate with pre-existing levels of plaque and periodontal disease (Hickey, Toth and Lindquist, 1982).

Prevention of periodontal infection in neutropenic patients depends upon early dental evaluation and good oral hygiene. Patients without neutrophils do not display the classic symptoms and signs of an acute inflammatory reaction (Peterson and Overholser, 1979); the presence and progression of the disease may therefore go unnoticed without careful dental examination (Overholser, *et al.*, 1982a). Dental evaluation and treatment prior to chemotherapy have been shown to reduce the septicaemia rate (Greenberg, *et al.*, 1982). Oral chlorhexidine mouth washes (0.1–0.2%), continued throughout the neutropenic period, have been shown to be effective in reducing gingivitis and mucositis in patients receiving treatment for acute leukaemia (McGaw and Belch, 1985) and those undergoing BMT (Ferretti, *et al.*, 1987). Chlorhexidine is bacterostatic against Gram-positive and Gram-negative organisms

and has also been shown to have anti-fungal activity *in vitro* although no effect on *Candida* colonization *in vivo* has been demonstrated (Sharon, *et al.*, 1977). Manipulation of teeth and gums has been shown to produce transient bacteraemias in normal subjects; brushing of teeth has therefore been regarded as a controversial issue in neutropenic patients, particularly in the presence of inevitably co-existent thrombocytopenia. It does not appear, however, that an increased risk of systemic infection arises from maintenance of these routine dental measures throughout chemotherapy and subsequent periods of neutropenia (Peterson, *et al.*, 1981).

When advanced periodontal disease is encountered in leukaemic or aplastic patients dental extractions can often be safely performed (Overholser, *et al.*, 1982b). Thrombocytopenic patients ($< 50 \times 10^9/l$) should have platelets available for transfusion. Granulocytopenic patients usually require antibiotic cover. In patients about to receive myelosuppressive chemotherapy the extractions should be performed approximately three days before therapy to allow about ten days of healing. Any exacerbation of periodontal disease during or immediately following chemotherapy, however, should be treated conservatively. Teeth should not be extracted until peripheral blood neutrophil and platelet counts are reconstituted due to the high risk of infection, bleeding and poor wound healing. Local gingival cellulitis may respond to metronidazole (Barrett, 1987). If fever is associated, treatment with systemic broad spectrum antibiotics (e.g. a combination of an aminoglycoside with a ureidopenicillin) should be commenced.

In general, severely immunocompromised patients require an uncomplicated and atraumatic oral hygiene regimen (Carl, 1986). Intermediate restorative dental treatment should be performed in advance where possible. Surgical manipulation should be avoided until the bone marrow has reconstituted.

Pulp and periapical disease

Pulpal pathology is invariably infectious in nature and may account for 5–10% of oral complications of chemotherapy (Overholser, 1986). Infection spreads in an apical direction and may involve periapical alveolar bone. Such infection may lie dormant in immunocompetent subjects but may become acute when host resistance is diminished. Prevention of pulpal infection and its complications are preferable to treatment during periods of myelosuppression. Early pulpal pathosis is reversible and conservative dental restorative treatment is appropriate. Advanced pulpal pathosis is irreversible. Ideally tooth extraction or endodontic treatment is indicated prior to commencement of chemotherapy. If infection is encountered after chemotherapy, or has spread beyond the pulp into surrounding alveolar bone, treatment with systemic broad spectrum antibiotics is required until neutrophil recovery occurs.

Acute necrotizing ulcerative gingivitis (ANUG)

ANUG is an opportunistic infection frequently seen in young adults in stressful situations (Goldhaber and Giddon, 1964). It comprises a small proportion of oral infective complications following cancer chemotherapy but has been particularly reported in association with treatment for Hodgkin's disease (Sonis, Sonis and Lieberman, 1978). It is thought to be caused by a symbiotic combination of a fusiform bacillus (*Fusobacterium dentum*) and a spirochete (*Borrelia vincentii*) (Greenberg, 1984). Treatment should be by maintenance of good oral hygiene and penicillin in neutropenic patients or patients with leukaemia. Local surgical debridement should be carried out following immune recovery.

Systemic and invasive bacterial infection

The oral cavity is a significant source of bacteraemia in patients with acute leukaemia (Greenberg, *et al.*, 1982). A wide variety of pathogens may cause sepsis following the breakdown of mucosal barriers (Brown, 1984). Colonization of the oral cavity with enterobacteria (e.g. *E. coli*, *Klebsiella*) or *Pseudomonas spp.* may precede severe infection in these patients (Johansen, Woods and Chauduri, 1979; Weibren, *et al.*, 1988). Hospitalization, coupled with broad spectrum antibiotic therapy, creates conditions which favour oral colonization with enterobacteria and enterococci (Wahlin and Holm, 1988). Administration of chemotherapy or the presence of specific disease states *per se* seems

to have little effect on oral colonization patterns. Pseudomonas may cause severe bacteraemic shock or may invade local tissue resulting in oropharyngeal ulceration and facial cellulitis (Weibren, *et al.*, 1988). *Staphylococcus epidermis* and *Streptococci*, both normal mouth commensal organisms, may be pathogenic in neutropenic patients (Brown, 1984). Oral ulceration from chemotherapy has been shown to predispose to streptococcal septicaemia, particularly from *Streptococcus mitis*, an inhabitant of normal buccal mucosa (Cohen, *et al.*, 1983). Increasing severity and duration of mucositis, as associated with BMT conditioning, increases the risk of streptococcal bacteraemia (Bostrom and Weisdorf, 1984).

Patterns of colonization and infection vary geographically between cancer treatment centres. The nature of prevalent organisms depend to a large extent on the use of prophylactic gut decontamination and mouthcare regimens. The introduction of regimens aimed at selectively eradicating Gram-negative organisms have been partially responsible for the dramatic rise in the number of Gram-positive organisms responsible for bacteraemia in neutropenic patients over the last decade (Kelsey, *et al.*, 1990a). Persistence of organisms at inaccessible sites, bacterial resistance to antiseptics and poor compliance with prophylactic antibacterial measures nevertheless ensures that immunocompromised patients are at continued risk of Gram-negative infections.

Viral infections

Herpes viruses form the majority of viral pathogens causing oropharyngeal infections in immunocompromised patients. In particular herpes simplex virus (HSV) is a common cause of oral cavity-associated morbidity following chemotherapy for haematological malignancy or BMT. Improved methods of detection have led to an increased awareness of the importance of these viruses as pathogens during periods of immune suppression.

Herpes simplex virus (HSV)

The incidence of oropharyngeal HSV infection following chemotherapy is between 10% and 40% (Meyers, *et al.*, 1982; Barrett, 1987) and may be higher following BMT (Pizzo, 1981). The vast majority of infections are reactivations of previously acquired, latent disease; fewer than 2% are thought to be primary infections (Meyers, Thomas and Flournoy, 1980). Patients who are seropositive for HSV prior to treatment are therefore at greatly increased risk of developing oral infection with the virus (Redding and Montgomery, 1989). Another major risk factor for HSV disease is the degree of immunosuppression that is induced. TBI, during BMT conditioning, is the most important promoter of HSV reactivation (Heimdal, *et al.*, 1989).

Although the majority of HSV infections are seen while patients are neutropenic, infection appears to be more directly associated with lymphopenia (Baglin, *et al.*, 1989). This is in keeping with proposed mechanism of T-lymphocyte-mediated immunity against HSV (Rand, *et al.*, 1977). Reactivation rarely occurs while chemotherapy is being administered. It has been suggested that anthracyclines and cytosine arabinoside, commonly included in anti-leukaemic chemotherapy protocols, directly inhibit viral replication (Lam, *et al.*, 1981).

Lesions of HSV infection usually appear within the first three weeks after BMT or cessation of chemotherapy (Kolbinson, 1988). Recognition of oropharyngeal HSV infection may be difficult in these periods of immuno-suppression. Lesions may be atypical in nature and appearance and may occur anywhere within the oral cavity (Montgomery, Redding and LeMaistre, 1986). Oral ulceration which yields positive cultures for HSV tends to be more severe, of longer duration and associated with more severe pain (Kolbinson, *et al.*, 1988). In addition, herpetic ulceration may form a portal of entry into the blood for bacterial flora colonizing the oral cavity. Fever may also be associated with oral HSV infection in its own right; muco-cutaneous HSV infection in neutro-penic patients is commonly associated with antibiotic-resistant fever (Baglin, *et al.*, 1989). The clinical course of oral HSV infection is variable. Lesions may be self-limiting despite on-going immunosuppression. Systemic spread of virus, though uncommon, may occur and may be associated with high mortality (Barrett, 1986). Viral oesophagitis or pneumonitis are the most likely sequelae.

The antiviral drug acyclovir (Zovirax, Wellcome) is effective against active HSV infection in immunocompromised patients (Selby, *et al.*, 1979). Latent virus, however, is not eliminated (Perna and Eskinazi, 1988). In active infection administration of acyclovir is associated with reduced duration of viral shedding and reduced pain of oral lesions. Toxicity and adverse reactions are minimal (Meyers, *et al.*, 1982). There has been recent interest in prophylactic use of acyclovir to prevent HSV infection in seropositive patients undergoing chemotherapy or BMT. Results have been encouraging. Intravenous acyclovir almost completely prevents oropharyngeal HSV infection post BMT and significantly reduces the infection rate following chemo-therapy (Hann, *et al.*, 1983; Redding and Montgomery, 1989). The mechanism of action may not actually be to prevent virus reacti-vation in the nerve root but to suppress appear-ance of clinically detectable lesions and associated symptoms at the mucosal site (Perna and Eskinazi, 1989). As a result acyclovir needs to be continued throughout the period of post-treatment immunosupression. Cessation of therapy prematurely is associated with rebound infection. Prophylactic acyclovir has also been shown to reduce the period of post-chemo-therapy neutropenia, possibly by preventing the direct myelosuppressive effect of HSV infection (Hann, *et al.*, 1983).

It is unclear whether the potential benefits of prophylactic systemic acyclovir therapy justify its cost. Oral acyclovir is cheaper than the intravenous preparation but is less effective as similar serum drug levels are not achieved (Redding and Montgomery, 1983). It has been suggested that prophylaxis is justified in HSV seropositive BMT recipients due to the greater risk of reactivation and subsequent morbidity than in those patients undergoing chemo-therapy in whom the degree of immuno-suppression is less profound (Barrett, 1986). Another potential disadvantage of prophylactic acyclovir administration is development of viral resistance. Resistance may emerge during the treatment of established oral HSV lesions although the significance is unclear (Gray, Wreghitt and Baglin, 1989). Resistant mutations, however, are most likely to occur in replicating virions. Prophylactic acyclovir, by suppressing viral replication, may therefore actually reduce the risk of resistance rather than encouraging it (Ambinder, *et al.*, 1984).

Fungal infections

The incidence of fungal infection in immuno-compromised patients, particularly those rendered neutropenic by chemotherapy or BMT, has increased over the last fifteen years (Ray, 1987). Oral fungal infections may occur in up to 40% of patients undergoing treatment for haematological malignancy (McElroy, 1984) and fungi may account for over 60% of oral pathogens isolated in these patients (Dreizen, *et al.*, 1986). As with bacterial infection, oral fungal infection in cancer patients is encouraged by the presence of neutropenia and mucositis. Broad spectrum antibiotic therapy and high-dose corticosteroids, which are commonly included in chemotherapy protocols, also encourage the proliferation of fungi in the oral cavity. *Candida albicans* is the most prevalent pathogen. *Candida tropicalis*, *Torulopsis glabrata* and *Aspergillus* species, particularly *fumigatus* and *flavus*, are also commonly identified.

Candida

Colonization of the oral cavity appears to be the starting point for infection. Colonization with *Candida spp.* occurs in the oral cavity in up to 80% of patients with leukaemia (Sharon, *et al.*, 1977) and is invariable after BMT (Kolbinson, *et al.*, 1988) although it may be transitory.

Candida infection may manifest initially as local lesions. Lesions may be typical in appearance with cream or white plaques and surrounding erythema. They may be extensive and painful in the severely immunocompromised patient. Spread into the oesophagus or lung may occur and direct invasion into the blood-stream, with resulting fungaemia and disseminated visceral infection, is not uncommon. The risk of systemic invasion by *Candida* is primarily dependent upon duration of neutropenia. However, duration of colonization and the number of body sites colonized are also important (Sandford, *et al.*, 1980). Systemic candidiasis occurs in 10–20% of patients with acute leukaemia and is associated with a high mortality (Peterson, *et al.*, 1981). Invasive *Candida* has been found at post-mortem examination in up to 40% of patients following BMT (Montgomery, Redding and LeMaistre, 1986). Interestingly, although *Candida albicans* is the commonest colonizing fungal pathogen

and accounts for the majority of local oro-pharyngeal infections, systemic invasion is more likely following colonization with *Candida tropicalis* (Sandford, *et al.*, 1980).

Good prophylaxis against *Candida* may be provided by oral non-absorbable anti-fungal agents such as nystatin or amphotericin B. These agents are commonly included in oral mouthcare regimens for patients undergoing chemotherapy or BMT. However, some patients find these preparations unpalatable. In addition, oropharyngeal candidal infection may occur despite good compliance with topical anti-fungal prophylaxis (Barrett, 1989). Excellent prophylaxis against both oro-pharyngeal and systemic candidal infection may be provided by daily oral administration of the triazole fluconazole (Diflucan, Pfizer Ltd.).

Early recognition and treatment of oro-pharyngeal *Candidiasis* is essential for minimizing systemic invasion. *Candida* infection must be included in the differential diagnosis of pharyngeal pain or ulceration in neutropenic patients. Fever or local lymphadenopathy are strong indications of invasive infection and systemic antifungal therapy is required. Fluconazole has been shown to be effective against oral and deep-seated *Candida* infection in neutropenic patients and is available as both oral and intravenous preparations (DeLord, Kelsy and Newland, 1989). Unfortunately fluconazole, unlike amphotericin B, has little activity against *Aspergillus* infection.

Aspergillus

Mortality and morbidity associated with *Aspergillus* infection in neutropenic patients is well recognized (Kelsey, *et al.*, 1990b). Local infections of the head and neck are less common than pulmonary infections but are difficult to diagnose due to the wide variety of symptoms and signs which may be present (Schubert, *et al.*, 1986). Delay in diagnosis and therapy increases subsequent morbidity and complicates management of these infections (Goering, Berlinger and Weisdorf, 1988).

Local aspergilloma may present as swelling of salivary glands or soft tissues, often mimicking lymphadenopathy or tumour. Sino-nasal disease is invasive. Infection often involves bone and blood vessels leading to destruction of facial tissues and potentially fatal bleeding. As with *Candida*, systemic invasion and visceral *Aspergillus* infection may occur.

Management relies on an early aggressive approach to diagnosis and a low threshold for empirical treatment with systemic antifungal agents such as intravenous amphotericin B. Sino-nasal *Aspergillus* infection can only be diagnosed early by detailed clinical and radiological examination. This should be undertaken if there is a high index of suspicion, such as antibiotic-resistant fever. Surgical resection of infected tissue is recommended in combination with intravenous anti-fungal therapy (Colman, 1985). Nevertheless, mortality from these infections is high, being 50–90%. The most important factor determining outcome is the recovery of bone marrow function with the return of circulating granulocytes. More recently, however, liposomal amphotericin B (AmBisome, Vestar Ltd) has been used with success to treat deep-seated *Aspergillus* infections in neutropenic patients without neutrophil recovery; liposomal amphotericin has the advantage of greater tissue penetration with dramatic reduction in nephrotoxicity but is considerably more expensive than conventional amphotericin. Itraconazole (Sporanox, Janssen) is effective against *Aspergillus* infections but is only available in the oral form and its bioavailability is inconsistent.

Oropharyngeal infections in states of chronic immunosuppression

The degree and nature of immunosuppression in long-term survivors of BMT and patients with chronic leukaemia is different from that seen during periods of severe neutropenia immediately following intensive chemotherapy. Neutrophil number and function may be adequate while humoral and cellular lymphocyte-associated defects may play a greater role in immunodeficiency (Kelsey, Lowdell and Newland, 1990).

Oropharyngeal infection with herpes viruses other than HSV are rare immediately post BMT but may manifest between two months to one year following transplantation. Herpes zoster infection occurs maximally around five months after BMT and can cause dermatomal lesions of the oro-facial region. As in patients with lymphoproliferative diseases, such as chronic

lymphocytic leukaemia, lymphoma and myeloma, zoster infection after BMT may be both severe and recurrent (Juel-Jensen, 1985). *Cytomegalovirus* (CMV) can be commonly detected in throat swabs from CMV sero-positive BMT recipients after marrow engraftment (Winston, *et al.*, 1984). Such excretion of CMV usually represents reactivation of latent virus but is not always associated with serious CMV disease. Oral lesions due to Epstein–Barr virus and HSV, manifesting as leukoplakia, have been reported up to one year following BMT (Birek, *et al.*, 1989).

Throat and sinus infections, particularly with capsulate bacteria such as *Haemophilus* and *Streptococcus pneumoniae*, may be responsible for up to 20% of late infections in BMT recipients (Meyers, 1986). Such infections are usually associated with defective synthesis of immunoglobulin, particularly IgG2 and IgA (Kelsey, Lowdell and Newland, 1990). Appropriate antibiotic therapy is usually effective in the short term but recurrent infections may respond to intravenous infusions of human immunoglobulin (Graham-Pole, *et al.*, 1988).

Patients with chronic leukaemia may be susceptible to oral candidal colonization and infection. This usually responds to topical non-adsorbable antifungal therapy or oral fluconazole. Chronic indolent oro-facial HSV infection has also been described in these patients (Barrett, 1988).

Peri-anal infection

The incidence of peri-anal and peri-rectal infections is increased in patients receiving treatment for haematological malignancy, being between 3% and 7% (Schimpff, Weirnick and Block, 1972). Peri-anal abscess may be a presenting feature of acute leukaemia (Slater, 1984). Patients with monocytic leukaemias (e.g. acute myeloid leukaemia FAB classification M4 or M5) are at greater risk than those with other types of malignancy. It has been suggested that this is associated with high muramidase levels in the serum of these patients which facilitates mucosal ulceration and thus secondary infection (Schimpff, Weirnick and Block, 1972).

It is thought that ano-rectal infections result from secondary infection of minor mucosal tears which results in cellulitis and possible abscess formation. Chemotherapy with subsequent neutropenia significantly increases the risk of both mucosal perforation and infection. Organisms ordinarily resident in the bowel are usually the causative pathogens; Gram-negative bacteria such as *Pseudomonas spp.* and *Eschericia coli* are the most prevalent isolates (Barnes, Sattler and Ballard, 1984). Problems which predispose to the formation of mucosal lesions, such as constipation and haemorrhoids, commonly precede the development of peri-anal infections although this is not always the case.

Patients with infected lesions present with peri-anal pain, induration, ulceration and possibly fever (Glenn, *et al.*, 1988). Fluctuance may be difficult to detect in the absence of circulating neutrophils as pus is not formed. Infection may spread rapidly along fascial planes leading to extensive local oedema and necrosis. Secondary bacteraemia is common and ano-rectal infection is considered to be an important source of septicaemic fever in neutropenic patients (Schimpff, *et al.*, 1972).

As with oropharyngeal infections, good resolution of peri-anal infection without serious morbidity depends on recovery of circulating neutrophils. While bone marrow recovery is awaited, systemic broad spectrum antibiotics, providing adequate anti-Gram negative cover, should be administered. Intravenous combination antibiotic therapy with an aminoglycoside plus ureidopenicillin, 4-quinolone or third generation cephalosporin is usually recommended. Additional cover against anaerobic bacteria may be provided by metronidazole. Surgical debridement during the cytopenic phase can be complicated by increased bleeding and poor wound healing. In addition, surgery has not been shown to prevent subsequent recurrence of ano-rectal infection (Glenn, *et al.*, 1988). Surgery may be necessary, and may in fact be life saving, if there is obvious fluctuance, progression of soft tissue infection or ongoing sepsis despite a trial of antibiotic therapy.

Summary

Infections of the oropharynx and peri-anal areas are important causes of morbidity and mortality in severely immunocompromised patients, such as those undergoing chemotherapy or bone marrow transplantation for haematological malignancy. In addition to significant local infection these areas provide a primary source of pathogens responsible for septicaemia and visceral invasion.

The oropharyngeal and peri-anal areas are predisposed to infection by mucosal damage, a direct result of chemotherapy and irradiation, and neutropenia which reduces host defence mechanisms. The presence of significant numbers of existing commensal organisms, as well as colonization with other potentially pathogenic organisms during patient hospitalization and treatment, is also of considerable importance.

Prevention of serious morbidity depends on awareness of the high risk of infection, the commonly atypical presentation of the disease and the tendency for systemic spread with subsequent high mortality. For oropharyngeal infections in particular, effective prophylaxis and a low threshold for introducing appropriate empirical antimicrobial therapy are the mainstays of management. Excepting specific indications surgical intervention should be avoided during periods of neutropenia. Even after institution of therapy, the major factor determining the outcome of oropharyngeal and peri-anal infections caused by bacteria or fungi in immunocompromised patients is recovery of circulating peripheral blood neutrophils.

References

Ambinder, R.F., Lietman, P.S., Burns, W.H. and Saral, R. (1984) Prophylaxis: a strategy to minimise antiviral resistance. *Lancet*, **i**, 1154–1155

Baglin, T.P., Gray, J.J., Marcus, R.E. and Wreghitt, T.G. (1989) Antibiotic resistance fever associated with herpes simples virus infection in neutropenic patients with haematological malignancy. *Journal of Clinical Pathology*, **42**, 1255–1258

Barnes, S.G., Sattler, F.R. and Ballard, J.O. (1984) Perirectal infections in acute leukaemia. *Annals of Internal Medicine*, **100**, 515–518

Barrett, A.P. (1986) A long term prospective clinical study of orofacial herpes simplex virus infection in acute leukaemia. *Oral Surgery, Oral Medicine, Oral Pathology*, **61**, 149–152

Barrett, A.P. (1987) A long-term prospective clinical study of oral complications during conventional chemotherapy for acute leukaemia. *Oral Surgery, Oral Medicine, Oral Pathology*, **63**, 313–6

Barrett, A.P. (1988) Chronic indolent orofacial herpes simplex virus infection in chronic leukaemia: a report of three cases. *Oral Surgery, Oral Medicine, Oral Pathology*, **66**, 387–390

Barrett, A.P. (1989) Recognition and management of invasive pharyngeal candidiasis in acute leukaemia. *Oral Surgery, Oral Medicine, Oral Pathology*, **67**, 275–278

Birek, C., Patterson, B., Maximew, W.C. and Minden, M.D. (1989) EBV and HSV infections in a patient who had undergone bone marrow transplantation: Oral manifestations and diagnosis by *in situ* nucleic acid hybridisation. *Oral Surgery, Oral Medicine, Oral Pathology*, **68**, 612–7

Bostrom, B. and Weisdorf, D. (1984) Mucositis and alpha-streptococcal sepsis in bone marrow transplant recipients. *Lancet*, **i**, 112–1121

Bottomley, W.K., Perlin, E. and Ross, G.R. (1977) Antineoplasic agents and their oral manifestations. *Oral Surgery*, **44**, 527–534

Brown, A.E. (1984) Neutropenia, fever and infection. *American Journal of Medicine*, **76**, 421–428

Carl, W. (1986) Oral manifestations of systemic chemotherapy and their management. *Seminars in Surgery and Oncology*, **2**, 187–199

Cohen, J., Worsley, A.M., Goldman, J.M., Donelly, J.P., Catovsky, D. A. and Galton, D.A.G. (1983) Septicaemia caused by viridans Streptococci in neutropenic patients with leukaemia, *Lancet*, **ii**, 1452–1454

Colman, M.F. (1985) Invasive aspergillus of the head and neck. *Laryngoscope*, **95**, 898–899

DeLord, C., Kelsey, S.M. and Newland, A.C. (1989) Fluconazole for the treatment of systemic fungal infection in severely immunocompromised patients. *British Journal of Haematology*, **71**,(suppl. 1), 41

Dreizen, S., McCredie, K.B., Bodey, G.P. and Keating, M.J. (1986) Quantitative analysis of the oral complications of antileukaemia chemotherapy. *Oral Surgery, Oral Medicine, Oral Pathology*, **62**, 650–653

Ferretti, G.A., Hansen, I.A., Whittenburg, K., Brown, A.T., Lillich, T.T. and Ash, R.C. (1987) Therapeutic use of chlorhexidine in bone marrow transplant patients. *Oral Surgery, Oral Medicine, Oral Pathology*, **63**, 683–687

Glenn, J., Cotton, D., Wesley, R. and Pizzo, P.A. (1988) Anorectal infections in patients with malignant diseases. *Reviews in Infectious Diseases*, **10**, 42–52

Goldhaber, P. and Giddon, D.B. (1964) Present concepts concerning the aetiology and treatment of acute nectrotising ulcerative gingivitis. *International Dental Journal*, **14**, 468–488

Goering, P., Berlinger, N.T. and Weisdorf, D.J. (1988) Agressive combined modality treatment of progressive sinonasal fungal infections in immunocompromised patients. *American Journal of Medicine*, **85**, 619–623

Goldman, H.M. and Cohen, D.W. (1973) *Periodontal therapy*. CV Mosby Co., St. Louis, p. 57

Graham-Pole, J., Camitta, B., Casper, J., Elfenbein, G., Gross, S., Herzig, R., Koch, P., Mahoney, D., Marcus, R., Munoz, L., Pick, T., Spruce, W., Steuber, P. and Weiner, R. (1988) Intravenous immunoglobulin may lessen all forms of infection in patients receiving allogeneic bone marrow transplantation for acute lymphoblastic leukaemia: a pediatric oncology group study. *Bone Marrow Transplantation*, **3**, 559–566

Gray, J.J., Wreghitt, T.G. and Baglin, T.P. (1989) Susceptibility to acyclovir of herpes simplex virus: emergence of resistance in patients with lymphoid and myeloid neoplasia. *Journal of Infection*, **19**, 31–40

Greenberg, M.S., Cohen, S.G., McKitrick, J.C. and Cassileth, P.A. (1982) The oral flora as a source of septicaemia in patients with acute leukaemia. *Oral Surgery*, **53**, 32–36

Greenberg, M.S. (1984) Acute necrotising ulcerative gingivitis. In: Burket's Oral Medicine, 8th edition, eds: M.A. Lynch, V.J. Brightman, M.S. Greenberg (J.B. Lippincott, Pennsylvania), pp. 178–181

Hann, I.M., Prentice, H.G., Blacklock, H.A., Ross, M.G.R., Brigden, D., Rosling, A.E., Burke, C., Crawford, D.H., Brumfitt, W. and Hoffbrand, A.V. (1983) Acyclovir prophylaxis against herpes virus infections in severely immunocompromised patients: randomised double blind trial. *British Medical Journal*, **287**, 384–388

Heimdal, A., Mattsson, T., Dahloff, G., Lonnquist, B. and Rigden, O. (1989) The oral cavity as a port of entry for early infections in patients treated with bone marrow transplantation. *Oral Surgery, Oral Medicine, Oral Pathology*, **68**, 711–716

Hickey, A.J., Toth, B.B. and Lindquist, S.B. (1982) Effect of intravenous hyperalimentation and oral care on the development of oral stomatitis during cancer chemotherapy. *Journal of Prosthetic Dentistry*, **47**, 188–197

Howard, R.J. (1983) Non-specific host defences in surgical cancer patients. *Current Problems in Cancer*, **7**, 1–39

Johanson, W.G., Woods, D.E. and Chauduri, T. (1979) Association of respiratory tract colonisation with adherence of Gram negative bacilli to epithelial cells. *Journal of Infectious Diseases*, **139**, 667–673

Juel-Jensen, B.E. (1985) *Virecella zoster* virus infections: chicken pox and zoster. In: Oxford Textbook of Medicine, eds: D.J. Weatherall, J.G.G. Ledingham, D.A. Warrell (Oxford University Press, UK), pp. 5.57–5.61

Kelsey, S.M., Collins, P.W., DeLord, C., Weinhart, B. and Newland, A.C. (1990a) A randomised study of teicoplanin plus ciprofloxacin versus gentamicin plus piperacillin for the empirical treatment of fever in neutropenic patients. *British Journal of Haematology*, (in press)

Kelsey, S.M., Van der Walt, J., Doran, H. and Newland, A.C. (1990b) *Pulmonary aspergillosis* in leukaemia patients. *Journal of Clinical Pathology*

Kelsey, S.M., Lowdell, M. W. and Newland, A.C. (1990) IgG Subclass levels and immune reconstitution after T cell depleted allogeneic bone marrow transplantation. *Clinical and Experimental Immunology*

Kolbinson, D.A., Schubert, M.M., Flournoy, N. and Truelove, E.L. (1988) Early oral changes following bone marrow transplantation. *Oral Surgery, Oral Medicine, Oral Pathology*, **66**, 130–138

Lam, M.T., Pazin, G.J., Armstrong, J.A. and Ho, M. (1981) Herpes simplex infection in acute myelogenous leukaemia. *Cancer,* **48**, 2168–2171

McElroy, T.H. (1984) Infection in the patient receiving chemotherapy for cancer: oral considerations. *Journal of the American Dental Association,* **109**, 454–456

McGaw, W.T. and Belch, A. (1985) Oral complications of acute leukaemia: Prophylactic impact of a chlorhexidine mouth rinse regimen. *Oral Surgery, Oral Medicine, Oral Pathology,* **60**, 275–280

Meyers, J.D., Flournoy, N. and Thomas, E.D. (1980) Infection with herpes simplex virus and cell mediated immunity after marrow transplant. *Journal of Infectious Diseases,* **142**, 338–346

Meyers, J.D., Wade, J.C., Mitchell, C.D., Saral, R., Lietman, P.S., Durack, D.T., Levin, M.J., Segreti, A.C. and Balfour, H.H. (1982) Multicentre collaborative trial of intravenous acyclovir for treatment of muco-cutaneous herpes simplex virus infection in the immuno-compromised host. *American Journal of Medicine,* **73**, 229–235

Meyers, J.D. (1986) Infection in bone marrow transplant recipients. *American Journal of Medicine,* **81** (suppl. 1A), 27–38

Montogemery, M.T., Redding, S.W. and LeMaistre, C.F. (1986) The incidence of oral herpes simplex virus infection in patients undergoing cancer chemotherapy. *Oral Surgery, Oral Medicine, Oral Pathology,* **61**, 238–242

Overholser, D.C., Peterson, D.E., Williams, L.T. and Schimpff, S.C. (1982a) Periodontal infection in patients with acute nonlymphocytic leukaemia. *Archives of Internal Medicine,* **142**, 551–554

Overholser, C.D., Peterson, D.E., Bergman, S.A. and Williams, L.T. (1982b) Dental extractions in patients with acute non-lymphocytic leukemia. *Journal of Oral and Maxillofacial Surgery,* **40**, 296–298

Overholser, D.C. (1986) Oral complications of cancer and its therapy. In: *Comprehensive Textbook of Oncology,* eds: A.R. Moossa, M.C. Robson and S.C. Schimpff (Williams and Wilkins, Baltimore) pp. 431–442

Perna, J.J. and Eskinazi, D.P. (1988) Treatment of oro-facial herpes simplex infections with acyclovir: a review. *Oral Surgery, Oral Medicine, Oral Pathology,* **65**, 689–692

Peterson, D.E. and Overholser, C.D. (1979) Dental management of leukaemic patients. *Oral Surgery,* **47**, 40–42

Peterson, D.E. and Overholser, C.D. (1981a) Increased morbidity associated with oral infection in patients with acute nonlymphocytic leukaemia. *Oral Surgery,* **51**, 390–393

Peterson, D.E., Overholser, C.D., Schimpff, S.C., Williams, L.T. and Newman, K.A. (1981b) Relationship of intensive oral hygiene to systemic complications in acute nonlymphocytic leukaemia. *Proceedings of the American Federation for Clinical Research,* **29**, 440

Pizzo, P.A. (1981) Infectious complications in the child with cancer. *Journal of Pediatrics,* **98**, 341–354

Rand, K.H., Rasmussen, L.E., Pollard, R.B., Arvin, A. and Merigan, T.C. (1977) Cellular immunity and herpes virus infections in cardiac transplant patients. *New England Journal of Medicine,* **296**, 1372–1377

Ray, T.L. (1987) Oral Candidiasis. *Dermatologic Clinics,* **5**, 651–662

Redding, S.W. and Montgomery, M.T. (1989) Acyclovir prophylaxis for oral herpes simplex virus infection in patients with bone marrow transplants. *Oral Surgery, Oral Medicine, Oral Pathology,* **67**, 680–683

Sandford, G.R., Merz, W.G., Wingard, J.R., Charache, P. and Saral, R. (1980) The value of fungal surveillance cultures as predictors of systemic fungal infections. *Journal of Infectious Diseases,* **142**, 503–509

Schimpff, S.C., Young, V.M., Greene, G.H., Vermeulen, G.D., Moody, M.R. and Wiernik, P.H. (1972) Origin of infection in acute nonlymphocytic leukaemia. *Annals of Internal Medicine,* **77**, 707–714

Schimpff, S.C., Wiernick, P.H. and Block, J.B. (1972) Rectal abcesses in cancer patients. *Lancet,* **ii**, 844–847

Schubert, M.M., Peterson, D.E., Meyers, J.D., Hackman, R. and Thomas, E.D. (1986) Head and neck aspergillosis in patients undergoing bone marrow transplantation. *Cancer,* **57**, 1092–1096

Selby, P.J., Jameson, B., Watson, J.G., Morgenstern, G., Powles, R.L., Kay, H.E.M., Thornton, R., Clink, H.M., Prentice, H.G., Ross, M.G., Corringham, R. and Hoffbrand, A.V. (1979) Parenteral acyclovir therapy for herpes virus infection in man. *Lancet,* **ii**, 1267–1270

Sharon, A., Bericevsky, I., Ben-Aryeh, H. and Gutman, D. (1977) The effect of chlorhexidine mouth rinses on oral Candida in a group of leukaemic patients. *Oral Surgery,* **44**, 201–205

Slater, D.N. (1984) Perianal abcess: have I excluded leukaemia? *British Medical Journal,* **289**, 1682

Sonis, S.T., Sonis, A.L. and Lieberman, A. (1978) Oral complications in patients receiving treatment for malignancies other than of the head and neck. *Journal of the American Dental Association,* **97**, 468–472

Wahlin, Y.B. and Holm, A.K. (1988) Changes in the oral microflora in patients with acute leukaemia and related disorders during the period of induction therapy. *Oral Surgery, Oral Medicine, Oral Pathology,* **65**, 411–417

Weibren, M.J., Forgeson, G., Helenglass, G., Jameson, B. and Powles, R. (1988) Unusual presentation pseudo-monas infection. *British Medical Journal,* **297**, 1034–1035

Winston, D.J., Ho, W.G., Champlin, R.E. and Gale, R.P. (1984) Infectious complications of bone marrow trans-plantation. *Experimental Haematology,* **12**, 205–215

12

Infections complicating bone marrow transplantation

T.R.F. Rogers and S. Selwyn

Introduction and historical background

Bone marrow transplantation (BMT) has become established as a therapeutic option for a variety of leukaemias, aplastic anaemia, thalassaemia, congenital immunodeficiencies and inborn errors of metabolism (see Table 12.1). In 1990 over 4000 BMTs were undertaken in 20 European countries with an equal distribution of allogeneic vs autologous transplants (Gratwohl, 1991). This achievement is a tribute to the pioneering studies carried out in the 1950s. These demonstrated, initially in animals and subsequently in man, that survival was possible after an otherwise lethal dose of irradiation by virtue of an intravenous infusion of bone marrow (Thomas, *et al.*, 1975). A major factor that has made BMT feasible is tissue typing which identifies the extent of HLA and ABO blood group match between donor and recipient. This helps to prevent or mitigate the effects of graft-versus-host disease (GVHD), the clinical features of which include skin rash, profuse diarrhoea, hepatitis and most seriously interstitial pneumonitis.

Of comparable importance for success is the conditioning of the patient before the transplant, in order to prevent rejection of the donor marrow. For leukaemic patients this includes the use of cyclophosphamide and total body irradiation with the aim of eradicating any residual tumour. For non-malignant disorders cyclophosphamide or busulphan are normally used. From their earliest transplant experience Thomas, *et al.* (1975) reported survival rates of

Table 12.1 Bone marrow transplants reported in Europe 1990*

Disease	No. of transplants	
	Allogeneic	*Autologous*
Leukaemia:		
Acute myeloid	494	388
Acute lymphatic	483	284
Chronic myeloid	546	80
Lymphoma	98	818
Solid tumour	5	377
Myelodysplasia	86	4
Severe aplastic anaemia	136	0
Inborn error	32	0
Thalassaemia	117	0
Severe immunodeficiency	26	0
Total	2023	1951

* Adapted from Gratwohl (1991).

50% for aplastic anaemia and less than 30% for acute leukaemia. They pointed out the differences in results achieved between their unit and those of others which appeared to relate to the conditioning regimen used and the supportive care provided.

It is clear from these early observations that the causes of failure of the transplant procedure fell into three categories: infection, GVHD or relapse of the underlying malignancy. One such study highlighted the frequency with which infection occurred as well as its role in accounting for early fatality (Solberg, *et al.*, 1971): a total of 50 different infections were encountered in 11 patients who had received allogeneic transplants. The most prominent pathogens were Gram-negative enteric bacilli and *Candida albicans*. There were six deaths due to infection, five of which were within the first six weeks following transplant. Only the most basic precautions were taken to prevent infection in these patients. As a result of their experience the authors emphasized the importance of exogenously acquired organisms, in addition to the patients' own resident flora, as causes of infection, and pointed to the future need for continuous microbiological surveillance, strict protective isolation and intestinal decontamination in the early stages after transplantation.

Throughout the 1970s and 1980s there was a rapid accumulation of data on infectious complications of BMT and a clear pattern has emerged in relation to the different time periods before and after the transplant as shown in Figure 12.1 (Winston, *et al.*, 1978; Meyers and Atkinson, 1983; Zaia, 1983; Rogers, 1988; Wingard, 1990).

Risk factors and patterns of infection during BMT

Pre-transplant

The majority of patients referred for BMT have a haematological malignancy, and will already have undergone remission induction chemotherapy (RIT). As a result, these patients are demonstrably immunosuppressed. For example, Rogers, *et al.* (1986) found that circulating immunoglobulin (Ig) levels of leukaemic patients were only 60% of expected values. Patients with aplastic anaemia will be neutropenic pre-BMT ($<1 \times 10^9$/l), while infants with congenital immunodeficiency may have impaired T-lymphocyte function. Indeed the initial presentation in any of these underlying diseases may be opportunistic infection. Winston, *et al.* (1978) encountered 25 infections in 17 of 60 patients with either aplastic anaemia or leukaemia during their hospitalization before

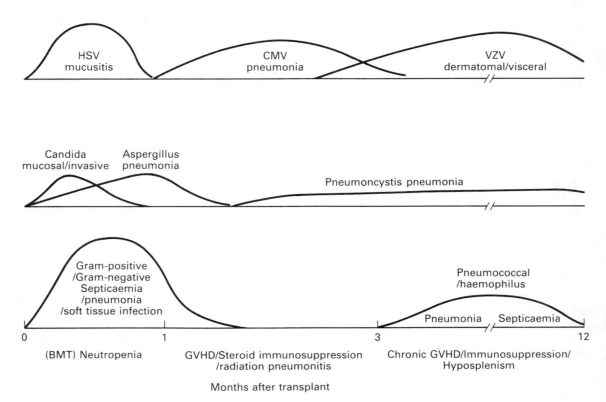

Figure 12.1 Temporal relationship of opportunistic infections to risk factors associated with bone marrow transplantation

BMT. The majority of these episodes were localized infections due to Gram-negative bacteria, and although only two post-transplant deaths could be attributed to pre-transplant infections they reported a higher incidence of early fungal deaths in association with pre-transplant infection.

It is clearly important to carry out a full physical examination of the patient prior to or on admission to hospital. X-ray examination of the chest and nasal sinuses may reveal covert infection, and atypical features would not be surprising in view of the patient's inability to mount an effective immune response to the infecting organism. Serological testing for evidence of latent infection with cytomegalovirus (CMV) as well as tests for hepatitis B and human immunodeficiency virus (HIV) infection should be undertaken routinely as many of these patients will already have received multiple transfusions and have an increased risk of acquisition of these viruses as a consequence. A summary of measures recommended in preparation for BMT is given in Table 12.2.

Table 12.2 Measures to be taken before transplant to prevent infectious complications

1. Full physical examination
   - (a) To detect signs of infection of oropharynx, chest, skin, etc.
   - (b) To include dental examination for caries/root abscesses

2. X-ray examination of chest, sinuses, teeth

3. Microbiological screen
   - (a) For potential pathogens, e.g. *P. aeruginosa*, *Enterobacter* spp, *Candida* spp in oropharynx, stool, urine
   - (b) Serological studies for CMV and HSV antibody, human immunodeficiency virus antibody, hepatitis B virus surface antigen

4. Insertion of Hickman catheter using full aseptic technique (antibiotic prophylaxis not indicated)

5. Initiate oral and topical chemoprophylaxis regimens*

6. Nurse in single-room protective isolation
   - (a) Attendant staff wash hands with alcoholic chlorhexidine prior to entry to room, and don plastic apron and gloves on each visit
   - (b) Clean cooked food and sterile drinks in dietary regimen

7. Marrow donor: full physical examination and 3(b) as above

* See text and Table 4.

Post-transplant

The neutropenic period

The conditioning regimen invariably precipitates acute bone marrow failure which is manifest as profound neutropenia within a few days of the transplant. This state can be expected to last for the ensuing three weeks or longer until engraftment has occurred. The association between neutropenia and opportunistic infection in leukaemic patients was first clearly demonstrated by Bodey, *et al.* (1966). Many subsequent studies have confirmed this observation, and in particular the increased incidence of Gram-negative infections in this situation (Storring, *et al.*, 1977). These include localized soft tissue infections, septicaemia and pneumonia.

The principal reservoir from which these infections arise is the oro-gastro-intestinal tract, and the responsible bacteria may be either members of the patient's resident flora, or organisms that have been acquired from sources within the transplant unit. The acquisition of the latter potentially pathogenic organisms, with colonization of the oropharynx or stomach, is likely to be facilitated by the prior administration of broad spectrum systemic antibiotics or the use of antacids or H-2 receptor antagonists which suppress gastric acid production. Colonization of the bowel by toxigenic *Clostridium difficile* may also be attributable to disturbance of the resident flora by antibiotics, and associated gastrointestinal symptoms have been reported in children undergoing BMT (Rogers, *et al.*, 1981).

Table 12.3 shows the distribution of organisms reported to have caused septicaemia in several transplant units over the past decade. It can be seen that there has been a significant increase in Gram-positive sepsis rates. Most viridans streptococcal septicaemias probably originate from the oropharynx as a complication of mucositis. Cohen, *et al.* (1983) were the first to record this association in 10 neutropenic leukaemic patients; 7 of 10 streptococcal isolates were *Streptococcus mitis*. Symptoms were, however, considered mild and although all patients had fever, the only other dominant physical sign was pharyngitis. However Guiot, *et al.* (1990) have reported an adult respiratory distress type syndrome associated with streptococcal septicaemia. Similarly Valteau, *et al.*

Table 12.3 Blood culture-isolates from bone marrow transplant patients 1973–1987

Centre	U.C.L.A.	City of Hope National Medical Center	Seattle	Westminster Hospital
Period of Survey (Reference)	1973–76 (Winston, et al., 1978)	1976–82 (Zaia, 1983)	1981–84 (Bowden and Meyers, 1985)	1985–87 (Barnes and Rogers, 1987, 1988)
Gram-negative	**26**	**19**	**18**	**9**
Pseud. aeruginosa	9	6	4	5
Esch. coli	5	4	10	1
Klebsiella spp.	7	3	—	—
Other aerobes	5	6	—	3
Anaerobes	—	—	4	—
Gram-positive	**6**	**34**	**49**	**49**
Staph. aureus	4	9	4	2
Coag. neg. staph.	—	11	35	21
Streptococcus spp.	2	9	—	16
Diptheroids	—	2	1	1
Clostridium spp.	—	1	—	1
Others	—	2	9	8
Fungi	**16**	**2**	**10**	**3**
Cand. albicans	—	—	—	3
Cand. tropicalis	—	—	—	—
Cand. spp.	13	2	10	—
Aspergillus spp.	2	—	—	2+
Trichosporon	1	—	—	—
Total isolates/patients	50*/57	55/170	79/365	61*/84

+ Mixed fungaemia. * Episodes of bacteraemia.

(1991) report a high rate of streptococcal sepsis in their patients leading to a 12% mortality; no specific risk factors were identified in this study.

The universal increase in coagulase-negative staphylococcal (CNS) infections has been firmly linked to the widespread use of Hickman catheters for long-term vascular access (Moosa, *et al.*, 1991). In 1980 Bjeletich and Hickman described their experience of using these catheters in 585 patients. They reported an overall infection rate related to their use of only 3%. However, they had earlier noted a far higher incidence in BMT (Hickman, *et al.*, 1979). In a series of 75 patients, one or more episodes of septicaemia occurred while the catheter was *in situ*, and in 7 patients the catheter had to be removed because of persistent septicaemia despite antibiotic therapy. Removal of the catheter led to the recovery from the episode of septicaemia in 5 of the 7 patients. It has recently become evident that coagulase-negative staphylococci – the most frequent group associated with catheter infection – may be spread by cross-infection on the transplant unit (Oppenheim, *et al.*, 1989) and detailed epidemiological studies confirm this view (Hedin and Hambraeus, 1991).

Antibiotic-resistant corynebacteria and other Gram-positive bacteria, as well as *Candida* spp. appear to be particularly associated with persistent catheter-related sepsis (CRS). Further experience in different age groups suggests that there is a higher incidence of CRS in children, perhaps as a consequence of more frequent handling of the catheter itself or the skin exit site (Barnes and Rogers, 1987). Darbyshire and colleagues (1985) also observed a high frequency of coagulase-negative staphylococcal infections in their catheterized children, although the majority of episodes were successfully treated with antibiotics, and mechanical problems were, in fact, more often responsible for catheter removal. Endoscopy may also be a risk factor for CNS sepsis: Bianco, *et al.* (1990) encountered 9 cases of bacteraemia occurring within 24 hours of performing gastrointestinal endoscopy. Concurrent administration of prednisone for GVHD was regarded as a related risk factor.

As might be expected, recurrent episodes of sepsis are seen in patients who suffer prolonged periods (>3 weeks) of neutropenia. The initial infective episodes, which are often streptococcal, tend to progress to sepsis due to anti-biotic-resistant bacteria and ultimately to fungal infection. Another contributory factor to white cell depletion is pre-treatment of the donor bone marrow with monoclonal antibodies directed against the T-lymphocytes implicated in GVHD, in order to reduce the incidence and severity of this major complication. However, the use of this technique has led to an increasing number of patients with delayed or failed engraftment. Moreover, Pirsch and Maki (1986) found a significant increase in invasive fungal infections in patients receiving T-cell depleted transplants, particularly in the group whose donors were HLA-mismatched. This pattern of emerging fungal infection – notably due to *Candida albicans* (Goodrich, *et al.*, 1991), *Aspergillus* spp. or a combination of these – has also been found in other large transplant units (Meyers and Atkinson, 1983).

Candida infections usually originate from endogenous sources, whereas Aspergillus is exogenously acquired and several dramatic outbreaks of nosocomial aspergillosis have been attributed to heavy contamination of the patients' environment with fungal spores (Rogers and Barnes, 1988). Structural work adjacent to the bone marrow unit or faulty ward air conditioning have most often been implicated in these outbreaks, where patients were not maintained in a filtered air environment. However, Ruutu, *et al.* (1987) emphasized the risks of using inadequately maintained air filtration systems. They reported that over a one-year period there were eight cases of aspergillosis, including four patients in single room isolation with high efficiency particulate air (HEPA) filtration. Repair of the filter mechanism quickly led to a cessation of the outbreak.

Removal of patients from a protective environment may well lead to undue exposure to airborne fungal spores. This may occur for example when it is necessary to take the patient to theatre for placement of a catheter or to admit him to the intensive care unit for mechanical ventilation. Support for this view comes from the report of Allo, *et al.* (1987) who observed nine cases of *Aspergillus flavus* skin infection with two deaths due to dissemination. All nine infections followed insertion of Hickman catheters in operating rooms in which the air supply was unduly contaminated with fungal spores. An unusual case of aspergillosis was reported by Hamadeh, *et al.* (1988) where marijuana, smoked by the patient was shown to be the source of the organism. It is of interest that the majority of cases reported from the United States have been due to *A. flavus* whereas those from Western Europe are most often due to *A. fumigatus*; this may relate to the different climatic conditions which favour one or other species. Rarely, other fungi (Table 12.3) are a cause of local or disseminated infection during this time period. For example, a case of *Pseudoallescheria boydii* pneumonia was reported by Guyotat, *et al.* (1987) with a fatal outcome, autopsy revealing disseminated infection.

Herpes simplex virus reactivation will occur in about 70% of seropositive BMT patients as a result of acute immunosuppression (Saral, 1985). In seronegative patients the frequency of herpetic infection is considerably lower than this. Most cases arise within the first four weeks after BMT, and are usually manifest as painful oral mucositis, although genital herpes infections have also been reported in this setting. Prentice (1983) noted that active herpes simplex infection was often complicated by prolongation of the period of neutropenia, presumably as a result of virus-induced marrow suppression. On rare occasions the infection extends into the oesophagus. Ulceration of these mucosal surfaces undoubtedly provides a portal of entry for bacteria into the tissues and the circulation, and the association with streptococcal infection has already been referred to.

Clinically evident reactivation of other herpes viruses, notably cytomegalovirus (CMV), has been recorded infrequently during the neutropenic period. Infections with a number of respiratory and gastrointestinal viruses, including adenoviruses, enteroviruses (Biggs, *et al.*, 1990) and rotaviruses (Willoughby, *et al.*, 1988), can also cause considerable morbidity at this time and are especially frequent in children (Wasserman, *et al.*, 1988). Townsend, *et al.* (1982) reported an outbreak of coxsackie A1 gastroenteritis among adult BMT recipients, and six out of seven of those affected subsequently died compared to only one of the seven non-infected patients. It was felt that the virus infection had an important contributory role in the six fatal cases. Respiratory syncytial virus (RSV) may cause penumonia with severe illness (Hertz, *et al.*, 1989). Nosocomial transmission of the virus can be facilitated by carriage on hands of

members of staff on the BMT unit (Martin, *et al.*, 1988).

Haemorrhagic cystitis is a frequent and troublesome early complication which has been considered to be a side-effect of cyclophosphamide use. However, viruses have more recently been regarded as playing a contributory role. Thus urinary excretion of adenoviruses (Miyamura, *et al.*, 1987) and BK papovaviruses (Drummond, *et al.*, 1987; Arthur, *et al.*, 1988) has coincided with the development of haemorrhagic cystitis. Attention was originally drawn to the pathogenic role of the BK group by O'Reilly, *et al.* (1981) who associated viral excretion with hepatic dysfunction but this has not been substantiated.

Clinical presentations and management of infection during neutropenia

The development of a 'significant' episode of fever (i.e. 38 °C for ≥ 2 h) is an almost inevitable occurrence in the neutropenic transplant patient. This normally occurs initially at least in the absence of localized signs of infection. A full physical examination of the patient is necessary to exclude any infected focus such as the indwelling catheter exit site. Ecthyma gangrenosum is a rare but pathognomonic cutaneous feature of Pseudomonas septicaemia. Endotoxic shock is a clear manifestation of septicaemia, typically due to aerobic Gram-negative rods. As reported earlier more recent studies highlight the emergence of Gram-positive septicaemias, which are more likely to occur as a complication of oral mucositis or I.V. catheter infection; however, we have frequently observed *Staph. epidermidis* septicaemia in the absence of any obvious primary focus, and have assumed that the Hickman catheter tip has become 'infected'. Occasionally the subcutaneous tunnel through which the catheter passes is obviously inflamed and is acting as the source of septicaemia. The possibility of infective endocarditis should be considered when a patient develops a cardiac murmur in the face of staphylococcal septicaemia (Martino, *et al.*, 1990).

A non-infective basis for the fever should also be sought. Apart from such obvious causes as drug and transfusion reactions, the most likely explanation is acute GVHD. In this condition fever may precede the appearance of the rash with its characteristic distribution. In addition, of course, GVHD and infection can occur simultaneously. In an attempt to distinguish these two processes from each other several serological markers have been evaluated. Walker, *et al.* (1984a) undertook serial measurements of the acute phase reactant C-reactive protein (CRP) and found that the serum CRP concentrations were significantly increased in response to bacterial infection. By contrast, the levels were normal or only slightly raised in documented episodes of GVHD and viral infection. They and others (De Bel, *et al.*, 1991) have concluded that this test is of value in the diagnosis and management of bacterial infections. Some earlier studies had suggested that immunoglobulin (Ig) E elevation was a useful serum marker of acute GVHD, but Walker, *et al.* (1984b) in a study of 25 BMT patients found that IgE levels were also raised in infection, and therefore had poor discriminative value. The results of the studies of Walker, *et al.* conflict with a more recent report in which it was argued that the use of these two tests together was helpful in distinguishing infection from GVHD, since the authors observed no elevation of IgE values during infection in their 38 patients (Saarinen, *et al.*, 1987). Another potentially helpful serum marker is neopterin, a macrophage product, the levels of which are elevated in viral infection or acute GVHD but not specifically in response to bacterial infection (Bron, *et al.*, 1988).

Few comprehensive studies of empirical antibiotic therapy in neutropenic BMT patients have been performed. This is largely because the approach to management has parallelled that employed in non-transplant neutropenic patients. More recently Barnes and Rogers (1987) have evaluated a frequently prescribed ureidopenicillin + aminoglycoside combination. In initial febrile episodes there was a 50% response rate, but this contrasted with poorer responses in recurrent episodes of fever. They concluded, on the basis of the pattern of documented infections, that the predominance of resistant coagulase-negative staphylococci together with the emergence of fungi in the later stages of neutropenia accounted for the deteriorating response to these antibiotics. On the basis of these findings they advocated the use of a staged approach to empirical therapy which should be particularly suited to the transplant patient. In a follow-up study in which vancomycin + ceftazidime was given where initial therapy failed, or in patients with second or subsequent episodes of fever, a significant improvement in the response rate was achieved. Whether an anti-staphylococcal agent should be incorporated into the initial empirical antibiotic regimen continues to be the subject of debate. Menichetti and colleagues (1988) evaluated the glycopeptide teicoplanin as a component of an empirical regimen in 34 BMT patients. The 90% response rate observed in Gram-positive bacteraemias was largely attributed to the use of teicoplanin which might be a suitable alternative to vancomycin. In patients who have fever persisting for >96 hours the possibility of fungal infection has to be considered seriously. The clinical features are variable although there may be clinical and radiological evidence of pulmonary involvement (Mori, *et al.*, 1991). Recent advances have been made with serological tests to detect circulating fungal antigens (Rogers, *et al.*, 1990) which, when present would support the administration of potentially toxic antifungal drugs such as amphotericin. The study protocol of Barnes and Rogers (1988) incorporated early amphotericin B therapy. Two-thirds of patients who were deemed to have a fungal infection on clinical grounds only, responded to empirical amphotericin B. The recent availability of liposomal amphotericin B in the UK, has enabled clinical studies to be undertaken. Preliminary results suggest there is significantly less toxicity associated with this formulation of the drug although it is considerably more expensive.

Another controversial issue is the role of granulocyte transfusions as an adjunct to antibiotic therapy (Clift and Buckner, 1984). While some studies in neutropenic patients have confirmed their therapeutic efficacy when given in adequate concentrations, others have been unable to reproduce these beneficial results in BMT patients (Winston, *et al.*, 1982). A particular hazard is the transmission of CMV in unscreened transfusions. Our approach is to restrict the use of granulocyte transfusions to patients most likely to benefit namely those with documented Gram-negative septicaemia who are not responding to 'appropriate' antibiotics, and who are likely to remain neutropenic for some days. In this situation a chronic granulocytic leukaemia donor may be sought in order to provide an adequate yield of neutrophils. Another strategy that is currently still at an experimental stage is the use of intravenous immune globulin which has a high titre of antibodies to Gram-negative pathogens such as *Pseudomonas aeruginosa*. A similar approach would be to use antiserum rich in anti-endotoxin antibody.

It is now clear that antibiotic-resistant fever may also be due to herpes simplex virus infection – even in the absence of oro-pharyngeal herpetic lesions (Baglin, *et al.*, 1989). Where cultures are positive for HSV and more clearly, when herpetic mucositis is clinically evident, acyclovir therapy is indicated. Several studies have demonstrated how effective acyclovir is either intravenously or by the oral route in reducing the duration of symptoms and viral shedding (Meyers, *et al.*, 1982; Shepp, *et al.*, 1985).

Preventive measures during neutropenia

It will be apparent from the preceding section that the neutropenic period represents a major risk for life-threatening infection to the transplant patient. A recent exciting development has been the production of recombinant granulocyte/macrophage colony stimulating factor (G-CSF and GM-CSF). Early clinical trials in autologous BMT suggest that the duration of neutropenia can be significantly reduced (Brandt, *et al.*, 1988; Hermann, *et al.*, 1990; Vose, *et al.*, 1991). The trend in these studies has been towards a reduction in intercurrent infections as a result of accelerated bone marrow recovery. Further studies are needed to establish the value and safety of this new therapy.

Various studies over the years have attempted to identify the most cost-effective methods of prevention. Early recognition of the principal sources and routes of acquisition of infection led to the combined approaches of giving oral prophylactic antibiotics to suppress the resident (endogenous) flora of the bowel while maintaining the patient in a protective environment to provide a barrier to organisms from exogenous sources. Over the past decade the protocols that have proved to be effective in conventionally treated leukaemic patients have been employed also for use in the BMT patient. These have been reviewed and elsewhere (Hann and Prentice, 1984; Rogers, 1985, 1991;

Warren, 1992). The results of trials of chemo-prophylaxis that have included BMT patients suggest that some reduction in infection rates can be obtained by giving either a non-absorbable regimen such as neomycin + colistin (NEOCON) or co-trimoxazole + colistin. However both of these regimens have major deficiencies; NEOCON is poorly tolerated and does not confer any systemic protection, while the incidence of co-trimoxazole resistance has steadily increased; furthermore there is experimental evidence that co-trimoxazole impairs bone marrow engraftment (Golde, *et al.*, 1978) thereby prolonging the duration of neutropenia. An alternative choice is one of the new quinolones such as ciprofloxacin, norfloxacin or ofloxacin, which despite their broad spectrum of activity do not alter the resident bowel flora in an unfavourable way, and by leaving the anaerobic flora intact (Reeves, 1986) should promote the 'colonization resistance' conferred by these commensals. As yet there are insufficient data in BMT to advocate the routine use of a quinolone for chemoprophylaxis although the results of preliminary studies indicate a significant protective effect against Gram-negative bacterial infection (De Pauw, *et al.*, 1990; Menichetti, *et al.*, 1989; Gluckman, *et al.*, 1991), but an obvious concern must be that drug resistance will rapidly emerge and undermine the value of this drug for the therapy of infection. Already emergent resistance during the treatment of *Pseudomonas aeruginosa* infection has been observed (Azadian, *et al.*, 1987) as have resistant CNS colonizing patients receiving ciprofloxacin (Kotilainen, *et al.*, 1990). The value of currently used oral antifungal agents is rather less clear. While the topically active non-absorbed polyenes, amphotericin B and nystatin, suppress the resident yeasts in the bowel they afford no systemic protection. Ketoconazole is an orally administered systemic antifungal primarily active against *Candida* and some related yeasts. This drug has been evaluated in neutropenic patients as a prophylactic agent, and although a significant reduction in the incidence of oral candidiasis (Hann, *et al.*, 1982a) and in intestinal colonization (Benhamou, *et al.*, 1991) was seen, there was inadequate evidence of protection against invasive candidiasis. Subsequent pharmaco-kinetic studies have revealed that there is reduced absorption of ketoconazole in these severely immunocompromised patients (Hann, *et al.*, 1982b). A further problem with the use of this drug in BMT is an unfavourable interaction with cyclosporin A (Shepard, *et al.*, 1986) which is a widely used immunosuppressive agent; failure to recognize this interaction may increase the risk of nephrotoxicity as a result of excessive serum cyclosporin levels. Itraconazole is a more promising antifungal as it is more active against *Aspergillus* spp., and a recently developed improved formulation of the drug may overcome the initial bioavailability problems that were encountered. There is some controversy over whether itraconazole has a similar interaction with cyclosporin A (Kwan, *et al.*, 1987). The results of prophylactic trials are awaited with interest. Conneally, *et al.* (1990) report a significantly reduced incidence of cases of aspergillosis in patients receiving nebulized amphotericin B. This was compared to the incidence in a historical group of BMT patients. Further evaluation of this mode of administration of fungal chemoprophylaxis is warranted. Other established components of antibacterial and antifungal regimens include the topical application of chlorhexidine in order to suppress resident skin and oro-pharyngeal flora. The benefits to be obtained from this tedious practice have not been clearly demonstrated, although one detailed study of oral decontamination did suggest that streptococcal septicaemia rates could be reduced in this way (Ferretti, *et al.*, 1987). With regard to food we advocate the use of freshly cooked meals, ideally, prepared by kitchen staff on the transplant unit. This includes the consumption of 'sterile' canned foods that could be prepared by microwave heating. Animal studies that were conducted some years ago indicated that the maintenance of a germ-free or gnotobiotic 'patient' reduced the risk of GVHD, and it is interesting that in a recent analysis of risk factors in over 2000 patients (Gale, *et al.*, 1987), the use of co-trimoxazole chemoprophylaxis was a factor significantly (p value < 0.04) associated with a reduced incidence of GVHD.

Most patients undergoing BMT will be placed in a single room and be nursed with protective isolation precautions. Our current policy is for staff to wear a disposable plastic apron, gloves and hat, but not a mask, when attending the patient. There is controversy over the microbiological efficacy and cost effectiveness of using laminar air flow rooms that incorporate HEPA filtration (Armstrong, 1984). However, it is clear that this strict environment significantly reduces the rate of acquisition of Aspergillus (Barnes and Rogers, 1989) while it is less clear whether there is a reduction in bacterial or other infections (Navari, *et al.*, 1984; Skinhoj, *et al.*, 1987). The provision of HEPA filtered rooms is a desirable goal for all BMT patients, but is likely to be limited by financial constraints. As part of the microbiological monitoring of patients during this period it is popular to obtain surveillance cultures from various skin sites, oropharynx, stool and urine (Daw, *et al.*, 1990). Early detection of persistent colonization by resistant Gram-negative bacteria especially *Pseudomonas aeruginosa* provides valuable information since there is a correlation with subsequent infection with the same bacterial species (Wingard, *et al.*, 1986). In the case of yeasts, colonization by *C. albicans* appears to have poor predictive value for development of invasive infection, while the reverse is the case for *C. tropicalis* (Sandford, *et al.*, 1980). We believe surveillance on a twice weekly basis is justified where the specimens taken are limited to throat, stool, urine and indwelling vascular catheter site.

The use of acyclovir chemoprophylaxis against HSV reactivation during the first four weeks post-transplant is justified on the clinical basis that mucositis and fever, often in the absence of oropharyngeal lesions, are frequently-occurring manifestations of infection; but also on rare occasions a disseminated infection, with encephalitis, may ensue. Furthermore several trials have established that acyclovir is very effective when given prophylactically. Initial studies were with intravenous acyclovir (Saral, *et al.*, 1981; Shepp, *et al.*, 1985) but oral administration of the drug has been found to provide comparable rates of protection (Gluckman, *et al.*, 1983; Wade, *et al.*, 1984). Because some patients may not tolerate oral medicines soon after the transplant, and as acyclovir has poor bioavailability some still advocate the intravenous route (Shepp, *et al.*, 1987) although this is considerably more expensive. There has been recent concern over the isolation of acyclovir-resistant strains of HSV from patients with pneumonia (Ljungman, *et al.*, 1990); when tested *in vitro* these were also resistant to ganciclovir but sensitive to foscarnet.

In seronegative patients the incidence of

HSV infection is sufficiently low that acyclovir prophylaxis is not necessary.

Infections following bone marrow engraftment

Once bone marrow recovery is established and the patient is no longer neutropenic, the incidence of bacterial and fungal infections greatly reduces, so that the preventive measures recommended in the previous section are no longer necessary. Nevertheless, when persistent GVHD requires continuation of immunosuppressive therapy the risk of aspergillus infection is high, so that chemoprophylaxis with itraconazole is recommended. Serum drug levels should be monitored to ensure that protective concentrations are obtained (Tricot, *et al.*, 1987).

Interstitial pneumonitis (IP) is the major complication of BMT occurring during this time period. It is characterized clinically by dyspnoea, hypoxaemia accompanied by interstitial lung infiltrates seen on X-ray. During the first year following allogeneic BMT about 40% of patients will develop IP. Wingard, *et al.* (1988) reported 166 cases of IP occurring in 386 consecutive transplants; further analysis revealed that half the cases occurred between 21 and 80 days post BMT. With regard to aetiology, 50% were idiopathic, 36% due to CMV, while 5% were due to *Pneumocystis carinii*. Sullivan, *et al.* (1986) categorized their cases as 'early' or 'late'; CMV accounted for 42% of early cases, while in 198 patients, all of whom had chronic GVHD and had survived to beyond 100 days post BMT, there were 31 episodes of IP including: 7 idiopathic, 6 CMV and 6 *P. carinii*.

Risk factors for the development of IP include the type of conditioning regimen used pre-BMT and the presence of GVHD. These are probably co-factors for the development of CMV pneumonia. There is now good experimental evidence that CMV pneumonia has an immunopathological basis (Grundy, *et al.*, 1987) which would explain why antiviral therapy has been inadequate. In support of this hypothesis is the finding that there is a lower incidence of CMV pneumonia (6%) after autologous BMT, which is generally not complicated by GVHD (Reusser, *et al.*, 1990). The serological status of the marrow recipient is the most important determinant of the risk of CMV

infection. CMV seropositivity before transplant is associated with an incidence of post-transplant infection of 60 to 70% (Guyotat, *et al.*, 1987b) compared to a figure of *c.* 35% in patients who have not had a previous CMV infection, that is, are seronegative before transplant, and are receiving unscreened blood products (Paulin, *et al.*, 1986). Once CMV infection occurs, as evidenced by active virus shedding in bronchoalveolar lavage samples or by viraemia, the chances of pneumonia developing subsequently are considerably increased (Ruutu, *et al.*, 1990; Meyers, Ljungman and Fisher, 1990).

It is not clear whether the serological status of the donor influences the rate at which infection occurs but there is evidence that immune donors protect CMV-seropositive patients from developing pneumonia (Grob, *et al.*, 1987); the reason for this is unclear.

The approaches to management of CMV pneumonia have been reviewed (Meyers, 1988; Prentice, 1989; Winston and Gale, 1991). Until recently drug therapy was found to be ineffective: vidarabine, acyclovir and interferon have all proved disappointing. But ganciclovir, a nucleoside analogue related to acyclovir, is considered to be more promising since it has greater activity *in vitro* against CMV. But, when given in dosages ranging from 2.5 to 15 mg/kg/d, for 14 days or longer, response rates have been surprisingly poor, and the majority of treated patients died from respiratory failure (Faulds and Heel, 1990). Immunotherapy with intravenous CMV hyperimmune globulin (CMV Ig) has also been evaluated as an alternative therapy with variable results being reported in the literature (Meyers, 1988; Saral, 1991; Gale and Winston, 1991). However, the best results have been obtained with a combination of these treatments. Schmidt, *et al.* (1988) used a regimen of ganciclovir (10 mg/kg/d for 21 days, followed by maintenance with 5 mg/kg/d) plus CMV Ig (500 mg/kg alternate days, then 500 mg/kg/week maintenance) and had satisfactory responses in 11 of 13 patients. The mechanism of action of CMV Ig is poorly understood: rather than having a direct antiviral effect it is thought to block the host's damaging T-lymphocyte responses on the lung.

Despite these encouraging results with treatment of CMV pneumonia, it is recognized that a better approach would be to prevent primary or reactivation CMV infection from occurring.

Over the past five years much progress has been made in achieving this goal. In order to protect seronegative patients from exposure to the virus, studies have been undertaken where exclusively seronegative blood products have been given and the efficacy of this approach has been confirmed (Mackinnon, *et al.*, 1988; Bowden, *et al.*, 1986, 1987). Another approach that has been successful is the use of leucocyte depleted platelets and CMV-negative red cells when given for transfusion purposes (Bowden, *et al.*, 1991a).

More recently Bowden, *et al.* (1991b) evaluated the role of CMV Ig as prophylaxis in seronegative patients who had seropositive marrow donors; although there was a reduced rate of virus excretion and viraemia the incidence of CMV pneumonia was no different from the control group of patients who did not receive CMV Ig. The same group conducted a large trial of CMV Ig prophylaxis and achieved a significant reduction in incidence of interstitial pneumonia even though the reduction in CMV pneumonia was not so impressive. Another important finding in this study was a reduction in the incidence of acute GVHD in Ig recipients (Sullivan, *et al.*, 1990). Of note was the fact that most of the patients in this study were CMV seropositive before transplant. It is clear from studies which have analysed the association of risk factors for acute and chronic GVHD that CMV seropositivity, and subsequently infection in the patient, is a significant risk factor (Bostrom, *et al.*, 1988, 1990).

The use of chemoprophylaxis has also been evaluated. Meyers, *et al.* (1988) found that acyclovir ($500 \, \text{mg/m}^2$/d from day -5 to day $+30$) reduced the incidence of CMV pneumonia to 19% compared to 31% in the control group. Recognizing that ganciclovir is more active against CMV than acyclovir even though it is more likely to cause bone marrow suppression, Schmidt, *et al.* (1991) devised a strategy for ganciclovir prophylaxis of CMV pneumonia which appears to be very effective. Patients underwent BAL and tests for CMV by immunofluorescence and culture at day 35 post-transplant. Those with evidence of CMV shedding were given ganciclovir or standard treatment. There was a reduction in incidence of CMV pneumonia from 12/17 standard care group to 5/20 in the ganciclovir group.

Extrapulmonary CMV infection may involve the brain, intestine, liver, kidneys or other organs (Petersen, 1991). Studies of responses to chemotherapy are few; however, Reed, *et al.* (1990) experienced poor responses to ganciclovir in cases of CMV gastroenteritis.

Recommendations for management of CMV infection are summarized in Table 4.

Pneumocystis carinii is recognized to be a potential cause of interstitial pneumonitis during this period; however, co-trimoxazole is very effective as prophylaxis against this organism. Our policy is to give all patients co-trimoxazole once their neutrophil count is $>1 \times 10^9$/l until day $+150$. For those who do not tolerate the drug, pentamidine given as an aerosol is a suitable alternative although it is unpleasant for the patient to take.

Late infections

It is recognized that patients continue to be susceptible to opportunistic infections up to one year post-BMT and beyond. This is because full immunological recovery, which might be expected by one year, is often delayed by the need for immunosuppression for chronic GVHD. A variety of complications have been recorded during this period (Deeg, Storb and Thomas, 1984). The major infectious complications are due to varicella-zoster virus (VZV) and capsulated strains of *Streptococcus pneumoniae* and *Haemophilus influenzae*.

About 50% of patients will develop VZV infection by 6 months. This usually presents as localized dermatomal zoster; however, more severe infections due to visceral dissemination occasionally occur and the Seattle group in an early study reported a mortality of 8% overall (Deeg, Storb and Thomas, 1984). Treatment with acyclovir has reduced the risk of morbidity; for most cases oral therapy is fully effective (Ljungman, *et al.*, 1989), but in more severe infections intravenous therapy is warranted.

Should patients with latent VZV infection, as evidenced by the presence of antibody to the virus before transplant, be given prophylactic acyclovir? Certainly clinical trials have shown this to be very effective but it requires prolonged administration of the drug. This has raised concerns about the development of acyclovir resistance, so that the preferred approach is not to give prophylaxis but to treat cases promptly as they arise (Perren, *et al.*, 1988).

Table 12.4 Overview of management of infection following bone marrow transplantation

	Example of recommended regimen	Reference	Comment
1 Neutropenic period			
(a) Oral chemoprophylaxis	neomycin + colistin or quinolone (+ colistin)	Warren, *et al.*, 1990	screen stools for quinolone resistant enterobacteria
	chlorhexidine applied to oropharynx	Ferretti, *et al.*, 1987	
	fluconazole or itraconazole	Tricot, *et al.*, 1987	screen for resistant *C. krusei* and *C. glabrata*
	acyclovir	Shepp, *et al.*, 1987	
(b) Initial empirical therapy of fever (>38 °C)	ureidopenicillin + aminoglycoside or ceftazidime (+ vancomycin)	Barnes and Rogers, 1988	
(c) Empirical therapy for persistent fever (>96 h)	amphotericin B		
2 Post-marrow engraftment			
(a) CMV prophylaxis:			
(i) seronegative recipient	CMV seronegative blood products	Bowden, *et al.*, 1986	(CMV Ig not indicated)
(ii) seropositive recipient	acyclovir or ganciclovir	Meyers, *et al.*, 1988 Schmidt, *et al.*, 1988	(screen blood or BAL for reactivation of infection at day 35)
(b) Pneumocystis prophylaxis	co-trimoxazole to day 150	Wingard, *et al.*, 1988	(prophylaxis not given during neutropenia)
(c) CMV therapy	ganciclovir + CMV immunoglobulin	Schmidt, *et al.*, 1988	(establish diagnosis by detection of CMV in BAL)
3 Late infections			
(a) VZV infection therapy	acyclovir	Locksley, *et al.*, 1985	
(b) Chemoprophylaxis during chronic GVHD therapy	penicillin/amoxycillin		give co-amoxyclav if resistant *H. influenzae* prevalent

Epstein–Barr virus is known to reactivate frequently in the course of marrow transplantation and while occasionally it has been considered to be a cause of hepatitis, generally it is not a major pathogen. Rarely, however, in the particular case of HLA-mismatched transplants lymphoid malignancy has developed and been shown to be due to E–B virus (Shapiro, *et al.*, 1988; Zutter, *et al.*, 1988).

In patients with chronic-GVHD, who require continuation of immunosuppressive therapy there is evidence of selective deficiency of immunoglobulins IgA and IgG subclass 2 (Rogers, *et al.*, 1986; Sheridan, *et al.*, 1990). Another 'late' consequence of chronic-GVHD is splenic atrophy (Kahls, *et al.*, 1988). These represent important risk factors for infections

with pneumococcus and *H. influenzae* – the most important of which are pneumonia and septicaemia. Our policy is to give such patients long-term prophylactic penicillin, or in the case of children less than 8 years of age amoxycillin.

Future developments

The indications for BMT are likely to expand in future years. In order to prevent infections and related complications occurring, research is likely to be focused on several key areas namely (i) the use of growth factors to accelerate recovery of bone marrow failure in the immediate post-transplant period; (ii) chemotherapeutic and immunological methods to prevent CMV and interstitial pneumonia and (iii) prevention of chronic GVHD thereby reducing the risk of related opportunistic infections. The prospects for the attainment of these goals over the next decade are good!

References

Allo, M.D., Miller, J., Townsend, T. and Tan, C. (1987) Primary cutaneous aspergillosis associated with Hickman intravenous catheters. *New England Journal of Medicine*, **317**, 1105–1108

Ambrosino, D.M. (1991) Impaired polysaccharide responses in immunodeficient patients: relevance to bone marrow transplant patients. *Bone marrow Transplantation*, **7** (suppl. 3), 48–51

Armstrong, D. (1984) Protected environments are discomforting and expensive and do not offer meaningful protection. *American Journal of Medicine*, **76**, 685–689

Arthur, R.R., Shah, K.V., Charache, P. and Saral, R. (1988) BK and JC virus infections in recipients of bone marrow transplants. *Journal of Infectious Diseases*, **158**, 563–569

Atkinson, K., Dodds, A.J., Concannon, A.J. and Biggs, J.C. (1987) The development of the acquired immunodeficiency syndrome after bone-marrow transplantation. *Medical Journal of Australia*, **147**, 510–512

Aulitzky, W.E., Schulz, T.F., Tilg, H., Niederwiesser, D., Larcher, K., Ostberg, L., Scriba, M., Martindale, J., Stern, A.C., Grass P., *et al.* (1991) Human monoclonal antibodies neutralizing cytomegalovirus (CMV) for prophylaxis of CMV disease: report of a phase I trial in bone marrow transplant recipients. *Journal of Infectious Diseases*, **163**, 1344–7

Azadian, B.S., Bendig, J.W.A. and Samson, D.M. (1986) Emergence of ciprofloxacin-resistant *Pseudomonas aeruginosa* after combined therapy with ciprofloxacin and amikacin. *Journal of Antimicrobial Chemotherapy*, **17**, 771

Baglin, T.P., Gray, J.J., Marcus, R.E. and Wreghitt, T.G. (1989) Antibiotic resistant fever associated with herpes simplex virus infection in neutropenic patients with haematological malignancy. *Journal of Clinical Pathology*, **42**, 1255–1258

Barnes, R.A. and Rogers, T.R. (1989) Control of an outbreak of nosocomial aspergillosis by laminar air-flow isolation. *Journal of Hospital Infection*, **14**, 89–94

Barnes, R.A. and Rogers, T.R. (1988) Response rates to a staged antibiotic regimen in febrile neutropenic patients. *Journal of Antimicrobial Chemotherapy*, **22**

Barnes, R.A. and Rogers, T.R. (1987) An evaluation of empirical antibiotic therapy in febrile neutropenic patients. *British Journal of Haematology*, **66**, 137–140

Benhamou, E., Hartmann, O., Nogu'es, C., Maraninchi, D., Valteau, D. and Lemerle, J. (1991) Does ketoconazole prevent fungal infection in children treated with high dose chemotherapy and bone marrow trans-

plantation? Results of a randomized placebo-controlled trial. *Bone Marrow Transplantation*, **7**, 127–31

Bianco, J.A., Pepe. M.S., Higano, C., Appelbaum, F.R., Mcdonald, G.B. and Singer, J.W. (1990) Prevalence of clinically relevant bacteremia upper gastrointestinal endoscopy in bone marrow transplant recipients. *American Journal of Medicine*, **89**, 134–136

Biggs, D.D., Toorkey, B.C., Carrigan, D.R., Hanson, G.A. and Ash, R.C. (1990) Disseminated echovirus infection complicating bone marrow transplantation. *American Journal of Medicine*, **88**, 421–425

Bjeletich, J. and Hickman, R.O. (1980) The Hickman indwelling catheter. *American Journal of Nursing*, **80**, 62–65

Bodey, G.P., Buckley, M., Sathe, Y.S. and Freirich, E.J. (1966) Quantitative relationships between circulating leukocytes and infection in patients with acute leukemia. *Annals of Internal Medicine*, **64**, 328–340

Bostrom, L., Ringdén, O., Jacobsen, N., Zwaan, F. and Nilsson, B. (1990) A European multicenter study of chronic graft-versus-host disease: the role of cytomegalovirus serology in recipients and donors – acute graft-versus-host disease, and splenectomy. *Transplantation*, **49**, 1100–1105

Bostrom, L., Ringdén, O., Sundberg, B., Linde, A., Tollemar, J. and Nilsson, B. (1988) Pretransplant herpesvirus serology and acute graft-versus-host-disease. *Transplantation*, **46**, 548–552

Bowden, R.A., Slichter, S.J., Sayers, M.H., Mori, M., Cays, M.J. and Meyers, J.D. (1991a) Use of leukocyte-depleted platelets and cytomegalovirus-seronegative red blood cells for prevention of primary cytomegalovirus infection after marrow transplant. *Blood*, **78**, 246–50

Bowden, R.A., Fisher, L.D., Rogers, K., Cays, M. and Meyers, J.D. (1991b) Cytomegalovirus (CMV)-specific intravenous immunoglobulin for the prevention of primary CMV infection. *Journal of Infectious Diseases*, **164**, 483–7

Bowden, R.A., Sayers, M., Gleaves, C.A., Banaji, M., Newton, B. and Meyers, J.D. (1987) Cytomegalovirus seronegative blood components for the prevention of primary cytomegalovirus infection after marrow transplantation. Consideration for blood banks. *Transfusion*, **27**, 478–481

Bowden, R.A., Sayers, M. and Fluornoy, N. (1986) Cytomegalovirus immune globulin and seronegative blood products to prevent primary cytomegalovirus infection after marrow transplantation. *New England Journal of Medicine*, **314**, 1006–1010

Brandt, S.J., Peters, W.P., Atwater, S.K., Kurtzberg, J., Borowitz, M.J., Jones, R.B., Shpall, E.J., Bast, R.C. Jr, Gilbert, C.J. and Oette, D.H. (1988) Effect of recombinant human granulocyte-macrophage colony-stimulating factor on hematopoietic reconstitution after high-dose chemotherapy and autologous bone marrow transplantation. *New England Journal of Medicine*, **318**, 869–876

Bron, D., Wouters, A., Barekayo, I., Snoeck, R., Stryckmans, P. and Fruhling, P. (1988) Neopterin: a useful biochemical marker in the monitoring of allogeneic bone marrow transplantation. *Acta. Clin. Belg.*, **43**, 120–126

Bufill, J.A., Lum, L.G., Caya, J.G., Chitambar, C.R., Ritch, P.S., Anderson, T. and Ash, R.C. (1988) Pityrosporum folliculitis after bone marrow transplantation. *Annals of Internal Medicine*, **108**, 560–563

Carrigan, D.R., Drobyski, W.R., Russler, S.K., Tapper, M.A., Knox, K.K. and Ash, R.C. (1991) Interstitial pneumonitis associated with human herpesvirus-6 infection after marrow transplantation. *Lancet*, **338**, 147–9

Clift, R.A. and Buckner, C.D. (1984) Granulocyte transfusions. *American Journal of Medicine*, **76**, 631–636

Cohen, J., Donnelly, J.P., Worsley, A.M., Catovsky, D., Goldman, J.M. and Galton, D.A.G. (1983) Septicaemia caused by viridans streptococci in neutropenic patients with leukaemia. *Lancet*, **ii**, 1452–1454

Conneally, E., Cafferkey, M.T., Daly, P.A., Keane, C.T. and McCann, S.R. (1990) Nebulized amphotericin B as prophylaxis against invasive aspergillosis in granulocytopenic patients. *Bone Marrow Transplantation*, **5**, 403–406

Darbyshire, P.J., Weightman, N.C. and Speller, D.C.E. (1985) Problems associated with indwelling central venous catheters. *Archives of Disease in Childhood*, **60**, 129–134

Daw, M.A., MacMahon, ?. ?. and Keane, C.T. (1988) Surveillance cultures in the neutropenic patient. *Journal of Hospital Infection*, **12**, 251–261

de Bel, C., Gerritsen, E., de Maaker, G., Moolenaar, A. and Vossen, J. (1991) C-reactive protein in the management of children with fever after allogeneic bone marrow transplantation. *Infection*, **19**, 92–96

Deeg, H.J., Storb, R. and Thomas, E.D. (1984) Bone marrow transplantation: a review of delayed complications. *British Journal of Haematology*, **57**, 185–208

De Pauw, B.E., Donnelly, J.P., De Witte, T., Nováková, I.R.O. and Schattenberg, A. (1990) Options and limitations of long-term oral ciprofloxacin as antibacterial prophylaxis in allogeneic bone marrow transplant recipients. *Bone Marrow Transplantation*, **5**, 179–182

Drummond, J.E., Shah, K.V., Saral, R., Santos, G.W. and Donnenberg, A.D. (1987) BK virus specific humoral and cell mediated immunity in allogeneic bone marrow transplant (BMT) recipients. *Journal of Medical Virology*, **23**, 331–344

Faulds, D. and Heel, R.C. (1990) Ganciclovir. *Drugs*, **39**, 597–638

Ferretti, G., Ash, R.C., Brown, A.T., Largent, B.M., Kaplan, A. and Lillich, T.T. (1987) Chlorhexidine for prophylaxis against oral infections and associated complications in patients receiving bone marrow transplants. *Journal of American Dental Association*, **114**, 461–467

Gale, R.P., Bortin, M.M., van Bekkum, D.W., Biggs, J.C., Dicke, K.A., Gluckman, E., Good, R.A., Hoffman, R.G., Kay, H.E.M., Kersey, J.H., Marmont, A., Masaoka, T., Rimm, A.A., van Rood, J.J. and

Zwann, F.E. (1987) Risk factors for acute graft versus host disease. *British Journal of Haematology*, **67**, 397–406

Gale, R.P. and Winston, D. (1991) Intravenous immunoglobulin in bone marrow transplantation. *Cancer*, **68**, 1451–1453

Gluckman, E., Roudet, C., Hirsch, I., Devergie, A., Bourdeau, H., Arlet, C. and Perol, Y. (1991) Prophylaxis of bacterial infections after bone marrow transplantation. A randomized prospective study comparing oral broad-spectrum nonabsorbable antibiotics (vancomycin-tobramycin-colistin) to absorbable antibiotics (ofloxacin-amoxicillin). *Chemotherapy*, **37** (suppl. 1), 33–38

Gluckman, E., Lotsberg, J., Devergie, A., *et al.* (1983) Prophylaxis of herpes infections after bone-marrow transplantation by oral acyclovir. *Lancet*, **2**, 706–708

Goldberg, N.S., Ahmed, T., Robinson, B., Ascensao, J. and Horowitz, H. (1989) Staphylococcal scalded skin syndrome mimicking acute graft-vs-host disease in a bone marrow transplant recipient. *Archives of Dermatology*, **125**, 85–87

Golde, D.W., Bersch, N. and Quan, S.G. (1978) Trimethoprim and sulphamethoxazole inhibition of haematopoiesis in *in vitro*. *British Journal of Haematology*, **40**, 363–367

Goodrich, J.M., Reed, E.C., Mori, M., Fisher, L.D., Skerrett, S., Dandliker, P.S., Klis, B., Counts, G.W. and Meyers, J.D. (1991) Clinical features and analysis of risk factors for invasive candidal infection after marrow transplantation. *Journal of Infectious Diseases*, **164**, 731–40

Gratwohl, A. (1991) Bone marrow transplantation activity in Europe 1990. *Bone Marrow Transplantation*, **8**, 197–201

Grob, J.P., Grundy, J.E., Prentice, H.G., *et al.* (1987) Immune donors can protect marrow transplant recipients from severe cytomegalovirus infections. *Lancet*, **i**, 774–776

Grundy, J.E., Shanley, J.D. and Griffith, P.D. (1987) Is cytomegalovirus interstitial pneumonitis in transplant recipients an immunopathological condition? *Lancet*, **ii**, 996–999

Guiot, H.F., Peeters, W.G., van den Broek, P.J., van der Meer, J.W., Willemze, R. and van Furth, R. (1990) Respiratory failure elicited by streptococcal septicaemia in patients treated with cytosine arabinoside (letter). *European Journal of Haematology*, **44**, 267–268

Guyotat, D., Piens, M.A., Bouvier, R. and Fiere, D. (1987a) A case of disseminated Scedosporium apiospermum infection after bone marrow transplantation. *Mykosen*, **30**, 151–156

Guyotat, D., Gilbert, R., Chomel, J., Archimaud, E., Bossard, S., Maupas, J., Fiere, D. and Aymard, M. (1987a) Incidence and prognosis of cytomegalovirus infections following allogenic bone marrow transplantation. *Journal of Medical Virology*, **23**, 393–400

Hamadeh, R., Ardehali, A., Locksley, R.M. and York, M.K. (1988) Fatal aspergillosis associated with smoking contaminated marijuana, in a marrow transplant recipient. *Chest*, **94**, 432–433

Hann, I.M. and Prentice, H.G. (1984) Infection prophylaxis in the patient with bone marrow failure. *Clinics in Haematology*, **13.3**, 523–547

Hann, I.M., Prentice, H.G., Corringham, R., Blacklock, H.A., Keaney, M., Shannon, M., Noone, P., Gascoigne, E., Fox, J., Boesen, E., Szawatkowski, M. and Hoffbrand, A.V. (1982a) Ketoconazole versus nystatin plus amphotericin B for fungal prophylaxis severely immunocompromised patients. *Lancet*, **i**, 826–829

Hann, I.M., Prentice, H.G., Keaney, M., Corringham, R., Blacklock, A., Fox, J., Gascoigne, E. and Van Cutsem, J. (1982b) The pharmacokinetics of ketoconazole in severely immunocompromised patients. *Journal of Antimicrobial Chemotherapy*, **10**, 489–496

Hedin, G. and Hambraeus, A. (1991) Multiply antibiotic-resistant Staphylococcus epidermidis in patients, staff and environment – a one-week survey in a bone marrow transplant unit. *Journal of Hospital Infection*, **17**, 95–106

Herrmann, F., Schulz, G., Wieser, M., Kolbe, K., Nicolay, U., Noack, M., Lindemann, A. and Mertelsmann, R. (1990) Effect of granulocyte-macrophage colony-stimulating factor on neutropenia and related morbidity induced by myelotoxic chemotherapy. *American Journal of Medicine*, **88**, 619–624

Hertz, M.I., Englund, J.A., Snover, D., Bitterman, P.B. and McGlave, P.B. (1989) Respiratory syncytial virus-induced acute lung injury in adult patients with bone marrow transplants: a clinical approach and review of the literature. *Medicine*, **68**, 269–281

Hickman, R.O., Buckner, C.D., Clift, R.A., Sanders, J.E., Stewart, P. and Thomas, E.D. (1979) A modified right atrial catheter for access to the venous system in marrow transplant recipients. *Surgery, Gynecology and Obstetrics*, **148**, 871–875

Hirsch, R., Burke, B.A. and Kersey, J.H. (1984) Toxoplasmosis in bone marrow transplant recipients. *Journal of Pediatrics*, **105**, 426–428

Hyatt, D.S., Young, Y.M., Haynes, K.A., Taylor, J.M., McCarthy, D.M. and Rogers, T.R. (1992) Rhinocerebral mucormycosis following bone marrow transplantation. *Journal of Infection*, **24**, 67–71

Kahls, P., Panzer, S., Kletter, K., Minar, E., Stain-Kos, M., Walter, R., Lechner, K. and Hinterberger, W. (1988) Functional asplenia after bone marrow transplantation: a late complication related to extensive chronic graft-versus-host disease. *Annals of Internal Medicine*, **109**, 461–464

Kibbler, C.C., Smith, A., Hamilton-Tutoit, S.J., Milburn, H., Pattinson, J.K. and Prentice, H.G. (1987) Pulmonary cryptosporidiosis occurring in a bone marrow transplant patient. *Scandinavian Journal of Infectious Diseases*, **19**, 581

Kotilainen, P., Nikoskelainen, J. and Huovinen, P. (1990) Emergence of ciprofloxacin-resistant coagulase-negative staphylococcal skin flora in immunocompromised patients receiving ciprofloxacin. *Journal of Infectious Diseases*, **161**, 41–44

Kwan, J.T., Foxall, P.J., Davidson, D.G., Bending, M.R. and Eisinger, A.J. (1987) Interaction of cyclosporin and itraconazole. *Lancet*, **2**, 282

Ljungman, P., Ellis, M.N., Hackman, R.C., Shepp, D.H. and Meyers, J.D. (1990) Acyclovir-resistant herpes simplex virus causing pneumonia after marrow transplantation. *Journal of Infectious Diseases*, **162**, 244–248

Ljungman, P., Lönnqvist, B., Ringđen, O., Skinhöj, P. and Göosta Gahrton for the Nordic Bone Marrow Transplant Group (1989) A randomized trial of oral versus intravenous acyclovir for treatment of herpes zoster in bone marrow transplant recipients. *Bone Marrow Transplantation*, **4**, 613–615

Locasciulli, A., Bacigalupo, A., Vanlint, M.T., Tagger, A., Uderzo, C., Portmann, B., Shulman, H.M. and Alberti, A. (1991) Hepatitis C virus infection in patients undergoing allogeneic bone marrow transplantation. *Transplantation*, **52**, 315–318

Locksley, R.M., Flournoy, N., Sullivan, K.M. and Meyers, J.D. (1985) Infection with varicella-zoster virus after marrow transplantation. *Journal of Infectious Diseases*, **152**, 1172–1181

Mackinnon, S., Burnett, A.K., Crawford, R.J., Cameron, S., Leask, B.G.S. and Sommerville, R.G. (1988) Seronegative blood products prevent primary cytomegalovirus infection after bone marrow transplantation. *Journal of Clinical Pathology*, **41**, 948–950

Martin, M.A., Bock, M.J., Pfaller, M.A. and Wenzel, R.P. (letter) (1988) Respiratory syncytial virus infections in adult bone marrow transplant recipients. *Lancet*, **i**, 1396–1397

Martino, P., Micozzi, A., Venditti, M., Gentile, G., Girmenia, C., Ravah, R., Santilli, S., Alessandri, N. and Mandelli, F. (1990) Catheter related right-sided endocarditis in bone marrow transplant recipients. *Review of Infectious Diseases*, **12**, 250–257

Martino, P., Gentile, G., Caprioli, A., Baldassarri, I., Donelli, G., Arcese, W., Fenu, S., Micozzi, A., Venditti, M. and Mandelli, F. (1988) Hospital-acquired cryptosporidiosis in a bone marrow transplantation unit. *Journal of Infectious Diseases*, **158**, 647–648

Menichetti, F., Felicini, R., Bucaneve, G., et al. (1989) Norfloxacin prophylaxis for neutropenics undergoing bone marrow transplantation. *Bone Marrow Transplantation*, **4**, 489–492

Menichetti, F., Del Favero, A., Bucaneve, G., Aversa, F., Baldelli, F., Falicini, R., Terenzi, S.A. and Pauluzzi, F. (1988) Teicoplanin in empirical combined antibiotic therapy of bacteraemias in bone marrow transplant patients. *Journal of Antimicrobial Chemotherapy*, **21** (suppl. A), 105–111

Meyers, J.D., Ljungman, P. and Fisher, L.D. (1990) Cytomegalovirus excretion as a predictor of cytomegalovirus disease after marrow transplantation: importance of cytomegalovirus viremia. *Journal of Infectious Diseases*, **162**, 373–380

Meyers, J.D. (1988) Management of cytomegalovirus infection. *American Journal of Medicine*, **85** (suppl. 2A), 102–106

Meyers, J.D., Reed, E.C., Shepp, D.H., Thornquist, M., Dandliker, P.S., Vicary, C.A., Fluornoy, N., Kirk, L.E., Kersey, J.H., Thomas, E.D. and Balfour, H.H. (1988) Acyclovir for prevention of cytomegalovirus infection and disease after allogeneic marrow transplantation. *New England Journal of Medicine*, **318**, 70–75

Meyers, J.D. and Atkinson, K. (1983) Infection in bone marrow transplantation. *Clinics in Haematology*, **12**, 791–811

Meyers, J.D., Wade, J.C., Mitchell, C.D., *et al.* (1982) Multicenter collaborative trial of intravenous acyclovir for treatment of mucocutaneous herpes simplex virus infection in the immunocompromised host. *American Journal of Medicine*, **73** (suppl. 1A), 229–235

Miyamura, K., Minami, S., Matsuyama, T., Kodera, Y., Yamauchi, T., Tahara, T., Sao, H., Morishima, Y. and Yokomaku, S. (1987) Adenovirus-induced late onset hemorrhagic cystitis following allogeneic bone marrow transplantation. *Bone Marrow Transplantation*, **2**, 109

Moosa, H.H., Julian, T.B., Rosenfeld, C.S. and Shadduck, R.K. (1991) Complications of indwelling central venous catheters in bone marrow transplant recipients. *Surgery, Gynecology and Obstetrics*, **172**, 275–279

Mori, M., Galvin, J.R., Barloon, T.J., Gingrich, R.D. and Stanford, W. (1991) Fungal pulmonary infections after bone marrow transplantation: evaluation with radiography and CT. *Radiology*, **178**, 721–726

Navari, R.M., Buckner, C.D., Clift, R.A., *et al.* (1984) Prophylaxis of infection in patients with aplastic anaemia receiving allogeneic marrow transplants. *American Journal of Medicine*, **76**, 564–572

Oppenheim, B.A., Hartley, J.W., Lee, W. and Burnie, J.P. (1989) Outbreak of coagulase negative staphylococcus highly resistant to ciprofloxacin in a leukaemia unit. *British Medical Journal*, **299**, 294–297

O'Reilly, R.J., Lee, F.K., Grossbard, E., Kapoor, N., Kirkpatrick, D., Dinsmore, R., *et al.* (1981) Papovavirus excretion following marrow transplantation: incidence and association with hepatic dysfunction. *Transplantation Proceedings*, **13**, 262–266

Pariente, E.A., Goudeau, A., Dubois, F., Degott, C., Gluckman, E., Devergie, A., Brechot, C., Schenmetzler, C. and Bernuau, J. (1988) Fulminant hepatitis due to reactivation of chronic hepatitis-B virus infection after allogeneic bone marrow transplantation. *Dig. Dis. Sci.*, **33**, 1185–1191

Paulin, T., Ringdén, O., Lönnquist, B., Wahren, B. and Nilsson, B. (1986) The importance of pre bone marrow transplantation serology in determining subsequent cytomegalovirus infection. *Scandinavian Journal of Infectious Diseases*, **18**, 199–209

Perren, T.J., Powles, R.L., Easton, D., Stolle, K. and Selby, P.J. (1988) Prevention of herpes zoster in patients by long-term oral acyclovir after allogeneic bone marrow transplantation. *American Journal of Medicine*, **85** (suppl. 2A), 99–101

Petersen, E.A. (1991) Extrapulmonary cytomegalovirus disease in transplant patients. *Transplantation Proceedings*, **23** (suppl. 1), 13–16

Peterson, M.W., Pratt, A.D. and Nugent, K.M. (1987) Pneumonia due to *Histoplasma capsulatum* in a bone marrow transplant recipient. *Thorax*, **42**, 698–699

Pirsch, J.D. and Maki, D.G. (1986) Infectious compli-

cations in adults with bone marrow transplantation and T-cell depletion of donor marrow. *Annals of Internal Medicine*, **104**, 619–631

Prentice, H.G. (1989) Prophylaxis and treatment of cytomegalovirus infections in the bone marrow transplant recipient. *Journal of Antimicrobial Chemotherapy*, **23** (suppl. E), 23–30

Prentice, H.G. (1983) Use of acyclovir for prophylaxis of herpes infections in severely immunocompromised patients. *Journal of Antimicrobial Chemotherapy*, **12** (suppl. B), 153–159

Ranson, M.R., Oppenheim, B.A., Jackson, A., Kamthan, A.G. and Scarffe, J.H. (1990) Double-blind placebo controlled study of vancomycin prophylaxis for central venous catheter insertion in cancer patients. *Journal of Hospital Infection*, **15**, 95–102

Reed, E.C., Myerson, D., Corey, L. and Meyers, J.D. (1991) Allogeneic marrow transplantation in patients positive for hepatitis B surface antigen. *Blood*, **77**, 195–200

Reed, E.C., Wolford, J.L., Kopecky, K.J., Lilleby, K.E., Dandliker, P.S., Todaro, J.L., McDonald, G.B. and Meyers, J.D. (1990) Ganciclovir for the treatment of cytomegalovirus gastroenteritis in bone marrow transplant patients: a randomized placebo-controlled trial. *Annals of Internal Medicine*, **112**, 505–510

Reeves, D.S. (1986) The effect of quinolone antibacterials on the gastrointestinal flora compared with that of other antibacterials. *Journal of Antimicrobial Chemotherapy*, **18** (suppl. D), 89–102

Reusser, P., Fisher, L.D., Buckner, C.D., Thomas, E.D. and Meyers, J.D. (1990) Cytomegalovirus infection after autologous bone marrow transplantation: occurrence of cytomegalovirus disease and effect on engraftment. *Blood*, **75**, 1888–1894

Rogers, T.R. (1991) Prevention of infection during neutropenia. *British Journal of Haematology*, **79**, 544–549

Rogers, T.R., Haynes, K.A. and Barnes, R.A. (1990) Value of antigen detection in predicting invasive pulmonary aspergillosis. *Lancet*, **336**, 1210–1213

Rogers, T.R. (1988) Infective complications of bone marrow transplantation. *Current Opinion in Infectious Diseases*, **1**, 616–624

Rogers, T.R. and Barnes, R.A. (1988) Prevention of airborne fungal infection in immunocompromised patients. *Journal of Hospital Infection*, **11** (suppl. 1A), 15–20

Rogers, T.R., Riches, P.G., Walker, S.A. and Joshi, R. (1986) Changes in immunoglobulin levels and implications for immunoglobulin therapy to prevent infection following bone marrow transplantation. In, *Clinical use of intravenous immunoglobulin* (A. Morell, U.E. Nydegger, eds), Academic Press, London

Rogers, T.R. (1985) Prevention of infection in neutropenic bone marrow transplant patients. In, *Antibiotics and Chemotherapy* H. Schonfeld, F.E. Hahn, eds, vol. 33, pp. 90–113, Karger Basel

Rogers, T.R., Petrou, M.A., Lucas, C., *et al.* (1981) Spread of Clostridium difficile among patients receiving non-absorbable antibiotics for gut decontamination. *British Medical Journal*, **283**, 408–409

Ruutu, P., Ruutu, T., Volin, L., Tukaianen, P., Ukkonen, P. and Hovi, T. (1990) Cytomegalovirus is frequently isolated in bronchoalveolar lavage fluid of bone marrow transplant recipients without pneumonia. *Annals of Internal Medicine*, **112**, 913–916

Ruutu, P., Valtonen, V., Tittanen, L., Elonen, E., Volin, L., Veijalainen, P. and Ruutu, T. (1987) An outbreak of invasive aspergillosis in a haematologic unit. *Scandinavian Journal of Infectious Diseases*, **19**, 347–352

Saarinen, U.M., Strandjord, S.E., Warkentin, P.I., Cheung, N.V., Lazarus, H.M. and Coccia, P.F. (1987) Differentiation of presumed sepsis from acute graft-versus-host disease by C-reactive protein and serum total IgE in bone marrow transplant recipients. *Transplantation*, **44**, 540–546

Sandford, G.R., Merz, W.G., Wingard, J.R., Charache, P. and Saral, R. (1980) The value of fungal surveillance cultures as predictors of systemic fungal infections. *Journal of Infectious Diseases*, **142**, 503–509

Saral, R. (1991) The role of immunoglobulin in bone marrow transplantation. *Transplantation Proceedings*, **23**, 2128–2132

Saral, R. (1985) Viral infections in bone marrow transplantation recipients. *Plasma Therapy and Transfusion Technology*, **6**, 275–284

Saral, R., Burns, W.H., Laskin, O.L., Santos, G.W. and Leitman, P.S. (1981) Acyclovir prophylaxis of herpes simplex virus infections: a randomized double-blind controlled trial in bone marrow transplant recipients. *New England Journal*, **305**, 63

Schmidt, G.M., Horak, D.A., Niland, J.C., Duncan, S.R., Forman, S.J. and Zaia, J.A. (1991) A randomized, controlled trial of prophylactic ganciclovir for cytomegalovirus pulmonary infection in recipients of allogeneic bone marrow transplant; The City of Hope-Stanford-Syntex CMV Study Group. *New England Journal of Medicine*, **324**, 1005–1011

Schmidt, G.M., Kovacs, A., Zaia, J.A., *et al.* (1988) Ganciclovir/immunoglobulin combination therapy for the treatment of human cytomegalovirus-associated interstitial pneumonia in bone marrow allograft recipients. *Transplantation*, **46**, 905–907

Schwebke, J.R., Hackman, R. and Bowden, R. (1990) Pneumonia due to *Legionella micdadei* in bone marrow transplant recipient. *Review of Infectious Diseases*, **12**, 824–828

Shapiro, R.S., McClain, K., Frizzera, G., Gajl-Peczalska, K.J., Kersey, J.G., Blazan, B.R., Arthur, D.C., Patton, D.F., Greenberg, J.S., Burke, B., Ramsay, N.K.C., McGlove, P. and Filipovich, A.H. (1988) Epstein–Barr virus associated B-cell lymphoproliferative disorders following bone marrow transplantation. *Blood*, **71**, 1234–1243

Shepard, J.H., Canafax, D.M., Simmons, R.L. and Najarian, J.S. (1986) Cyclosporine-ketoconazole: a potentially dangerous drug-drug interaction. *Clinical Pharmacology*, **5**, 468

Shepp, D.H., Dandliker, P.S., Fluornoy, N. and Meyers, J.D. (1987) Sequential intravenous and twice daily oral acyclovir for extended prophylaxis of herpes simplex virus infection in marrow transplant patients. *Transplantation*, **43**, 654–658

Shepp, D.H., Newton, B.A., Dandliker, P.S., Fluornoy, N. and Meyers, J.D. (1985) Oral acyclovir therapy for mucocutaneous herpes simplex virus infections in immunocompromised marrow transplant recipients. *Annals of Internal Medicine*, **102**, 783–785

Shepp, D.H., Dandliker, P.S., Fluornoy, N. and Meyers, J.D. (1985) Once-daily intravenous acyclovir for prophylaxis of herpes simplex virus reactivation after marrow transplant. *Journal of Antimicrobial Chemotherapy*, **16**, 389

Sheridan, J.F., Tutschka, P.J., Sedmak, D.D. and Copelan, E.A. (1990) Immunoglobulin G subclass deficiency and pneumococcal infection after allogeneic bone marrow transplantation. *Blood*, **75**, 1583–1586

Siegert, W., Henze, G., Wagner, J., Rodloff, A., Zimmermann, R., Malchus, R., Schwerdtfeger, R., Reichelt, A., Graft, K. and Hugn, D. (1988) Invasive *Trichosporon cutaneum (beigelii)* infection in a patient with relapsed acute myeloid leukemia undergoing bone marrow transplantation. *Transplantation*, **46**, 151–153

Skinhoj, P., Jacobsen, N., Hoiby, N. and Faber, V. (1987) Strict protective isolation in allogeneic bone marrow transplantation: effect on infectious complications, fever and graft versus host disease. *Scandinavian Journal of Infectious Diseases*, **19**, 91–96

Solberg, C.O., Meuwissen, H.J., Needham, R.N., Good, R.A. and Matsen, J.M. (1971) Infectious complications in bone marrow transplant patients. *British Medical Journal*, **1**, 18–23

Storring, R.A., Jameson, B., McElwain, T.J., Wiltshaw, E., Spiers, A.S.D. and Gaya, H. (1977) Oral non-absorbed antibiotics prevent infections in acute non-lymphoblastic leukaemia. *Lancet*, **ii**, 837–840

Sullivan, K.M., Kopecky, K.J., Jocom, J., Fisher, L., Buckner, C.D., Meyers, J.D., Counts, G.W., Bowden, R.A., Petersen, F.B., Witherspoon, R.P., Budinger, M.D., Schwartz, R.S., Appelbaum, F.R., Clift, R.A., Hansen, J.A., Sanders, J.E., Thomas, E.D. and Storb, R. (1990) Immunomodultory and antimicrobial efficacy of intravenous immunoglobulin in bone transplantation. *New England Journal of Medicine*, **323**, 705–712

Sullivan, K.M., Meyers, J.D., Fluornoy, N., Storb, R. and Thomas, E.D. (1986) Early and late interstitial pneumonia following human bone marrow transplantation. *International Journal of Cell Cloning*, **4** (suppl. 1), 107–121

Thomas, E.D., Storb, R., Clift, R.A., Fefer, A., Johnson, F.L., Neiman, P.E., *et al.* (1975) Bone-marrow transplantation. *New England Journal of Medicine*, 832–843

Townsend, T.R., Bolyard, E.A., Yolken, R.H., Beschorner, W.E., Bishop, C.A., Burns, W.H., *et al.* (1982) Outbreak of coxsackie A1 gastroenteritis: a complication of bone-marrow transplantation. *Lancet*, **i**, 820–823

Tricot, G., Joosten, E., Boogaerts, M.A., Van de Pitte, J.

and Cauwenbergh, G. (1987) Ketoconazole vs itraconazole for antifungal prophylaxis in patients with severe granulocytopenia: preliminary results to two nonrandomized studies. *Reviews of Infectious Diseases*, **9** (suppl. 1), 594–599

Valteau, D., Hartmann, O., Brugieres, L., Vassal, G., Benhamou, E., Andremont, A., Kalifa, C. and Lemerle, J. (1991) Streptococcal septicaemia following autologous bone marrow transplantation in children treated with high-dose chemotherapy. *Bone Marrow Transplantation*, **7**, 415–419

Vose, J.M., Bierman, P.J., Kessinger, A., Coccia, P.F., Anderson, J., Oldham, F.B., Epstein, C. and Armitage, J.O. (1991) The use of recombinant human granulocyte-macrophage colony stimulating factor for the treatment of delayed engraftment following high dose therapy and autologous hematopoietic stem cell transplantation for lymphoid malignancies. *Bone Marrow Transplantation*, **7**, 139–143

Wade, J.C., Newton, B., Fluornoy, N. and Meyers, J.D. (1984) Oral acyclovir for prevention of herpes simplex virus reactivation after marrow transplant. *Annals of Internal Medicine*, **100**, 823

Walker, S.A., Rogers, T.R., Riches, P.G., White, S. and Hobbs, J.R. (1984a) Value of serum C-reactive protein measurement in the management of bone marrow transplant recipients. Part I: early transplant period. *Journal of Clinical Pathology*, **37**, 1018–1021

Walker, S.A., Rogers, T.R., Perry, D., Hobbs, J.R. and Riches, P.G. (1984b) Increased serum IgE concentrations during infection and graft versus host disease after bone marrow transplantation. *Journal of Clinical Pathology*, **37**, 460–462

Warren, R.E., Wimperis, J.Z., Baglin, T.P., Constantine, C.E. and Marcus, R. (1990) Prevention of infection by ciprofloxacin in neutropenia. *Journal of Antimicrobial Chemotherapy*, **26** (suppl. F), 109–123

Wasserman, R., August, C.S. and Plotkin, S.A. (1988) Viral infection in pediatric bone marrow transplant patients. *Pediatric Infectious Diseases*, **7**, 109–115

Willoughby, R.E., Wee, S.-B. and Yolken, R.H. (1988) Non-group A rotavirus infection associated with severe gastroenteritis in a bone marrow transplant patient. *Pediatric Infectious Diseases Journal*, **7**, 133–135

Wingard, J.R. (1990) Advances in the management of infectious complications after bone marrow transplantation. *Bone Marrow Transplantation*, **6**, 371–383

Wingard, J.R., Mellits, E.D., Sostrin, M.B., *et al.* (1988) Interstitial pneumonitis after allogeneic bone marrow transplantation. *Medicine*, **67**, 175–186

Wingard, J.R., Dick, J., Charache, P. and Saral, R. (1986) Antibiotic-resistant bacteria in surveillance stool cultures of patients with prolonged neutropenia. *Antimicrobial Agents and Chemotherapy*, **30**, 435–439

Winston, D.J. and Gale, R.P. (1991) Prevention and treatment of cytomegalovirus infection and disease after bone marrow transplantation. *Bone Marrow Transplantation*, **8**, 7–11

Winston, D.J., Ho, W.G., Lin, C.-H., Bartoni, K., Budinger, M.D., Gale, R.P. and Champlin, R.E. (1987) Intravenous immune globulin for prevention of cytomegalovirus infection and interstitial pneumonia after bone marrow transplantation. *Annals of Internal Medicine*, **106**, 12–18

Winston, D.J., Ho, W.G. and Gale, R.P. (1982) Therapeutic granulocyte transfusions for documented infections. *Annals of Internal Medicine*, **97**, 509–515

Winston, D.J., Pollard, R.G., Ho, W.G., Gallagher, J.G., Rasmussen, L.E., Nan-Yang, S., Lin, C.H., Gossett, T.G., Merigan, T.C. and Gale, R.P. (1982) Cytomegalovirus immune plasma in bone marrow transplant recipients. *Annals of Internal Medicine*, **97**, 11–18

Winston, D.J., Gale, R.P., Meyer, D.V., Young, L.S. and the U.C.L.A. Bone Marrow Transplantation Group. (1978) Infectious complications of human bone marrow transplantation. *Medicine*, **58**, 1–31

Yoshikawa, T., Suga, S., Asano, Y., Nakashima, T., Yazaki, T., Sobue, R., Hirano, M., Fukuda, M., Kojima, S. and Matsuyama, T. (1991) Human herpesvirus-6 infection in bone marrow transplantation. *Blood*, **78**, 1381–1384

Zaia, J.A. (1983) Infections. In *Clinical Bone Marrow Transplantation*, K.G. Blume, L.D. Petz, eds, pp. 131–176. New York: Churchill Livingstone

Zutter, M.M., Martin, P.J., Sale, G.E., Shulman, H.M. Fisher, L., Thomas, E.D. and Durnam, D.M. (1988) Epstein–Barr virus lymphoproliferation after bone marrow transplantation. *Blood*, **72**, 520–529

13

Granulocyte transfusions

J.K.M. Duguid and A.C. Newland

Introduction

Episodes of profound granulocytopenia are commonly seen in patients receiving intensive chemotherapy for haematological malignancy and other types of cancer. The incidence of infection in these patients is high and it is a major cause of morbidity with a 10–25% mortality (*Lancet*, Editorial 1980). The incidence of infection increases markedly once the white cell count falls below $1 \times 10^9/l$, and is particularly severe when the neutrophils are less than $0.5 \times 10^9/l$ (Bodey, *et al.*, 1966). In those patients whom granulocytopenia is persistent and marrow recovery not imminent, the use of granulocyte transfusions therefore appears a rational treatment choice. Its efficacy, however, is not well established (Alavi, *et al.*, 1977; Vogler and Winton, 1977). One of the main problems encountered in the use of granulocyte transfusions is that of obtaining sufficient cells. In healthy adults the daily turnover of granulocytes is $1 \times 10''$ cells, each with a survival of only a few hours. During infection the daily turnover may be increased as much as eight-fold (Marsh, *et al.*, 1967). Provision of an adequate granulocyte dose from single units of blood is therefore impractical. However, large doses of granulocytes can be obtained by leucapheresis. Early work by Freireich, *et al.* (1964) using granulocytes collected by leucapheresis from patients with chronic granulocytic leukaemia (CGL) showed clinical improvement in more than 50% of infected neutropenic patients.

Subsequent studies have shown that granulocyte transfusions can be used successfully to prevent and treat infections in neutropenic animals and to aid in treating infections in man. Despite these findings the use of granulocyte transfusions in treating these patients remains controversial, mainly because the causes of and responses to infection in these patients are multifactorial. The results from trials are conflicting making the interpretation of the clinical efficacy of granulocyte transfusions difficult. The EORTC Study (1983) administered granulocytes with empiric antibiotic therapy as initial treatment in the febrile neutropenic patient. The overall response (70%) was not significantly different from that of the control group. This contrasts with two other studies which showed a significant improvement in response ($P < 0.05$) when granulocyte transfusions were administered in patients with documented infections (Klastersky, 1979; Vogler and Winton, 1977).

This, taken in association with the known hazards to both donor and recipient, the difficulty in collecting adequate numbers of granulocytes and the time and cost involved has meant that the regular use of granulocyte transfusions has not become established in clinical practice. Despite these disadvantages granulocyte transfusions can be used successfully to prevent and treat infections and (in selected patients) may have a place in the treatment of patients with neutropenia.

Indications for granulocyte transfusions

Animal studies have shown that granulocyte transfusions have a beneficial effect when given to nonimmunized neutropenic animals with experimental infections (Hollingsworth, *et al.*, 1956; Epstein, *et al.*, 1969; Dale, *et al.*, 1975; Epstein, *et al.*, 1974; Popovic, *et al.*, 1977). Granulocytes transfused into immunized (previously transfused) animals do not show the same beneficial result (Appelbaum, *et al.*, 1977). As the majority of neutropenic patients who require granulocyte support will have been previously transfused, it is therefore difficult to predict in this group of at risk patients who will benefit from granulocyte transfusions.

The likelihood of a neutropenic patient becoming infected has been shown by Bodey, *et al.* (1966) to be directly related to the severity and duration of granulocytopenia. Once granulocyte levels are less than $0.2 \times 10^9/l$ for a prolonged period the incidence of infections increases markedly. Within this group of patients there is some indication as to which patients are likely to benefit from granulocyte transfusions (Table 13.1) given in conjunction with effective antimicrobial therapy (Higby and Burnett, 1980).

An important consideration is the prognosis of the underlying disease (Foon and Gale, 1982) and the likelihood of a prolonged period of aplasia. If bone marrow recovery is imminent or the primary condition unresponsive then granulocytes are not indicated. When their use is being considered, appropriate antibiotic therapy should in most cases be used for at least 24–48 hours first. Certain types of infection appear to be more responsive to granulocyte infusions, these include Gram-negative septicaemia unresponsive to appropriate antibiotics, pneumonia and cellulitis. Granulocyte transfusions have not been shown to benefit patients with non-bacterial infections or fever of unknown origin. However, their empirical early use in Gram-negative shock may be beneficial.

Two other groups of patients may also be considered, septic neonates with agranulocytosis in conjunction with antibiotics (Laurenti, *et al.*, 1981; Christensen, *et al.*, 1982; Laing, *et al.*, 1983) and also patients with chronic granulomatous disease during septic episodes (Bueschler and Gallin, 1982).

Granulocyte collection

Selection of donors The collection of sufficient granulocytes for transfusion purposes in general requires the use of a cell separator. The use of this equipment is associated with certain recognized hazards including the possible use of drugs, therefore extra care must be taken in the selection of granulocyte donors.

Ideally donors should have donated whole blood on at least one occasion previously and most countries have guide-lines for their selection and care. These obviously vary, but at a minimum should include the following:

(i) Prior to becoming a granulocyte donor a full medical examination should be undertaken by a medical officer familiar with the operation of cell separators; this should include a chest X-ray, and also an ECG for donors over 40 years of age.
(ii) A full blood count, prothrombin time and partial thromboplastin time, together with an estimation of total serum proteins, albumin and immunoglobulin concentration should be undertaken.
(iii) The donors ABO and Rh grouping and also their HLA type should be determined.
(iv) In view of the recognized increased risk of transmission of cytomegalovirus (CMV) infection by granulocyte transfusions (Winston, *et al.*, 1980a; Hersman, *et al.*, 1982) the CMV antibody status of potential granulocyte donors should be checked. This should be repeated at each donation to exclude seroconversion.
(v) Screening tests for HBsAg, Hepatitis C and for HIV1 must be performed at each collection.
(vi) Fully informed written consent should be obtained prior to each donation.

Recommendations are made by some countries

Table 13.1 Indications for granulocyte transfusions in neutropenic patients

Granulocytopenia ($<0.5 \times 10^9/l$)
Disease responsive to chemotherapy
Prolonged period of aplasia likely
Failure to respond to adequate and appropriate
    antibiotic therapy for 24–48 hours
Gram-negative septicaemia with 'shock'
Cellulitis, necrotic ulceration or pneumonia with
    septicaemia

as to the maximum number of granulocyte donations to be made by an individual donor annually. In the UK this is 12 donations a year (DHSS, 1978). Any donors giving the maximum number of times should have a full medical examination annually. At each donation a full blood count should be performed, a white cell count greater than $4.0 \times 10^9/l$ being essential.

Relations and friends of patients requiring granulocyte donations often request that they should be donors. Increased care must be taken in selecting from this group of people, and the same selection criteria as outlined above must apply. The physician in charge must also ensure that no undue moral pressure is being put on these potential donors. On no account should a relative who may be considered as a bone marrow donor for the patient be used as a granulocyte donor.

Methods of collection A variety of techniques exist for the collection of granulocytes. These range from time-consuming manual methods to the use of cell separators. The latter fall into two main categories, those that work on a filtration principle and those that separate granulocytes by centrifugation. In an attempt to obviate the need for expensive cell separators an attempt to use healthy bone marrow as a source of granulocytes has been made (Aghai, 1983). This technique met with limited success and, as it involves multiple marrow aspirations, donor acceptability is understandably low.

Centrifugal cell separators Two main types of centrifugal cell separator exist, separation being obtained either with an intermittent, or a continuous, flow of blood. The first widely used cell separator, the Haemonetics Model 30 (Haemonetics Corporation, Braintree, Massachusetts, USA) is an intermittent flow cell separator. Blood in combination with a fixed ratio of anticoagulant enters the centrifuge bowl, the heavy cellular elements are packed at the periphery of the bowl by the centrifugal force, displacing plasma and lighter cellular elements towards a centrally placed outlet port. Separated elements, granulocytes, are collected through the exit port until red cells reach this port when centrifugation is stopped and red cells and plasma are returned via a reinfusion bag to the donor during the next centrifugation cycle (Huestis, *et al.*, 1975). This original

machine although still widely used, requires continuous operator attention and has been replaced by the Haemonetics V50 which provides more automated operation and incorporates a variety of donor safety features. This newer model though based on the same principles as its predecessor is easier to operate and has the facility of being able to draw and return blood through a single venepuncture. Intermittent flow machines have the disadvantage that they require a relatively large extra-corporeal volume, though the provision of centrifuge bowls of varying sizes (325 ml, 225 ml and 125 ml) help to minimize this. However, hypotension and syncope are more commonly encountered with this type of machine. An increased incidence of citrate toxicity is also encountered as large volumes of citrated blood are returned to the donor at the end of each draw cycle. The time taken for each procedure is also longer than with other centrifugal methods, particularly if a single venepuncture is used.

Continuous flow cell separators These operate on a differential density centrifugation principle, separation of packed cells and plasma allowing the granulocyte buffy coat to be concentrated at the interface. Granulocytes can then be removed through an outlet port whilst the remainder of the blood is continuously returned to the donor through a second venepuncture. The IBM 2997 (COBE Laboratories Inc. Lakewood, Colorado, USA) continuous flow cell separator is widely used, it automatically positions the interface so that it is visible to the operator who adjusts the rate of the blood pumps to achieve an optimal collection, though only partially automated this machine includes a variety of safety features and warning devices. A more fully automated machine the Cobe Spectra has recently been introduced and is replacing the IBM 2997. A further continuous flow machine, the Fenwal CS 3000 (Fenwal Laboratories, Deerfield, Illinois, USA) is fully automated and operates on a unique principle, that of constant centrifugal asynchrony thereby allowing the use of a seal-less apheresis kit. Continuous flow machines have the advantage of operating with only a small extra-corporeal volume. They do, however, require two venepunctures which can be a disadvantage, and may be unacceptable to some donors. Operator skill is required to obtain an optimal granulocyte collection from these machines.

Filtration leucapheresis This technique of leucapheresis depends on the adherence of granulocytes to nylon fibres from which they can then be eluted. Machines work on a continuous flow technique and the donor has to be heparinized. Filtration leucapheresis was initially widely used as it was considered to be easier and more efficient than centrifugal methods. However due to an increased number of donor risks and the numerous modifications introduced to the detriment of granulocyte yield and function it is not used nowadays.

Gravity leucapheresis This method is based on the collection of sequential whole units of anti-coagulated blood. Each unit is centrifuged and platelet rich plasma is removed, a sedimenting agent such as hydroxy ethyl starch (HES) is then added to the packed red cells and gravity sedimentation occurs. The red cells and plasma are returned to the donor and the granulocyte rich buffy coat is retained.

Though apparently simple to perform this technique is time-consuming and prone to problems. A maximum of six units can be removed at one session and though it has been recommended that two units can be removed at a time (Djerassi, 1977) this leads to a large extra-corporeal volume and its attendant problems. This technique is, however, useful if granulocytes are required for neonates with septicaemia and depleted bone marrow granulocyte reserves; the small dose of granulocytes required in these circumstances can be obtained by gravity sedimentation of a single unit of blood within 24 hours of collection. Despite its apparent simplicity it has been calculated (Aisner, *et al.*, 1981) that this is the most expensive way to collect granulocytes.

Random donor buffy coats Buffy coats separated from fresh units of blood by centrifugation can be used as a source of granulocytes. It is difficult to provide an adequate dose of granulocytes by this means. Pooled random donor buffy coats also carry an increased risk of virus transmission and increase the likelihood of the patient developing HLA, granulocyte and platelet alloimmunization. They have the advantage, however, of being readily available from most transfusion centres.

Risks to the donor There is a morbidity and a mortality associated with granulocyte donation. Fortunately complications are rare, but in order to prevent or alleviate them it is important that careful monitoring of each donation procedure is undertaken. Staffing should be of sufficient number and ability to cope with any emergency. Ideally a cardiac arrest facility should be immediately available.

There are various recognized risks associated with any cytapheresis procedure including granulocyte donation. They may occur at the time of the donation, or later (Table 13.2). The incidence of adverse reactions varies according to the type of cell separator being used.

Immediate risks Commonly occurring risks comprise such occurrences as haematomas, vasovagal reactions, citrate toxicity and chills.

Haematomas are a common complication of any cytapheresis procedure. Leakage of blood into tissue at the venepuncture site occurs but is only serious if superinfection, serious haemorrhage or subsequent thrombosis result. Vasovagal reactions occur commonly during routine blood donation but are described as showing an increased incidence in leucapheresis donors (Sandler and Nusbacher, 1982). The donor is normally aware of the reaction, becomes pale, anxious, nauseated and hyperventilates. Appropriate action at this stage can prevent syncope or seizure. These reactions are commonest during removal of the first aliquot of blood using an intermittent flow cell separator, probably because these machines require a large extra-corporeal volume (ECV) of blood for their operation. Care should be taken that the ECV does not exceed 15% of the donor's blood volume. Modern fully automated inter-

Table 13.2 Hazards to the donor of granulocyte collection

Frequent	
Immediate	Vasovagal reaction
	Haematoma
	Citrate toxicity
	Chills
Less common	Haemorrhage
	Haemolysis
	Allergic reaction
	Air embolism
Delayed	Infection and septicaemia
	Reactions to HES
	Lymphocyte depletion

mittent flow cell separators warn the operator if a safe ECV is being exceeded. Vasovagal reaction can be aborted by rapid infusion of saline or return of the donor's blood. Care must be taken if the latter manoeuvre is undertaken not to induce the added complications of citrate toxicity.

Citrate toxicity results if the rate of reinfusion is fast or if the citrate content of the anticoagulant is high. The donor complains of circumoral and peripheral paraesthesia, chest discomfort and nausea. Hyperventilation may occur leading to frank tetany. Symptoms are due to a fall in ionized calcium and are avoided by using slow reinfusion rates and lower concentrations of citrate. It is inadvisable to try and correct the problem by using intravenous calcium as this may cause clotting in the extracorporeal circuit or severe arrhythmia in the donor.

Chills result from cooling of the blood whilst in the extra-corporeal circuit. As rapid infusion of cold blood is known to cause cardiac arrest, care should be taken to avoid this complication. A high ambient temperature and the use of a blood warmer on the return line in a two arm procedure will help. The donor should be kept warm throughout the procedure.

Risks which rarely occur include haemorrhage, haemolysis, allergic reactions, air embolism, cardiac failure, cardiac arrest, drug effects and the effects of complement activation. Severe allergic reactions consisting of asthma, dyspnoea, urticaria and angiodema have been reported. Sensitization to ethylene oxide gas used for sterilization purposes has been implicated in some of these cases (Leitman, *et al.*, 1986).

Drugs may be administered prior to donation or during the donation itself, and may affect the donor adversely. Attempts to raise a donor's white cell count prior to leucapheresis include the administration of steroids. Dexamethasone is the most commonly used preparation and whilst not associated with the more serious side-effects of steroid medication its administration may be associated with headache, fever, fatigue and arthralgia. Hydroxy ethyl starch (HES) used as a rouleaux-forming agent to aid red cell sedimentation has a mild anticoagulant effect. It can also cause skin reactions at the site of reinfusion and haemodynamic changes which may precipitate cardiac failure.

Activation of complement is mainly associated with filtration leucapheresis. Some evidence suggests it occurs in intermittent flow leucapheresis, but this has not been proved (McCleoud and Sassetti, 1981). Activation of complement particularly the production of C5a leads to leucostasis and particularly margination of granulocytes in the pulmonary vasculature which could lead to pulmonary dysfunction in both donor and recipient.

Delayed risks of leucapheresis though infrequent can be serious, and are often related to the frequency of donation. Included in this group of risks are septicaemia, accumulation of HES and lymphocyte depletion.

Infection may be localized to the site of venepuncture when it is usually related to the length of time that a needle remains *in situ*. More serious infections and septicaemia may result from the use of contaminated intravenous solutions or administration sets. A careful record of the batch number of all solutions and administration sets should be kept.

HES may persist in the circulation for several months (Ring, *et al.*, 1980), and it has been associated with hepatitis and renal toxicity. The use of a reducing dosage regime, if frequent leucapheresis is planned, limits accumulation and persistence in the circulation. Lower molecular weight formulations of HES are undetectable in the circulation six days post leucapheresis and are associated with good granulocyte yields.

Lymphocytes are lost during granulocyte donations. A six-cycle donation using an intermittent flow cell separator is associated with a loss to the donor of 3.5×10^9 lymphocytes (Koepke, *et al.*, 1981). Newer continuous flow equipment is associated with lower lymphocyte losses (Strauss, *et al.*, 1983). The extent of this loss of lymphocytes is increased with frequency of donation and appears to be most marked in the B-cell population. The implications for the donor's immune response are unknown but donors who develop a lymphopenia (lymphocytes $< 1 \times 10^9$/l) should be excluded from further donation.

Granulocyte yields Obtaining an effective therapeutic dose of granulocytes is one of the main limitations of granulocyte transfusion therapy. The satisfactory dose per transfusion is between $1 - 5 \times 10^{10}$ granulocytes for an adult patient. Care in the selection of donors, the type of machine used and the efficiency of the machine operators are important factors in the determination of granulocyte yields. Satisfactory yields are rarely obtained by gravity leucapheresis and a large number of random buffy coats are required for a satisfactory transfusion dose of granulocytes. The donor's initial white cell count is obviously a factor in determining the eventual yield and donors with a low white count ($<4.0 \times 10^9$/l) should be excluded. Patients with chronic granulocytic leukaemia and a high white count were at one time frequently used as a source of granulocytes for transfusion but an increased number of recipient reactions were reported and anxieties about engraftment have led to a decrease in their use.

Centrifugal cell separators are relatively inefficient collectors of granulocytes. Granulocyte specific gravity is very close to that of red cells causing the former to sediment in the red cell layer leaving the buffy coat relatively rich in lymphocytes. In order to overcome this various techniques have been used to improve granulocyte yields (Table 13.3).

Corticosteroid administration Administration of corticosteroids to the donor causes an increase in the granulocyte count. Three mechanisms are responsible for this:

(i) an increased release of granulocytes from the bone marrow reserve pool
(ii) a shift of marginated granulocytes to the circulating pool
(iii) inhibition of the passage of granulocytes out of the circulation (Mischler, 1977)

Table 13.3 Techniques to improve granulocyte yields during leucapheresis

Agent used	Method of use	Mode of action
Dexamethasone	Taken by donor	Release of granulocyte from marrow, shift from marginated pool, and inhibition of migration of granulocytes out of circulation
HES Dextrans Plasmagel	Added continuously to blood in cell separator	Promote rouleaux formation

Recommended corticosteroid regimes are prednisone 40–60 mg orally or dexamethasone 6–12 mg given 10–12 hours prior to donation.

Rouleaux-forming agents The addition of a rouleaux-forming agent to blood in the input line of a cell separator improves the separation between white and red cells and hence the yield of granulocytes. Hydroxy ethyl starch (HES) is the most widely used agent. Its effect on granulocyte yield is not solely due to increased sedimentation as it appears to have an effect independent of ESR increase in some cell separators (Mischler, 1982). HES use is associated with some side-effects, these are usually minimal and less than those reported to occur with the other rouleaux-forming agents, Dextrans and Plasmagel. Plasmagel is a modified fluid gelatin which, though widely used in some countries, is associated with frequent allergic reactions and less satisfactory granulocyte yields.

Yields can be further enhanced by using a combination of centrifugal and filtration techniques. Though higher yields are obtained the increased donor time required makes this unacceptable. The use of donations from two or more donors at a time is another way of providing increased dosages.

Granulocyte function

In order for granulocyte transfusion to be effective the function of granulocytes must be maintained. The final test of the granulocyte function is the patient's clinical response, but the contribution of granulocyte transfusions to individual patients recovery is often difficult to assess. One-hour post transfusion increments have been used as an indicator of granulocyte viability, but in view of the small changes likely to be encountered this presents technical problems. Furthermore by using Indium labelled granulocytes it has been shown that, 30 minutes, migration to sites of infection has occurred and margination in the liver and spleen takes place which does not clear for 24 hours (Dutcher, *et al.*, 1981) suggesting that one-hour post transfusion increments are of limited value as an indicator of *in vivo* function. Post transfusion recovery and intravascular survival of granulocytes collected using a continuous flow centrifugal technique have been shown to be normal (McCullough, *et al.*, 1976; Lin, *et al.*, 1980). It has also been shown (Price and Dale, 1977, 1978) that granulocytes collected by intermittent flow centrifugal techniques have normal post transfusion recovery, good migration into skin chambers and a half-life in the blood of 4.1 hours. Cells collected by filtration leucapheresis are activated, have poor function and are rapidly cleared. They should no longer be used.

Collection of granulocytes using cell separators could theoretically damage the granulocytes by centrifugal forces and also by contact with foreign surfaces. Intermittent flow cell separators subject granulocytes to higher centrifugal forces and contact with foreign surfaces is more prolonged than with continuous flow cell separators. Granulocytes collected this way have been shown to undergo degranulation (Blumberg, *et al.*, 1978) and to show reduced phagocytosis of staphylococcus aureus (Martin, *et al.*, 1983).

Anticoagulation affects granulocyte function and therefore influences function not only in machine collected granulocytes but also random donor buffy coat preparations and gravity leucapheresis collections. ACD and CPD anticoagulants maintain chemotaxis best, particularly if granulocytes are not used immediately. Little other data is available on *in vivo* and *in vitro* function of granulocytes obtained by manual techniques.

Prior to administration granulocytes should be irradiated to prevent graft versus host disease; doses recommended vary between 15 Gy and 50 Gy but even at higher doses some lymphoid function may remain. No effect on *in vitro* granulocyte function has been demonstrated (Button, *et al.*, 1981).

Cells from patients with chronic granulocytic leukaemia collected by centrifugal techniques show some *in vitro* changes but this is compensated for by the large numbers usually collected. *In vivo* studies show that these cells migrate to sites of infection and ingest organisms (Eyre, *et al.*, 1970).

Granulocyte storage

Ideally granulocytes should be transfused as soon after collection as possible. Limited storage is possible however. Leucapheresis products should not be stored for more than 24 hours as collection is often technically an 'open' process, with the risk of bacterial contamination. The ideal temperature for storage has not been established. Granulocytes stored between 1–6 °C for 24 hours show morphological changes and reduction in 'in vitro' function. When transfused, circulating numbers are reduced and poor migration into skin abrasions occurs (Glasser, 1979). Chemotactic function is impaired at 24 hours and severely impaired at 48 hours though these changes are less in granulocytes collected by continuous flow techniques, and stored at 20–24 °C. McCullough, *et al.* (1983) showed that granulocytes collected from whole blood or by centrifugal cell separation could be stored for 8 hours at 20–24 °C without impairment of their ability to circulate or migrate to skin windows, suggesting that this is the optimal storage time and temperature for granulocytes.

Following cryopreservation of granulocytes there is a mean recovery of 58% with bacteriocidal activity of 72% in samples stored in liquid nitrogen for up to eight months (Richman, 1983). *In vivo* effects of these cryopreserved granulocytes are not known. In general, however, the technique is too cumbersome and time consuming for widespread use.

Administration

It is difficult to lay down strict guidelines for the transfusion of granulocytes as techniques of collection and storage influence the likely response to transfusion. Granulocytes should be infused through a standard blood giving set without a microfilter. As the incidence of reactions to granulocyte infusions correlates with the infusion rate, this should be about 1×10^{10} granulocytes per 30 minutes though this also depends on the volume to be infused.

Compatibility testing Some sort of compatibility testing is required prior to granulocyte transfusion. In view of the presence of a significant number of contaminating red cells, ABO and Rh compatibility is recommended. If however the patient is highly immunized and requires HLA matched transfusions then ABO and Rh grouping can be ignored if red cell contamination is kept to a minimum. Repeated granulocyte transfusions are associated with a high incidence of alloimmunization, this incidence is increased if platelet transfusions are given as well (Pegels, *et al.*, 1982).

Correlation between alloimmunization and transfusion has not been clearly demonstrated, probably due to the use of antibody detection techniques of limited sensitivity. Dahlke, *et al.* (1980) however, demonstrated, using an immunofluorescence test for neutrophil specific antibodies, a correlation with poor post-transfusion increments, increased reactions and unsatisfactory clinical response. The use of Indium-labelled granulocytes has shown that in alloimmunized patients, shown by the presence of lymphocytotoxic antibodies, normal granulocyte migration to sites of infection does not occur (Dutcher, *et al.*, 1981; McCullough, *et al.*, 1981).

Current recommendations for compatibility testing therefore are that an ABO, Rh and HLA compatible donor should be used; red cell cross-matching and a lymphocytotoxic screening test should be performed. If this latter is positive HLA matched donors should be used. Only if clinically indicated need immunofluorescent cross-matching for granulocyte and lymphocyte specific antigens be undertaken.

Dosage and frequency Recommendations for the dosage of granulocytes vary, the minimum daily dose should be 1×10^{10} (Higby and Burnett, 1980; International Forum, 1980). This dosage should be given daily for a minimum of 4 days until infection resolves or the pre-transfusion neutrophil count consistently exceeds 0.4×10^9/l. If there is no, or a poor response, daily granulocyte transfusions may be continued for 7 days before abandoning or modifying the regime. At this stage consideration of twice daily infusions should be made if donors are available. Patients need to be carefully monitored as reactions are common and may indicate the development of alloimmunization and thus impaired response.

Irradiation Patients receiving granulocyte transfusions are likely to be severely immunocompromized and there is a significant risk of acquiring graft versus host disease (GVHD) from any transfused blood products. This is particularly the case in allogeneic and autologous bone marrow transplantation and in patients with severe aplastic anaemia undergoing immunosuppressive therapy, the outcome is invariably fatal. The risk is related to the presence of viable T-lymphocytes in the product infused. If granulocytes from donors with CGL are used there is a more serious risk of engraftment with CGL although this may be temporary. Both these problems can be alleviated if prior to transfusion all blood products are irradiated. A dose of 15 Gy is recommended. Impairment of granulocyte function by ionizing radiation does occur but is dose dependent and not significant until doses exceed 50 Gy.

Use of granulocyte transfusions

Therapeutic granulocyte transfusions There are no clear guidelines for the therapeutic use of granulocyte transfusions. The only group of patients in whom granulocytes have been shown to improve survival are those who are neutropenic with a documented septicaemia (Graw, *et al.*, 1972; Vogler and Winton, 1977; Herzig, *et al.*, 1977; Klastersky, 1979). Benefits of granulocyte transfusions for neutropenic patients with fungal or viral infections have not been proved and use in the former in conjunction with amphotericin B may cause acute respiratory distress (Wright, *et al.*, 1981).

Therapeutic granulocyte transfusions may be undertaken in patients with proven bacterial infection and persistent neutropenia who fail to respond to optimal antibiotic therapy after 48 hours. Positive culture results are the best evidence of proven infection, however, strong clinical evidence such as a skin abcess or X-ray changes consistent with pneumonia may sometimes be the only indicator of infection. Account of previous chemotherapy and bone marrow examination will indicate whether early bone marrow recovery is likely. Persistent fever together with continuing positive bacterial cultures and progressive clinical signs together with shock are evidence of non-response to antibiotics. Therapeutic granulocyte transfusions should be instituted in these patients. Granulocytes should be given as outlined previously and antibiotic choice and dosage may need to be changed according to results of cultures, sensitivity testing and drug levels.

Their use, however, must be tempered with caution. Among the many major complications is the frequent development of lymphocytotoxic antibodies with subsequent refractoriness to both further granulocytes and platelets as well as the development of cytomegalovirus infection. In the young patient, in whom bone marrow transplantation is a therapeutic option, future effective treatment may be jeopardized (Klastersky, 1979).

Prophylactic granulocyte transfusions The use of prophylactic granulocyte transfusions to prevent infection in known neutropenic patients appears an attractive proposition. Studies to date on bone marrow transplant recipients (Clift, *et al.*, 1978; Navari, *et al.*, 1984; Winston, *et al.*, 1980b) and during remission induction for acute leukaemia (Schiffer, *et al.*, 1979; Strauss, *et al.*, 1981; Winston, *et al.*, 1981) have shown no benefit in terms of preventing septicaemia nor on remission rates, remission duration or mortality. Infections due to organisms such as Proprionobacteria, Klebsiella and alpha haemolytic streptococci were more common in the group receiving prophylactic granulocytes as was the incidence of CMV infection. The incidence of alloimmunization was high leading to the abandonment of one study because of problems in providing concomitant platelet support. The evidence to date indicates that there is no place for the use of prophylactic granulocyte transfusions in the treatment of neutropenic patients.

Assessment of response Assessment of response to granulocyte transfusions is difficult, it should be looked for predominantly in signs of clinical improvement, laboratory measurements are only occasionally of help. Clear indicators of a satisfactory clinical response to granulocyte transfusions are resolution of fever and resolution of pulmonary infiltrates or other localized infections. Stabilization of a downhill course or improvement in such parameters as state of alertness, appetite or height of fever are also signs suggesting a response to granulocyte transfusions.

Laboratory evidence of response is not easy to obtain. An increase in granulocyte count is unlikely, the dose of granulocytes transfused is really too small to be measurable, and ideally for transfused granulocytes to be effective they should be concentrated at the site of infection rather than in the circulation. A measurable increase in granulocytes is more likely to reflect bone marrow recovery than transfused granulocytes. Negative blood cultures (which were previously positive) are however a definitive laboratory sign of a response to granulocyte transfusion.

Hazards of granulocyte transfusions Granulocyte transfusions pose hazards to both donor and recipient. The former have already been discussed and the latter mentioned in the previous section. Recipient reactions may occur at the time of transfusion or some time later (Table 13.4).

Immediate reactions A form of respiratory distress syndrome with rapid deterioration of respiratory function, dyspnoea, pulmonary infiltration on X-ray and deterioration in arterial oxygenation is well described in patients receiving granulocyte transfusions. A variety of causes are postulated including fluid overload, granulocyte sequestration, interaction of granulocytes and circulating endotoxin donor lymphocytotoxic antibodies or infusion of aggregated granulocytes with pulmonary embolization. An interaction between Amphotericin B and granulocyte transfusions has also been suggested (Wright, *et al.*, 1981). Severe pulmonary reactions can be kept to a minimum if care is taken in the selection of donors and in the collection, handling and transfusion of granulocytes. Premedication of recipients who have had previous reactions, with antihistamines and corticosteroids should be routine.

Alloimmunization Despite exposure to multiple antigens alloimmunization following granulocyte transfusion is not inevitable. If antibodies develop they can be responsible for febrile reactions and pulmonary infiltrates. The development of HLA and specific anti-granulocyte antibodies is associated with transfusion reactions, poor post transfusion increments, and alterations in the circulating kinetics and the antimicrobial effects of granulocyte transfusion. These problems can be partially avoided by using ABO and HLA compatible donors, and testing for lymphocytotoxic antibodies prior to each transfusion.

Table 13.4 Hazards to recipients of white cell transfusions

Febrile reactions
Pulmonary reactions
Alloimmunization (ABO, HLA, platelet or neutrophil specific)
Infection (esp. CMV)
Graft versus host disease

Should antibodies be detected an HLA matched donor should be used and a lymphocyte or granulocyte cross-match performed.

Infection transmission Certain infections can be transmitted by transfusion of any blood components. Hepatitis B, Hepatitis C, Human Immunodeficiency Virus (HIV1) and syphilis should all be screened for routinely. Donors at risk of HIV2 virus should be excluded. Toxoplasmosis and malaria have been transmitted by granulocyte transfusions and Epstein-Barr virus can also theoretically be transmitted.

The most serious frequently encountered infection transmission associated with granulocyte transfusions is cytomegalovirus (CMV). This virus is transmitted by transfusion of viable leucocytes and is an important cause of morbidity and mortality in immunocompromised patients. Screening of donors and the use of only CMV antibody negative donors is a means of decreasing transmission of this infection.

Graft versus host disease (GVHD). The development of GVHD is related to the transfusion of allogeneic T-lymphocytes capable of proliferation. The disease occurs most commonly in the severely immunocompromised patient. Its incidence, morbidity and mortality related to granulocyte transfusions is unknown. Most of these patients are receiving other products which could be responsible and the clinical syndrome is difficult to diagnose as it is often seen in conjunction with other intercurrent infections (especially CMV). When it has been described following red cell or platelet transfusion the clinical course is often severe and the outcome fatal. The treatment of GVHD is unsatisfactory but prevention by irradiating granulocytes prior to transfusion is possible. A dose of 15 Gy is generally sufficient to prevent lymphocyte proliferation and all granulocytes for transfusion should receive irradiation at this dose prior to use.

Summary

The demand for granulocyte transfusions has declined in recent years. The expense and time involved in collection coupled with difficulties in obtaining adequate numbers of granulocytes and conflicting reports of their efficacy has led to this decline. Granulocyte transfusions can

be, however, of benefit in profoundly neutropenic patients with documented Gram-negative septicaemia. Other manoeuvres may need to be considered to speed bone marrow recovery. It has been suggested that lithium carbonate may reduce the period of leucopenia (Lyman, *et al.*, 1980) and the use of granulocyte colony-stimulating factors will have a part to play, although in myeloid leukaemia the latter may also stimulate the disease process.

Increased usage and benefit of granulocyte transfusions would occur if more advanced technology was developed allowing for maximum granulocyte yields in a short time. Cryopreservation of granulocytes would also offer significant advantages. Until these techniques are available the risks incurred in using granulocyte transfusions with the long-term effects on future patient care must be considered in conjunction with any benefits that are likely to accrue. General guidelines for their use cannot be made and each patient must be considered individually.

References

Aghai, E. (1983) Normal bone marrow as a source of granulocytes for transfusion. *Transfusion*, **23**, 496–499

Aisner, J., Schiffer, C.A., Daley, P.A. and Bucholz, D.H. (1981) Evaluation of gravity leucapheresis and comparison with intermittent centrifugation leucapheresis. *Transfusion*, **21**, 100–106

Alavi, J.B., Root, R.K., Djerassi, I., *et al.* (1977) A randomised clinical trial of granulocyte transfusions for infection in acute leukaemia. *N. Eng. J. Med.*, **196**, 706–711

Appelbaum, F.R., Trapain, R.J. and Graw, R.G. (1977) Consequences of prior alloimmunisation during granulocyte transfusion. *Transfusion*, **17**, 460–464

Blumberg, N., Genco, P., Katz, A. and Bare, J. (1978) Collection of granulocytes for transfusion. The effect of collection methods on cell enzyme release. *Vox Sang*, **35**, 207–214

Bodey, G.P., Buckley, B.A., Sathe, Y.S. and Freirich, E.J. (1966) Quantitative relationships between circulating leucocytes and infections in patients with acute leukaemia. *Annals of Internal Medicine*, **64**, 328–340

Bueschler, E.S. and Gallin, J.I. (1982) Leucocyte transfusions in chronic granulomatous disease. *N. Eng. J. Med.*, **307**, 800–803

Button, L.N., De Wolf, W.C., Newburger, P.E., *et al.* (1981) The effects of irradiation on blood components. *Transfusion*, **21**, 409–426

Christensen, R.D., Rothstein, G., Austall, H.B. and Bybee, B. (1982) Granulocyte transfusions in neonates with bacterial infection, neutropenia and depletion of mature marrow neutrophils. *Paediatrics*, **70**, 106

Clift, R.A., Saunders, J.E., Thomas, E.D., Williams, B. and Buckner, C.D. (1978) Granulocyte transfusions for the prevention of infection in patients receiving bone marrow transplants. *N. Eng. J. Med.*, **298**, 1052–1057

Dahlke, M.B., Keashen, M.A., Alari, J.B., Koch, P.A. and Okpara, R.A. (1980) Response to granulocyte transfusion in the alloimmunized patient. *Transfusion*, **20**, 555–558

Dale, D.C., Reynolds, H.Y., Pennington, J.E., Elin, R.J., Pitts, T.W. and Graw, R.G. (1975) Granulocyte transfusion therapy of experimental Pseudomonas pneumonia. *Journal of Clinical Investigation*, **54**, 664–671

Department of Health and Society Security (1992) *Code of practice for the clinical use of blood cell separators.* London, HMSO

Djerassi, I. (1977) Gravity leucapheresis – a new need for collection of transfusable granulocytes. *Experimental Haematology*, **5** (suppl. 1), 139–143

Dutcher, J.P., Schiffer, C.A. and Johnston, G.S. (1981) Rapid migration of Indium labelled granulocytes to sites of infection. *N. Eng. J. Med.*, **304**, 586–589

EORTC International antimicrobial project group (1983) Early granulocyte transfusion in high risk febrile neutropenic patients. *Schweiz. Med. Wochenschr.*, **113** (suppl. 14), 46–48

Epstein, R.B., Clift, R.A. and Thomas, E.D. (1969) The effect of Leucocyte transfusions on experimental bacteriaemia in the dog. *Blood*, **34**, 782–790

Epstein, R.B., Waxman, F.J., Bennett, B.T. and Anderson, B. (1974) *Pseudomonas septicaemia* in neutropenic dogs. I. Treatment with granulocyte transfusion. *Transfusion*, **14**, 51–57

Eyre, H.J., Goldstein, I.M., Perry, S. and Graw, R.J. (1970) Leucocyte transfusions: Function of transfused granulocytes from donors with chronic myelocytic leukaemia. *Blood*, **36**, 432–442

Foon, K.A. and Gale, R.P. (1982) Controversies in the therapy of acute myelogenous leukaemia. *Am. J. Med.*, **7**, 963–972

Freireich, E.J., Levin, R.H., Whang, J., Carbone, P.P., Bronson, W. and Morse, E.E. (1964) The function and fate of transfused leucocytes from donor with chronic myelocytic leukaemia in leukopenic recipients. *Am. N.Y. Acad. Sci.*, **113**, 1081–1089

Glasser, L. (1979) Functional considerations of concentrates used for clinical transfusions. *Transfusion*, **19**, 1–6

Graw, R.G., Herzig, G., Perry, S. and Henderson, E.S. (1972) Granulocyte transfusion therapy: Treatment of septicaemia due to Gram-negative bacteria. *N. Eng. J. Med.*, **287**, 367–371

Hersman, J., Meyers, J.D., Thomas, E.D., Buckner, C.D. and Cliff, R. (1982) The effect of granulocyte transfusions upon the incidence of cytomegalovirus. Infections after allogeneic bone marrow transplantation. *Annals of Internal Medicine*, **96**, 149–152

Herzig, R., Herzig, G., Graw, R.G., Bull, M.I. and Ray,

K.K. (1977) Efficacy of granulocyte transfusion therapy for gram-negative sepsis: A propsective randomised controlled study. *N. Eng. J. Med.*, **196**, 701–705

Higby, D.J. and Burnett, D. (1980) Granulocyte transfusions current status. *Blood*, **55**, 2–8

Hollingsworth, J.W., Finch, S.C. and Beeson, P.B. (1956) The role of transfused leucocytes in experimental bacteriaemia of irradiated rats. *Journal of Laboratory and Clinical Medicine*, **48**, 227–236

Huestis, D.W., Goodsite, L.M., Price, M.J. and White, R.F. (1975) Granulocyte collection with the Haemonetics blood cell separator. In *leucocytes: separation, collection and transfusion* J.M. Goldman, R.L. Lowenthal (eds), 208–219, London, Academic Press

International Forum (1980) Granulocyte transfusions: established or still an experimental therapeutic approach? *Vox Sang*, **38**, 40–56

Klastersky, J. (1979) Granulocyte transfusions as a therapy and prophylaxis of infection in neutropenic patients. *Eur. J. Cancer*, **15** (suppl.), 15–22

Koepke, J.A., Parks, W.M., Gocken, J.A., Klee, G.G. and Strauss, R.G. (1981) The safety of weekly plateletpheresis: Effect on the donors lymphocyte population. *Transfusion*, **21**, 59–63

Laing, I.A., Boulton, F.E. and Hume, R. (1983) Polymorphonuclear leucocyte transfusion for the treatment of sepsis in the newborn infant. *J. Paediat.*, **98**, 118–123

Lancet, Editorial (1980) Infection complicating severe granulocytopenia. *Lancet*, **1**, 25

Laurenti, F., Ferro, R., Isacchi, G., Perero, A., Sarignour, P.G., Malagnino, F., Palermo, D., Mandelli, F. and Bucci, G. (1981) Polymorphonuclear leucocyte transfusion for the treatment of sepsis in the newborn infant. *Journal of Paediatrics*, **98**, 118–123

Leitman, S.F., Boltansky, H., Alter, H.J., Pearson, F.C. and Kaliner, M.A. (1986) Allergic reactions in healthy plateletpheresis donors caused by sensitisation to ethylene oxide gas. *N. Eng. J. Med.*, **315**, 1192–1196

Lin, A., Smith, J., Porter, R., et al. (1980) Developmental studies of granulocyte collection using the Fenwal CS-3000 blood cell separator. *Transfusion*, **20**, 638–639

Lyman, G.H., Williams, C.C. and Preston, D. (1980) The use of lithium carbonate to reduce infection and leukopenia during systemic chemotherapy. *N. Eng. J. Med.*, **302**, 257–260

Marsh, J.C., Boggs, D.Q., Cartwright, G.E. and Wintrobe, M.M. (1967) Neutrophil kinetics in acute infection. *Journal of Clinical Investigation*, **46**, 1943–1953

Martin, S., Ghoneim, A.T.M., Robinson, E.A.E. and Child, J.A. (1983) Comparison of the effect of filtration leucapheresis and discontinuous flow cell centrifugation leucapheresis on granulocyte microbial function. *Journal of Clinical Pathology*, **36**, 586–590

McCleoud, B.C. and Sassetti, R.J. (1981) Effects of centrifugation leucapheresis with hydroxyethyl starch on the complement system of granulocyte donors. *Transfusion*, **21**, 403–411

McCullough, J., Weiblen, B., Deinard, A.R., et al. (1976) *In vitro* function and post transfusion survival of granulocytes collected by continuous flow centrifugation and by filtration leucapheresis. *Blood*, **38**, 315–326

McCullough, J., Weiblen, B.J., Clay, M.E. and Forstrum, L. (1981) Effect of leucocyte antibodies on the fate *in vivo* of indium[111] labelled granulocytes. *Blood*, **58**, 164–170

McCullough, J., Weiblen, B.J. and Fine, D. (1983) Effects of storage of granulocytes on their fate *in vivo*. *Transfusion*, **23**, 20–24

Mischler, J.M. (1977) The effect of corticosteroids on mobilisation and function of neutrophils. *Experimental Haematology*, **5** (suppl. 1), 15–32

Mischler, J.M. (1982) *Pharmacology of hydroxyethyl starch*. Oxford University Press, Oxford

Navari, R.M., Buckner, C.D., Clift, R.A., *et al.* (1984) Prophylaxis of infection in patients with aplastic anaemia receiving allogeneic marrow transplants. *American Journal of Medicine*, **76**, 564–572

Pegels, J.G., Bruynes, E.C.E., Engelfreit, C.P. and Kr Vonem, A.E.G. (1982) Serological studies in patients on platelet and granulocyte substitution therapy. *British Journal of Haematology*, **52**, 59–68

Popovic, V., Schaffer, R. and Poporic, P. (1977) Granulocyte transfusions in recovery of neutropenic rats from induced E. Coli toxicaemia. *Experimental Haematology*, **5**, 166–170

Price, T.H. and Dale, D.C. (1977) Neutrophil transfusion: The effect of collection technique and storage on *in vivo* chemotaxis. *Blood*, **50** (suppl. 1), 309

Price, T.H. and Dale, D.C. (1978) Neutrophil transfusion: The effect of storage and of collection method on neutrophil blood kinetics. *Blood*, **51**, 789–798

Richman, C.M. (1983) Prolonged cryopreservation of human granulocytes. *Transfusion*, **23**, 508–511

Ring, J., Sharkhoff, D. and Richter, W. (1980) Using HES in man. *Vox Sanguinis*, **39**, 181–185

Sandler, S.G. and Nusbacher, J. (1982) Health risks of leucapheresis donors. *Haematologia*, **15**, 57–69

Schiffer, C.A., Aisner, J., Daly, P.A., Schinpff, S.C. and Wiernik, P.H. (1979) Alloimmunisation following prophylactic granulocyte transfusion. *Blood*, **54**, 766–774

Strauss, R.G., Connett, J.E., Gale, R.P., *et al.* (1981) A controlled trial of prophylactic granulocyte transfusions during initial induction chemotherapy for acute myelogenous leukaemia. *N. Eng. J. Med.*, **305**, 597–603

Strauss, R.G., Huestis, D.W., Wright, D.G. and Hester, J.P. (1983) Lymphocyte and platelet depletion by mechanical apheresis. *Journal of Clinical Apheresis*, 158–165

Vogler, W.R. and Winton, E.F. (1977) The efficacy of granulocyte transfusions in neutropenic patients. *Am. J. Med.*, **63**, 548–555

Winston, D.J., Ho, W.G., Howell, L.L., Miller, M.J., Mickey, R., Martin, W.J., *et al.* (1980a) Cytomegalovirus infections associated with leucocyte transfusions. *Annals of Internal Medicine*, **93**, 671–675

Winston, D.J., Ho, W.G., Young, L.S. and Gale, R.P. (1980b) Prophylactic granulocyte transfusions during human bone marrow transplantation. *American Journal of Medicine*, **68**, 893–897

Winston, D.J., Ho, W.G. and Gale, R.P. (1981) Prophylactic granulocyte transfusions during chemotherapy of acute non-lymphocytic leukaemia. *Annals of Internal Medicine*, **94**, 616–622

Wright, D.G., Robichaud, K.J., Pizzo, P.A. and Deisseroth, A.B. (1981) Lethal pulmonary reactions associated with the combined use of amphotericin B and leucocyte transfusions. *N. Eng. J. Med.*, **304**, 1185–1189

Part Three

Infection Hazards in Relation to Blood Products

14

Standard blood transfusion services processes: Special requirements of different patients particularly at risk

P. Flanagan, S. Ramskill and E.A.E. Robinson

Introduction

During the past 20 years, intensive research and technical advances have resulted in remarkable improvement in transfusion supportive care which has significantly contributed to the increased survival now achievable in patients with leukaemia, aplastic anaemia and malignant disease. The combined efforts of transfusion centres, hospital laboratories and clinical users of donor blood and its components to promote safer transfusion practices now prevent what were the commonest forms of adverse transfusion reactions, namely pyrogenic reactions, circulatory overload, haemolytic reactions and bacterial contamination of donations. The net effect of this achievement has been to focus attention on the need to prevent the transmission of infective agents by transfusion. Despite the extension of precautionary measures introduced in the last decade, no blood product should ever be prescribed without considering the possibility that infection may be transmitted.

Recent changes in medical practice have also exacerbated the problem, as the severity of some transfusion transmitted infections depend in part on the immunocompetence of the recipient. Transfusion replacement therapy in patients with impaired immune responses, can

Table 14.1 Infections that can be transmitted by transfusion of blood or its components

Transfusion transmitted disease	
Hepatitis A virus (HAV)	
Hepatitis B virus (HBV)	
Hepatitis Non-A, Non-B (NANB)	
HIV (AIDS)	can be transmitted by cell free fractions
Parvovirus (HPVLV)	
Syphilis	
Brucellosis (undulant fever)	
Bacterial contamination	
Cytomegalovirus (CMV)	
Epstein–Barr virus (EBV)	usually only transmitted by cellular blood fractions
HTLVI (Human T-cell leukaemia virus)	
Malaria	
Chagas' disease (American Trypanosomiasis)	
Babesiosis (Nantucket fever)	only rarely transmitted by blood transfusion
Toxoplasmosis	
Trypanosomiasis (African sleeping sickness)	

occasionally result in an overwhelming and sometimes fatal infection with cytomegalovirus.

The advent of blood component therapy, whereby a single donation may be used to provide up to three different blood components means that an infective agent in one donation may potentially be transmitted into several recipients. Conversely, because some blood products are produced from the fractionation of a large number of pooled plasma donations, a recipient may be exposed to infective agents from multiple blood donors. This is of particular concern in the preparation and administration of coagulation factor concentrate where pools of plasma composed of many thousands of individual donations are used as the raw material for the preparation of the concentrate. Table 14.1 lists the infections that can be transmitted by transfusion of blood or its components.

One of the principal aims of modern transfusion practice is to attempt to reduce the risk of disease transmission and this can be achieved in a variety of ways, namely:

(i) The introduction of appropriate selection criteria for blood donors
(ii) The introduction of standardized donor sessional procedures
(iii) The screening of individual blood donations for specific diseases
(iv) Treatment of the blood component or product by physical or chemical means to reduce or eliminate the potential infectivity of the product.

General considerations

Donor selection

Blood donors should be in good health with no recent illnesses or symptoms that may produce an increased likelihood of them carrying an infective agent that may be transmitted by blood transfusion. In view of this the diseases most likely to be transmitted by transfusion will be those either with a long presymptomatic incubation period or those with a prolonged asymptomatic phase or carrier state, these being exemplified by hepatitis B virus infection which remains the classical model for transfusion transmitted viral disease. An understanding of the epidemiology of such transmissible agents will help to define the specific

donor selection criteria that will aim to exclude donors who are most likely to harbour an individual infection. Within the United Kingdom these criteria are laid down in *Guidelines for the Blood Transfusion Services in the United Kingdom* (DoH, 1992).

It has been recognized for many years that payment of blood donors significantly increases the risk of transmission of viral disease, most notably post transfusion hepatitis and HIV infection. In 1975 the World Health Organization (WHO) recognizing this recommended that each country should aim to achieve national self-sufficiency in blood and blood products from volunteer non-remunerated donors. This concept has recently been re-iterated by a European Economic Community (EEC) Directive. Alter (1972) demonstrated that the risk of post-transfusion hepatitis increased following transfusion of blood from commercial sources. This work was subsequently confirmed by other investigators (Seef, 1977). Despite the introduction of sensitive screening tests for HBV, blood collected from paid donors still has an excessive risk of transmitting both hepatitis B virus (HBV) and Non-A Non-B (NANB) disease. This was illustrated in a particular region of the USA when the introduction of an HBV screening programme together with a switch to a predominantly volunteer blood donor programme decreased the incidence of post-transfusion hepatitis requiring hospitalization from one in 117 blood recipients to one in 734 (Goldfield, 1978). It has also been unequivocally proved that pooled plasma derivatives originating from paid plasma donors carry much higher risks of transmitting infectious diseases. This was highlighted by the transmission of hepatitis and now by the transmission of the Human Immunodeficiency Virus (HIV) infection to haemophiliacs exposed to Factor VIII concentrate prepared from paid plasma donors.

The problem with monetary inducement is that it attracts the wrong sort of blood donors. The amounts offered are usually not enough to interest the majority of healthy, economically secure people but are an incentive for people from low socio-economic groups. This constitutes a danger both for the paid donors, who are prone to be bled too often and who may be inclined to hide contraindications to blood or plasma donation and for the recipient who is more exposed to transmissible disease. An integrated national non-profit system for the collection of whole blood and plasma is the best guarantee for a rational use of all resources and for the safety of both donors and recipients, i.e. for the safest source of blood, the first requirement is a voluntary non-remunerated blood donor system.

All transfusion services need to produce specific donor selection guidelines to reduce the potential for disease transmission. The specific criteria for individual diseases are considered later in this chapter. However if such guidelines are to be effective considerable effort must be made to educate the donor population and to produce practical procedures for identifying and deferring donors, who are felt unsuitable. This may involve the use of simple questionnaires, and also include a requirement for the donor to indicate that they have read and understood the most important criteria. The very nature of blood donor clinics are such that extensive individual questioning is impractical and the available evidence indicates that strict adherence to simple rules is most likely to be effective.

Blood collection and storage

Although there is a potential for many bacterial infections to be transmitted by blood transfusion, there are several factors that make this a very uncommon occurrence. These include the exclusion of febrile donors, the bacteriostatic effects of the citrate in the anticoagulant, the effects of storage at 4 °C upon most human pathogens, and possibly bactericidal components in the blood.

The introduction of commercially produced plastic blood collection packs prefilled with anticoagulant has greatly reduced the potential for introduction of bacterial infection during blood collection and processing. These packs are prepared to a high standard under stringent quality assurance conditions and can then be subjected to sterilization prior to final packaging. These measures have virtually eliminated bacterial contamination of transfusion fluids. The introduction of multipack systems has permitted a variety of blood components to be produced within a closed system thereby eliminating a further potential source of introduction of bacteria. Despite these measures external contamination of the collection pack can still occur and is usually consequent upon pinhole leaks or tears within the pack. It is therefore important that the standard procedures used at blood donor sessions should include simple checks for defects both before and after donation. Fatalities have been reported following the transfusion of infected blood consequent upon pinhole leaks (Habibi, *et al.* 1973).

It is impossible to guarantee sterility of the skin surface prior to venepuncture, even when the greatest care is taken to avoid contamination. However when a normal donation of blood is mixed with a relatively small amount of anticoagulant any organisms present are usually killed, so that stored blood is normally sterile. Nevertheless a strict aseptic technique should be employed using a collection pack with an integral needle.

Consideration also needs to be given to the conditions in which blood is stored and transported. Within the United Kingdom it is recommended that following donation, blood should be transferred to a refrigerated container at 4 °C and care should be taken to maintain the blood as near as possible to this temperature during processing. The one exception to this is for donated units that are destined for platelet concentrate production when it is recommended that blood is kept at 22 °C until the platelet concentrate has been prepared, but that this period of storage at 22 °C should not exceed 8 hours. In general it is accepted that most bacteria grow poorly at 4 °C. However occasionally stored units of blood may yield a growth of cryophilic organisms such as pseudomonas, coliforms and achromobacter. These organisms may multiply at 4 °C resulting in endotoxic production, citrate consumption and subsequent coagulation and haemolysis of the blood. Transfusion of such blood can be rapidly fatal due to endotoxic shock, one of the rarest but most devastating complications of blood transfusion. This rare situation aside, refrigerated blood components are less likely to support bacterial growth than are those components such as platelet concentrate and granulocytes, which are routinely stored at 22 °C. This is particularly important with regard to component production that involves 'open' processing techniques, i.e. involve entering the blood pack, and hence raising the potential for bacterial contamination. This includes processes such as laboratory-based red cell filtration and platelet pooling. It is recommended that such processing is undertaken within the sterile environment of a laminar flow cabinet. However the shelf life of products produced in this way is reduced to 24 hours for red cells but only 6 hours for components to be stored at room temperature. This places significant limitation on the use of such products. It is possible that the use of sterile docking devices which enable a connection to be made between two separate plastic tubes without endangering sterility may overcome many of these problems.

Blood for transfusion should be kept in designated refrigerators which have a temperature recording device and an audible alarm. It is important that all hospital transfusion laboratories have written procedures for the release of blood from refrigerators and that these should be followed by all staff. If a patient requires more than one unit of blood, only one unit should be taken to the bedside at any one time. Blood which is removed from the refrigerator for more than 1 hour but not used should not be subsequently transfused (McClelland, 1988). Finally consideration should be given to the means by which blood is transfused. It is recommended that a single unit of red cells should be transfused within 4 hours, and that the giving set used for blood transfusion should be changed at least every 24 hours.

Laboratory screening tests

Remarkable technical advances have been made over the past two decades to ensure that the risk of disease transmission by blood transfusion is minimized. Such developments are epitomized by a comparison of the crude attempts to prevent hepatitis B virus transmission in the early 1970s using immunoelectrophoresis for the detection of hepatitis B surface antigen (HBsAg) in blood donors to the sophisticated and sensitive commercial enzyme immunoassays used in the contemporary laboratory. These advances progressed rapidly with the recognition of the causative pathogen of AIDS in the 1980s, and the need to quickly stem the fears that transfusion services would be seriously compromised without effective screening tests for human immunodeficiency virus (HIV). Such tests were successfully introduced in the United Kingdom in 1985.

The criteria used for selecting suitable screening methods in blood banks must take into account the need for mass, rapid, sensitive and specific serological analysis. In today's trans-fusion service it is essential to attract and bleed large numbers of donors. Most centres process several hundred donations daily, some over a thousand. Testing needs to be done quickly in order to obtain the full benefit of the limited life-span of cellular products; particularly as demands are continually increasing in modern clinical practice.

The assays developed must also be of the highest order of sensitivity, a term in this context which refers to detection of the largest number of true positive donations. This is generally evaluated by challenging competing tests against extensive panels of known positive sera. Nevertheless, however sensitive a screening test for antibody is shown to be, it does not alter the fact that a small proportion of blood donors may be infectious while exhibiting a negative screen result. With individuals recently infected with HIV for instance antibody may not appear in the host for several weeks. Thus assays which will look directly for viral antigens or specific gene sequences are constantly being sought, and will hopefully at some stage, be applicable to blood bank screening.

In one particular area antigen screening has always applied, and that concerns hepatitis B virus. This virus is unique as it produces excessive amounts of surface antigen in the host, which in most cases is easily detectable in serum. Reference standards for HBsAg indicate a thousand-fold increase in sensitivity through progressive generations of screening tests, up to the present day when less than 1 ng/ml can be detected. These improvements have exposed more HBsAg positive donors, but it must be said that there are diminishing returns with each new generation of tests, because the vast majority of HBsAg carriers have levels far in excess of these amounts.

With all laboratory assays involving a variety of human and animal reagents there are likely to be false positive reactions. In terms of transfusion screening, tests which give high numbers of non-specific reactions are unacceptable. Not only do they result in the loss of potentially usable units of blood, but they also require elaborate confirmation testing procedures to clarify results, thus wasting valuable reagents and staff time. The administrative work involved in dealing with many false positive units of blood can lead to an increased risk of errors occurring and this may be disastrous for the recipient and for the reputation of the transfusion service. Modern tests increasingly use reagents consisting of monoclonal antibodies and manufactured peptides from recombinant DNA technology to reduce the likelihood of false reactions.

Most of the serological markers that transfusion centres look for can be detected by a variety of techniques. From a historic viewpoint the simplest assays were immunodiffusion techniques, initially used for HBsAg and antibody to the surface antigen (anti-HBs). Immunoelectropheresis was at the time a major advance, improving the speed and sensitivity of the screening process. Complement fixation was commonly used to test donors for reagin antibody, a non-specific marker for syphilis, although many found it unsuitable for mass screening.

These early methods were superseded by agglutination tests, either involving inert particles such as latex and carbon, or chemically treated red cells, any of which could be coated with immune reactants and used to great effect to detect serological markers. Haemagglutination tests were particularly successful in screening for HBsAg. Not only were the tests rapid and specific but they were also able to detect low levels of antigen (10–12 ng/ml).

With the ever increasing use of microtitre plates, solid-phase assays utilizing the ability of plastic to bind proteins were soon developed and a new generation of techniques evolved.

Radioimmunoassay (RIA) became the routine screening test for HBsAg in many transfusion centres in the early 1980s, using solid-phase HBsAg capture principles which resulted in high gamma counts generated by I^{125}-labelled anti-HBs.

However, the disadvantages of radioisotope labelled tests, with their short shelf-life and questionable safety, have caused a general move towards enzyme immunoassays (EIA). These techniques have now established a firm foothold in the modern transfusion screening laboratories. A variety of sandwich assays are available for HBsAg in which the radio-labelled antibody of RIA is replaced by an enzyme: anti-HBs conjugate and the signal generated is colour produced by the enzyme chromogenic substrate.

In October 1985 all transfusion centres in the UK began testing for anti–HIV, and a range of commercial EIA tests were available to choose

from. Most of these assays were and still are, based upon the detection of anti-HIV captured on to an antigen coated solid-phase. Originally viral lysates were utilized as an antigen source, but many of the latest tests have progressed to the use of specific HIV peptides prepared by molecular biological techniques. This is particularly so with the current assays used for the detection of both anti-HIV1 and anti-HIV2.

In September 1991, routine testing for antibody to hepatitis C virus, a specific marker for non-A non-B hepatitis was introduced in UK transfusion centres. The available screening tests utilize EIA methodology in microtitre plates (Ortho Diagnostics), or with plastic beads (Abbott Diagnostics), coated with synthesized viral protein.

One of the great advantages of RIA and EIA methods is the fact that the signal generated as the end-point of the test can be read objectively, removing the possibility of errors associated with manual reading, particularly when confronted with weak positives. Indeed the printouts produced by gamma-counters or spectrophotometers serve as a permanent record of the result obtained on each donation. This has become an essential element of the elaborate quality control mechanisms now applied in blood screening laboratories. Add to this the application of robotic samplers, automated ELISA processing and computer analysis to validate test controls and interpret results then one has some idea of the current state of the art in transfusion microbiology. However, even with rapidly advancing technology, concern has been expressed that the increasing number of microbiological tests performed on each blood donation adds to the complexity of the transfusion centre's operation, creating potential sources of error (Bove, 1990).

Specific diseases

Hepatitits B

World-wide, hepatitis B infection is one of the most important causes of acute and chronic liver damage, liver cirrhosis and primary hepatocellular carcinoma. Transmission is possible by parenteral, sexual or vertical (mother to child) routes. The frequency of infection differs considerably in different parts of the world. In western Europe as well as the United States and Australia, the incidence is relatively low. In these areas only 0.1% to 0.5% of the population are viral carriers, in contrast to areas of Asia, Africa and South America where this frequency rises to anywhere between 5 and 15%.

In infected persons the virus is found in most body fluids, and its presence in blood or blood components is not affected by storage at 4 °C or by the long-term freezing of plasma.

The incidence of post transfusion hepatitis B has been dramatically reduced by a combination of donor exclusion and testing for HBsAg. In some countries individuals with a history of hepatitis or jaundice are permanently excluded from blood donation. However within the UK donors are accepted so long as a minimum of 12 months have passed since the infection, and of course so long as the test for HBsAg proves negative. The incubation period for hepatitis B is up to 6 months and this is the time period used for deferral of individuals who may be deemed at high risk of developing the infection. This includes individuals who have been in close contact with cases of hepatitis and also those who have undergone a form of skin piercing procedure (tattooing, ear piercing, acupuncture and electrolysis) which is a recognized form of disease transmission. The tendency to the use of sterile disposable instruments for skin piercing procedures has significantly reduced if not eliminated, the risk of transmission by such means but currently it is not felt appropriate to relax the above rules. Individuals who have suffered needlestick injuries are also deferred from donating for 6 months, this is however increased to 9 months if hepatitis B immunoglobulin has been administered since it is now recognized this may prolong the incubation period of the disease.

Blumberg's historic discovery of the 'Australia antigen' in 1965 revolutionized our understanding of hepatitis B infection. It was later renamed HBsAg. Prince (1968) demonstrated a relationship with hepatitis and it was also shown that carriers of the antigen were likely to pass on the disease to recipients of their blood.

HBsAg is derived from the outer protein shell of the 42 nm Dane particle (the intact virus) where it is produced in great excess. It is consistently found in high levels in the serum of persons with acute or chronic hepatitis B infection, as well as in subjects who are healthy long-term carriers of the virus. Surface antigen therefore acts as an admirable indicator of donors who may unknowingly be hazardous to recipients of their blood.

After infection with the virus it may be two to six months before the onset of any symptoms and HBsAg usually appears four to eight weeks in advance of such symptoms. The duration of antigenaemia varies, but persistence for more than six months signifies that the chronic carrier state has developed. The disappearance of HBsAg and the subsequent emergence of its corresponding antibody (anti-HBs) denotes the recovery phase of hepatitis B. However the serologically inert period between the presence of these two markers (the diagnostic window) disguises the fact that blood may still be infectious.

The Dane particle contains a complex core which has a specific core antigen (HBcAg), and although this antigen is never naturally found free in serum, it may be released from intact HBV by detergent treatment. An additional serum antigen, the 'e' antigen is also associated with HBV and its presence in serum reflects active viral replication and is indicative of high infectivity. Indeed blood from an HBsAg positive and HBeAg positive carrier is the most infectious material for the transmission of hepatitis B containing up to 500 μg/ml of viral protein, and the injection of just a few microlitres is sufficient to transmit the disease (De Groote, 1987).

Antibody to the core antigen (anti-HBc) usually appears about two to four weeks after HBsAg is first detected but before symptoms are seen in the subject. Anti-HBc titres rise continuously during acute HBV infection but in the chronic disease a steady high titre is maintained.

With such an array of serological markers, the issue of how best to screen for HBV in blood may become confused, but while the concept of a single first-line screening test predominates, HBsAg is considered to be the most appropriate target for the exclusion of potentially infectious donors.

In 1972, following the lead of the USA, an advisory group to the NHS recommended that HBsAg should be introduced for blood donation. Subsequent reports from this committee have recommended increasing the sensitivity of screening tests in an effort to detect low level antigen carriers. Current guidelines in use (*DoH Guidelines for Transfusion Services in the*

UK, 1992) specify a minimum detection level of 1 iu/ml of HBsAg for screening tests. Despite this, current tests fail to identify a small proportion of infectious units. It has been debated for some years whether anti-HBc screening should be used as an additional test to reduce further the incidence of post transfusion hepatitis B (PTHB). (Hoofnagle, 1978; Tedder, 1980). The arguments for and against this are well known in transfusion circles. The test would pick out donors in the window phase between loss of HBsAg and the appearance of anti-HBs. It is also recognized, however, that if anti-HBc testing were introduced it would result in many harmless units from immune donors being discarded, unless tests for anti-HBs are also performed. Even if such measures were introduced PTHB would not be completely eradicated. Driss (1989) reported the presence of HBV DNA in five of 247 French blood donors who had no detectable HBsAg by contemporary methods. Only one of the five had anti-HBc. It is currently felt that anti HBc screening cannot be justified within the UK.

At the present time screening for HBsAg in the UK is performed using a variety of commercial EIA 'sandwich' assays. Each of these assays performs well detecting well below the required 0.5 iu/ml.

Over the last 5 years the frequency of HBsAg positive blood donors in the Yorkshire region was as low as one in 48,000 when accounting for all donations taken. When considering first-time donors who have never before been tested, this rises to one in 4,600 (0.02%). This rate is somewhat less than the frequency seen in the past by other workers in the UK (i.e. 0.1 to 0.2% [Wallace, *et al.*, 1975; Barbara, *et al.*, 1983]). This may reflect regional variations, but it should be borne in mind that the overall situation may have changed since 1985 when the exclusion criteria brought in to reduce the chances of HIV transmission by transfusion included the high risk groups who are also more likely to carry HBV.

As a general policy of the transfusion service, once it is confirmed that a donor is a carrier of HBsAg, tests for further HBV markers are performed, either at the transfusion centre, or at a reference laboratory, to establish the serological profile and the probable clinical significance of the infection. The provision of a long-term programme to monitor the donor's con-

dition is made available, but whatever the outcome of this, it is made clear that the subject must be excluded from the donor panels to ensure the safety of blood supplies.

Human immunodeficiency virus (HIV) and AIDS

The Acquired Immune Deficiency Syndrome (AIDS) is a late manifestation of infection with HIV. AIDS was initially reported in the late 1970s and it was soon recognized that it could develop as a consequence of transfusion of blood and its products (Curran, 1984). The isolation in 1984 of a retrovirus, now known as HIV, by two groups of workers, Gallo in the United States and Montagnier from the Pasteur Institute, revolutionized our understanding of the disease and directly led to the development of tests for antibody to HIV.

It is now recognized that two distinct viruses can lead to the development of AIDS. These are known as HIV-1 and HIV-2. HIV-1 is the predominent form in most of the world, HIV-2 occurring predominantly in Western Africa, although small numbers of cases have been described elsewhere, including the United Kingdom (Evans, 1991).

HIV antibody usually develops 1–2 months following infection and then in most individuals persists. The disease is associated with a prolonged asymptomatic phase which may last several years. There is clear evidence that in the majority of individuals HIV antibody is not neutralizing and hence HIV antibody positivity can be used as a marker of potential infectivity.

Imagawa (1989) reported that in a group of high risk individuals HIV virus was detectable in lymphocytes for at least three years in the absence of detectable antibody. Although there is no conclusive evidence that such individuals are capable of transmitting HIV infection these results are of concern to transfusion services and justify the rigorous donor selection processes that have been developed to minimize the risk of HIV transmission. Antibody negative virus positive individuals have been described, apparently in the 'window period' prior to seroconversion (Salahuddin, *et al.*, 1984).

In the Western World the majority of cases of HIV infection and AIDS occur in individuals who have undertaken particular risk activities.

These risk activities form the basis of transfusion service exclusion criteria. In addition to excluding individuals known to be infected with HIV from donating, individuals who have undertaken such risk activities are asked not to donate. Currently the main risk categories recognized by UK transfusion services include, homosexual and bisexual men, intravenous drug abusers and prostitutes. The sexual partners of individuals falling into such groups are also excluded from donating, as are the sexual partners of haemophiliacs. One particular area of increasing concern is the recognition that heterosexual transmission of HIV may be increasing. Currently the majority of cases of heterosexually acquired infection reported within the UK, outside of the above risk groups, are attributable to heterosexual exposure abroad in countries where heterosexual transmission of HIV is the predominant means of spread (Noone, 1991). Currently UK transfusion services exclude donors who have had heterosexual contact with men or women living in Africa. It is likely that as the epidemiology of the disease changes worldwide that this particular exclusion category will require constant review. The nature of the exclusion categories outlined above present particular problems for transfusion services in view of the lack of privacy usually available at donor sessions. This can be overcome in a variety of ways, these must include education of the donor population. Details of the exclusion categories can be sent with the donor invitation and details can be displayed outside of the donor venue. These procedures will allow the donor to self-defer without facing potential embarrassment at the donor sessions. It has been suggested (Contreras, 1985) that in addition donors should be given a facility to indicate confidentially that their blood should not be used for transfusion. Currently within the United Kingdom blood donors are asked to read a notice outlining the exclusion categories and to sign a form indicating that they have read and understood the contents of the notice. This form also acts as a consent form for the HIV antibody test that is carried out on all blood donations.

HIV antibody testing of blood donations in the UK commenced in October 1985. A variety of test formats are available but within the United Kingdom enzyme immunoassays have been the method of choice. The majority of EIAs have been based on an antiglobulin technique, but the preferred method in the UK was a competitive inhibition EIA developed in the UK (Mortimer, 1985). This latter assay had the advantage of good sensitivity with a high level of specificity thus resulting in the generation of few false positive results.

Early EIAs for HIV antibody were based on purified viral lysate as the captive antigen for HIV antibody. More recently these tests have been refined and current assays utilize a combination of core and envelope antigens that have been genetically engineered. Assays are now being produced that are based on synthetic peptides as antigens.

The majority of these assays were designed to detect antibody to HIV-1, the predominant form of infection outside of West Africa. HIV-1 antibody assays cross-reacted to a variable extent with HIV-2 antibody but do not detect all HIV-2 infected individuals. HIV-2 infection has been reported within the UK (Evans, 1991) and one blood donor from Western Africa has been identified. Assays have now been developed that are designed to detect both HIV-1 and HIV-2 antibody. These are all EIAs and have been used routinely within the UK since June 1990.

Despite the improved specificity of current assays a positive result in a low risk population such as blood donors is poorly predictive of the presence of true antibody. Hence although screening assays are of value in preventing the transfusion of HIV antibody positive blood donations, the results of such assays alone should not be used as the basis of donor counselling. Reactive specimens from donors should be submitted to reference laboratories for confirmatory testing, and donors contacted only when the results are known. The Western Blot is the accepted confirmatory test within the United States. This test is an antiglobulin test in which antibody to specific viral proteins is detected. Within the United Kingdom confirmatory testing is based on a variety of assays of different format and tests are now available to distinguish clearly HIV-1 infection from HIV-2. Currently within the UK very few HIV antibody positive donors are identified. Approximately one in 75,000 donors are confirmed as positive, and one in 25,000 when only new donors are considered. Although these figures indicate that the risk of

HIV transmission by transfusion is very low it is recognized that a small risk of transmission persists. Within the US it has been estimated that the risk of transmission of HIV by blood that is antibody negative is in the order of one in 150,000 donations (Cumming, 1989), in the UK where the incidence of HIV antibody positivity is much lower, the risk has been calculated as one in a million donations.

Assays for HIV antigen are now available. HIV antigen is not detectable in most infected healthy individuals and so is not a suitable alternative to HIV antibody testing for transfusion services. However, in some individuals undergoing seroconversion following infection antigen is detectable for some days prior to antibody (Stromer, 1988). The question has been raised as to whether HIV antigen testing should be undertaken in addition to HIV antibody testing, but current opinion is that this would not significantly reduce the risk of transmission and that concentration on more effective donor exclusion and more sensitive antibody tests is likely to be more effective (Jullien, 1988).

Non A, Non B hepatitis

Post transfusion hepatitis has long been recognized as an important complication of blood transfusion. The development of diagnostic tests for the causative agents of hepatitis A and B have clearly indicated that another agent is responsible for the majority of cases of post-transfusion hepatitis, and this has been called Non A, Non B hepatitis (NANBH). Until recently the investigation and prevention of NANBH has been hampered by the absence of specific diagnostic tests, the diagnosis being essentially one of exclusion. Recently, however, using molecular biological techniques scientists at the Chiron corporation have succeeded in producing an assay system that appears to be capable of detecting the major causative agent of NANB hepatitis (Kuo, 1989) and this agent has been called the hepatitis C virus (HCV).

The majority of cases of transfusion transmitted NANBG are asymptomatic and detectable only by sequential alanine amniotransferase (ALT) levels following transfusion. Seventy-five per cent of cases are anicteric. Prospective studies have demonstrated however that up to 50% of cases may have evidence of chronic liver disease at 12 months and that

a proportion of these will go on to develop hepatic cirrhosis (Berman, 1979). The incidence of post-transfusion NANBH varies in different parts of the world. Studies in the United Kingdom (Collins, 1983), Australia (Cossart, 1982) and Sweden (Widell, 1988) have shown levels of 2% or lower, whereas in the United States up to 12% of transfusions have been shown to result in NANBH (Koziol, 1986). The recipients of coagulation factor concentrates are particularly at risk of developing NANBH. Prior to the introduction of routine heat treatment of Factor VIII concentrate almost all recipients of NHS concentrate developed NANBH (Kernoff, 1985). Recent studies have however demonstrated that effective heat treatment reduces this risk almost to zero.

The frequency of NANBH and the evidence demonstrating the tendency to develop chronic liver disease aroused concern, particularly in the United States and, in the absence of specific viral markers, methods to reduce the extent of the problem were sought. Evidence has clearly shown an increased incidence of NANBH in the recipients of transfusion from paid blood donors when compared with that from voluntary non-remunerated donors (Aach, 1981). The epidemiology of transfusion transmitted NANBH shows many similarities with that of hepatitis B and HIV. It is likely that the tightening of donor selection criteria introduced to reduce the incidence of transfusion transmitted HIV, will also have had an impact on the incidence of NANBH. Unfortunately no prospective studies are available to confirm this. Within the United States two studies appeared to demonstrate a relationship between donor ALT level (Aach, 1981) and hepatitis B core antibody (Anti-HBc) (Koziol, 1986) and the subsequent development of NANBH in the recipient. These two factors have been shown to be additive. It was estimated that the introduction of ALT testing and anti-HBc testing as 'surrogate' markers for NANBH in the United States would result in a reduction in the incidence of NANBH by around 50% but with a significant loss of donor units.

Surrogate testing by these methods was introduced in the USA in November 1986. It was felt that the American data may not be entirely valid within the volunteer donor population in the UK where the apparent incidence of NANBH is much lower and this combined with concern over the financial cost and loss of donor units involved in testing meant that surrogate testing has not been carried out within the UK (Anderson, 1988).

The recent developments leading to the detection of the hepatitis C virus (HCV) have created renewed interest within transfusion services world wide. An innovative approach by Chiron Laboratories using recombinant techniques resulted in the detection of part of the viral genome of what is now known as HCV (Choo, 1989). An assay for the detection of HCV antibody (anti-HCV) was produced and is now available commercially. The initial assays were based on a single protein (C-100) grown in yeasts. Work showed a good correlation between patients with chronic NANBH and the presence of anti HCV. Approximately 80% of patients with chronic NANBH have detectable anti-HCV although interestingly antibody is seen in only a proportion of patients with acute resolving disease (Kuo, 1989). These first generation tests have now been superseded by assays capable of detecting a number of different viral antigens, including structural core epitopes. Within the UK, approximately 0.4% of donors are reactive in the anti-HCV test.

A number of supplementary testing systems are now available. Immunoblot systems, such as the Recombinant Immunoblot Assay (RIBA) are capable of detecting antibody to a number of viral antigens; these techniques are broadly analogous to the Western Blot confirmatory assay for HIV antibody. The polymerase chain reaction (PCR) is capable of detecting HCV RNA. PCR testing has the advantage that it is capable of detecting viral antigens, and hence should correlate more closely with the ability to transmit HCV infection by transfusion. Preliminary evidence indicates however a very close correlation between PCR and RIBA tests which indicate that both may be satisfactory for confirmatory testing in the transfusion field. Approximately 10% of EIA reactive donor sera will be confirmed by RIBA and PCR. Donor screening is invariably associated with the generation of false positive results. However the predictive value for the current anti-HCV test taken in conjunction with the relatively high prevalence of anti-HCV EIA reactive donors is likely to pose significant logistical problems for transfusion services. Routine anti-HCV screening

of blood donations has already commenced in many countries and became mandatory in September 1991. The delay between exposure to the virus and development of detectable antibody is, on average, about six months (Kuo, 1989). This long 'window period' and the sensitivity of current assays suggest that a proportion of infectious donors will not be detected. In view of this the AABB has continued to use the surrogate tests in addition to anti-HCV testing. These concerns have also created debate with regard to the advisability of excluding anti-HCV positive plasma donations from plasma pools for fractionation. The FDA has advised that anti-HCV testing of plasma for fractionation cannot be justified on the basis that removal of possible neutralizing antibody may have a deleterious effect on the safety of its products, whereas an opposite view has been taken by the French Regulatory bodies (Finlaysen, 1990). There is however clear evidence that effective heat treatment of factor VIII concentrate can eliminate NANBH transmission. Moreover there is evidence that PCR testing of treated concentrates may be capable of predicting infectivity in this setting (Garson, 1990).

Human T-lymphotrophic virus (HTLV-1)

HTLV-1 is a transforming retrovirus that has been shown to be closely associated with two distinct diseases, namely tropical spastic paraparesis (TSP) and adult T-cell leukaemia/lymphoma (ATLL). A closely related virus, HTLV-2, has also been described. This was first isolated from cultured lymphocytes of a patient with T-cell hairy cell leukaemia (Kalyanaraman) but no definite aetiological relationship has been established.

HTLV-1 is an intracellular pathogen, proviral DNA being incorporated with the DNA of infected lymphocytes.

HTLV-1 infection has been shown to be endemic in south-west Japan, and also prevalent within areas of the Caribbean, Africa and South America. Within the United Kingdom the majority of cases of HTLV-1 associated disease have been reported in migrants from endemic areas, particularly the Caribbean (Tosswill, 1990). However a case of ATLL in a white British male has been reported (Wyld, 1990).

Infection with HTLV-1 is associated with

antibody formation and a prolonged clinically asymptomatic phase. It is now recognized that only a proportion of infected individuals will go on to develop clinically significant disease. This asymptomatic phase may be as long as 10–30 years. In Japan the lifetime risk of ATLL developing in carriers may be as low as 6% in perinatally acquired infection (Tsui, 1990). Hence although HTLV-1 infection may be associated with serious clinical sequelae the relationship between infection and the development of disease is not as clear cut as in HIV infection, the other transfusion transmitted retrovirus.

There is convincing evidence from Japan that HTLV-1 can be transmitted by transfusion (Sato, 1986). Up to 70% of recipients of HTLV-1 antibody positive blood will seroconvert following transfusion. Leucocyte transfer is necessary for infection to be transmitted and the injection of cell-free serum is not associated with seroconversion. In this context HTLV-1 behaves in a similar fashion to CMV in that transmission is only associated with the transfusion of cellular elements of the blood.

ATLL has not yet been described following the transfusion of HTLV-1 antibody positive blood. This may be a consequence of the long asymptomatic phase of HTLV-1 infection. There are however well documented cases of the development of TSP following transfusion acquired infection. In these cases the latent period between transfusion and the onset of symptoms has been unusually short, in the region of 16–20 weeks (Desgranges 1990).

Several HTLV-1 screening assays are now available (Kline, 1991). These are based on either an EIA or a particle agglutination format. Confirmatory assays using Western Blot PCR and RIPA (Radio Immunoprecipitation) are also available. The availability of these assays, along with clear evidence from Japan (Inaba, 1988) that HTLV-1 transmission by transfusion can be largely eliminated by the introduction of antibody screening have raised questions for transfusions services. In 1988 routine testing of blood donations for HTLV-1 antibody was introduced in the United States. Studies from Europe have shown a low seroprevalence within the donor population (*see* Lancet editorial 1991) and in the UK the prevalence has been reported as 0.00036% (Salker, 1990). The low prevalence along with

the evidence that HTLV-1 infection is largely confined to migrants from endemic areas has led to the suggestion that screening in the UK should concentrate on the Black donor population (Brennan, 1991). Selective screening may appear attractive whilst infection remains restricted to that 'at risk' population. Recent studies from the United States have shown an increasing incidence of HTLV infection in intravenous drug abusers (Robert-Giroff, 1986). This taken in conjunction with the recent description of ATLL in a white British male may be seen to challenge the possible effectiveness of a screening system based on racial origin. The question of UK donor screening for HTLV-1 infection is likely to increase in the near future and as indicated in a Lancet editorial on this topic a decision cannot be deferred indefinitely (Lancet, 1991).

Syphilis

Syphilis is a sexually transmitted disease caused by the delicate spirochaetal organism *Treponema pallidum*. The viability of this spirochaete out of the body is feeble – it is a strict parasite and dies rapidly in water, is very sensitive to drying, is readily killed by heat and dies more slowly (2–3 days) in the cold (0–4 °C) (Mackie and McCartney, 1960).

Transfusion transmitted syphilis was a well documented occurrence prior to the Second World War, but in the last 25 years only a few cases have been recorded (Chambers, *et al.*, 1969; Risseew-Appel and Kothe, 1983), these involving the use of fresh blood products.

The prime reason for this dramatic drop in incidence is considered to be the refrigeration of citrated blood at 4–6 °C which has become the standard practice since the 1950s. This now enables storage of whole blood and red cell components for up to five weeks. In most cases three days of refrigeration are sufficient to kill any spirochaetes in a unit of blood, however a reports state that survival has been observed for five days or more (Garretta, 1977, Van der Sluis, *et al.*, 1985) and Van der Sluis suggested that survival rate depends upon the number of organisms present in the donor blood.

As the temperature of storage is a major factor in the destruction of the spirochaete and so in the elimination of transfusion syphilis, it follows that the fresher the blood that is used, the greater the risk of transmission from an infected unit. Certainly no case of *T. pallidum* has yet been reported following the transfusion of stored blood. It has also been accepted that *T. pallidum* cannot survive for any length of time in plasma at −20 °C.

Serological tests for syphilis vary widely but all depend upon the detection of antibodies to the *T. pallidum* organism which develops 2–4 weeks after exposure. The type of test available to the syphilis testing laboratories can be broadly divided into 2 groups – those that use the Treponemal organism as an antigen source and the non-specific tests that use cardiolipin antigen. For many years transfusion services in the UK used the relatively insensitive cardiolipin tests but the efficacy of such methods are debatable (International Forum, 1981). More recently Treponemal pallidum haemagglutination (TPHA) has been widely adopted and has eliminated many of the sensitivity and specificity problems associated with previous practices.

The frequency of positive reacting donors is about one in 34,000 in the Yorkshire Region. The practice at most centres is to refer positive sera to specialist laboratories for full confirmation and follow-up tests. Although there are doubts about the need to screen blood donors for syphilis, most workers agree that testing should be maintained, at least for the present. It has been suggested that only fresh blood components require the test, but Seidl in a recent review (1990) maintains that syphilis screening should be regarded as a cheap surrogate test for HIV carriers in the window phase of infection. Certainly the medico-legal position leaves little room for choice and until this changes, all donors will continue to be tested.

Malaria and other tropical diseases

In endemic areas malarial transmission by blood transfusion is a constant risk and it has been suggested that the most effective method to prevent this problem is to treat the donor prophylactically with chloroquine 48 hours prior to the donation or to give the transfusion recipient a single dose of chloroquine at the time of the transfusion (Bruce-Chwatt, 1974). In temperate zones, such as the United Kingdom, transfusion transmitted malaria occurs infrequently but sensible precautions should be taken to prevent its occurrence. Malarial parasites can remain viable in blood stored for at least a week but are usually only transmitted by blood stored for under five days. Transmission occurs only by transfusion of cellular blood components. Currently within the United Kingdom individuals who have recently visited endemic malarial areas are allowed to continue to donate immediately following their return so long as they remain well and have no history of febrile illness whilst abroad. However for a 12-month period following return the plasma from such donations is used for fractionation only, and cellular blood components are not used for transfusion. This 12-month period is extended to three years for individuals who originate from or have been resident in endemic areas for three months or longer, and for individuals with a history of malaria. This donor deferral policy is effective when properly applied. However the increasing tendency for individuals to travel on holiday to endemic malarial areas means that a significant number of red cell units may be unnecessarily discarded. In one UK region as many as 5.8% of red cell units were discarded representing a loss of approximately 12,000 donations annually (Wells, 1986). It has been suggested that the selective use of malarial antibody testing along with a reduced exclusion period may be equally effective in reducing malarial transmission without losing as many red cell units.

Two different formats of malarial antibody testing are available. Indirect immunofluorescence tests and EIA based assays. The latter form is more amenable to use in transfusion centres. The availability of suitable malaria antigen is a potential restriction on the suitability of such tests. Currently only *Plasmodium falciparum* antigen is readily available *in vitro*, and the success of such testing is then dependent on cross-reacting between this and other malarial species.

African trypanosomiasis and leishmaniasis have rarely been transmitted by transfusion (Wolfe, 1975). However in Latin America the transmission of Chagas disease by blood transfusion is a serious problem. *Trypanosoma cruzi* is frequently present in the blood of people with chronic infection and transmission of the parasite by transfusion may lead to an acute or chronic incurable and even fatal illness in the recipient. Hence individuals who have visited areas of South or Central America where this disease is endemic, should be permitted to donate only plasma for fractionation purposes.

In endemic areas a screening programme for detection of antibodies to *Trypanosoma cruzi* may be employed, or the parasite can be destroyed by the addition of 125 mg crystal (gentian) violet to a unit of stored blood.

Cytomegalovirus

Human Cytomegalovirus (CMV) is a DNA virus belonging to the Herpes family and is one of the most common viruses to be found in man. Antibody frequencies, which indicate previous CMV infection, range from 40% in the highly industralized countries of Europe and North America to 100% in some 'third world' countries (Bayer and Tegtmeier, 1976). The incidence of seropositive blood donors in the UK is between 50 and 60%. According to Barbara (1983) antibody levels, in a London population, increase with age at an approximate 1% seroconversion rate per year up to the age of 55.

Although CMV is a ubiquitous agent, it generally carries little in the way of disease in healthy people, and is regarded as a significant infection only in the immunosuppressed or immunocompromised. In these groups it can result in considerable morbidity and mortality. Blood products with a reduced risk of CMV transmission are required only in specific clinical settings and these are outlined later in the chapter.

As with all herpes viruses, CMV is able to persist indefinitely in a latent state following infection. This latency is attributed to viral DNA integrating with the host genome, and the reticuloendothelial system has been implicated as a site of viral persistence during the latency period. Although the mechanism is not well understood, latent virus may be reactivated when immunity is compromised or in response to allogenic stimulus (Schoecter, 1972; Cheung and Lang, 1977). Recovery of CMV from the leucocytes of infected patients (Lang, 1975) suggests that lymphocytes or granulocytes are the most likely hosts of the viral agent, an important consideration in terms of transmission by transfusion and the relative hazards of different components.

In an attempt to reduce the problem of CMV transmission in these groups screening for cytomegalovirus has become routine practice in the transfusion service although some workers, as an alternative, have advocated the use of leucocyte-depleted cellular components to reduce the risk of transmission (International Forum, 1984). The former option presents a particular problem with CMV as the only practical way of screening at this time involves serological testing for antibody, which is present in over 50% of the UK donor population. This of course precludes the omission of seropositive donors from the blood panels. Fortunately this is unnecessary as only selected groups of recipients are at risk and seronegative donations may be directed towards these cases. At our centre a small proportion of red cell components are screened for CMV as well as all the platelet products which are to a large extent, used to support the local bone marrow transplant patients.

Over the past few years numerous techniques have been adopted for CMV screening, including complement fixation, haemagglutination, latex agglutination and EIA methods. Latex agglutination is widely used because of its speed and simplicity, and also the fact the IgM as well as IgG antibodies are detected. Whether both are required is not clear. IgG is regarded as necessary, because although it indicates a previous infection, it serves to highlight carriers of latent virus which may reactivate in the recipient. IgM presence suggests a recent infection in a donor which is more likely to be active, and therefore is probably more likely to transmit CMV. However, IgM positive donations do not account for all the infections transmitted by transfusion (Beneke, *et al.*, 1984). While the position remains unclear it may be safer to use an assay that will detect both, although some recent work (Koerner, *et al.*, 1990) suggests that IgG tests are sufficiently sensitive to detect both active and latent infections.

The development of commercial EIA tests has enabled centres to introduce CMV assays with the advantages of objective reading and data reduction by computer analysis. Whichever test is used, CMV seropositive blood donors remain on the blood panel and their donations continue to act as valuable contributions to routine transfusion procedures.

Hazards of different blood components and requirements for 'at risk' patients

Product related risks

Whenever transfusion of blood components or blood products is considered, the potential therapeutic benefits must be balanced against the risk involved. Where a choice of product is possible then that which has a clearer safety record should always be chosen.

In considering the risks related to different components and products a clear distinction needs to be made between blood components derived from individual donations, and blood products that are derived from fractionation of plasma pools containing many thousands of donations.

Increasing emphasis on quality assurance within modern transfusion services should ensure that blood components are not issued for transfusion until all of the required testing has been completed and the results are satisfactory. In situations where fresh blood or its components are required more rapid screening tests may be employed but these should meet the necessary sensitivity standards. Despite rigorous donor selection and the appropriate use of screening tests it is not possible to remove entirely the risk of disease transmission, although the risk can be reduced to an acceptable level. This potential risk should always be considered before prescribing a transfusion product for a patient.

Although there is evidence that modern leucocyte depleting filters can prevent transmission of CMV and HTLV-1 by transfusion, it is not possible to treat cellular components by physical or chemical means to destroy any viruses present. However Alter and co-workers (1988) have reported experimental data on the use of photochemical methods that may prove effective in this regard.

Blood products prepared by fractionation of large volume plasma pools can prevent particular problems with regard to viral transmission. The nature of the blood product and the method of fractionation are important determinants of the risk.

Human albumin solution (HAS) has a proved safety record. This is in part due to the pasteurization of the final product by heating at 60 °C for 10 hours. Intramuscular immunoglobulin products, when prepared by cold ethanol fractionation are also considered safe and there is no evidence of transmission of HIV or hepatitis by these products. The factors believed to be important in ensuring viral inactivation include the pH, temperature and alcohol concentration of the Cohn Cold ethanol process.

Intravenous immunoglobulin preparations have been associated with reports of NANBH (Lane, 1983; Lever, 1985; Ochs, 1985) but there are no convincing reports of HIV transmission by these products. The importance of method of manufacture is demonstrated by one report in which NANBH developed in patients receiving IV immunoglobulin but IM immunoglobulin preparations derived from the same plasma pool did not transmit the disease (Lever, 1984).

Coagulation factor concentrates, used in the treatment of haemophiliacs, have been clearly demonstrated to be associated with transmission of HBV, NANBH and HIV. The use of products prepared from volunteer plasma donor pools, combined with the use of sensitive screening tests both on the individual donations as well as on the final pool, can provide some degree of protection. However, concern about disease transmission has prompted the development of alternative methods to protect the recipient. The risk of HBV transmission can be eliminated in patients undergoing regular treatment by active immunization with hepatitis B vaccine (Crosnier, 1981). The development of viral inactivation processes has dramatically reduced the risk of transmission of HIV and NANBH. Heat treatment has been used extensively and there is debate over whether treatment in the liquid phase (wet) or lyophilized phase (dry) is more effective. Currently Factor VIII prepared at the BioProducts Laboratory utilizing plasma from volunteer UK donors is treated at 80 °C for 72 h in the dry state and appears to be highly effective (Study Group of UK Haemophilia Directors, 1988). Newer products utilizing a combination of immunoaffinity purification and solvent/detergent processes are also now available. It is important to ensure that each new process is rigidly evaluated to ensure patient safety, and there is evidence that PCR testing may be valuable in this setting (Garson, 1990).

The immunocompromised patient

In the last 15 years tremendous advances have been made in the fields of cancer and leukaemia chemotherapy, organ transplantation and neonatal care of the premature infant. Linking these patients together is the need for intensive supportive care and their compromised immune status either iatrogenically induced or due to immaturity. Much of the supportive care involves replacement therapy with specific blood components. It is now recognized that some of these blood components can transmit CMV infection which is a major cause of mortality and morbidity within this immuno-compromised patient group. The source of infection is believed to be latently infected white cells, hence any blood component that contains significant numbers of viable leuco-cytes could potentially transmit the virus.

CMV was first recognized as a transfusion problem by Kaarianen in 1966 when viruria was demonstrated in a patient with an infectious-mononucleosis-like syndrome which developed in up to 15% of open heart surgery cases. Subsequently many cases of transfusion acquired CMV were reported and Prince, *et al.* (1971) in the USA demonstrated a post-transfusion infection rate of about 7% from a single unit of blood. However CMV has never been regarded as a serious transfusion hazard in immunocompetent recipients, a conclusion drawn from the relatively small number of symptomatic cases reported in the literature. The two main groups of patient in which CMW transmission is most clearly associated with significant disease are organ transplant recipients and premature infants.

In transplant patients CMV infection can arise not only from transfusion but also from the donated graft, and also by reactivation of latent infection in the recipient. The study by Bowden and colleagues (1986) has shown that the use of seronegative blood products is highly effective in the prevention of primary CMV infection in seronegative patients who receive marrow transplants from seronegative donors. However, although this study also suggested that seronegative patients with seropositive donors do not benefit from receiving seronegative blood products, the numbers were too small to be conclusive on this point. These workers also emphasized how logistically difficult it was to provide CMV seronegative blood products on the scale required for this study the 51 patients involved required more than 6,000 units of CMV seronegative blood products during the 18 months' period of the trial.

Yeager (1981) demonstrated significant morbidity and mortality rates in premature low-birthweight neonates who acquired CMV infection from transfusion. The risk was greater in the infants of CMV antibody negative mothers with infants of birthweight less than 1,200 g. Other workers have not confirmed these findings (Tegtmeier, 1988; Preiksaitis, *et al.*, 1988).

Ideally all white cell-containing blood products should be screened for the presence of CMV antibody prior to transfusion to these groups of patients, particularly if the recipient is CMV antibody negative. When CMV anti-body screening is not available it is possible to reduce the risk of transmission by depleting components of white cells prior to transfusion. It has been shown that by using frozen re-constituted red cells the incidence of post-transfusion CMV infection can be reduced (Sutherland, 1984). It follows that other measures such as the use of filtered red cells, dextran sedimented red cells or washed red cells should also have some effect in reducing the CMV transmission risk. Platelet transfusions are a little more difficult to provide as white cell poor preparations. If multiple random platelet transfusions are used, the recipient is exposed to more chances of meeting the virus than if single donor platelets are used. Special techniques have to be employed to reduce the level of white cell contamination in this type of concentrate (Robinson, 1984).

Granulocyte tranfusions obviously carry the highest risk of transmitting CMV infection and the only protection that can be provided for the 'at risk' recipient is to select CMV antibody negative donors. With the advent of granulo-cyte transfusions for the management of neonatal septicaemia, transmission of CMV is a likely sequel unless seronegative donors are used for this highly susceptible group of patients.

References

Aach, R.D., Lander, J.J., Sherman, L.A., Miller, W.V., Kahn, R.A., Gitnick, G.L., *et al.* (1978) Transfusion transmitted viruses: interim analysis of hepatitis among transfused and non-transfused patients. In, *Viral hepatitis: A contemporary assessment of etiology, epidemiology, pathogenesis and prevention*, G.N. Vyas, S.N. Cohen and R. Schmid, (eds), pp. 383–396. Philadelphia, Franklin Institute Press

Aach, R.D., Szmuness, W., Mosley, J.W., Hollinger, F.B., Kahn, R.A., Stevens, C.E., Edwards, V.M. and Werch, J. (1981) Serum alanine aminotransferase of donors in relation to the risk of Non-A, Non-B hepatitis in recipients. *The New England Journal of Medicine*, **304**, 989–994

Adler, S.P. (1989) *Transfusion*-acquired CMV infection in premature infants. **29**, 278–279

Alter, H.J., Morel, P.A., Dorman, B.P., Con Smith, G., Creagan, R.P., Weisenhahn, G.P., *et al.* (1988) Photochemical decontamination of blood components containing hepatitis B and Non-A Non-B virus. *Lancet*, **2**, 1446–1450

Alter, H.J., Purcell, R.H., Shih, J.W., Melpolder, J.C., Houghton, M., Choo, Q. and Kuo, G. (1989) Detection of antibody to Hepatitis C virus in prospectively followed transfusion recipients with acute and chronic Non-A, Non-B hepatitis. *The New England Journal of Medicine*, **321**, 1494–1500

Alter, H.J., Holland, P.V., Purcell, R.H., Lander, J.J., Feinstone, S.M., Morrow, A.G., *et al.* (1972) Post transfusion hepatitis after exclusion of commercial and hepatitis B antigen-positive donors. *Annals of Internal Medicine*, **77**, 691–699

Barbara, J.A.J. (1983) 'Cytomegalovirus' page 75. In, *Microbiology in Blood Transfusion*, Institute of Medical Laboratory Sciences monograph. Bristol, John Wright & Sons Ltd

Barbara, J.A.J., Howell, D.R. and Monchnaty, P.Z. (1983) HBsAg detection rates in the blood donor population. RIA and RPHA compared by parallel screening. In, R. Hopkins and S.E. Field (eds), *Proceedings of Hepatitis Workshop*. Stirling, Sept. 1982

Bayer, W.L. and Tegtmeier, G.E. (1976) The blood donor: detection and magnitude of cytomegalovirus carrier states and the prevalence of cytomegalovirus antibody. *Yale Journal of Biology and Medicine*, **49**, 5–12

Beneke, J.S., Tegtmeier, G.E., Alter, H.J., Luetkemeyer, R.B., Solomon, R. and Bayer, W.L. (1984) Relation of titers of antibodies to CMV in blood donors to the transmission of cytomegalovirus infection. *Journal of Infectious Diseases*, **150**, 883–888

Berman, M., Alter, H.J., Ishak, K.G., Purcell, R.H. and Jones, E.A. (1979) The chronic sequelae of Non-A, Non-B hepatitis. *Annals of Internal Medicine*, **91**, 1–6

Blumberg, B.S., Alter, H.J. and Visnich, S. (1965) A 'new' antigen in Leukaemia sera. *Journal of the American Medical Association*, **191**, 541–546

Bove, J.R. (1990) Testing in the years ahead: New pressures and new concerns. *Transfusion*, **30**, 63–69

Bowden, R.A., Sayers, M., Flournay, N., Newton, B., Banaji, M., Donnal, Thomas, E. and Meyers, J.D. (1986) Cytomegalovirus immune globulin and sero-negative blood products to prevent primary cytomegalovirus infection after marrow transplantation. *The New England Journal of Medicine*, **314**, 1006–1010

Brennan, M., Barbara, J. and Contreras, M. (1990) Screening for HTLV-1. *The Lancet*, **336**, 1517

Bruce-Chwatt, L.J. (1974) Transfusion Malaria. *Bulletin of the World Health Organization*, **50**, 337

Cameron, C.H. (1983) What's in a nanogram? *Transfusion Microbiology*, **4**, 8–10

Chambers, R.W., Foley, H.T. and Schmidt, P.J. (1969) Transmission of Syphilis by fresh blood components. *Transfusion*, **9**, 32–34

Cheung, K.S. and Lang, D.J. (1977) Transmission and activation of cytomegalovirus with blood transfusion: a mouse model. *Journal of Infectious Disease*, **135**, 841–845

Choo, Q., Kuo, G., Weiner, A.J., Overby, L.R., Bradley, D.W. and Houghton, M. (1989) Isolation of a cDNA clone derived from a blood borne Non-A, Non-B viral hepatitis genome. *Science*, **244**, 359–362

Collins, J.A., Bassendine, M.F., Codd, A.A., Collins, A., Ferner, R.E. and Jones, O.F.W. (1983) Prospective study of post-transfusion hepatitis after cardiac surgery in a British Centre. *The British Medical Journal*, **287**, 1422–1424

Contreras, M., Hewitt, P.E., Barbara, J.A.J. and Mochnaty, P.Z. (1985) Blood donors at risk of transmitting the acquired immune deficiency syndrome. *British Medical Journal*, **290**, 749–750

Cossart, Y.E., Kirsh, S. and Ismay, S.L. (1982) Post transfusion hepatitis in Australia. *Lancet*, **1**, 208–213

Crosnier, J., Jungers, P., Courouce, A.M., Laplanche, A., Benhamoll, E., Dego, F. *et al.* (1981) Randomized placebo controlled trial of hepatitis B surface antigen vaccine in French haemodialysis units. *Lancet*, **1**, 797–800

Cunming, P.D., Wallace, E.L., Schorr, J.B. and Dodd, R.Y. (1989) Exposure of patients to Human Immunodeficiency virus through the transfusion of blood components that test antibody negative. *The New England Journal of Medicine*, **321**, 941–946

Curran, J.W., Lawrence, D.N., Jaffe, H. *et al.* (1984) Acquired Immunodeficiency Syndrome (AIDS) associated with transfusions. *The New England Journal of Medicine*, **310**, 69–75

De Groote, J.J. (1987) Therapeutic measures after hepatitis B virus infection: post-exposure prophylaxis. *Postgraduate Medical Journal*, **63** (suppl. 2), 33–39

Dept of Health and Social Security (1972) *Revised report of the Advisory Group on testing for the presence of Australia (hepatitis associated) antigen and its antibody*. HMSO, London

Dept of Health (1989) *Guidelines for the Blood Transfusion Services in the United Kingdom*. HMSO, London

Desranges, C., Winter, C., Delzant, G. Screening for HTLV-1. *Lancet*, **336**, 1517

Driss, F., Boboc, B., Zarski, J.P., Carls, M.J., Pol, S., Eme, D., Ekindjian, D.G., Courouce, A.M., Brechot, C., Berthelot, P. and Nalpas, B. (1989) An epidemiological and clinical study of Transaminase levels and hepatitis B antibodies in 1,100 blood donors. *Vox Sanquinis*, **57**, 43–48

Evans, B.G., Gill, O.N., Gleave, S.R., Mortimer, P.P. and Parry, J.V. (1991) HIV-2 in the United Kingdom – A review. *Communicable Disease Reports*, **1**, R19–R23

Finlayson, J.S. and Tankersley, D.L. (1990) Anti-HCV screening and plasma fractionation: the case against. *Lancet*, **335**, 1274

Garretta, M., Paris-Haemlin, A., Muller, A. and Vaisman, A. (1977) Syphilis et transfusion sanguine. *Revue Francais Transfusion immuno-haematolgie*, **20**, 287–308

Garson, J.A., Preston, F.E., Makris, M., Tuke, P., Ring,

C., Machine, S.J. and Tedder, R.S. (1990) Detection by PCR of hepatitis C virus in factor VIII concentrates. *Lancet,* **335,** 1473–1474

Goldfield, M., Bill, J. and Colismo, F. (1978) The control of transfusion-associated hepatitis. In viral hepatitis, G.N. Vyas, S.N. Cohen., R. Schmid, (eds) pp. 404–414. *Franklin Institute Press*, Philadelphia

Guidlines for the Blood Transfusion Services in the United Kingdom (1989) HMSO, London

Habibi, B., Klenknecht, D., Vachon, F., Cavalier, J. and Salmon, C. (1973) Le choc transfusionnel par contamination bacterienne du sang conserve. Analyse de 25 observations. *Revue Francaise Transfusion,* **14,** 41

Hoofnagle, J.H. (1990) Post transfusion hepatitis B. *Transfusions,* **30,** 384–386

Imagawa, D.T., Moon, H.L., Wolinsky, S.M., Sano, K., Morales, F., *et al.* (1989) Human Immuno-deficiency virus type 1 infection in homosexual men who remain seronegative for prolonged periods. *The New England Journal of Medicine,* **320,** 1458–1462

Inaba, S., Sat, H., Okochi, K., Fukada, K., Takakura, F., Tokinega, K., *et al.* (1988) Prevention of transmission of human T-Lymphotropic virus type 1 (HTLV-1) through transfusion, by donor screening with antibody to the virus. *Transfusion,* **29,** 7–11

International Forum (1981) Does it make sense for blood transfusion services to continue to time-honoured syphilis screening with cardiolipin antigen? *Vox Sanquinis,* **41,** 183–192

International Forum (1984) Transfusion-transmitted CMV infections. *Vox-Sanquinis,* **41,** 387–414

Jullien, A.M., Courouce, A., Richard, D., Favre, M., Hefrere, J. and Halibi, B. (1988) Transmission of HIV by blood from seronegative donors. *Lancet* 1248–1249

Kaarianen, L., Klemol, E. and Paloheimo, J. (1966) Rise of Cytomegalovirus antibodies in an infectious-mononucleosis-like syndrome after transfusion. British Medical Journal, **1,** 1270–1272

Kalyanaraman, V.S., Sarngattharan, M.G., Robert-Giroff, M., Miyoshi, I., Blayney, D., Golde, D. and Gallo, R.C. (1982) A new subtype of human T cell leukaemia virus (HTLV-11) associated with a T-cell variant of hairy cell leukaemia. *Science,* **218,** 571–573

Kernoff, P.B.A., Lee, C.A., Karayiannis, P. and Thomas, H.C. (1985) High risk of Non-A, Non-B hepatitis after a first exposure to volunteer of commercial clotting factor concentrates: effects of prophylactic immune serum globulin. *British Journal of Haematology,* **60,** 469–479

Kline, R.L., Brothers, T., Halsey, N., Boulos, R., Lairmore, M.D. and Quinn, T.C. (1991) Evaluation of enzyme immunoassays for antibody to human T-lympho-tropic viruses type 1/11. *Lancet,* **337,** 30–33

Koerner, K., Kilian, D., Zimmerman, B., Nebel-Schickel, H. and Horn, J. (1990) Comparison of four different ELISA's and indirect immunofluoresence for screening of blood donors for antibodies to Cytomegalovirus. *Biotest Bulletin,* **4,** (vol. 2) 119–123

Koziol, D.E., Holland, P.V., Alling, D.W., Melpolder, J.C., Solomon, R.E., Purcell, R.H., *et al.* (1986) *Annals of Internal Medicine,* **104,** 488–495

Kuo, G., Choo, Q.-L., Alter, H.J., Gitnick, G.L., Redeker, A.G., Purcell, R.H., *et al.* (1989) An assay for circulating antibodies to a major etiologic virus of human Non-A, Non-B hepatitis. *Science,* **244,** 362–364

Lancet Editorial (1990) HTLV-1-A screen too many? *Lancet,* **336,** 1161–1162

Lane, R.S. (1983) Non-A Non-B, hepatitis from intra-venous immunoglobulin. *Lancet,* **2,** 974–975

Lang, D.J. (1975) Cytomegalovirus and Epstein–Barr virus infections in *Transmissible diseases and blood transfusion.* Greenwalt and Jamieson (eds) and published by Grune and Stratton (NY) pp. 153–169

Lever, A.M.L., Webster, A.D.B., Brown, D. and Thomas, H.C. (1985) Non A, non B, hepatitis after intravenous immunoglobulin. *Lancet,* **1,** 587

Lever, A.M.L., Webster, A.D.B., Brown, D. and Thomas, H.C. (1984) Non A, non B hepatitis occurring in agammaglobulinaemic patients after intravenous immunoglobulin. *Lancet,* **2,** 1062–1064

Mackie, T.J. and MacCartney, J.E. (1960). Spirochaetes in *Handbook of Bacteriology.* R. Cruikshank, (ed.) and published by Livingstone (Edinburgh) p. 709

McClelland, D.B.L. (ed.), (1988), in, Handbook of transfusion medicine. HMSO, London

Mortimer, P.P., Parry, J.V. and Mortimer, J.V. (1985) which anti-HTLV III/LAV assays for screening and confimatory testing? *Lancet,* **2,** 877–878

Noone, A., Gill, O.N., Clarke, S.E. and Porter, K. (1991) Travel, heterosexual intercourse and HIV-1 infection. *Communicable Disease Reports,* **1,** R39–R43

Ochs, H.D., Fischer, S.H., Virant, F.S., Lee, M.L., Kingdon, H.S. and Wedgewood, R.J. (1985) Non-A, non-B hepatitis and intravenous immunoglobulin. *Lancet,* **1,** 404–405

Preiksaitis, J.K., Brown, L. and Mackenzie, M. (1988) Transfusion-acquired cytomegalovirus infection in neonates. *Transfusion,* **28,** 205–209

Prince, A.M. (1968) An antigen detected in blood during the incubation period of serum hepatitis. *Proceedings of the National Academy of Sciences. (USA),* **60,** 814–821

Prince, A.M., Smuzness, W., Millian, S.J. and David, D.S. (1971) A serological study of cytomegalovirus infection associated with blood transfusion. *New England Journal of Medicine,* **284,** 1125–1131

Risseew-Appel, I.M. and Kothe, F.C. (1983) Transfusion syphilis: a case report. *Sexually-transmitted Diseases,* **10,** 200–201

Robert-Guroff, M., Weiss, S.H. and Giron, J.A. (1986) Prevalence of antibodies to HTLV-1-11 and -111 in intravenous drug abusers from an AIDS endemic region. *The Journal of the American Medical Association,* **255,** 3133–3137

Robinson, E.A.E. (1984) Single donor granulocytes and platelets. In *Clinics in Haematology* 13, W.L. Bayer (ed.), pp. 185–216, W.B. Saunders, London

Salahuddin, S.Z., Groopman, J.E., Markham, P.D., Sarngadharan, M.G., Redfield, R.R., McClane, M.F., *et al.* (1984) HTLV-111 in symptom free seronegative persons. *Lancet,* **ii,** 1418–1420

Salker, R., Tosswill, J.H.C., Barbara, J.A.J., Runganga,

J., Contreras, M., Tedder, R.S., Parra-Mejia, N. and Mortimer, P.P. (1990) HTLV1/11 antibodies in UK blood donors. *Lancet,* **336**, 317

Sato, H. and Okochi, K. (1986) Transmission of human T-cell leukaemia virus (HTLV-1) by blood transfusion: demonstration of proviral DNA in recipients blood lymphocytes. *International Journal of Cancer,* **37**, 395–400

Schoechter, G.P., Soehlen, F. and McFarland, W. (1972) Lymphocyte response to blood transfusion in man. *New England Journal of Medicine,* **287**, 1169–1173

Seef, L.B., Zimmerman, H.J., Wright, E.C., Finkelstein, J.D., Garcia-Pont, P. and Greenlee, H.B. (1977) Randomized, double blind controlled trial of the efficacy of immune serum globulin for the prevention of post-transfusion hepatitis. *Gastroenterology,* **72**, 111–121

Seidl, S. (1990) Syphilis screening in the 1990s. *Transfusion,* **30**, 773–775

Stramer, S.L., Heller, J.S., Coombs, R.W., Ho, D.D. and Allain, J.P. (1988) Transmission of HIV by blood transfusion. *The New England Journal of Medicine,* **319**, 513–517

Study Group of the U.K. Haemophilia Centre Directors (1988) Effect of dry heating of coagulation factor concentrates at 80 °C for 72 hours on transmission of non-A, non-B hepatitis. *Lancet,* **ii**, 814–816

Sutherland, S. (1984) Is cytomegalovirus a problem for the transfusion service? *Transfusion Microbiology,* **5**, 3–7

Tedder, R.S., Cameron, C.H., Wilson-Groome, R., Howell, D.R., Colgrove, A. and Barbara, J.A.J. (1980) Contrasting patterns and frequency of antibodies to the surface, core and e antigens of hepatitis B virus in blood donors and in homosexual patients. *Journal of Medical Virology,* **6**, 323–332

Tegtmeier, G.E. (1988) The use of cytomegalovirus screened blood in neonates. *Transfusion,* **28**, 201–203

Tosswill, J.H.C. and Parry, J.V. (1989) HTLV-1 in English Patients. *Lancet,* **ii**, 328

Tsuji, Y., Doi, H., Yamabe, T., Ishimaru, T., Miyaomoto, T. and Hino, S. (1990) Prevention of mother to child transmission of human T-lymphototropic virus type-1. *Paediatrics,* **86**, 11–17

Van der Sluis, J.J., ten Kate, F.J.W., Vusevski, V.D., Kothe, F.C., Aelbers, G.M.N. and Van Eijk, K.V.W. (1985) Transfusion syphilis, survival of *Treponema pallidum* in stored donor blood. *Vox Sanquinis,* **49**, 390–399

Wallace, J., Barr, A. and Milne, G.R. (1975) Which techniques should be used to screen blood donations for hepatitis B surface antigen. *British Medical Journal,* **2**, 412–414

Watson, J.G. (1983) Problems of infection after bone-marrow transplantation. *Journal of Clinical Pathology,* **36**, 683–692

Wells, L.J. and Ala, F.A. (1985) Malaria and blood transfusion. In: *Proceedings of the British Blood Transfusion Society* (Oxford 1985), PO2-1, pp. 80

Widell, A., Sundstrom, G., Hansson, B.G., Fex, G., Moestrup, T. and Nordenfelt, E. (1988) Relation between donor transaminase and recipient hepatitis Non-A, Non-B in Sweden. *Vox Sanquinis,* **54**, 154–159

Wolfe, M.S. (1975) Parasites other than malaria, transmissible by blood transfusion. In *Transmissible disease and blood transfusion*, T.J. Greenwalt and G.A. Jameson (eds), Grine and Stratton, New York

Wyld, P.J., Tosswill, J.H.C., Mortimer, P.P. and Weber, J.N. (1990) *British Journal of Haematology,* 149–150

Yeager, A.S., Grumet, F.C., Hafleigh, E.B., Arvin, A.M., Bradley, J.S. and Prober, C.G. (1981) Prevention of transfusion acquired cytomegalovirus infections in newborn infants. *Journal of Paediatrics,* **98**, 281–287

15

Hepatitis, AIDS and blood

A.J. Zuckerman

The importance of viral infections which are transmissible by blood and blood products has been acknowledged for many years, and significant and successful advances have been made in the control of hepatitis B. The significance of cytomegalovirus infection in immunocompromised recipients of blood, the recognition of human T-cell leukaemia viruses and the emergence of the human immuno-deficiency viruses stress that blood-related viral infections remain a vital challenge to preventive medicine.

The emphasis in this chapter is on hepatitis B since this provides a model for prevention of a transfusion-associated viral infection by careful selection and serological screening of blood donors and individual blood units before separation and preparation of plasma factors from large pools. An additional line of defence is provided by prophylactic immunization of persons at risk.

Viral hepatitis

Viral hepatitis is caused by at least six different viruses, hepatitis A (infectious or epidemic hepatitis), hepatitis B (serum hepatitis), and a possible variant of hepatitis B (HBV2), hepatitis D virus (the delta agent), hepatitis C, and an epidemic form of enterically transmitted hepatitis caused by a recently identified virus, hepatitis E. Viral hepatitis is a recognized major public health problem occurring in all parts of the world.

Hepatitis B and co-infection with the delta virus, and infection with hepatitis C may lead to persistent infection (the carrier state) and may progress to chronic liver disease, which may be severe. There is now firm evidence of an aetio-logical association between hepatitis B virus and hepatocellular carcinoma, one of the ten most common malignant tumours world-wide.

Hepatitis B

Much has been written about the epidemiology of hepatitis B. The infection is spread by blood to blood contact including inapparent pene-tration of the mucosa and skin, by the sexual route and perinatally. The importance of this infection is stressed by a reservoir of carriers estimated to number at least 300 million world-wide and by progression to serious chronic liver disease including hepatocellular carcinoma in a proportion of patients.

Hepatitis B virus (HBV)

Hepatitis B virus is a spherical double-shelled 42 nm particle clearly identifiable in serum by its distinct morphology by electron microscopy (Figure 15.1), whereas the small 22 nm particles and the tubular structures are non-infectious surplus virus coat protein. Double-stranded DNA has been isolated from circulating virus and also from the viral cores extracted from the nuclei of infected hepatocytes. The DNA

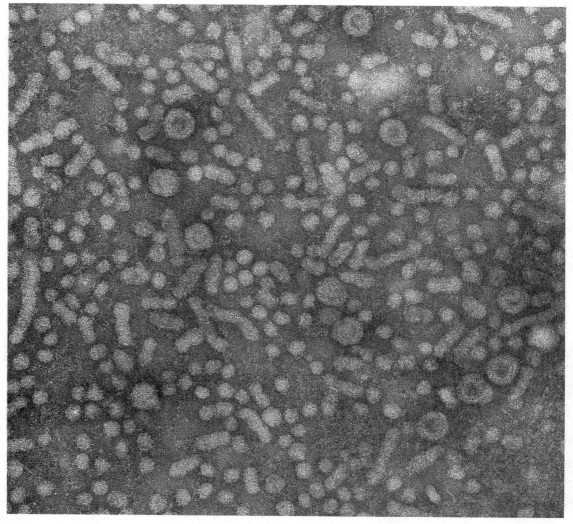

Figure 15.1. Electron micrograph showing the double-shelled 42 nm hepatitis B virus particles, the small 22 nm spherical particles of hepatitis B surface antigen and the tubular forms

consists of circular nucleic acid molecules with a molecular weight of about $2 \times 3 \times 10^6$ and approximately 3,200 nucleotides in length containing single-stranded gaps of 600–2100 nucleotides. The entire DNA of hepatitis B virus has been cloned in *E. coli*, in yeast (*Saccharomyces cerevisiae*) and also in several strains of mammalian cells.

Initial studies of HBV were hampered by the inability to cultivate the virus *in vitro* and were essentially limited to biochemical analysis of purified virions and viral antigens, and to serological and histological investigations of clinical infections. Molecular cloning of the viral genome provided better analytical methods and resulted in the determination of the entire necleotide sequence. Analysis of the nucleotide sequence revealed four open reading frames (Figure 15.2), regions of the genome which code for proteins.

Prior to the sequencing of the HBV genome, the amino acid sequence of both the amino- and carboxyl-termini of the major hepatitis B surface antigen (HBsAg) polypeptide had already been determined and it was therefore possible to locate the gene for this polypeptide

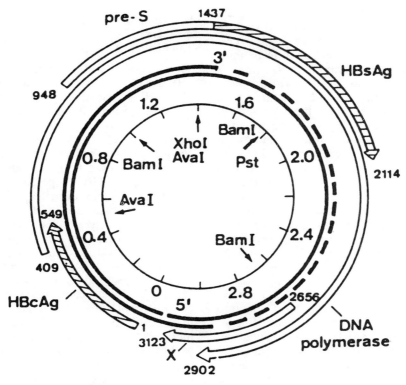

Figure 15.2. The molecular structure of the genome of hepatitis B virus

within one of the open reading frames. Part of the open reading frame was not represented in the HBsAg polypeptide and was designed pre-S as it was assumed that these sequences were cleaved off a larger precursor polypeptide after translation. The pre-S region is therefore subdivided into pre-S1 and pre-S2. Sequences in pre-S2 appear to encode a viral-cell receptor, but the function of the pre-S1 region, which is variable between the different HBV subtypes, is not yet established.

The product of the C gene is the hepatitis B core antigen (HBcAg). Both the core polypeptide expressed in *E. coli* and the native polypeptide from the virus particle may be converted by proteolytic digestion to *e* antigen. Hepatitis B *e* antigen may exist as two or three antigenically distinct polypeptides of slightly different size and the precise relationship of these to one another and to HBcAg remains to be determined. The protein kinase activity detected in the hepatitis B virion resides in the core antigen which appears to be self-phosphorylating.

The largest open reading frame overlaps the other three, and codes for the polymerase responsible for the replication of the viral genome. Viral DNA replication is believed to proceed via an RNA intermediate; domains within the putative translation product of this gene share amino acid homology with the reverse transcriptase of retroviruses and with the polymerases of caulimonviruses, plant DNA viruses which also replicate via an RNA intermediate.

The predicted gene product of the X gene, is a small polypeptide of approximately 150 amino acids. Although evidence has recently been obtained that this gene is expressed during infection resulting in antibody response, the function of the protein appears to be transactivation.

Hepatocellular carcinoma

Although primary liver cancer is rare in Europe and North America, it is very common in many areas of the world including tropical Africa and

South-East Asia and it is therefore among the 10 most common human cancers. Review of many studies shows a highly significant excess of markers of hepatitis B infection in patients with hepatocellular carcinoma. Hepatitis B is ubiquitous in areas of the world where macronodular cirrhosis and primary liver cancer are common and where the development of the carrier state occurs most frequently. It has been suggested that an important factor in the aetiological association between hepatitis B infection and liver cancer may well be an early age of infection. Indeed, in geographical regions where the prevalence of macronodular cirrhosis and primary liver cancer is high, infection with hepatitis B virus and the carrier state occur most frequently in early life, before the defence immune mechanisms have fully developed, and as many as 20% or more of the apparently healthy population may be carriers. It seems likely, therefore, that persistent hepatitis B infection occurs before the onset of chronic liver damage. Another possibility is that persistent infection with hepatitis B virus leads to cirrhosis and that carcinoma then arises from regenerative nodules by mechanism in which the virus itself is not involved. However, this sequence does not explain liver cancer associated with persistent hepatitis B infection is about 20–30% of patients in the absence of cirrhosis. More recent laboratory studies have demonstrated integration of hepatitis B viral DNA into the host chromosomal DNA molecules. In addition, several cell lines which produce hepatitis B antigen in culture have been derived from primary liver cell tumours and at least one cell line is heterotransplantable with the production of tumours, which are histologically similar to liver cancer and which produce HBsAg. There are several animal viruses which are phylogenetically related to human hepatitis B (the hepadnaviruses). At least two of these viruses, the woodchuck hepatitis B virus and the duck hepatitis B virus cause primary liver cancer in their respective hosts and there are reports of hepatocellular carcinoma in infected ground squirrels. In man it is possible that liver cancer is the cumulative result of several cofactors including genetic and hormonal factors, mycotoxins, chemical carcinogens and other environmental factors, and that hepatitis B virus acts either as a carcinogen or a cocarcinogen in persistently infected hepatocytes.

Screening of blood donors for serological markers of hepatitis B virus infection and history of hepatitis

The discovery of the hepatitis B surface antigen (HBsAg) and its specificity for the hepatitis B virus (HBV) has made possible the serological diagnosis of hepatitis B. It has also permitted identification of almost all donors whose blood is capable of transmitting hepatitis B to susceptible (seronegative) recipients via transfusion. The detection of individuals whose blood contains HBV is possible since the non-infectious HBsAg particles are produced in large quantity and released in excess of HBV into the serum by infected hepatocytes during acute and chronic hepatitis B; in the former for a limited period, and in the latter for a prolonged period. HBV coexists with HBsAg in varying ratios in different individuals. Strongly HBsAg positive serum can contain as many as 10^{12}–10^{14} particles/ml. The HBV/HBsAg ratio may be as high as $1:200$. Current sensitive methods for HBsAg can detect concentrations as low as 10^8 particles/ml. Other serological markers have been associated with high or low HBV/HBsAg ratios but the detection of HBsAg, regardless of the acute or chronic nature of the infection, is strong evidence that viable HBV is present unless inactivating procedures or materials have been applied. A number of prospective studies of transfused patients have documented a significant decrease of up to 85–90% in the incidence of hepatitis B following the transfusion of blood, all of which was negative for HBsAg using sensitive serological tests such as radioimmunoassay and enzyme immunoassay. A progressive decrease in cases of post-transfusion hepatitis (PTH) has been observed paralleling the use of tests with increasing sensitivity to detect HBsAg. Despite the use of the most sensitive tests to detect HBsAg positive blood, some cases of hepatitis B continue to occur (approximately 10% of the PTH in the USA remains hepatitis B despite the elimination of all blood positive for HBsAg by RIA). These cases of hepatitis B PTH represent either failure of sensitive tests for HBsAg to detect blood containing hepatitis B during hospitalization by means other than the transfusion of blood.

HBsAg testing has resulted in the identification of groups of prospective blood donors with high prevalences of HBsAg ('high-risk donors'). (The term 'paid' donor has been applied to groups who often donate blood in return for the direct payment of money.) In practice, 'high-risk' donors are those whose socio-economic status, place of employment or life-style greatly increase the likelihood of their transmitting hepatitis B to recipients of their blood. Hepatitis B as well as hepatitis C transmitted by 'high risk' donors remain significant problems. 'High-risk' donors should be identified and, where possible, prevented from donating blood. Steps to identify such donors and to prevent the transfusion of their blood may provide the most effective means, other than specific serological testing, to reduce further the risk of PTH due to HBV. That there is an increased prevalence of 'subdetectable' HBV positive donors among 'high-risk' groups has been supported by the increased prevalence of HBeAg (a marker of increased infectivity) among such groups at all levels of detectable HBsAg when compared to controls (Table 15.1).

The risk of hepatitis B PTH increases when there is:

1 Inadequate testing for HBsAg
2 Failure to identify and exclude blood from 'high-risk' donors
3 Large numbers of units of blood transfused into a single patient

4 Transfusion of blood products or plasma derivatives produced from large pools of plasma.

Specific serological tests for HBsAg can only be expected to prevent hepatitis B transmission, and not hepatitis either from sources other than the tested blood or due to other viruses.

Antibody to HBsAg (anti-HBs) Actively acquired antibody to HBsAg (anti-HBs) appears during convalescence in the sera of individuals recovering from or recovered from hepatitis B. Only a small percentage of persons fail to make anti-HBs, during convalescence (5–15%). Tests for anti-HBs can be positive, however, often at low levels, in the sera of some chronically infected individuals. When examined for specificity, anti-HBs in this latter group is most often heterotypic (directed to HBsAg determinants other than those present on the HBsAg circulating in the same individual).

Despite the possibility of HBV coexisting in sera positive for anti-HBs, complexed with excess anti-HBs, especially during early convalescence from hepatitis B, the transfusion of blood containing anti-HBs does not carry an increased risk of hepatitis B to the recipient.

Table 15.1 Transfusion-transmitted viruses study (1974–1979, USA)

	%	Hepatitis B	Non-A, non-B hepatitis
1 Recipients	429	1 (0.2%)	34 (7.9%)
Control	414	0	9 (2.2%)
2 Recipients	506	2 (0.4%)	22 (4.3%)
Control	522	1 (0.2%)	12 (2.3%)
3 Recipients	392	8 (2.1%)	68 (17.4%)
Control	370	0	17 (4.6%)
4 Recipients	206	4 (1.9%)	32 (15.5%)
Control	282	0	8 (2.8%)
Total			
Recipients	1533	15 (1.0%)	156 (10.2%)
Control	1588	1 (0.06%)	46 (2.9%)

Notes

1 The risk of non-A, non-B hepatitis in hospital patients was 2–6 times greater for transfused patients
2 72% (range 47–82%) of the risk of hepatitis could be attributed to blood transfusion
3 The lowest attack rate was with volunteer blood obtained primarily from middle-class Caucasian donors. Most of the blood used in hospitals with the highest attack rates was obtained from low socio-economic groups, including family and friends of patients, and until 1976 from paid blood donors
4 It is emphasized that in virtually every study in the USA where volunteer and commercial blood were compared directly in the same population of recipients, the risk of hepatitis in recipients of paid donors was 2.5 times higher. For example, among 2,079 patients in five studies in the USA (1970–1978), the risk of hepatitis in those receiving only volunteer blood was 6.9% compared to 27.5% risk in those receiving paid donor blood

Screening of blood products and blood components for markers of hepatitis B virus infection

All individual units of blood prior to utilization of its components and all individual units of plasma prior to pooling for the purpose of either manufacturing into plasma derivatives or quality control laboratory reagents should be negative for HBsAg by the most sensitive and practical test available. Similarly, individual sera used to produce quality control laboratory reagents should be negative for HBsAg. Testing intermediate samples from plasma pools for the presence of HBsAg should be done to identify inadvertent HBV contamination due to inadequate HBsAg testing of individual plasma units since dilution alone often will not result in a negative HBsAg test on pools contaminated with HBS/HBsAg even if some units contain anti-HBs. If possible, 'high-risk' donors should be identified and interdicted from donating blood or plasma. Blood components, derived from the blood of 'low-risk' individuals and properly tested for HBsAg pose the same small risk of hepatitis B as the units of blood from which they were prepared. Plasma derivatives themselves can be classified as 'low risk' or 'high risk' depending upon their method of manufacture, the size of the plasma pool and the population from which the plasma was obtained. Testing of the final products for HBsAg does not provide meaningful information. Negative tests for HBsAg on 'high risk' final products do not ensure that they are free of infectious HBV. Similarly, positive tests for HBsAg on 'low risk' (pasteurized) products do not indicate the presence of infectious HBV. This is accounted for by the differential distribution of HBV and HBsAg during the manufacture of plasma derivative and the ability or inability of a particular derivative to withstand procedures which can inactivate HBV.

Human normal immunoglobulin, when prepared by cold-ethanol fractionation (Cohn-Oncley process) from plasma negative for HBsAg by a sensitive method, appears not to transmit hepatitis B. Human normal immunoglobulin, however, contains detectable HBsAg and transmits hepatitis B when it is either made, from plasma pools contaminated with HBsAg or when it is manufactured by a method other than the Cohn-Oncley process, e.g. ammonium sulphate precipitation.

Products such as Factor VIII(AHF) and Factor IX clotting factors (II, VIII, IX, X) may transmit hepatitis B to susceptible recipients, despite HBsAg testing of plasma, presumably because it is prepared from plasma pools consisting of a thousand or more individual plasma donations. Therefore, such materials should be administered only to those congenitally deficient in the respective factors after the application of approved inactivation procedures and to recipients who had been immunized against hepatitis B.

Passive immunization

Hepatitis B immunoglobulin is prepared from pooled plasma with high titre of hepatitis B surface antibody and it may confer temporary passive immunity under certain defined conditions. The major indication for the administration of hepatitis B immunoglobulin is a single acute exposure to hepatitis B virus, such as occurs when blood containing surface antigen is inoculated, ingested or splashed onto mucous membranes and the conjunctiva. The optimal dose has not been established but doses in the range of 250–500 i.u. have been used effectively. It should be administered as early as possible after exposure and preferably within 48 hours, usually 3 ml (containing 200 i.u. of anti-HBs per ml) in adults. It should not be administered seven days following exposure. It is generally recommended that two doses of hepatitis B immunoglobulin should be given 30 days apart.

Results with the use of hepatitis B immunoglobulin for prophylaxis in babies at risk of infection with hepatitis B virus are encouraging if the immunoglobulin is given as soon as possible after birth or within 12 hours of birth, and the chance of the baby developing the persistent carrier state is reduced by about 70%. More recent studies using combined passive and active immunization indicate an efficacy approaching 90%. The dose of hepatitis B immunoglobulin recommended in the newborn is 1–2 ml (200 i.u. of anti-HBs per ml).

Active immunization

Immunization against hepatitis B is required for groups which are at an increased risk of acquiring this infection. These groups include infants born to carrier mothers, individuals requiring repeated transfusions of blood or blood products, prolonged in-patient treatment, patients who require frequent tissue penetration or need repeated access to the circulation, patients with natural or acquired immune deficiency and patients with malignant diseases. Viral hepatitis is an occupational hazard among health care personnel and the staff of institutions for the mentally-retarded and in some semi-closed institutions. High rates of infection with hepatitis B occur in narcotic and other drug abusers, homosexuals and prostitutes. Individuals working in high endemic areas are also at an increased risk of infection. Women in areas of the world where the carrier state in that group is high are another segment of the population requiring immunization in view of the increased risk of transmission of the infection to their offspring. Infants born to carrier mothers, young infants, children and susceptible persons living in certain tropical and sub-tropical areas where present socio-economic conditions are poor and the prevalence of hepatitis B is high should also be immunized.

Hepatitis B vaccines

The plasma-derived hepatitis B vaccines which meet the WHO requirements have been shown to be safe and effective and free of the risk of transmission of bloodborne viruses.

Polypeptide vaccines

Hepatitis B polypeptide vaccines contain specific hepatitis B antigenic determinants of the major non-glycosylated peptide I of the surface antigen with a molecular weight of 22–24,000 and its glycosylated form. The individual polypeptides of the surface antigen are immunogenic, and the purified 25,000 and 30,000 molecular weight polypeptides are effective antigens. Clinical trials of the polypeptide micelle vaccine are in progress.

Production of hepatitis B vaccines by r-DNA techniques

Recombinant DNA techniques have been used for expressing hepatitis B surface antigen and core antigen in prokaryotic cells (*Escherichia coli*) and in eukaryotic cells, such as mutant

mouse LM cells, HeLa cells, COS cells, CHO cells and yeast cells (*Saccharomyces cerevisiae*).

Recombinant yeast hepatitis B vaccines have undergone extensive evaluation by clinical trials. The results indicate that this vaccine is safe, antigenic and free from side-effects (apart from minor local reactions in a proportion of recipients). The immunogenicity is similar to that of the plasma-derived vaccine. Recombinant yeast hepatitis B vaccines have now been licensed for use in all countries.

Hybrid virus vaccines

Potential live vaccines using recombinant vaccinia virus have been constructed for hepatitis B and other viruses. Foreign viral DNA is introduced into the vaccinia DNA by construction of chimaeric genes. This is accomplished by homologous recombination in cells since the large size of the genome of vaccinia virus (185,000 base pairs) precludes *in vitro* gene insertion. A chimaeric gene consisting of vaccinia virus promoter sequences ligated to the coding sequence for the desired foreign protein is flanked by vaccinia virus DNA in a plasmid vector.

The recloned vaccinia virus containing HBsAg sequences has been used successfully for 'priming' experimental animals. At present, however, there is no accepted laboratory marker of attenuation or of virulence of vaccinia virus for man, either in the host directly inoculated with the virus or after several passages in the same species. Alterations in the genome of vaccinia virus which are concomitant with the selection of recombinants may alter the virulence of the virus. Changes in host range or tissue tropism of vaccinia viruses may also occur.

The advantages of vaccinia virus recombinant as a vaccine include low cost, ease of administration by multiple pressure or by the scratch technique, vaccine stability, long shelf-life, and the possible use of polyvalent antigens. The adverse reactions with vaccinia virus are well documented and their incidence and severity must be carefully weighed. There are also reports of spread of current strains of vaccinia virus to contacts and this may present difficulties. Other recombinant viruses as vectors are being explored, and in particular the oral adenovirus vaccine strains which have been in use for some 20 years.

Novel hepatitis B vaccines using hybrid particles

More recent developments include the use of hepatitis B surface antigen in a particulate form by expressing the proteins in mammalian cells. In-phase insertions of variable length and sequence of another virus (poliomyelitis virus type I) were made in different regions of the S gene of hepatitis B virus. The envelope proteins carrying the surface antigen and the insert is assembled with cellular lipids in the cultured mammalian cells after transfection. The inserted polio neutralization peptide was found to be exposed on the surface of the hybrid envelope particles and induced neutralizing antibodies against poliovirus in mice immunized experimentally. The expression and secretion of hybrid envelope particles by the established cell lines may thus provide an efficient system for the production of potential new vaccines.

Another potentially excellent carrier vehicle for human and veterinary vaccines in addition to hepatitis B, is the use of the core particles of HBV. The advantage of the core structure as a particle includes its ability to induce antibody with approximately 100-fold greater efficiency than the surface antigen particle, and an ability to augment T-helper cell function. The feasibility of this approach was recently demonstrated with synthetic and biosynthetic peptides of foot and mouth disease virus (FMDV) after fusion to hepatitis B core.

Chemically synthesized hepatitis B vaccines

The development of chemically synthesized polypeptide vaccines offers the advantage of producing chemically uniform, safe and cheap viral immunogens to replace many current vaccines which often contain large quantities of irrelevant microbial antigenic determinants, proteins and other material additional to the essential immunogen required for the induction of a protective antibody. The preparation of antibodies against viral proteins using fragments of chemically synthesized peptides mimicking viral amino acid sequence is now a possible and attractive alternative approach in immunoprophylaxis.

Successful mimicking of determinants of HBsAg using chemically synthesized peptides in linear and cyclical forms has been reported by several groups of investigators. Peptides have been synthesized which retain biological function and appropriate secondary structure, even though they have a limited sequence homology with the natural peptide or are much smaller.

Various other studies also confirm that selected overlapping peptides corresponding to relevant epitopes of hepatitis B surface antigen may be useful as synthetic vaccines when combined with adjuvants.

Hepatitis D virus (the delta agent)

Delta virus is a defective, transmissible virus which requires multiplication of hepatitis B virus for its own replication. The agent is unique among human viruses and consists of spherical particles measuring 35–37 nm in diameter, with the internal component containing the delta antigen surrounded by an outer protein coat of hepatitis B surface antigen. The genome of this virus is very small, consisting of a single stranded circular RNA with a molecular weight of 500,000.

Serological studies indicate a world-wide distribution of hepatitis D in association with hepatitis B virus. The infection is epidemiologically important in Italy, the Middle East (the Gulf States and Saudi Arabia), eastern Europe, parts of Africa and particularly in a number of regions of South America. Epidemics with high mortality have been described in South America in association with hepatitis B. Delta infection is associated with acute and chronic hepatitis, always in the presence of hepatitis B, and superinfection in a carrier of hepatitis B virus often leads to exacerbation of severe hepatitis.

The mode of transmission of hepatitis D is similar to the parenteral spread of hepatitis B, so that serological evidence of infection is found most frequently in Western Europe and North America in multi-transfused individuals such as patients with haemophilia and in drug addicts. Non-percutaneous spread probably also occurs. Immunization against hepatitis B will also protect against infection with the delta agent.

Parenteral non-A, non-B hepatitis

Non-A, non-B hepatitis is clearly unrelated to any recognized viruses. The infection has been transmitted experimentally to chimpanzees. Although specific laboratory tests for identifying this new type of hepatitis are not yet available and the diagnosis can only be made by exclusion, there is considerable information on the epidemiology and some of the clinical features of this infection.

Non-A, non-B hepatitis has been found in every country in which it has been sought and it shares a number of epidemiological and clinical features with hepatitis B. This form of hepatitis has been most commonly recognized as a complication of blood transfusion, and in countries where all blood donations are screened for hepatitis B surface antigen by very sensitive techniques non-A, non-B hepatitis may account for as many as 90% of all cases of post-transfusion hepatitis (Table 15.2). Outbreaks of non-A, non-B hepatitis have also been reported after the administration of blood-clotting factors VIII and IX. Non-A, non-B hepatitis has occurred in haemodialysis and other specialized units, among drug addicts and after accidental inoculation with contaminated needles and other sharp objects. In several countries a significant number of cases are not associated with transfusion and such sporadic cases of non-A, non-B hepatitis account for 10–25% of all adult patients with recognized viral hepatitis. The route of infection or the source of infection cannot be identified in many of these patients.

Table 15.2 Transfusion-transmitted viruses study (USA)

Attack rate of non-A, non-B hepatitis and volume of blood transfused

1 unit	6.9%
2–3 units	10.5%
4–5 units	11.0%
6–15 units	12.0%

Notes

1 The lack of linear relationship between volume of transfusion and risk of hepatitis, observed previously in other studies, is believed to be due in part to secondary neutralization of the virus by specific antibodies present in some of the units

2 Adjustment of the effect of alanine aminotransferase (ALT) level in the donor in this study showed that the highest attack rates of 37–42% were in recipients of at least 1 unit of blood with ALT > 45 iu/litre attack rates of 5–8% with ALT < 45 iu/l

Thus the effect of the volume of transfusion is associated only indirectly with the development of post-transfusion hepatitis

Three prospective studies in the USA and one in Japan (1975–1979), using volunteer blood screened for hepatitis B surface antigen, revealed an incidence of hepatitis ranging from 7–12%. In another prospective study in the US Army the incidence of post-transfusion hepatitis was 17%. In each of these studies, over 90% of cases of hepatitis were attributed to non-A, non-B hepatitis. Prospective studies of post-transfusion hepatitis since 1980, conducted primarily in patients undergoing open-heart surgery in The Netherlands, Sweden, Australia, Spain and Italy, showed an incidence ranging from 3% in Australia to 55% in Japan. The proportion of cases attributed to non-A, non-B hepatitis ranged from 78–100%.

Clinical, epidemiological and experimental studies in several laboratories indicate that non-A, non-B hepatitis may be caused by two and possibly more than two infectious agents. Clinical evidence is based on the observation of multiple attacks of hepatitis in individual patients. Epidemiologically, short-incubation and long-incubation forms of non-A, non-B hepatitis have been described. The incubation period, however, does not appear to be a reliable index for differentiating between the two non-A, non-B types of hepatitis, and it is likely that differences in the incubation period represent differences in the infective dose. Experimental evidence for the existence of at least two distinct non-A, non-B hepatitis viruses has been obtained from cross-challenging experimental transmission studies in chimpanzees, but final confirmation must await the development of specific laboratory tests and the identification and characterization of the virus(es).

A report has been published on the finding of reverse transcriptase in association with the parenterally-transmitted forms of non-A, non-B hepatitis. Peak reverse transcriptase activity was found at the 1.14 g/ml fraction in a sucrose gradient and inoculation of this fraction into susceptible chimpanzees induced infection. The enzyme is distinguished from cellular DNA polymerases and it is not inhibited by actinomycin D (which inhibits DNA-dependent DNA synthesis). The enzyme is sensitive to RNAse with endogenous template primer. These results suggest that these viruses bear similarities to retroviruses, but independent confirmation of these findings is not yet available. The description of a membrane-coated virus replicating in chimpanzee liver cell cultures after inoculation with an infectious non-A, non-B hepatitis serum is now known to be due to an indigenous contaminant chimpanzee virus.

Although in general the illness is mild and often subclinical or anicteric, severe hepatitis with jaundice does occur and the infection is a significant cause of fulminant hepatitis. There is considerable evidence that the infection may be followed in many patients, by prolonged viraemia and the development of a persistent carrier state. Studies of the histopathological sequelae of acute non-A, non-B hepatitis infection revealed that chronic liver damage, which may be severe, may occur in as many as 40–50% of the patients.

Hepatitis C and other hepatitis viruses

Whereas hepatitis A and hepatitis B have been known for centuries, hepatitis C, a form of non-A, non-B hepatitis, has recently been identified and cloned. Delta hepatitis is now well established and the identification of hepatitis F and non-B non-C hepatitis is close.

Non-A, non-B hepatitis (NANBH) Apart from non-viral causes, the viral aetiology of NANBH includes the parenterally borne, blood borne infection which has now been identified as hepatitis C virus (HCV). There is evidence of unknown or as yet unidentified NANBH viruses and of the recently cloned enteric water-borne NANBH, now called hepatitis E virus (HEV).

The importance of NANBH is evident. It is spread in the same way as HBV: by blood products, from mother to infant, and by percutaneous spread, including sexual contact. The incubation period ranges from 2–26 weeks. In general, NANBH and HCV are mild infections; most are anicteric and therefore not recognized, but individual cases may be severe. Doctors and microbiologists should not be misled by the mild clinical features of NANBH because 50% of cases associated with blood transfusion progress to chronic liver disease, including chronic active hepatitis cirrhosis. There is evidence that in some regions, NANBH is associated with primary hepatocellular carcinoma.

Sporadic hepatitis presents a different feature. In a survey of about 750,000 people in West London during the 1970s, of the patients who had been tested comprehensively serologically, 58% suffered from HAV, 27% from HBV and, by exclusion, 13% were diagnosed as having NANBH. Follow-up of these cases of sporadic NANBH indicated that most recovered completely – only 10% progressed to chronic liver disease.

HCV cloning

An exciting recent advance has been the cloning of HCV – a single stranded RNA virus related to both the flaviviruses and the pestiviruses and intermediate between them. The first strain to be cloned in the United States is now referred to as HCV-1, but since then there have been at least five other isolates.

The antibody response to these different antigens of HCV is important. Antibody is not detected until late in convalescence and depends greatly on which antigen is used. For instance, with C100 antigen, antibody is not usually detected until 12 weeks into convalescence. With other antigens, such as C33 or C22, the gap between clinical symptoms and convalescence begins to close, whereas with 5.1.1 it is rather late. This does not solve the problem of how to diagnose an acute or recent HCV infection, as the response to these antigens differs from patient to patient.

Tests for HCV antibody

There are several licensed tests for antibody to HCV: the problem is that as they identify two different blood donor populations, there is considerable overlap. Samples identifiable by both tests initially represented only 30–50% of what we believe are true positives. We therefore do not have a confirmatory test (the only way to decipher this complex situation), only supplementary tests. At present, we rely on repeated positive samples. However, the positive group can be divided into two main categories. In the high risk group, ELISA positives are much more likely to be positive, and although there are two supplementary (not confirmatory) tests, the ELISA tends to be reasonably specific.

In the low risk group, such as healthy blood donors, the specificity of these licensed tests is not good; some confirmation with supplementary tests is needed. Supplementary testing is becoming extremely important.

The recombinant immunoblot assay (RIBA) is expensive but elegant. There are two versions. RIBA I contained only two of the several antigens – $C100_3$ (expressed in yeast) and 5.1.1 (expressed in *E. coli*). These are not entirely satisfactory but are a step in the right direction. RIBA II, introduced later, is more satisfactory and includes four antigens, so that it is much more likely to pick up antibodies. RIBA III has just been introduced and RIBAs will certainly be important supplementary tests.

Looking at HCV and blood, and transfusion-associated infection in the context of tests which have been rapidly introduced into clinical practice, we see that they do not solve the problem. Seventy-five per cent of patients with transfusion associated hepatitis have received blood which contains anti-HCV antibody and are RIBA positive, but 25% of HCV infection was transmitted by anti-HCV negative carriers. At the same time, 80% of RIBA positive donors (i.e. based on a very sensitive test) did transmit the infection. Of the 20% who did not transmit, there are two possibilities – either the donor was not infectious or the recipients were immune to the infection. We have no way of assessing immunity to HCV. Furthermore, it is becoming evident that RIBA negative donors seldom transmit the infection, so this appears to be a very good test.

However, persistence of antibody to HCV generally indicates viraemia: it is not a protective antibody but an indicator of infection as assessed by the polymerous chain reaction by detection of RNA. For the time being at least, it has to be accepted that anti-HCV antibody donor or an anti-HCV antibody patient is infectious. Antibody does not indicate lack of infectivity.

Another important and surprising feature is that in the United States, 20–40% of acute viral hepatitis is now caused by NANBH. However, blood transfusion contributes to only 5% of these cases. Drug abuse is responsible for 35% of HCV cases. It is of great concern to microbiologists and the professions that medical and dental work is responsible for 2% of NANBH in the United States. Heterosexual exposure and multiple partners are responsible for 7%. However, most cases are of unknown source, so that

much work still needs to be done; screening blood donors does not solve the problem of HCV.

Regarding the seroprevalence of HCV among blood donors, a highly selected healthy population, the prevalence in urban communities is greater than in rural, as would also be expected with HBV. In general, however, if this is based on the first generation anti-HCV tests, that is a common carrier state among blood donors. If these samples are examined by a supplementary test, the false positive rate is 50% or more. This is confirmed in various countries.

A remarkable feature of HCV is the chronic liver state associated with it. A proportion of well-selected patients respond to treatment with α-interferon.

Another recent and important observation concerns the presence of infectivity, which at present is assessed only by measuring RNA in serum. Surprisingly, of those who have antibody to HCV, up to 45% have RNA in the serum, and the proportion rises to 60–70% if looking only at those positive by RIBA. The intermediate RIBA readings are problematic but HCV RNA is found in up to 47% of individuals in whom antibody to HCV is not detected. The state of play with these tests is hardly satisfactory.

Complicating the issue further, apart from the variance of HCV in different strains, there are probably other NANBH viruses awaiting identification. Experimental, sequential and cross-challenge studies indicate that there are at least two different viruses. There is also evidence that autologous challenge is ineffective. We are clearly dealing with more than one NANBH parenterally transmitted infection.

Hepatitis E virus (HEV) was only recently cloned. This is an extremely important infection, initially referred to as epidemic non-A hepatitis and described in Asia, the Middle East, North Africa, Mexico and found in many travellers returning to Britain. As with HAV, the infection is transmitted by contaminated water, contaminated shellfish and the like. Its importance is that although it is generally an acute, self-limiting infection, and usually cholestatic in form, it is very severe in pregnancy, with mortality of 17–35%. Although at first sight under the electron microscope it resembles HAV, it is in fact totally different from it. The high mortality it causes in pregnancy makes it a most important infection.

Routing diagnostic tests for HEV are urgently required. A prevention strategy needs to be developed, and a vaccine is needed.

Hepatitis B provides much new, and disconcerting, information concerning the identification and emergence of HBV variants and mutants. A survey carried out in Italy since 1982, of children and adults successfully immunized against HBV who have developed high titres of protective antibody, astonishingly showed that 2.8% of 1,590 vaccinated contacts, either born to carrier mothers or contacts of carriers and who had high titres of HBV surface antibody, developed HBV infection. This finding, between 1982–87, was so difficult to believe that it was not published until 1990.

Why did this infection occur? It is now recognized that there are at least 10 strains of HBV. They have one common determinant, known as *a*; an antibody to *a* is the protective, neutralizing antibody.

How to explain infection in fully immunized subjects? The only way is to assume that something has gone wrong with the *a* determinant. Polyclonal assays indicated that the *a* determinant did not exist in these subjects; the panel of the Royal Free Hospital School of Medicine's monoclonal antibodies showed that only part of the *a* determinant was lost or that it was sequestered. Subsequently, when the virus strains were sequenced, a single stable mutation was found in position 587 of the nucleotide sequence of the surface antigen which resulted in an amino acid substitution from glycine to arginine in position 145.

As a result, the virus was able to replicate in immunized subjects. We now have evidence that this escape mutant is present in Singapore, Japan, Brunei, Germany, the USA and the UK. This is a potentially major development of escape HBV mutants infecting immunized subjects.

Thus, although HBV is far from new, it presents new challenges.

HBV vaccines

The duration of immunity given by vaccination is now known. If it is based on the rate of decline of antibody to the *a* determinant, it depends on the level of titre of antibody response induced.

With a high titre antibody response, the antibody can be expected to decline over a period of 24–36 months and will probably persist for up to five years. In low responders, with antibody titres of 100–200 milli-international units, antibody usually declines after 1–2 years. This does not necessarily mean that these individuals are susceptible to HBV, because cell-mediated immunity may be important.

There is not yet any uniform policy on booster immunization against HBV but my personal recommendation is that it should be repeated, particularly in those at high risk, every 3–5 years. For many years, the level of antibody titre to HBV accepted as protective was 10 milli-international units. That figure is now regarded as insufficient. The minimum acceptable level is at least 50; 80–100 is desirable.

There are no side-effects or any risk of acquiring infection with currently or previously licensed HBV vaccines which meet WHO requirements.

With those who have not responded after three inoculations, there is still good reason to give a fourth injection, provided the first three were given in a correct site, the deltoid or the anterolateral aspect of the thigh. If the patient was inoculated in the buttocks, the whole course of immunization must be repeated. If there is no response after the fourth dose, the matter should be left. It is hoped that the new generation of HBV vaccines will overcome the problem of non-responsiveness, present in 5–15% of healthy individuals. Non-responsiveness is an enormous problem and better vaccines against HBV are needed.

In light of the fact that travellers are returning to Britain with HEV, pooled human immunoglobulin prepared, for example, in places outside endemic areas may be protective; batches in the UK, for example, do not contain antibody to HEV. The antibody content of immunoglobulin prepared in endemic areas is being investigated and is expected to offer passive protection provided there is enough antibody.

The Acquired Immunodeficiency Syndrome

Since the recognition of the acquired immunodeficiency syndrome (AIDS) in 1981, infection with the human immunodeficiency viruses

(HIV) has become a major public health problem with estimates by the World Health Organization of infection of up to 10,000,000 people world-wide in 1988. The clear differences between the patient groups in industrialized countries in North America, Europe and Australia and the developing countries in Africa include the high proportion of homosexual males, intravenous drug abusers and recipients of blood clotting fractions (haemophiliacs) before the introduction of screening of blood in 1985, and heterosexual and perinatal infections in tropical Africa.

The human immunodeficiency virus has been detected in blood, semen and saliva. Modes of transmission include sexual contact, parenteral exposure to blood and blood products, and directly from an infected mother to child during the perinatal period. In the industrialized countries intravenous drug abuse, and its accompanying problems associated with the sharing of contaminated syringes and needles, represent a major mode of transmission of the virus. In the developing world, however, this represents a minor risk factor. On the other hand, the use of unsterilized syringes and needles outside the health programme and the use of unsterilized instruments for tattooing and for scarification poses a risk of trans-

mission. There is no evidence that the virus is spread through social contact with an infected individual, including contacts in a family setting, schools or other groups living or working together. Large prospective studies on health care workers in contact with the blood of infected patients through penetrating needle injuries or mucosal exposure have documented only a few cases of infection. There is no evidence of transmission by blood-sucking insects. The virus is not transmitted by food or water, swimming pools or toilet seats, coughing or sneezing or casual contact.

Studies of recipients of blood transfusions who developed AIDS show a long interval between exposure to the infection and onset of the disease. Mean intervals of 12 months in children and 29 months in adults have been noted. Estimates based on mathematical models suggest even longer incubation periods. The clinical outcome of known infection with HIV within a period of 2–5 years of observation is that approximately two-thirds will have no evidence of ill health; the remaining one-third will develop illness varying in severity from mild to very serious.

The human immunodeficiency virus

Retroviruses are RNA viruses which encode an RNA-directed DNA polymerase (reverse transcriptase), which synthesizes a double-stranded DNA intermediate (the provirus) from a single-stranded virion RNA. The provirus subsequently becomes integrated into the chromosomal DNA of the host cell and serves as a template for viral genomic and mRNA transcription by the RNA of the cell.

Retroviruses are divided taxonomically into three groups: the oncoviruses, the lentiviruses (the slow viruses, the prototype of which is visna virus of sheep) and the spumaviruses (the foamy viruses), which are not pathogenic. Four major classes of human retroviruses are recognized:

1 T-cell lymphotropic C type oncoviruses associated with leukaemia and lymphoma
2 T-cell lymphotropic lentivirus which causes AIDS, now named the human immunodeficiency virus types 1 and 2. The morphology of the virus is shown in Figure 15.3
3 Foamy viruses, which are apparently non-pathogenic

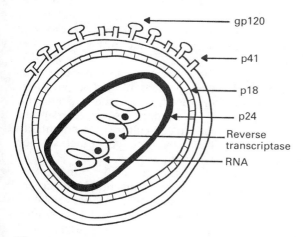

Figure 15.3. The anatomy of HIV (after Dr H. Gelderblom). The virus particle consists of a lipid bilayer in which the envelope protein is incorporated with the transmembrane pedicle (gp 31) and the protruding knob-like structures (gp 120). The core which contains the RNA genome and reverse transcriptase is surrounded by two membranes, an outer layer (p 18) and an inner membrane (p 24)

4 Endogenous genetic elements related to C-type oncoviruses and expressed as non-infectious C type particles.

Note that simian lentiviruses (SIV), which are related to HIV, have been identified in old world monkeys which are non-pathogenic in African vervets and mangabeys but which cause immune deficiency (SAIDS) in rhesus macaques. HIV-2 is more closely related structurally and antigenically to SIV and HIV-2 causes AIDS and AIDS-related disease in man.

CD4 protein – the receptor of HIV

The CD4 molecule is the receptor for HIV. Thus cells which can be identified by HIV are identified by immunofluorescence for CD4 with anti-CD4 monoclonal antibodies or have detectable mRNA for CD4.

HIV can infect any cell expressing CD4 on the cell surface including T-lymphocytes, 10–20% of circulating monocytes, 5–10% of circulating B-cells and a variable proportion of fixed tissue macrophages. However, some cells which do not express CD4 as assessed by surface fluorescence are permissive for HIV and these include glial cells in the central nervous system. Glial cells and some cells in the gut have detectable CD4 mRNA and can be infected in culture. However, infection of the brain *in vivo* involves principally the non-glial, non-neuronal macrophages and microglial cells, and the precise mechanisms involved in HIV lesions in the CNS require elucidation.

Provision of safe blood and blood products

The initial measures which were recommended in 1983 for increasing the safety of blood and blood products included education of the public and blood donors about AIDS, self-exclusion of donors 'at risk' of AIDS, exclusion of donors who belong to high-risk groups and the avoidance of non-essential use of blood and blood products. Screening of blood donors and individual units of blood for IgG antibody to HIV were introduced in 1985 and antibody-positive units of blood were not used. Donor education and exclusion of high-risk groups

continue at the same time. The introduction of appropriate heat treatment in the production of blood factors VIII and IX has apparently eliminated the risk of transmission of HIV by these products.

Current serological screening tests for HIV are based on evidence of IgG antibodies to structural viral components and the fact that such persons are persistently infected with the virus and are infective. However, negative antibody screening results in infected persons may occur because of the 'window phase' (during the early phase of infection) of 2–12 weeks or longer when virus is present before antibodies develop; antibody may decline in titre late during the clinical illness, and more important in practice antibody may not be detectable in 2–5% of infected persons although virus may be isolated from these individuals.

In order to circumvent these difficulties, the development of other screening test procedures has been undertaken and the detection of virus and viral antigens may become more important. Although, except under the circumstances outlined above carriers of HIV have antibodies, often to high titre, to the main core protein (p24) and the main cleaved product of the envelope protein (p41), the earliest antibody response is of the IgM class. IgM antibodies to HIV are found alone transiently during the fourth and fifth weeks after infection. This antibody is preceded by viraemia and by the presence of the core antigen. Core antigen is usually found in the circulation for up to four weeks after exposure (and often during the development of clinical symptoms of AIDS). Assays for these markers as screening procedures have at present limited application. Virus isolation procedures are cumbersome and although enzyme immunoassay virus capture assay techniques in cell cultures are potentially attractive, these are not yet practical nor suitable for screening.

Similarly, specific reverse transcriptase assays are expensive and unsuitable as screening procedures. Several DNA probes are being evaluated for their ability to detect integrated viral sequences in cells, but this approach must circumvent low signal-to-noise ratios since in most cases only very few cells are infected with HIV. Methods to amplify significantly the viral signal must therefore be developed before rapid screening of blood donors can be established in practice.

Antiviral drugs

Considerable knowledge of the mode of replication of HIV presents opportunities for the development of drugs which will act on selective and specific targets, for example on reverse transcriptase. Azidothymidine (AZT) is used now clinically, and 2′, 3′ dideoxycytidine is under trial. Other selective nucleoside analogues are being evaluated.

Glycosidase inhibitors have been identified and naturally occurring glucosidase inhibitor alkaloids of plant origin which act on the development of the major glycoprotein (gp 120) of HIV are under study. Other approaches are being developed.

Prospects for AIDS vaccines

The development of AIDS vaccines is beset with difficulties because antibodies to the structural components of the virus are present in infected persons often to high titre, the surface envelope of the virus is subject to variation, and because of the lack of suitable animal models.

Inactivated lentivirus vaccines (CAEV and visna virus) resulted in a more severe disease on challenge with live virus. Inactivated HIV vaccines may induce immunosuppression and preparation requires high containment facilities.

Non-pathogenic virus produced by gene deletion may be reverse transcribed into DNA copies and be integrated into the host genome, or the virus may recombine with endogenous retroviral sequences restoring pathogenicity, or recombine with proto *onc* genes generating acute tumour virus or it may activate cellular *onc* genes.

Recombinant vaccines including hybrid vaccinia viruses and vaccines produced to date by rDNA techniques have been disappointing so far. The construction of hybrid particles and the use of novel epitope presentation may result in immunogenic preparations. Chemically synthesized peptides and anti-idiotype antibodies are under development.

Any candidate vaccine must be subjected to meticulous evaluation and premature unsubstantiated claims may have a serious impact on other immunization programmes. Because of the lengthy incubation period of 5–8 years it is unlikely that an HIV vaccine will be generally available for another 5–10 years.

Further reading

Clarke, B.E., Newton, S.E., Carrol, A.R., Francis, M.J., Appleyard, G., Syred, A.D., Highfield, P.E., Rowlands, D.J. and Brown, F. (1987) Improved immunogenicity of a peptide epitope after fusion to hepatitis B core protein. *Nature*, **330**, 381–384

Delpeynoux, F., Chenciner, N., Linn, A., Malpiece, Y., Blondel, B., Crainic, R., Werf, van der S. and Streeck, R.E. (1986) A poliovirus neutralization epitope expressed on hybrid hepatitis B surface particles. *Science*, **233**, 472–475

Greenaway, P.J. and Farrar, G.H. (1987) Prospects for an AIDS vaccine. *Microbiology Digest*, **4**, 26–39

Langley, D. and Spier, R.E. (1988) Is a vaccine against AIDS possible? *Vaccine*, **6**, 3–5

Moss, B., Smith, G.L., Gerin, J.L. and Purcell, R.H. (1984) Live recombinant vaccinia virus protects chimpanzees against hepatitis B. *Nature*, **311**, 67–68

Petricciani, J.C., Cust, I.D., Hoppe, P.A. and Krijnen, H.W. (eds) (1987) *AIDS: the safety of blood and blood products*. John Wiley and Sons, Chichester

World Health Organization (1988) *Viral Hepatitis*. Technical Report Series, Geneva

Zuckerman, A.J. (1987a) Tomorrow's hepatitis B vaccines. *Vaccine*, **5**, 165–167

Zuckerman, A.J. (1987b) The development of novel hepatitis B vaccines. *Bulletin of the World Health Organization*, **63**, 275–275

Zuckerman, A.J. (1988) Viral hepatitis and liver disease. Alan R Liss, Inc., New York

16

Human Immunodeficiency Virus (HIV) and haemophilia

B.T. Colvin

Prevalence of HIV infection in haemophilia

It is known that approximately 1,200 patients with haemophilia in the UK have been infected by HIV, the vast majority being those with haemophilia A (factor VIII deficiency). Most of these infections were due to the transfusion of contaminated large pool factor VIII concentrates between 1980 and 1985 and while commercial material imported from the USA was the major source of infection there is no doubt that NHS-derived concentrates were also implicated (AIDS Group of UK Haemophilia Centre Directors, 1986). Long-term British self-sufficiency in factor IX production has been one reason for the much lower incidence of anti-HIV antibodies in haemophilia B but it also seems that the fractionation methods used in the production of this material are capable of removing the majority of contaminating HIV (Ludlam, et al., 1985). Few patients with von Willebrand's disease have been infected because either blood products were avoided during the critical period (Mannucci, et al., 1977) or cryoprecipitate derived from single NHS donations was given in preference to large pool concentrates (Colvin, Collier and Craske, 1987), until superseded by safe effective concentrates containing adequate amounts of von Willebrand factor (Pasi, et al., 1990; Cumming, et al., 1990). Reports on HIV infection of the sexual partners of HIV positive haemophiliacs have indicated an overall transmission rate of up to 10% (Jones, et al., 1985; Laurian, Peynet

and Verroust, 1989) all the seroconversions in Laurian's study taking place in couples who did not use condoms. By late 1991 notifications of AIDS cases in haemophilia sufferers in the UK had reached 272 of whom 196 had died. Not surprisingly the severely affected patients have borne the brunt of the epidemic but those with mild haemophilia, once infected, have been just as much at risk of illness and death.

Towards the end of 1984 reports of the heat inactivation of HIV in factor VIII concentrates were published (Levy, Mitra and Mozen, 1984) soon to be followed by evidence that heat treated concentrates do not transmit HIV (Mosseler, et al., 1985; Rouzioux, et al., 1985). By October 1985 all blood donations in the UK were being tested for anti-HIV antibodies and the policy of donor selection by questionnaire and laboratory testing followed by the viral inactivation of pooled concentrate eliminated the risk of HIV transmission by this route. The spread of HIV infection to the haemophilia community has therefore been contained and no new sero-conversions have occurred in the UK since the mid-1980s.

Table 1 shows the distribution of positive anti-HIV tests among patients with various haemostatic defects treated at the Royal London Hospital Haemophilia Centre.

Natural history

The course of HIV infection in patients with haemophilia largely mirrors the experience

Table 16.1 Distribution of positive anti-HIV tests at the Royal London Hospital Haemophilia Centre

Haemophilia A

Severe		Mild	
Positive	Negative	Positive	Negative
31	23	9	91

Haemophilia B

Positive	Negative
1	24

von Willebrand's Disease

Positive	Negative
0	21

of the condition in other high risk groups. A glandular fever-like illness associated with initial exposure has been reported (Tucker, *et al.*, 1985), as have the features of persistent generalized lymphadenopathy, AIDS-related complex and fully developed AIDS. The problems of herpes zoster, candidiasis, seborrhoeic dermatitis, folliculitis, molluscum contagiosum, fungal skin infection, sinusitis, septicaemia, pneumocystis pneumonia, toxoplasmosis, lymphoma and the neuropsychiatric complications of AIDS have become all too familiar to specialists in haemophilia (Lee, *et al.*, 1990) although Kaposi's sarcoma remains extremely rare (McCormick, *et al.*, 1987).

Other viral infections

Donor selection and hepatitis B vaccination have virtually eliminated new hepatitis B infection in haemophilia but before these advances the majority of patients showed evidence of former exposure to the virus and some remained HBe antigen positive. It is interesting to note that of the four Royal London Hospital patients who have been anti-HIV and HBe antigen positive three have developed AIDS while only 13 of the 41 anti-HIV positive patients have done so overall. The prevalence of non-A, non-B hepatitis in patients treated with large pool concentrates before the advent of heat treated concentrates was 100% (Kernoff, *et al.*, 1985) and whether chronic infections from this source will influence progression to AIDS may never become clear.

Cytomegalovirus (CMV) infection is no more prevalent in haemophiliacs than in the general population but it may nevertheless contribute to HIV disease progression. Webster, *et al.* (1989)

studied 108 HIV seropositive patients with haemophilia and reported that the age adjusted risk of CDC group IV disease in CMV seropositive patients was 2.5 times the CMV seronegative group.

Thrombocytopenia

Idiopathic thrombocytopenic purpura (ITP) associated with haemophilia has been particularly worrying because of the potential danger of life threatening haemorrhage when the platelet count falls below $50 \times 10^9/l$ (Ragni, *et al.*, 1990). Patients with both severe haemophilia and mild thrombocytopenia can remain well for long periods whatever treatment is used.

Age

The most definite prognostic feature to emerge from the study of the AIDS epidemic in the haemophilia population has been the effect of age (Goedert, *et al.*, 1989). They and others have shown quite clearly that the risk of AIDS increases with age and for the 1,219 subjects they studied the figures were:

Age	*AIDS development*
Years	*8-year cumulative rate (%)*
1–17	13.3
18–34	26.8
35–70	43.7

HLA status

It has also been shown that the possession of HLA A1 B8 DR3 carries a higher risk of seroconversion and progression to AIDS in patients with haemophilia (Steel, *et al.*, 1988) although the reason for this is not clear and other reports have produced different findings (Fabio, *et al.*, 1990).

Summary

Most reports have so far suggested that progression has been slower in the haemophilia community than for others at risk (Anderson, 1989) and an overall incidence of AIDS of 20% in the UK by early 1991 in a group exposed to infection between six and ten years ago seems to support this view. Nevertheless new cases of illness continue to accumulate and there is no reason to be optimistic about the overall prognosis than there was at the beginning of the epidemic.

Laboratory investigation

While the cause of AIDS remained unknown there was no alternative to the continuation of treatment for haemophilia A and during this period monitoring of patients was restricted to routine haematological tests combined with CD4 counts which were often expressed as a CD4/CD8 ratio. Skin tests were also performed in some centres but have the disadvantage that they are not very convenient for long-term follow up. As soon as anti-HIV tests became available screening was undertaken, often using previously stored samples and by the time the ethical importance of testing by consent had been established the majority of those at risk had been informed of their results, sometimes without the opportunity for appropriate counselling. More recently the value of the detection of antigen and antibody to individual HIV proteins has been recognized, the core protein p24 having assumed particular importance. There is evidence in haemophilia, as elsewhere, that loss of anti-p24 antibody is associated with re-emergence of HIV antigen and that the sequence of events carries a poor prognosis (Allain, *et al.*, 1987; Pedersen, *et al.*, 1987). Study of the Edinburgh cohort (Cuthbert, *et al.*, 1990) has provided some support for the measurement. of $\beta2$ microglobulin. These additional investigations have not however proved to be more valuable in patient assessment and treatment planning than the more traditional lymphocyte subset analysis that has been available since the beginning of the epidemic (Phillips, *et al.*, 1991).

The following list illustrates the investigations likely to be useful in the management of HIV infection in haemophilia:

Haemoglobin concentration
Total white cell count
Platelet count
Total lymphocyte count
CD4 cell count
CD8 cell count
Anti-HIV (global)
Anti-p24
HIV antigen
Skin tests

Staff safety

Haemophilia Centre staff routinely use venepuncture to treat their patients and obtain samples for investigation. In addition patients are not infrequently admitted to the wards for surgery while external bleeding, although uncommon, does occur, especially after injury. Fortunately a number of studies have demonstrated the extremely low risk of HIV transmission in these situations, even after needle-stick injury or splashing of blood or body fluids (Marcus, 1988).

Precautions

A code of practice is clearly worthwhile to minimize the chances of an accident (Advisory Committee on Dangerous Pathogens, 1990). The rules adopted at the Royal London Hospital Haemophilia Centre may be summarized as follows.

Only competent staff are allowed to perform venepunctures and handle the blood samples of patients with haemophilia. Needles must never be resheathed and must be disposed of safely in puncture-proof bins. Personal contact with blood and body fluids should be avoided and gloves and simple protective clothing should be used for this purpose. Cuts, grazes or other breaks in the skin should be covered by waterproof dressings. Face protection is not usually necessary and admission to a side ward is only advisable when a patient is bleeding externally or is producing copious volumes of fluid such as vomit, sputum or diarrhoea.

It has been shown that there is a significant risk of intraoperative exposure to blood for all surgical personnel (Gerberding, 1990) and there is support for the practice of double gloving and the increased use of waterproof garments and face shields in the operating theatre especially as patients with haemophilia may also represent a risk for hepatitis B and C transmission.

It is advisable to mark all samples from patients with haemophilia with High Risk labels, whatever their HIV status and proper bagging of samples and request forms is essential before delivery to the laboratory. Centrifugation should be performed in sealed buckets but there is no need to use safety cabinets for routine laboratory procedures. Mouth pipetting must, of course, be absolutely forbidden and it may be useful to batch High Risk samples where this is possible. Proper arrangements must be made for the disposal of contaminated waste on the ward, in the clinic and in the laboratory and appropriate solutions made up to deal with accidental spillages and to clean contaminated surfaces and laboratory equipment. Any wounds should be encouraged to bleed and be washed in hot, soapy water and any accidents must be reported immediately to a designated safety officer.

No testing of laboratory staff should be performed without written consent but it may be advantageous to staff who have been involved in an accident to have blood taken and stored for subsequent analysis if desired.

Zidovudine prophylaxis

There is still doubt concerning the value of prophylactic zidovudine after occupational exposure to HIV. Despite the lack of scientific evidence of benefit and the potential short and long-term side-effects of zidovudine, its use should be considered after accidental exposure to HIV and hospitals should have clearly defined systems for making advice and the drug available immediately at all times, including nights and weekends (Jeffries, 1991).

Patient management

Effective treatment for haemophilia became widely available following the introduction of cryoprecipitate in 1965. The production of freeze-dried large pool concentrates permitted the development of home treatment programmes in the early 1970s which were then extended to offer 'comprehensive care' (Kasper and Dietrich, 1985). This concept involves a hospital led, community-based system in which specialists from many disciplines cooperate to offer a wide range of services. Nursing staff and social workers have always played a key role in this work and many haemophilia centres have appointed their own staff, sometimes with help of the Haemophilia Society (Colvin, *et al.*, 1977).

General advice and support

As soon as the risk of HIV infection among patients with haemophilia was appreciated the comprehensive care system was adapted to the changing need. This resulted in an enormous increase in the time spent by doctors, nurses and social workers in explaining the latest available information and giving their patients appropriate support. Counsellors were appointed and the Haemophilia Society issued regular bulletins. The Society also launched a successful campaign for government recognition of the needs of the haemophilia community which was followed by litigation which now has largely been resolved.

As soon as a test for HIV became available the first priority was to identify those who had been infected and to give the most accurate available prognosis. For home treatment patients, rules were formulated for the prevention of needle injuries in family members, the covering of wounds and the avoidance of spillage of blood and other body fluids together with advice on the treatment of contaminated objects and the safe disposal of waste. Dental care may be best organized within a hospital setting. It is clear that the risk of transmission of HIV in a social context is very low (Friedland and Klein, 1987) and the recent report of probable HIV transmission from one child to another needs to be seen in this context (Simons and Rogers, 1993). The assessment and explanation of the risk of sexual transmission is much more difficult and although comparatively few cases of sexual transmission within the haemophilia community in the UK have been reported (Jones, *et al.*, 1985) the risk clearly exists and the widely agreed rules on safer sex apply equally to seropositive patients with haemophilia. Tragically this advice must also include an explanation of the dangers of starting or extending a family, even where the female partner is sero-negative since infection could clearly be transmitted at the time of conception.

Where pregnancies have occurred termination has been offered but it is not uncommon for couples to continue with the pregnancy, partly for emotional reasons, but also because the vertical transmission rate from anti-HIV positive mothers is lower than originally predicted. Thus in the European Collaborative Study (1991) the transmission rate was approximately 15% although 26% of infected children developed AIDS by 12 months of age.

A number of children were infected by HIV due to concentrate infusion before 1985 although the use of cryoprecipitate for very young children, which was still widespread in the early 1980s limited the size of this problem. Some chidren have died, but for those who grow up normally, parents and haemophilia centre directors face the difficult question of what to tell them and when.

Decisions also have to be made concerning what to tell other family members, especially siblings and how to preserve confidentiality within the community. Schooling provides a good example of this difficulty. Many parents feel that the school should know of their child's condition but are understandably reluctant to risk the wide dissemination of this knowledge. There is indeed no obligation or necessity for the school to be informed because of the lack of evidence of the social spread of HIV. The discussion of the problems associated with sexual activity in the HIV positive adolescent with haemophilia is one of the most painful subjects that needs to be addressed.

Groups have been formed to discuss all these matters and to allow mutual support in addition to the more formal care provided by the haemophilia centres themselves and some staff support groups have also been formed.

Treatment

There are no unique features of the natural history of HIV infection in haemophilia which require a special approach to drug treatment. This was initially chiefly concerned with the management of opportunistic infection (Young, 1987) and there has been a steady improvement in the range of drugs available since the beginning of the epidemic.

The latent period

In the period between seroconversion and the development of AIDS there are a number of problems which arise commonly and respond to simple measures. Skin lesions such as seborrhoeic dermatitis, folliculitis and fungal infection can be quickly controlled with the help of a dermatologist and chronic sinusitis may require medical or surgical intervention. Shingles is very common and may be associated with a poor long-term prognosis (Melbye, *et al.*, 1987) but rarely becomes disseminated and can be treated with acyclovir in the usual way. Oral candidiasis responds rapidly to fluconazole although high doses may be required in the more advanced stages of disease. Episodes of quite severe bacterial infection may occur and usually respond well to appropriate antibiotic therapy but a growing number of patients with HIV infection are dying without achieving a formal diagnosis of AIDS.

AIDS

The most important AIDS defining illness seen in the haemophilia community has been pneumocystis pneumonia. The diagnosis is often clear clinically but diagnostic bronchoscopy can be performed with appropriate concentrate cover. Conventional treatment with high-dose intravenous cotrimoxazole, is used, oral treatment being substituted after a few days. Pentamidine is an alternative drug but must be given intravenously for haemophiliacs who must not receive intramuscular injections. By the time respiratory failure occurs it is often too late for ventilation to be successful and the intensive care of a patient with haemophilia presents considerable logistic difficulties because of the invasive nature of this approach. It is therefore very important to try to ensure that patients seek advice before they become seriously ill.

Fortunately it is increasingly uncommon to see cases of pneumocystis pneumonia because of the introduction of prophylaxis for those patients most at risk. Aerosolized pentamidine 300 mg is convenient to administer monthly to patients with CD4 counts below $0.2 \times 10^9/l$ (Leoung, *et al.*, 1990) and has few side-effects. Oral cotrimoxazole is an alternative but tends to be associated with an allergic skin rash and dapsone has also been used.

Oesophageal candidiasis usually responds to fluconazole if a high enough dose is used and this drug is also valuable in the management of cryptococcosis because it is effective and is well absorbed (Bozzette, *et al.*, 1991).

One of the most difficult aspects of the success of treating opportunistic infections in recent years has been the eventual development of lymphomas or HIV related neuropsychiatric disorders. These are difficult to manage from every point of view and result in much distress for patients, their relatives, friends and carers. Lymphomas have been very disappointing to treat but zidovudine has proved to be of some benefit in the neuropsychiatric disorders.

Zidovudine

When zidovudine was introduced (Fischl, *et al.*, 1987; Richman, *et al.*, 1987) it was used only to treat patients with AIDS. Since then the indications for its use have become more clearly defined and have been extended to mildly symptomatic (Fischl, *et al.*, 1990) and asymptomatic (Volberding, *et al.*, 1990) patients. The benefits have become clearer as time has passed (Moore, *et al.*, 1991), the dose used has been reduced with an associated reduction in toxicity and many haemophilia centres are now recommending zidovudine 500 mg daily in divided doses for those patients with a CD4 count below 0.5 or 0.2×10^9/l irrespective of their clinical condition.

The experience of a large British haemophilia centre has been summarized by Lim, Lee and Kernoff (1990b) while the neuropsychological outcome of zidovudine treatment has been addressed by Schmitt, *et al.* (1988).

The introduction of zidovudine has also made a major contribution to the management of the thrombocytopenia associated with HIV infection. When this problem was first described there was an understandable reluctance to give corticosteroids which were in any case comparatively ineffective. High dose intravenous immunoglobulin and splenectomy were advocated (Beard and Savidge, 1988) but this approach is very expensive when factor concentrate replacement is taken into account. Zidovudine has proved to be very effective in standard doses in improving or normalizing the platelet count (Lim, Lee and Kernoff, 1990a). Another approach is the regular infusion of anti-D immunoglobulin (Gringeri, *et al.*, 1993) and splenectomy is now rarely necessary.

Bacterial infection and failure to thrive in children

The use of high dose intravenous immunoglobulin has been advocated for the prevention of bacterial infection in children with HIV infection and there is now some scientific evidence that the treatment is effective for those with initial CD4 counts above 0.2×10^9/l (National Institute of Child Health and Human Development Intravenous Immunoglobulin Study Group, 1991).

Pneumococcal vaccine has been advocated for the prevention of pneumococcal infection in children and adults with HIV infection (Shann, 1990).

The potential effect of factor concentrates

It has been suggested that factor VIII concentrates are in themselves immunosuppressive although there is no evidence that treatment for haemophilia in any way accelerates the clinical progress of HIV infection. As discussed earlier there is, if anything, a slower progression from seroconversion to AIDS in the haemophilia community for reasons which are not clear. A number of studies have shown that the decline in CD4 counts characteristic of HIV infection can be halted or delayed by the administration of monoclonal-antibody purified factor VIII concentrates (Seremetis, *et al.*, 1993). It is now accepted in the UK that high purity concentrates should be used for all HIV positive patients with haemophilia.

Summary

HIV infection has been a major tragedy for the haemophilia community and has affected approximately 25% of patients with haemophilia A in the United Kingdom. The natural history of the disease is the same as for other high risk groups save for the absence of Kaposi's sarcoma and the same methods are used for diagnosis, follow-up and treatment. Patients and their relatives need much support from a wide variety of health care professionals and the outlook for the length and quality of life has improved markedly since the epidemic began (Lee, *et al.*, 1991).

References

Advisory Committee on Dangerous Pathogens (1990) HIV – the causative agent of AIDS and related conditions – second revision of guidelines

AIDS Group of the United Kingdom Haemophilia Centre Directors (1986) Prevalence of antibody to HTLV-III in haemophiliacs in the United Kingdom. *British Medical Journal*, **293**, 175–176

Allain, J-P., Laurian, Y., Paul, D.A., Verroust, F., Leuther, M., Gazengel, C., *et al.* (1987) Long-term evaluation of HIV antigen and antibodies to p24 and gp41 in patients with haemophilia. *New England Journal of Medicine*, **317**, 1114–1121

Anderson, R. (1989) The AIDS epidemic in the UK; past trends and future projections. In, *HIV and AIDS*. UK Health Departments. Health Education Authority 24–30

Beard, J. and Savidge, G. F. (1988) High-dose intravenous immunoglobulin and splenectomy for the treatment of HIV related immune thrombocytopenia in patients with severe haemophilia. *British Journal of Haematology*, **68**, 303–306

Bozzette, S.A., Larsen, R.A., Chiu, J., Leal, M.A.E., Jacobsen, J., Rothman, P., *et al.* (1991) A placebo-controlled trial of maintenance therapy with fluconazole after treatment of cryptococcal meningitis in the acquired immunodeficiency syndrome. *New England Journal of Medicine*, **324**, 580–584

Colvin, B.T., Aston, C., Davis, G., Jenkins, G.C. and Dormandy, K.M. (1977) Regional co-ordinator for haemophilia in domiciliary practice. *British Medical Journal*, **2**, 814–815

Colvin, B.T., Collier, L.H. and Craske, J. (1987) A prospective study of cryoprecipitate administration: absence of evidence of virus infection. *Clinical and Laboratory Haematology*, **9**, 13–15

Cumming, A.M., Fields, S., Cumming, I.R., Wensley, R.T., Redding, O.M. and Burn, A.M. (1990) Clinical and laboratory evaluation of National Health Service factor VIII concentrate (8Y) for the treatment of von Willebrand's disease.. *British Journal of Haematology*, **75**, 234–239

Cuthbert, R.J.G., Ludlam, C.A., Tucker, J., Steel, C.M., Beatson, D., Rebus, S., *et al.* (1990) Five-year prospective study of HIV infection in the Edinburgh haemophiliac cohort. *British Medical Journal*, **301**, 956–961

European Collaborative Study (1991) Children born to women with HIV-1 infection: natural history and risk of transmission. *Lancet*, **337**, 253–260

Fabio, G., Smeraldi, R.S., Gringeri, A., Marchini, M., Bonara, P. and Mannucci, P.M. (1990) Susceptibility to HIV infection and AIDS in Italian haemophiliacs is HLA associated. *British Journal of Haematology*, **75**, 531–536

Fischl, M.A., Richman, D.D., Grieco, M.H., Gottlieb, M.S., Volberding, P.A., Laskin, O.L., *et al.* (1987) The efficacy of azidothymidine (AZT) in the treatment of patients with AIDS and AIDS-related complex. *New England Journal of Medicine*, **317**, 185–191

Fischl, M.A., Richman, D.D., Hansen, N., Collier, A.C., Carey, J.T., Para, M.F., *et al.* (1990) The safety and efficacy of zidovudine (AZT) in the treatment of subjects with mildly symptomatic human immunodeficiency virus type I(HIV) infection. *Annals of Internal Medicine*, **112**, 727–737

Friedland, G.H. and Klein, R.S. (1987) Transmission of the human immunodeficiency virus. *New England Journal of Medicine*, **317**, 1125–1135

Gerberding, J.J., Littel, C., Tarkington, A., Brown, A. and Schechter, W.P. (1990) Risk of exposure of surgical personnel to patients' blood during surgery at San Francisco General Hospital. *New England Journal of Medicine*, **322**, 1788–1793

Goedert, J.J., Kessler, C.M., Aledort, L.M., Biggar, R.J.,

Andes, W.A., White, G.C., *et al.* (1989) A prospective study of human immunodeficiency virus type I infection and the development of AIDS in subjects with haemophilia. *New England Journal of Medicine*, **321**, 1141–1148

Gringeri, A., Cattaneo, M., Santagostino, E. and Mannucci, P.M. (1993) Intramuscular anti-D immuno-globulins for home treatment of chronic immune thrombocytopenic purpura. *British Journal of Haematology*, **80**, 337–340

Jeffries, D.J. (1991) Zidovudine after occupational exposure to HIV. *British Medical Journal*, **302**, 1349–1351

Jones, P., Hamilton, P.J., Bird, G., Fearns, M., Oxley, A., Tedder, R., *et al.* (1985) AIDS and haemophilia: morbidity and mortality in a well defined population. *British Medical Journal*, **291**, 695–699

Kasper, C.K. and Dietrich, S.L. (1985) Comprehensive management of haemophilia. *Clinics in Haematology*, **14**, 489–512

Kernoff, P.B.A., Lee, C.A., Karayiannis, P. and Thomas, H.C. (1985) High risk of non-A non-B hepatitis after a first exposure to volunteer or commercial clotting factor concentrates: effects of prophylactic immune serum globulin. *British Journal of Haematology*, **60**, 469–479

Laurian, Y., Peynet, J. and Verroust, F. (1989) HIV infection in sexual partners of HIV seropositive patients with haemophilia. *New England Journal of Medicine*, **320**, 183

Lee, C.A., Phillips, A., Elford, J., Janossy, G., Griffiths, P. and Kernoff, P.B.A. (1990) Ten-year follow up of HIV infection in a haemophilic cohort. *British Journal of Haematology*, **75**, 623

Lee, C.A., Phillips, A.N., Elford, J., Janossy, G., Griffiths, P. and Kernoff, P.B.A. (1991) Progression of HIV disease in a haemophilic cohort followed for 11 years and the effect of treatment. *British Medical Journal*, **303**, 1093–1096

Leoung, G.S., Feigal, D.W., Montgomery, A.B., Corkery, K., Wardlaw, L., Adams, M., *et al.* (1990) Aerosolized pentamidine for prophylaxis against Pneumocystis carinii pneumonia. *New England Journal of Medicine*, **323**, 769–775

Levy, J.A., Mitra, G. and Mozen, M.M. (1984) Recovery and inactivation of infectious retroviruses added to factor VIII concentrates. *Lancet*, **ii**, 722–723

Lim, S.G., Lee, C.A. and Kernoff, P.B.A. (1990a) The treatment of HIV associated thrombocytopenia in haemophiliacs. *Clinical and Laboratory Haematology*, **12**, 237–245

Lim, S.G., Lee, C.A. and Kernoff, P.B.A. (1990b) Zidovudine treatment for anti-HIV positive haemo-philiacs. *Clinical and Laboratory Haematology*, **12**, 367–378

Ludlam, C.A., Steel, C.M., Cheingsong-Popov, R., Tucker, J., Tedder, R.S., Weiss, R.A., *et al.* (1985) Human T-lymphotropic virus type III (HTLV-III) infection in seronegative haemophiliacs after trans-fusion of factor VIII. *Lancet*, **ii**, 233–236

McCormick, A., Tillett, H., Bannister, B. and Emslie, J.

(1987) Surveillance of AIDS in the United Kingdom. *British Medical Journal*, **295**, 1466–1469

Mannucci, P.M., Ruggieri, Z.M., Pareti, F.I. and Capitanio, A. (1977) 1-Deamino-8-D-Arginine Vasopressin: a new pharmacological approach to the management of haemophilia and von Willebrand's disease. *Lancet*, **i**, 869–872

Marcus, R. and the CDC Cooperative Needlestick Surveillance Group (1988) Surveillance of health care workers exposed to blood from patients infected with human immunodeficiency virus. *New England Journal of Medicine*, **319**, 1118–1123

Melbye, M., Grossman, R.J., Goedert, J.J., Eyster, M.E. and Biggar, R.J. (1987) Risk of AIDS after herpes zoster. *Lancet*, **i**, 728–731

Mosseler, J., Schimpf, K., Auerswald, G., Bayer, H., Schneider, J. and Hunsmann, G. (1985) Inability of pasteurised factor VIII preparations to induce antibodies to HTLV-III after long term treatment. *Lancet*, **i**, 1111

Moore, R.D., Hidalgo, J., Sugland, B.W. and Chaisson, R.E. (1991) Zidovudine and the natural history of the acquired immune deficiency syndrome. *New England Journal of Medicine*, **324**, 1412–1416

National Institute of Child Health and Human Development Intravenous Immunoglobulin Study Group (1991) Intravenous immune globulin for the prevention of bacterial infections in children with symptomatic human immunodeficiency virus infection. *New England Journal of Medicine*, **325**, 73–80

Pasi, K.J., Williams, M.D., Enayat, M.S. and Hill, F.G.H. (1990) Clinical and laboratory evaluation of the treatment of von Willebrand's disease patients with heat treated factor VIII concentrate (BPL 8Y). *British Journal of Haematology*, **75**, 228–233

Pedersen, C., Nielsen, C.M., Vestergaard, B.F., Gerstoft, J., Krogsgaard, K. and Nielsen, J.O. (1987) Temporal relation of antigenaemia and loss of antibodies to core antigens to development of clinical disease in HIV infection. *British Medical Journal*, **295**, 567–572

Phillips, A.N., Lee, C.A., Elford, J., Janossy, G., Timms, A., Bofill, M., *et al.* (1991) Serial CD4 lymphocyte counts and development of AIDS. *Lancet*, **337**, 389–392

Ragni, M.V., Bontempo, F.A., Myers, D.J., Kiss, J.E. and Oral, A. (1988) Haemorrhagic sequelae of immune thrombocytopenic purpura in human immunodeficiency virus infected hemophiliacs. *Blood*, **75**, 1267–1272

Richman, D.D., Fischl, M.A., Grieco, M.H., Gottlieb, M.S., Volberding, P.A., Laskin, O.L., *et al.* (1987). The toxicity of azidothymidine (AZT) in the treatment of patients with AIDS and AIDS-related complex. *New England Journal of Medicine*, **317**, 192–197

Part Four

Infection and the Blood

17

Haematological aspects of malaria

Christine A. Facer

Introduction

Malaria remains, in spite of intensive world-wide efforts to reduce its transmission, the most serious and widespread protozoal infection of humans. A conservative estimate for those exposed to the risk of infection is more than 2.6 billion, a figure representing 55% of the world population (WHO, 1985). The total number of individuals with infections is unknown because of considerable under-reporting of diagnosed cases and the existence of asymptomatic infections. The WHO has estimated the global incidence of malaria to be 100 million cases per year. This figure has recently been challenged and a more realistic estimate for the year 1986 is 489 million clinical cases, including 234 million due to *Plasmodium falciparum*, of which at least 2.3 million are fatal (Table 1: Sturchler, 1988). Malaria is a major cause of mortality in childhood and at least one million die of the disease each year. Confounding this situation is the now widespread transmission in almost every endemic country of *P. falciparum* strains resistant to chloroquine and other antimalarial drugs.

As parasites of the blood for the majority of their complex life cycle, plasmodia induce marked haematological alterations and malaria remains the main cause of severe anaemia in children living in malaria endemic regions. At the genetic level, the high gene frequency for certain variant haemoglobins, such as HbS in malarious regions of the world, is attributed to the selective advantage of the heterozygote against the severe effects of falciparum malaria.

Tremendous advancement has been made in the past ten years in defining the molecular biology of the parasite and molecular interactions between parasite and host red cell. The aim of this chapter is to provide the reader with an updated appraisal of advances in our understanding of this disease with emphasis on the aforementioned topics.

Space does not permit consideration of developments in the production of malaria sub-unit vaccines, chemotherapy and drug resistance and the reader is referred to excellent reviews on these subjects (Nussenweig and Nussenweig, 1985; Mitchell, 1989; Lobel and Campbell, 1986).

Peripheral blood changes in malaria

The malaria parasite has a complicated life cycle involving many stages and natural transmission by anophelene mosquitoes (Figure 17.1). *P. falciparum* is the most widespread species and is responsible for a severe and frequently fatal disease. *P. vivax* is essentially cosmopolitan but predominates in the Indian sub-continent, Latin America, Turkey and China. Infection with this species results in an unpleasant and benign illness where complications are unusual and fatalities rare.

The haematologic abnormalities that invariably accompany infection with malaria include anaemia, thrombocytopenia, leukopenia, mild/moderate atypical lymphocytosis and splenomegaly. Most are correlated with the severity

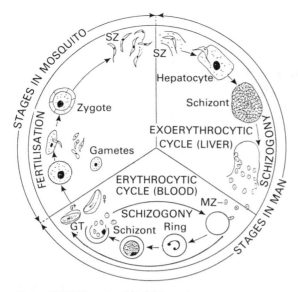

Figure 17.1 Life cycle of *P. falciparum*

Anaemia

Anaemia is an inevitable consequence of severe malaria because of the intravascular rupture of parasitized erythrocytes during schizogony and often accompanies other manifestations of the disease. Although the anaemia is normocytic the red cell morphology may be influenced by the nutritional status of the patient. Thus in malaria-endemic regions, it is not uncommon for patients to present with an associated microcytic or macrocytic component resulting from a co-existing iron or folic acid deficiency respectively (Facer and Jenkins, 1989).

The pathogenesis of the anaemia complicating malaria is complex and multifactorial (Table 17.2). An element of controversy surrounds the mechanisms of malarial anaemia over and above direct disruption of the red cell by the parasite and reports in the literature give conflicting results. This may well be a result in differences in the immune status of the patients investigated, or genetic diversity of host and parasite, or both. For example, results from

and duration of clinical illness with prolonged acute episodes of malaria producing the most severe changes. In addition, the abnormalities vary in degree according to the species of *Plasmodium*. Thus *P. falciparum* produces an anaemia of greater severity because of its ability to parasitize red cells of all ages (Table 17.1) and because of its high reproductive potential (more merozoites per schizont are produced than in the other species). As a result, untreated *P. falciparum* infections result in higher parasitaemias. The description that follows relates to changes associated with falciparum malaria: the consequences of *P. vivax*, *P. malariae* and *P. ovale* are generally much milder.

Table 17.2 Causes of anaemia in malaria

Mechanism	Importance
1. Haemolysis	
a. intravascular (lysis parasitized red cells)	+++
b. extravascular (peripheral erythrophagocytosis of parasitized and non-parasitized red cells)	++
2. Decreased erythropoiesis with dyserythropoietic changes	+
3. Splenic phagocytosis and/or pooling	+
4. Haemorrhage	+*
5. Anaemia of chronic disorders	+
6. Microangiopathy	?

* At sites of tissue schizogony, eg. brain, gastrointestinal tract

Table 17.1 The four major *Plasmodia* infecting humans

Species	Host cell	Disease	Prevalence ($\times 10^6$/year)	Deaths* ($\times 10^6$/year)
P. falciparum	Mature red cell (but reticulocyte preference)	Malignant tertian		
P. vivax	Reticulocyte	Benign tertian	489†	2.3
P. malariae	Mature red cell	Quartan		
P. ovale	Mature red cell	Tertian		

* Mostly attributed to *P. falciparum*
† Clinical cases including 234×10^6 due to *P. falciparum*

studies on non-immune Thai adults (Merry, et al., 1986) differ in many respects to those obtained from semi-immune Gambian children (Facer, Bray and Brown, 1979; Facer, 1980a, b; Abdalla and Weatherall, 1982; Jeje, Kelton and Blajchman, 1983) with regards to the incidence and relative importance of Coombs positivity and ineffective erythropoiesis (see below).

Haemolysis

Severe anaemia is defined as a haematocrit <20% (haemoglobin <4.4mmol/1 or <7.1g/dl) and patients presenting with this degree of anaemia (a common finding in children living in malaria-endemic regions) are at increased risk of morbidity and mortality and should be managed accordingly. The destruction of parasitized red cells is undoubtedly a prime factor in the aetiology of the anaemia and can be fully appreciated in those patients presenting with parasitaemias of >20% infected red cells (Figure 17.2a). However, the rate at which the anaemia develops, and its degree, usually exceeds that which can be accounted for by loss of parasitized erythrocytes alone (Devakul, Harinasuta and Kanakakorn, 1969; Srichaikul, 1973). In addition, anaemia frequently progresses for several days following clearance of parasites by antimalarials. These observations prompted the suggestion that a cohort of non-parasitized erythrocytes are destroyed (Facer, et al., 1979; Woodruff, Andsell and Pettitt, 1979; Facer, 1980a, b). The peripheral blood parasitaemia might not necessarily present a true picture of the total parasite burden since P. falciparum schizonts sequester within capillaries of the internal organs (see p. 283). However, when predictions take this into account, the estimated drop in haematocrit still falls short of that observed (Zuckerman, 1966). In addition, in experimental rodent malaria where the infecting Plasmodium species is known not to sequester (e.g. P. berghei), the degree of anaemia is again out of proportion to the parasitaemia (Seed and Krier, 1980). These observations in human and experimental animal malaria therefore suggest haemolysis of non-parasitized red cells, possibly by immune-mediated mechanisms.

Evidence for increased destruction of the non-parasitized erythrocyte compartment has come from the results of direct antiglobulin tests (DAT) and ^{51}Cr red cell survival studies. Red cell bound immunoglobulin and complement (C') components have been demonstrated either semi-quantitatively (using the DAT) (Facer, et al., 1979; Woodruff, et al., 1979; Abdalla and Weatherall, 1982) or quantitatively using a modified immunoradiometric assay (Jeje, et al., 1983). In the order of 50% of Gambian children were found to have a positive DAT and this was correlated with the presence of a P. falciparum parasitaemia (Facer, et al., 1979). In most cases red cell sensitization was with C3d alone or in combination with IgG and positivity persisted for several weeks following antimalarial treatment. In children presenting with acute infections, there was a significant statistical correlation with a positive DAT and concurrent anaemia although this was not confirmed in children with low-grade asymptomatic infections. A small percentage of children had a positive DAT for the haemolytically active C3b component (EC3b) and, not surprisingly, were severely anaemic and in haemolytic crisis with clear evidence for extravascular haemolysis in the peripheral blood films (Figure 17.2b). Erythrophagocytosis was by monocytes which possess complement receptors for C3b (CR1, CD35). Recovery from anaemia was accompanied by disappearance of C3b from the surface of red cells and appearance of haemolytically inactive C3d. The IgG sensitizing the erythrocytes was polyclonal with some predominance of the IgG2 and IgG4 subclasses (Facer, 1980a). One other observation to emerge was that sensitization of red cells with IgG1 correlated with the presence of anaemia. This high incidence of Coombs positivity in children living within the same endemic region was later confirmed by Abdalla and Weatherall (1982) although they were unable to correlate the positive results with the presence of anaemia. Further evidence for sensitization of non-parasitized red cells came from a study of a large group of Nigerian children with acute falciparum malaria (Jeje, et al., 1983). A statistically significant correlation was established between red cell associated IgG and the degree of anaemia, supporting the hypothesis that immunological mechanisms could be involved in the aetiology of the anaemia.

In contrast to the above studies, non-immune Thai adults with acute falciparum malaria were found to have a negative DAT and only low levels of IgG sensitization in the radiometric assay (Merry, et al., 1987). Likewise, a small

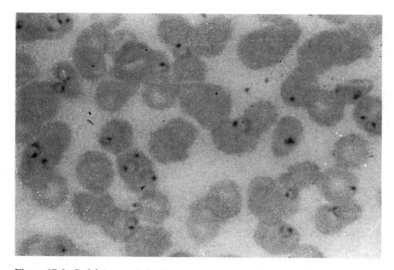

Figure 17.2a *P. falciparum* infection in a two-year-old Gambian child with acute malaria. Multiple invasion of red cells

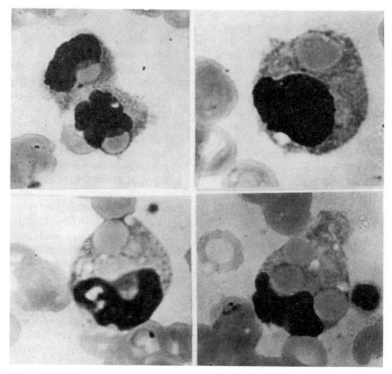

Figure 17.2b Extravascular haemolysis of non-parasitized red cells by monocytes in a patient with acute *P. falciparum* malaria. Red cells were sensitized with IgG, C3b, C4b and C3d

group of non-immune Caucasians with acute malaria were negative for red cell bound immunoglobulin and complement (Facer, unpublished observations). It is difficult to reconcile the differences between the African and Thai studies. However, one clue is found when analysing the data collectively – namely the age and immune status of the patients under investigation. The studies on semi-immune African children showed that DAT positively declines with increasing age (and increasing immunity to malaria) and that the occasional 10–15 year old presenting with an acute infection never had a positive DAT. Taken together with the data on adults, this suggests that a *negative* DAT may well be associated with the absence of previous exposure to malaria. In support of this suggestion was the observation that IgG eluted from the surface of DAT positive erythrocytes from Gambian children had specificity for schizont-related antigens of a West African strain of *P. falciparum* (Facer, 1980a). It is likely therefore that sensitization with IgG and C' represents either a Coombs and Cell Type II cytotoxic hypersensitivity (coating of cells with soluble malaria antigen followed by antibody and C') or Type III complex-mediated hypersensitivity. Certainly, when fresh normal erythrocytes are added to soluble malaria antigen-antibody complexes *in vitro*, they readily take up the complexes and give a strong positive reaction with anti-IgG and anti-C4 reagents (Facer, unpublished observations). Similarly, a 175kD *P. falciparum* antigen from culture supernatants was found to bind to intact normal erythrocytes in a manner that correlated with merozoite invasion into the erythrocytes (Camus and Hadley, 1985). It is interesting to note that over 85% of the total immune complex receptors (CR1, C3b receptors) reside on the surface of human red cells (Siegal, Liu and Gleicher, 1981) and play an important role in the clearance of immune complexes from the circulation (Sherwood and Virella, 1986). The positive DAT in malaria may represent such a mechanism in progress and a CR1 polymorphism might be an alternative explanation for frequency differences in DAT positivity between populations.

Evidence for increased red cell destruction comes from ^{51}Cr survival studies most of which have shown a dramatic reduction in red cell survival of compatible donor or autologous cells

following clearance of parasites which related to the severity of the anaemia prior to treatment (Rosenberg, *et al.*, 1973; Woodruff, *et al.*, 1979). In a more recent study (Phillips and Warrell, 1986) two interesting features were observed. First, the survival of radio-labelled compatible donor red cells was significantly shorter than that of autologous cells in patients recovering from falciparum malaria. One explanation for this surprising result is that the erythrocyte population within the patient's circulation (i.e. the autologous transfused cells) represent the survivors of a highly activated reticulo-endothelial clearance mechanism. A second feature of interest seen in some of the patients was a bi-phasic pattern of survival. This alluded to either the presence of two cell populations or, alternatively, an initial enhanced splenic clearance which later waned. A similar bi-phasic pattern of erythrocyte survival has been described in experimental trypanosomiasis (Jenkins and Facer, 1985).

Autoantibodies to red cell membrane components

The appearance of serum antibodies recognizing normal erythrocyte membrane antigens frequently follows infection with malaria although it is thought unlikely that they contribute to the aetiology of the anaemia. A detailed study in Gambian children failed to demonstrate the presence of antibodies with blood group specificity either in serum or in red cell eluates (Facer, 1980a). However, cold reacting serum IgM antibodies to the blood group I(i) system were demonstrated, but these were present only in low titres and were considered of no pathological significance (Facer, 1980a; Facer and Sangster, 1981).

An increase in the titre of naturally occurring anti-A and anti-B haemagglutinins and antibodies to the crypt T antigens have been described in acute malaria (Zouali, *et al.*, 1982). Likewise elevated heterophile antibodies to red cells of animal origin have also been documented (Greenwood, Herrick and Holborrow, 1970; Facer, unpublished observations). Elevated titres of autoantibodies to erythrocyte cytoskeletal polypeptides are produced in malaria infections as shown by Western blotting techniques (Berzins, Wahlgren and Perlmann, 1983; Sweeney and Facer, 1988). However, because of the intercellular localization of the polypeptides in question (e.g. spectrin) the autoantibodies are likely to be the result rather than the causes of haemolysis. However, the detection of antibodies reacting with a polypeptide of approximately 30 kD may be of some significance since this probably represents the major erythrocyte transmembrane sialoglycoprotein, glycophorin A, with the largest portion of the protein located on the exofacial surface of the red cell (Sweeney and Facer, 1988; Schetters, personal communication).

Antibodies to red cell band 3 polypeptides exist in low titres in the sera of healthy individuals (Lutz and Wipf, 1982) where they are thought to play a physiological role in the sequestration of senescent red cells since the senescent red cell antigen(s) is immunologically related to band 3 (Kay, *et al.*, 1983). Maturation of the *P. falciparum* schizont is accompanied by a premature 'ageing' of the red cell and, presumably, the appearance of red cell senescent membrane antigens. Evidence for this comes from the observation that normal human serum opsonizes schizonts for phagocytosis by monocytes taken from healthy individuals in an *in vitro* assay (H. Ginsburg, personal communication). Whether this is a result of increased expression of, or topographical changes in, the distribution of surface-exposed band 3 polypeptides, so allowing greater reactivity with anti-band 3 autoantibodies, remains to be seen. The increased titres of anti-band 3 serum antibodies found in malaria (Sweeney and Facer, 1980) may thus serve to remove parasitized red cells from the circulation in addition to their normal physiological role.

Splenomegaly

A decrease in haematocrit invariably accompanies splenic enlargement. The red cells accumulating in the large extra sinusoidal compartments of infiltrated spleens are subjected to reduced pH and low oxygen tensions which, in turn, increase both the osmotic fragility of the red cells and their cytoplasmic K^+/Na^+ ratio (see Jenkins and Facer, 1985, for review). Enlarged spleens also 'pool' red cells so depriving the circulation of a large volume of red cells at any one time. Infection with malaria stimulates a significant splenomegaly which is used to estimate the prevalence of malaria within African communities ('spleen rate').

However, the relative contribution of splenomegaly and splenic pooling to the anaemia of malaria remains uncertain.

Erythropoiesis

Normally when haemoglobin levels fall, the accompanying reduced oxygen tension stimulates erythropoietin production and release by the kidney which, in turn, stimulates the bone marrow into active erythropoiesis. However, despite low haemoglobin levels in malaria patients, marrow aspirates show little evidence of compensatory erythropoiesis. Two detailed reports show that erythroid precursors, in both children (Abdalla, Weatherall, Wickramasinghe and Hughes, 1980; Weatherall and Abdalla, 1982) and adults (Phillips, *et al.*, 1986) with acute falciparum malaria and anaemia, are normal or slightly reduced. The ineffective erythropoiesis could arise from a decreased erythropoietin production and/or failure of erythroid progenitors to respond to the hormone although this has been excluded in experimental malaria infections (see below).

Alternatively, the non-compensatory erythropoiesis in malaria may reflect defective iron re-utilization from degraded red cells arising from reticuloendothelial blockade. The observation of iron deposits in mononuclear cells of the bone marrow and spleen suggests a situation kinetically analogous to the anaemias of chronic disorders where the bone marrow becomes effectively starved of iron (Cartwright and Lee, 1975). A similar picture is also seen in other haemoprotozoal infections such as trypanosomiasis (Jenkins and Facer, 1985).

Bone marrows taken from severely anaemic (semi-immune) Gambian children with chronic infections and low reticulocyte counts also show multiple dyserythropoietic changes which include multinuclear erythroblasts, karyorrhexis and erythrophagocytosis (Abdalla, *et al.*, 1980). Haematinic deficiency (B12 or folate) was excluded as a cause of the dyserythropoiesis. More recently dyserythropoiesis has been documented in 73% of non-immune Thai adults with uncomplicated falciparum malaria. Interestingly, unlike the situation described above for Gambian children, the dyserythropoietic changes were *not* associated with severe anaemia, length of illness, parasitaemia or any other haematological variable, perhaps questioning the role of dyserythropoiesis in the development of anaemia (Phillips, *et al.*, 1986). The metabolic basis underlying the acquired dyserythropoiesis remains to be determined.

Dyserythropoiesis and ineffective erythropoiesis are not specific for falciparum malaria and both feature in *P. vivax* infections (Wickramasinghe, *et al.*, 1989) where their aetiology again remains uncertain. Unlike the situation observed in severe falciparum malaria the microvasculature of the marrow does not become obstructed by parasitized cells.

A recent detailed histological and ferrokinetic study in experimental murine malaria has provided some interesting and informative observations (Silverman, Schooley and Mahlmann, 1987). Mice were infected with *P. vinkei*, *P. berghei* or *P. chabaudi* and exposed to simulated high altitude in order to measure the erythropoietin response. All these species of plasmodia stimulated erythropoietin production during peak parasitaemia and this was further increased by the hypoxic exposure. The progressive defective erythropoietic activity of the bone marrow was instead found to result from a depletion of colony forming units – pluropotent stem cells (CFUs). The mechanism of stem cell depletion is unknown, although tumour necrosis factor (TNFα) has been implicated. TNFα inhibits adipocyte gene expression (Torti, *et al.*, 1985); cells which are major cellular components of stromal bone marrow and which an essential environment for renewal and differentiation of haemopoietic stem cells. Of relevance here, is the recent description of raised serum TNFα levels in patients with malaria (Scuderi, *et al.*, 1986). Since malaria parasites often sequester in the bone marrow and can directly stimulate TNFα production by resident macrophages (Bate, Taverne and Playfair, 1988), it is possible that local production of TNFα within the marrow may account for the ineffective erythropoiesis.

Malaria, iron and riboflavin

Iron deficiency is the most common micronutrient deficiency with the lowest non-haem iron stores in the human population being recorded in India, coastal Papua New Guinea and Burma (Oppenheimer, 1989). In attempts to prevent hypochromic microcytic anaemia, oral iron supplementation programmes have been introduced, mainly for children and pregnant mothers. However, current evidence indicates caution in such practices since iron supplementation may actually increase the likelihood of a subject developing patent malaria in endemic areas.

The immediate local availability of a large excess of iron for an intraerythrocytic parasite like *Plasmodium* would appear to obviate any influence of iron deficiency on the growth of the parasite and the clinical illness it produces. Nevertheless, several studies report increased malaria susceptibility following iron therapy (reviewed, Oppenheimer, 1989) in pregnant women (Byles and D'Sa, 1970) and in Somali nomads (Murray, *et al.*, 1978) where recrudescent malaria was seen in a proportion of individuals following oral iron supplementation. More recently, a prospective randomized, double-blind, placebo-controlled trial of iron supplementation in infancy was carried out in Papua New Guinea (Oppenheimer, 1989). Subsequent to a single dose of iron dextran (150 mg elemental iron) administered at two months of age, no significant difference in malaria rates was seen at the one week follow-up visit. However, malaria slide positivity and spleen rates were significantly higher in the iron treatment group at both the six- and twelve-month visits. No effect of iron on parasite densities was detectable at any time following iron supplementation. That the effects of iron were deleterious for a long period after administration differs from previous studies where only short-term adverse effects were reported. Although further controlled studies are clearly needed before making definite recommendations, given the results of this study, iron dextran prophylaxis to infants in malarious areas should be contraindicated.

In addition to children living in malaria-endemic regions, primiparous women form a group that appears to have a peculiarly lowered immunity to malaria (Brabin, 1983). Oral iron, a standard supplement in pregnancy, was found to result in higher rates of maternal perinatal malaria. In contrast, this effect was not seen in multiparous women. Since anaemia during pregnancy in the tropics is commonly attributed to malaria, treatment with iron may carry a definite risk especially for women in their first pregnancies.

How iron deficiency and iron administration interact with malaria remains uncertain. One hypothesis relates to the reticulocyte preference of *P. falciparum*. Reticulocytosis would be stimulated by administration of iron so enhancing the multiplication of parasites. Alternatively, iron administration, by increasing the saturation of transferrin (i.e. iron availability) may enhance parasite growth in a way similar to that described for bacteria and other micro-organisms (Weinberg, 1974). However, this theory implies that, since mature red cells lack transferrin receptors, then specific parasite encoded transferrin receptors must be inserted into the parasitized erythrocyte membrane. A recent report suggests that red cells infected with *P. falciparum* appear to acquire such transferrin receptors (Rodriguez and Jungery, 1986) although, to date, attempts to clone the gene responsible for this putative receptor have been unsuccessful. There is also evidence that desferrioxamine can modify malaria infections in animal models and inhibit the growth of *P. falciparum in vitro* (Raventos-Suarez, Pollack and Nagel, 1982), although a direct toxic effect of desferrioxamine has not been excluded.

One other micronutrient deficiency, that of riboflavin, has also been associated with protection against severe malaria, in animals and humans (Dutta, Pinto and Rivlin, 1985). An inverse relationship between riboflavin status and malarial parasitaemia occurs in both experimental rodent malaria and in infants with *P. falciparum* infections (Thurnham, *et al.*, 1983). Drugs that induce riboflavin deficiency in experimental animals (e.g. chlorpromazine and the tricyclic antidepressants) also show antimalarial properties (Dutta, *et al.*, 1985).

The mechanism(s) whereby riboflavin deficiency exerts antimalarial action remains uncertain. One possibility is that a deficiency results in a change in the structure and/or functional integrity of the red blood cell membrane. Lack of riboflavin reduces the level of polyunsaturated fatty acids in membrane phospholipids, and this would be expected to influence fluidity, permeability and binding properties not only in membranes of host cells but also in parasite membranes. New therapeutic approaches with metabolic inhibitors of riboflavin metabolism might be investigated for therapeutic potential as future antimalarial agents.

Thrombocytopenia

A classical feature of malaria is an accompanying marked thrombocytopenia (platelets $<150 \times 10^9/1$), so characteristic that in our laboratory it is used as an indicator of malaria in patients presenting with pyrexia of unknown origin. A low platelet count is seen in about 85% of patients with uncomplicated malaria and all patients with severe falciparum malaria (Devakul, Harinasuta and Reid, 1966; Kelton, *et al.*, 1983; Sorensen, Mickley and Schmidt, 1984; Phillips, *et al.*, 1986; Facer and Jenkins, 1989). Interestingly, the low platelet count has never been found to be related to any disturbance in haemostasis. The mean platelet volume is often raised confirming the presence of giant platelets on stained blood films and indicating the presence of activated platelets (Facer, unpublished observation). The thrombocytopenia occurs early in the illness and resolves within a few days of treatment, often with a rebound thrombocytosis of up to $580 \times 10^9/1$ (Horstmann, *et al.*, 1981). This feature, together with the observation of an inverse correlation between parasitaemia and the degree of thrombocytopenia, suggests a direct interaction between platelets and parasites.

The precise mechanism behind the thrombocytopenia, however, remains unclear. Decreased thrombopoiesis can be excluded since megakaryocytes in the marrow are normal or increased and actively budding (Srichaikul, Panikbutr and Jeumtrakul, 1967; Beale, Cormack and Oldrey, 1971). Immune mediated destruction of circulating platelets has been postulated. Malaria patients have elevated levels of platelet bound IgG with an inverse relationship between platelet count and level of platelet-associated immunoglobulin (Kelton, *et al.*, 1983; Sorensen, *et al.*, 1984).

Platelet hypersensitivity has been described in malaria (Essien and Ebhota, 1981) with enhanced platelet secretory activities and thromboxane B_2 production (Essien, *et al.*, 1984). The addition of infected *P. falciparum* erythrocytes to normal human platelets *in vitro* results in an enhanced platelet aggregation response to exogenous ADP and increased secretion of dense granules (Inyang, *et al.*, 1987). Platelets from malaria patients also show defects in both primary and secondary aggregation following addition of various agonists *in vitro* (Ospina, personal communication) which may indicate pre-activation of the platelets. C-reactive protein (CRP), an acute phase reactant protein reaching high serum levels in malaria infections (Ree, 1971), may adversely affect platelet function *in vivo* as a result of its known inhibitory effects on many platelet activities (Thomasson, *et al.*, 1973).

Malarial parasites (*P. vivax* and *P. yoelii*) have been viewed within platelets at the light and electron microscope level (Fajardo and Tallent, 1974). However whether this represents positive invasion by, or endocytosis (phagocytosis) of, merozoites into platelets remains uncertain. Whatever the route of entry, parasites fail to develop beyond the trophozoite stage (Perkash, Kelly and Fajardo, 1984).

White cell changes

Leucopenia is a common finding in both non-immune patients with falciparum malaria (Gunapala, *et al.*, 1990) and in semi-immune children living in malaria-endemic regions (Facer and Jenkins, 1989) where the white cell count is frequently as low as $1 - 2 \times 10^9/1$. Characteristically, during the first few days of a falciparum infection, the polymorphonuclear cells are raised and lymphocyte numbers low. However, progression of the infection results in reversal of this picture. A significant alteration in the subsets of circulating lymphocytes during the course of the disease is seen and can be found summarized in Tables 17.3 and 17.4.

Malaria-associated syndromes

Hyperreactive malarial splenomegaly (HMS)

The splenomegaly which normally accompanies acute clinical episodes of malaria regresses following treatment or resolution of the disease. In malaria endemic areas, the gradual slow acquisition of immunity to the disease in an individual is accompanied by a gradual decline in splenic size so that few adults ever present with enlarged spleens.

Persistent gross splenomegaly in an adult, for which there is no obvious explanation on clinical examination, is an abnormality that has been recognized for many years in certain parts of the tropics, notably Papua New Guinea and tropical Africa. Originally termed the tropical splenomegaly syndrome (TSS), the condition has now been renamed hyperreactive malarial splenomegaly (HMS) as a means of differentiating it from other forms of massive splenomegaly of unknown cause. Geographically HMS is only found in those areas where malaria is endemic and no one particular species of

Table 17.3 Leucocyte changes in malaria

Cell population	Observation
Total leucocytes	Reduced
Neutrophils	Moderate neutropenia, shift to the left, hypersegmentation of folate deficiency
Monocytes	Raised, vacuolation, erythro-phagocytosis, malaria pigment, haemosiderin
Eosinophils	Reduced. Eosinophilia occasionally following anti-malarials
Lymphocytes	Initial lymphopenia, then lymphocytosis
	Atypical lymphocytes
B cells	Markedly increased
T cells	Reduced. But increased proportion of CD8$^+$ cells
CD4:CD8	Normal or reversed

Table 17.4 Subset analysis of peripheral blood lymphocytes from patients with malaria and control donors

mAb	Ag cluster determinant	Patients (n = 18)	Controls (n = 18)
Leu 12	CD19 (B)	16.3 (11.2)	9.5 (5.5)
Leu 1	CD3 (T)	57.8 (20.7)	49.2 (6.3)
Leu 3a	CD4 (Th)	31.4 (19.4)	45.0 (9.6)
Leu 2a	CD8 (Ts)	17.5 (13.4)	9.2 (5.0)
anti-Tac	CD25 (T/B)	7.6 (4.6)	3.6 (1.9)
anti-HLA-DR	1a (B/T)	6.8 (2.4)	2.7 (0.7)
Leu 7	− (NK)	9.3	8.1 (3.4)
	CD4:CD8	1.7 (1.1)	2.0

Values are expressed as the mean percentage and standard deviation in parenthesis. All 18 patients had been clinically ill for <7 days.

Plasmodium has been implicated. There is considerable variation in the prevalence of the syndrome from region to region and highest prevalence rates (>50%) have been reported in Papua New Guinea and the island of Flores, Indonesia (Crane, 1981). By contrast, in tropical Africa, where the prevalence is considerably lower, HMS has an uneven (often tribal) distribution. In some areas of West Africa with high malarial endemicity, for example The Gambia, the condition is rare with a prevalence of approximately 1 : 1000 (Marsh and Greenwood, 1986).

Clinical picture

The clinical picture of HMS has been the subject of several reviews (Crane, 1986; Marsh and Greenwood, 1986; Greenwood, 1987) and will be dealt with only briefly here. The patient is typically a young adult with a long history of exposure to malaria. Criteria for the diagnosis of HMS are (i) massive splenomegaly (>10 cm below the coastal margin); (ii) elevation of serum IgM (>2 standard deviations above the local mean value); (iii) elevation of *Plasmodium* – specific IgM; (iv) a clinical and immunological response to antimalarial treatment. One other feature, hepatic sinusoidal lymphocytosis (see below), is often included. Severe and prolonged secondary infections, as a result of a neutropenia, accompany HMS and represent a major contribution to the high (50%) mortality rate.

Haematology and serology

Laboratory findings include chronic anaemia with a multifactorial aetiology (accelerated haemolysis, hypersplenism, hypovolaemia) and a pancytopenia. The marrow shows a compensatory haematopoiesis. Acute haemolytic episodes are common, although the DAT is not always positive during these periods and the mechanism of haemolysis remains unclear. Interestingly, malaria parasites are rarely demonstrated in blood films and other evidence for the presence of parasites, such as malaria pigment within reticuloendothelial cells, is also lacking.

Histopathological and immunological differences exist between cases studied in East and West Africa and in Papua New Guinea. For example, Nigerian patients have a greater incidence (80%) of hepatic sinusoidal lymphocytosis, although this feature is not considered pathognomic to sustain a diagnosis. Occasionally, the presence of lymphocytic infiltration has spuriously led to the diagnosis of chronic lymphocytic leukaemia (Fakunle, *et al.*, 1979). Most of the cells lining the hepatic sinusoids are T-lymphocytes (subset unknown) and there is some evidence for their sensitization to hepatic antigens (Greenwood and Fakunle, 1978). Despite this, hepatocytes appear histologically normal and cirrhosis is absent in HMS. Another regional difference is that in West African HMS there is a marked proliferation of B-lymphocytes not normally seen in cases from East Africa or Papua New Guinea.

Pathogenesis

The spleen is the major site of IgM production in HMS as evidenced by observations that IgM levels parallel spleen size and fall rapidly following splenectomy (Crane, 1986). High serum levels of immune complexes (of both malarial parasite and non-parasite origin) and IgM aggregates accompany the high IgM levels (Ziegler, 1973; Fakunle, *et al.*, 1979). Indeed the main cause of the splenomegaly is an activated reticuloendothelial system resulting from clearance of these complexes.

Recent studies have cast some light on the complicated pathogenesis of HMS (Figure 17.3). One question frequently addressed relates to the over-production of IgM. Certainly a malaria infection provides a powerful stimulus to immunoglobulin production because of the persistent and varying antigenic challenge, the presence of cross-reacting epitopes on malaria antigens, malaria-derived T-dependent and independent B-lymphocyte mitogens (Kataaha, Facer and Holborow, 1984; Kataaha, 1984) and, finally, reactivation of latent Epstein–Barr virus, itself a potent B-lymphocyte mitogen (Whittle, *et al.*, 1984; Gunapala, *et al.*, 1990). But what is the defect that results in HMS? The original hypothesis that this resides within the T-suppressor cell population (Fakunle and Greenwood, 1976) has now been supported by experimental data. Lymphocytes of the suppressor (CD8+) phenotype are normally markedly raised in acute *P. falciparum*

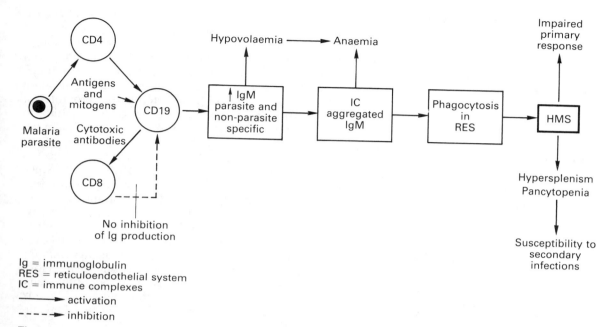

Figure 17.3 Possible pathways in the pathogenesis of HMS

infections (Table 17.4). However the reverse picture is seen in HMS (Hoffmann, *et al.*, 1984) supporting the concept of disturbed regulation of immunoglobulin production. In addition, the reduced numbers of CD8+ cells also demonstrate a functional defect. B-cells taken from HMS patients, when co-cultured with autologous CD4+ and CD8+ cells and mitogenically stimulated, produce significantly more IgM than those taken from village controls (Piessens, *et al.*, 1985). Furthermore, sera from Indonesian HMS patients contain complement-fixing antibodies that lyse CD8+ cells (Piessens, *et al.*, 1985), although these autoantibodies may well be a result rather than a cause of the enhanced IgM production. However, taken together, the above observations strongly support the hypothesis that the defective homeostatic mechanism in HMS resides within the suppressor cell population.

Genetic susceptibility

An underlying genetic susceptibility to develop HMS has always been suspected because of its limited geographical distribution, tribal prevalence and a familial tendency to develop the disease (Ziegler and Stuiver, 1972; Crane, 1981). However, early attempts to link HLA A and B locus antigens and HMS proved inconclusive (Crane, 1981). More recent tissue typing has revealed a significant association between severe HMS and HLA-DR2-related Class II antigens which may represent the determinants of immune responsiveness in HMS (Bhatia and Crane, 1985). More detailed HLA typing employing the sophisticated molecular techniques available today are obviously indicated.

Burkitt's lymphoma (BL)

The original description of lymphomas with a predilection for the jaw and ovaries of young African children was first made by Dennis Burkitt some 30 years ago. Since that time, significant progress has been made in describing the histological features of the lymphoma and linking its aetiology with the Epstein–Barr virus (EBV). However, the complex chain of events involved in the genesis of BL remains, to date, both uncertain and unclear, although recent studies have provided some insight as to how co-factors, in particular malaria, might be involved. With the unfolding of the various steps involved in BL pathogenesis, the tumour has assumed considerable importance as a model of multi-stage carcinogenesis in man. The role that malaria plays in this multi-stage process has recently been the subject of an extensive review (Facer and Playfair, 1989) and will only be summarized here.

Epidemiology

An interesting feature of BL is that it occurs in two forms, the classical endemic form (eBL; as described by Burkitt) found in equatorial Africa and Papua New Guinea, and the more recently recognized sporadic form (sBL) occurring world-wide. Both forms are clinically and histologically similar and surface marker analysis of biopsied tumour cells indicates that they both arise from cells arrested at a unique recognizable stage of B-cell differentiation. Furthermore, both eBL and sBL show uniformity in specific chromosomal translocations although fine molecular mapping shows that the chromosomal breakpoints do differ implying that eBL and sBL arise by different mechanisms (see below). One clear difference between the two lymphomas is that whereas 100% of eBL cases are associated with EBV, only 12% of sporadic cases show a similar association.

Endemic BL occurs at a rate of about one in 10,000 children per annum and shows a peak incidence between four and seven years of age. It represents not only the most common cancer of childhood in the tropics but is also the fastest growing tumour with a doubling time of 24 hours. Fortunately, this rapidity of growth is matched by the rapidity of response to cytotoxic drugs and prognosis is good. However, relapse may occur and the relapsed tumours, many of which evolve from a new clone of cells, are frequently resistant to chemotherapy.

Chromosomal translocations

All BL tumours show specific chromosomal rearrangements which are a prerequisite to the malignant transformation. Tumour cells show one of three characteristic translocations from chromosome 8 to a site on chromosome 12, 14 or 22 adjacent to the immunoglobulin genes for light chain κ, heavy chain and light chain λ respectively (Lenoir, *et al.*, 1982).

This translocation has important biological implications since the translocated part of chromosome 8 carries the cellular *c-myc* oncogene (which normally regulates cell differentiation and proliferation). The translocated *c-myc* gene thus comes into a position where it could be affected by the promoter of the active immunoglobulin gene, resulting in persistent and uncontrolled proliferation of the cell.

As mentioned above, there are differences in molecular detail between eBL and sBL which suggest that the two tumours have a different aetiology. For example, important new work has demonstrated that the translocated breakpoints are clustered 5' of the first *c-myc* exon on chromosome 8 in eBL. In contrast, in sBL, the breakpoint truncates the *c-myc* gene within the first intron or exon (Neri, *et al.*, 1988). However, despite these differences, both translocations result in deregulation of *c-myc* expression (see review by Facer and Playfair, 1989) with the same overall effect.

Co-factors

The complex pathogenesis of BL involves a multiplicity of different stages. At what stages are co-factors involved and how are they involved? Extensive epidemiological and some experimental evidence suggests that at least two co-factors are involved : EBV and malaria. The evidence implicating EBV is listed in Table 17.6. However, the virus is not *essential* for the development of BL as evidenced by the EBV-genome-negative cases of sBL. Since all eBL tumours are EBV-positive then it is possible that the other co-factor, malaria, may in some way selectively predispose individuals only to EBV-positive BL, possibly via an immunosuppression mechanism. Nevertheless if malarial immunosuppression is a key factor in the aetiology of eBL, then it must act in a different way from the drug-induced immunosuppression seen in renal transplant patients and in AIDS where immunosuppression is intense, yet Burkitt-type lymphomas are infrequent. Since EBV has a ubiquitous distribution (Henle and Henle, 1979) whereas the tumour is only found in remarkably well-defined geographical areas of high incidence, then the virus cannot act alone and additional interactive co-factors must be involved.

Table 17.5 Evidence linking malaria with the aetiology of endemic Burkitt's lymphoma

Epidemiological/Seroepidemiological

1. Endemic BL is only found in areas of holo- or hyper-endemic malaria
2. Within a given endemic area, BL is not found where (a) there are pockets of no malaria and (b) in urban areas
3. Within an endemic area, the distribution of BL is similar to that for HMS
4. Peak age incidence of BL closely follows that of severe falciparum malaria
5. Correlation between *P. falciparum* parasite rate and incidence of BL
6. Haemoglobin genotype AS may be under-represented in BL patients (to be confirmed)

Clinical/experimental

7. Post-mortem specimens from BL show heavy loading with malarial pigment
8. Experimental malaria infection of laboratory animals enhances the oncogenic potential of tumour viruses

Immunological

9. Malaria patients show impaired T-cell control of EBV
10. Lymphocytes from malaria patients spontaneously transform into proliferative immortal lymphoblastoid cell lines (EBV-positive)
11. Malaria antigens enhance normal lymphocyte transformation by EBV
12. Malaria antigens stimulate DNA synthesis in established EBV-positive lymphoblastoid cell lines

The role of malaria as an additional co-factor, perhaps working in concert with EBV, is supported largely from the geographical coincidence of eBL and holoendemic *P. falci-parum* malaria (Figure 17.4); a term used to describe intense and continuous malaria transmission throughout the year (Burkitt, 1969). Although this type of coincidence can never be taken as evidence for a causal relationship, malaria must be seriously considered as a major co-factor, not only from the convincing epidemiological data, but also from the clinical and laboratory evidence, and on its dramatic effects on the immune system being both immunostimulatory and immunosuppressive at the same time. Evidence implicating malaria as a co-factor has been extensively reviewed (Facer and Playfair, 1989) and is summarized in Table 17.5. It has been calculated that the overall effect of malaria is to increase the total incidence of eBL about 100-fold with all of this increase stemming from a rise in the number of EBV-positive tumours (Rickinson and Gregory, 1988).

In order to understand how malaria acts in the complex pathogenesis of the tumour, we need first to consider the origin of the lymphoma cell. Careful analysis of membrane characteristics of these cells indicates that the tumour phenotype precisely matches that of a normal subset of B-cell centroblasts from within the germinal centres of lymphoid tissue. Given this information, one proposal that follows is that the tumour represents a malignant proliferation arising from a single germinal centre centroblast (Gregory, *et al.*, 1987). Malarial infection is seen as a high risk factor

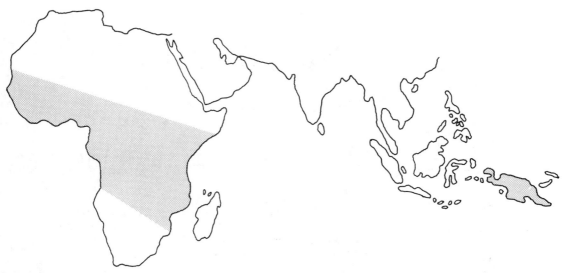

Figure 17.4 Geographical distribution of eBL is restricted to those areas where malaria is holoendemic

Table 17.6 Evidence implicating EBV as an aetiological agent in eBL

1. High titre of antibodies (and unique pattern of reactivity) to EBV antigens in all children with eBL
2. 98% of cases of eBL show multiple copies (up to 1,000) of the viral genome in each tumour cell
3. High titres (8–10 times greater than the local mean) of VCA antibodies in pre-Burkitt sera
4. EBV transforms B-lymphocytes *in vitro*
5. EBV transforms B-lymphocytes *in vivo* to produce polyclonal tumours in sub-human primates and immunosuppressed subjects

since it is known to induce chronic hyperactivity of germinal centres (see below) thereby increasing the chances of a chromosomal translocation.

How does malaria cause germinal centre hyperactivity? The asexual blood stage of the malaria parasite produces antigens containing characteristic repeat epitopes (Kemp, *et al.*, 1986) which act as T-cell independent antigens (as do most repeated antigens). Repeated epitopes stimulate centroblasts to proliferate so increasing the number of cell divisions and the chances of a genetic accident (Figure 17.5). EBV infection of a centroblast then follows. If the Burkitt lymphoma cell originates from an EBV-infected malaria antigen-stimulated centroblast, then it might be expected to produce low affinity IgM with specificity for a repeat epitope of a malaria polypeptide.

Other effects of malaria include disturbance of T-cell control of EBV in children or adults with acute (Whittle, *et al.*, 1984; Gunapala, *et al.*, 1990) and sub-clinical (Moss, *et al.*, 1983) malaria. A direct effect of this would be an increase in the number of EBV-infected B-cells within the lymphocyte population. The observation that *P. falciparum*-derived polypeptides are capable of enhancing lymphocyte transformation by EBV *in vitro* (Kataaha, *et al.*, 1984) adds additional weight for malaria as a co-factor.

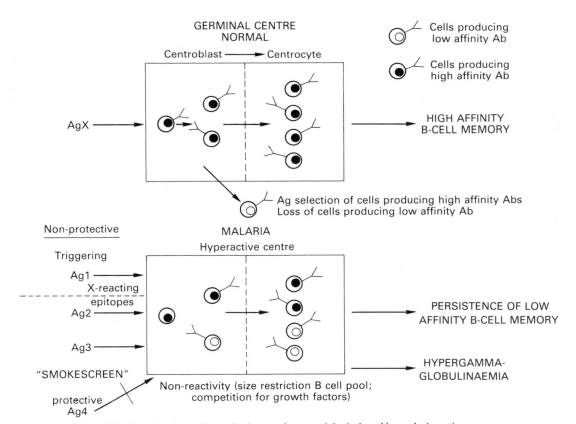

Figure 17.5 Polyclonal B-cell activation and germinal centre hyperactivity induced by malaria antigens

To summarize, there are at least three immunological roles for malaria as a co-factor: as a stimulator of polyclonal B-cell proliferation (including centroblasts); as a mediator of defective cell-mediated cytotoxicity to EBV; and last, but not least, as an enhancer of EBV-induced lymphocyte transformation (and, perhaps, EBV genome amplification). Children in equatorial Africa would experience all three effects during the frequent and protracted bouts of falciparum infection from the age of six months to around five years. One loose end still remains to be tied and that is why, in a population of individuals infected with both EBV and malaria, only a small number proceed to develop BL? The results of the prospective study in Uganda (de Thé, 1978) suggest that certain individuals are at special risk and evidence for a genetic predisposition should be more rigorously sought by applying today's more sophisticated technology. In addition, there is general agreement among tumour biologists that the observed incidence of all tumours world-wide is less than expected, implying that most potentially tumorogenic cells are destroyed at an early stage. From this one can speculate that a high percentage of children presenting with acute malaria will carry B-lymphocytes with malaria-induced chromosomal translocations (EBV + ?) but the majority of cells never survive to proliferate and form monoclonal tumours. Finally, the sera of children going on to develop eBL requires analysis of antibody titres to the various, now well-defined, malaria polypeptides available, and to see if these differ to titres found in the majority of age-matched controls living in the same malaria endemic region and subjected to the same intensity of malaria transmission.

Red cell polymorphisms in relation to malaria

A disease like malaria responsible for high morbidity and mortality over the millennia would be expected to select strongly for any genetic trait that reduces susceptibility. Thus various hereditary abnormalities of red cells are associated with complete or partial protection of individuals against infection with *P. vivax* and *P. falciparum*. The frequencies of such red cell abnormalities tend to be higher in areas endemic for malaria and this geographical correlation has been well documented and extensively reviewed (Luzzatto, 1979; Pasvol and Wilson, 1982). It is to be expected that within a local population, the selective advantage of protection against malaria would balance any disadvantage of the homozygous polymorphism. The following reviews the genetic red cell abnormalities associated with resistance to malaria and advances made in understanding the molecular and cellular mechanisms involved.

Haemoglobinopathies

Haemoglobin S

The high gene frequency of haemoglobin S in certain parts of Africa is a result of the selective advantage of balanced polymorphism (Allison, 1954). The carrier (AS) rate, seen as a broad band across Africa (Figure 17.6), is in the order of 10–30% of the population. It is evident that the presence of HbS does not prevent infection with *P. falciparum* but markedly reduces asexual blood parasitaemias resulting in decreased morbidity and mortality (particularly cerebral malaria) in the AS heterozygote (Luzzatto, Nivachuku-Jarrett and Reddy, 1970). In a group of Nigerian children lower *P. falciparum* parasite counts were found in sickle cell trait individuals, together with a lower average enlarged spleen index, than in normal children of the same age group (Willcox, *et al.*, 1983).

How does the presence of HbS within the red cell somehow protect against the severe effects of falciparum malaria? Attempts to explain the protective mechanisms at the cellular level were stimulated in the late 1970s following the development of short-term and continuous cultivation of *P. falciparum* within the laboratory (Trager and Jensen, 1976). By adding SS or AS erythrocytes to *P. falciparum* cultures and carefully monitoring physiological conditions, it became apparent that several protective factors were operational. First, although parasites invade and develop normally in AS erythrocytes under aerobic conditions, they become damaged if the oxygen tension is dropped to 5% (Friedman, 1979a; Pasvol and Wilson, 1982). In addition, accelerated sickling of cells containing parasite ring forms has been noted and the enhanced destruction of

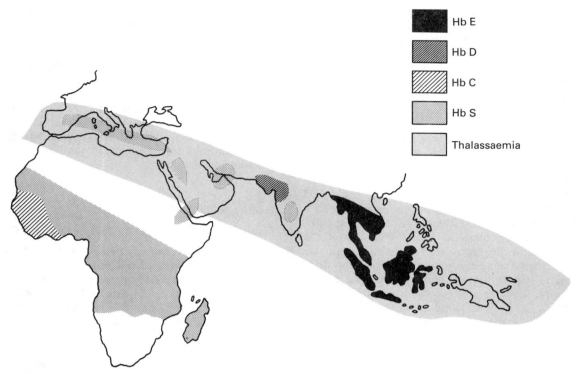

Figure 17.6 Geographical distribution of the haemoglobinopathies and thalassaemias. All overlap with the distribution of past and present malaria

parasitized red cells is probably one of the mechanisms responsible for which HbS carriers are afforded protection against *P. falciparum*. The mechanisms of parasite death in sickled AS and SS cells is not fully understood. Parasites in SS cells exhibit disruption of the parasitophorous vacuole and other membranes, probably due to the mechanical effects of polymerized haemoglobin (Friedman, 1979b) at low oxygen tensions. Since mature *P. falciparum* parasites (trophozoites and schizonts) are sequestered in tissues where the oxygen tension is low (5%) then it is these stages which might be damaged *in vivo*. However, since damaged parasites can also be seen in non-sickled AS cells taken from *in vitro* cultures (Pasvol, Weatherall and Wilson, 1978), then other more subtle mechanisms of a metabolic nature are implied. For example, at low oxygen tensions, the intracellular pH of the infected red cell drops considerably and this is accompanied by efflux of potassium from the cell (Friedman, *et al.*, 1979). Other characteristics

of the heterozygous AS erythrocyte may afford some protection against malaria. Thus the decreased deformability of infected and sickled cells, might result in their increased susceptibility to phagocytosis within splenic sinusoids.

Whether the metabolic and physical mechanisms discussed above are also effective against the other three species of human malarial parasite (*P. vivax*, *P. malariae* and *P. ovale*) remains unknown, since we are still unable to grow these species in continuous *in vitro*. cultivation in order to dissect their growth under defined conditions. However, since none of them show the convincing geographical coincidence exhibited by *P. falciparum* and HbS, then one suspects that there is little or no protective effect.

An interesting observation to have emerged in recent years is that parasites grown in erythrocytes containing HbS have a decreased response to chloroquine *in vitro* (Nguyen-Dinh and Parvin, 1986). When chloroquine sensitive parasites were grown in AA, AS or SS cells (*in vitro* at 18% O_2), chloroquine sensitivity was repeatedly diminished in SS cells showing an approximate six-fold decrease in sensitivity. The converse was also true in that one chloroquine-resistant isolate when grown in SS cells, became chloroquine-sensitive when grown in AA cells. The existence of HbS within a population can produce a false impression of chloroquine resistance in those epidemiological surveys which utilize *in vitro* screening tests. Whether the phenomenon applies *in vivo* remains to be established.

HbC, E and F

Evidence linking the other common haemoglobin disorders with protection against the severe effects of malaria has been less forthcoming. Haemoglobin C disease (HbC is another β chain variant) occurs commonly in West Africa, the carrier rate being highest in Ghana with an incidence of 16–28% (Figure 17.6). Further north, lower frequencies are found until, for example, in The Gambia, frequencies of only 1% are apparent (Facer and Brown, 1979a).

Despite the high frequencies of HbC in some African countries, there is no convincing data available in support of a protective effect of this haemoglobinopathy against malaria. For example, in a Liberian study, the number of patients with clinical *P. falciparum* malaria and the HbC trait was not significantly lower than in the normal patient population (Willcox, *et al.*, 1983). Nevertheless, before any valid conclusions can be made about this lack of association, a similar study needs to be performed in a country such as Ghana where the trait is present at a much higher frequency.

Culture of *P. falciparum* in cells containing HbC has revealed only minor effects on parasite multiplication as a result of a decrease in invasion and growth within AC and CC cells (Friedman, *et al.*, 1979; Pasvol and Wilson, 1982). These, all the same, might be important at an epidemiological level. In contrast to the heterozygous AS individual, HbC carriers are relatively healthy and, one might expect, therefore less selective pressure in order to maintain the gene frequency.

Yet another β chain variant, HbE (β26 Glu Lys), is found predominantly in malarious areas of South-East Asia. Here the β^E gene is only one of several mutant red cell genes and in some

areas, for example central Indochina, α and β thalassaemia and G6PD deficiency are so common that calculations suggest only 15% of the population has 'normal' red cells. Two early epidemiological studies compared the relative frequencies of HbE and *P. falciparum* infection in different parts of South-East Asia which resulted in contradictory conclusions (Flatz, Pik and Sundharagiati, 1964; Krauatrachue, *et al.*, 1969). Similarly, data from *in vitro* culture experiments have also led to differing conclusions, and HbE either decreased *P. falciparum* growth (Nagel, *et al.*, 1981) or had no effect (Santiyonont and Wilairat, 1981; Pasvol and Wilson, 1982). HbE is oxidatively unstable (Frisher and Bowman, 1975) and under conditions of between 5 and 20% oxygen tension, parasite growth decreased in proportion to the concentration of HbE (AA > AE > EE > EF; Vernes, *et al.*, 1986). The use of antioxodants partially reversed this situation indicating that at least some parasite death could be attributed to oxidant damage.

There is more convincing evidence for the protective effect of foetal haemoglobin F (HbF). Thus *P. falciparum* grown in cord blood cells or in cells from adults with hereditary persistence of HbF (HPFH), shows retarded growth (Pasvol, Weatherall and Wilson, 1977; Friedman, 1979a). Although the mechanisms behind this remain unknown, the effects of oxidant stress have been claimed (Friedman, 1979a). Given the apparent parasite growth-regulating effect of HbF as demonstrated *in vitro*, what are the implications at the population level? First, it would explain the prevalence of HPFH in malarious areas. It would also contribute towards the protection of infants against malaria during the first six months of life (in addition to the transplacental acquisition of maternal anti-malarial IgG). Finally, in many of the haemoglobinopathies (particularly thalassaemia) there is a clear retardation in the foetal to adult switch during the first five years of life at a time when morbidity and mortality from malaria is greatest.

Thalassaemia

The inherited defects of either α or β globin chain production (the α and β thalassaemias respectively) appear to co-incide where malaria was (Mediterranean) or still remains (West Africa, Middle East, Far East, India) endemic and in certain areas it can reach a high frequency with a carrier rate of between two and 10% (Weatherall, 1983). The frequency of α-thalassaemia exhibits an altitude and latitude dependent correlation with malarial endemicity in Melanesia which is not present for other unlinked polymorphisms in the same areas. β-thalassaemia may occur in association with structural haemoglobin variants, e.g. HbS, C or E, the latter an extremely common finding in South-East Asia with a clinical picture very similar to that of homozygous β thalassaemia.

Epidemiological observations imply that thalassaemia may well protect against the severe effects of malaria. One Liberian study found that children heterozygous for β-thalassaemia had lower *P. falciparum* parasitaemias and correspondingly lower morbidity and mortality. The percentage of patients presenting with clinical malaria and carrying the β-thalassaemia trait was less than that observed among the general population (5.5% against 9.0% respectively; Willcox, *et al.*, 1983).

The cellular mechanism(s) by which thalassaemia affords protection against clinical malaria has not been fully elucidated and, indeed, the mechanism may differ between the α and β condition. It has been suggested that the relative susceptibility of thalassaemic cells (α and β) to oxidant stress is responsible for the failure of parasites to survive within them under *in vitro* conditions of high oxygen tension (Friedman, 1979a) although at low oxygen tensions (5%) *P. falciparum* grows normally (Pasvol and Wilson, 1982). It is possible that components in the nutrient-rich medium used for *P. falciparum* culture may lead to 'masking' of the effects of oxidant stress which may be revealed with the use of a modified medium containing a markedly reduced content of glutathione and amino acids. This modification had been reported to unmask growth inhibition of *P. falciparum* in haemoglobin H disease and β-thalassaemia minor (Brockelman, *et al.*, 1987) but not in α-thalassaemic cells (Luzzi, personal communication). This may reflect a difference in the mechanisms whereby thalassaemia protects against malaria.

In an attempt to clear the controversy that exists concerning β-thalassaemia and protection against malaria disease, Roth and co-workers (1988) have used an animal model system and found that β-thalassaemia plays an inhibitory role in the growth of parasites *in vivo*. They utilized the recently described β-thalassaemic C57 BL/6J mice and infected them with *P. chabaudi*, a murine malaria parasite. Lower parasitaemias developed in the infected thalassaemic mice. Interestingly, mice in which the thalassaemia had been transgenically corrected with the human β^A-globin gene, infection with *P. chabaudi* proceeded as in normal mice, strongly implicating resistance associated with the thalassaemic condition. It must be emphasized however, that the thalassaemic condition in mice is comparable with a mild thalassaemia intermedia or pronounced β-thalassaemia trait in humans and thus only approximates the human carrier state of β-thalassaemia trait and is not identical to it.

An alternative immunological mechanism might explain the protective effect of β-thalassaemia and the lower parasitaemias observed in carriers of the trait. Erythrocytes taken from patients with β^0 and β^+ major and intermedia, have reduced amounts of membrane sialic acid (Kahane, *et al.*, 1980) resulting in exposure of underlying galactosyl residues. As a result, naturally occurring serum antigalactosyl IgG binds to these 'unmasked' cryptic antigenic sites in the circulation with subsequent phagocytosis of the thalassaemic cell by the reticuloendothelial system (Galili, *et al.*, 1983). Thus parasites growing within thalassaemic cells might be preferentially phagocytosed.

The high frequency of α-thalassaemia in areas of Papua New Guinea, Thailand and Africa, have been explained by the selective action exerted by malaria in these regions (Oppenheimer, *et al.*, 1984). The major genetic disorder of the South-West Pacific islands, is α^+-thalassaemia (deletion of one of the two α-globin genes), a condition which was virtually impossible to detect until the recent introduction of DNA probe technology. The newly emergent results clearly show that α-thalassaemia is the most prevalent haemoglobinopathy and indeed confirms its proposal as the most common genetic disorder of man (Haldane, 1949). Microepidemiological studies in Melanesia show that in highly malarious north coastal Papua New Guinea gene frequencies of almost 70% are found for α-thalassaemia. In the non-malarious highlands, this falls to under 5%. The α-gene frequencies show a remarkable parallelism to malarial endemicity (Hill, 1987). In this region, other haemoglobinopathies which might interact with α-thalassaemia are rare or absent, although a genetic trait affecting the red cell membrane, Melanesian ovalocytosis, is present and does influence resistance to malaria (see below).

Several attempts have been made to provide an explanation for the strong epidemiological coincidence between malaria and α-thalassaemia but possible protective mechanisms remain controversial.

As discussed above, the one possible mechanism whereby α-thalassaemia may protect against *P. falciparum* does not appear to rely on oxidant sensitivity of these cells but instead may reflect surface membrane differences on the thalassaemic cells. Preliminary studies have suggested that agglutination of parasitized α-thalassaemic cells with malaria immune serum (related to parasite-dependent neoantigens expressed on the red cell surface) may be greater than for normal parasitized cells (Luzzi and Pasvol, personal communication). Furthermore parasitized thalassaemic cells showed a high propensity for being phagocytosed by peripheral blood monocytes in an *in vitro* system (Yuthauong, *et al.*, 1988) as for β-thalassaemic erythrocytes (see above). Since thalassaemic erythrocytes also express more surface membrane HLA antigens than normal red cells, the possibility that cellular cytotoxicity involving Class I antigen and cytotoxic T-cells is involved requires investigation.

Finally, if the high frequencies of haemoglobinopathies are the result of selection by malaria, then in populations free of the disease, such genetic variants should be rare or absent. This is indeed the case for Icelandic and British populations with respect to α^+-thalassaemia. However, in certain tropical populations which have been exposed to more intense malaria than Melanesian islanders, the prevalence of α^+-thalassaemia is lower. It seems likely that this results from the higher frequencies of other more strongly selected variants in these areas such as HbS in Africa and HbC in South-East Asia.

Glucose-6-phosphate dehydrogenase deficiency

G6PD represents the most polymorphic locus known in man for which more than 300 alleles are known. That genetic variability at this locus relates to infection is suggested by the fact that some alleles are more frequent in malarious areas than can be accounted for by mutation alone. It was suggested some thirty years ago that the X-linked Gd- gene was selected by *P. falciparum* malaria (Allison, 1960) and since that time considerable evidence has accumulated to support the concept. This evidence has been in the form of geographical (Motulsky, 1960) and field data (Luzzatto, 1979) and, more recently, from malaria *in vitro* culture studies (Friedman, 1979a; Golenser, *et al.*, 1983; Roth, *et al.*, 1983; Yoshida and Roth, 1987).

G6PD- is common among the populations of present and past malaria-endemic regions. For example, Gd (A−), associated with 10–15% of normal red cell G6PD activity, is found in 10–20% of Negro populations. Similarly Gd Mediterranean B(−), associated with a more severe deficiency, is commonly found among Mediterranean, South-East Asian and South Pacific populations. It is generally accepted that malaria has been a major selective pressure for the spread of these common deficiency variants.

How can this apparent protection be explained at the cellular level? The comparative growth of *P. falciparum* in G6PD− and G6PD+ cells has provided several clues. The conclusion of most studies has been that *in vitro* G6PD− erythrocytes are invaded normally but that maturation of intracellular parasites is delayed and impaired resulting in a decreased parasitaemia over two to three growth cycles compared to that seen in the parallel G6PD+ cultures (Friedman, 1979a; Roth, *et al.*, 1983; Miller, Golenser and Spira, 1984; Usanga and Luzzatto, 1985; Mallinder and Facer, unpublished observations). One explanation for the decreased growth was the oxidant sensitivity of the G6PD− cells at the high (30%) O_2 tensions employed. However, decreased growth during the first few growth cycles was also observed at lower oxygen tensions of 17% (Luzzatto, Sodeinde and Martini, 1983; Roth, *et al.*, 1983). The difference in results may have been due to the use of less oxidant sensitive G6PD A- cells in the earlier work whereas both Roth, *et al.* (1983) and Luzzatto and colleagues (1983) employed the more oxidant sensitive G6PD− (Mediterranean) cells. Several explanations have been proposed to explain the relative protection against *P. falciparum* in girls heterozygous for G6PD deficiency but not in hemizygous G6PD(−) boys (Bienzle, *et al.*, 1972; Luzzatto, *et al.*, 1983). G6PD-deficiency, as mentioned earlier, is an X-linked trait. Thus female heterozygotes are mosaics in that they have two populations of red cells, one has normal enzyme activity and the other is deficient. Since males are hemizygous for the X-chromosome, all the red cells will be either G6PD deficient or not (Figure 17.7). When *P. falciparum* was grown in African G6PD deficient (A−) or Mediterranean deficient (B−) cells for more than three growth cycles, the parasite surprisingly improved its ability to multiply in the deficient cells. This adaptive change we now know is a result of up-regulation of a parasite-encoded G6PD gene (Hempelmann and Wilson, 1981; Usanga and Luzzatto, 1985; Yoshida and Roth, 1987; Roth and Schulman, 1988). The *P. falci-*

parum G6PD gene is only weakly active when the parasite grows in normal cells but the activity of the enzyme rapidly increased in G6PD− erythrocytes. This is an example of variant gene expression in response to the parasite's environment rather than selection of new parasite mutants. Sequences in the parasite genome hybridize with human G6PD cDNA (Yoshida and Roth, 1987).

The putative *P. falciparum* G6PD migrates as a slow-moving anodal band on starch gel electrophoresis (Hemplemann and Wilson, 1981; Yoshida and Roth, 1987) and also exhibits unique kinetic properties in that it has a higher affinity for its substrate (G6P and NADP) and could therefore be physiologically more active than its human equivalent.

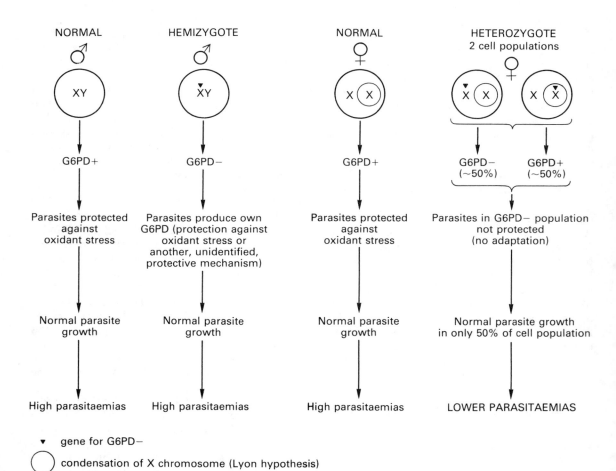

▼   gene for G6PD−

◯   condensation of X chromosome (Lyon hypothesis)

Figure 17.7 G6PD deficiency and protection against severe *P. falciparum* malaria

It seems clear therefore that the parasite can adapt to G6PD deficient red cells. However, the function of the parasite enzyme remains somewhat obscure. It should be remembered that both the parasite and the host red cell must be protected from oxidative stress otherwise parasite growth will be impaired. It is well documented that the principal role of red cell G6PD is to provide NADPH as a needed co-factor in the enzymatic reduction of oxidized glutathione (GSSH) (Eaton and Brewer, 1974). That parasite G6PD might similarly protect the deficient cell against oxidant stress was considered a possibility. Results showed an increase in resistance to the oxidant drug phenylhydrazine by parasites adapted to G6PD- (Mediterranean) cells as compared to unadapted ones, but still the parasite system remains four times more sensitive to the oxidant than normal (G6PD +) infected cells (Roth and Schulman, 1988). This probably relates to the fact that the amount of parasite-produced G6PD only reaches about 5% of the activity of normal red cells (Yoshida and Roth, 1987) and, although this may be physiologically more active, it is still not sufficient to give complete protection against oxidant stress. Alternatively, the role of parasite G6PD might not be related at all to oxidative stress resistance and may have another function.

The behaviour of *P. falciparum* in G6PD − cells described above, explains why hemizygous G6PD − males are not protected against severe malaria whereas heterozygous females are (Figure 17.7). In the female mosaic, parasites have a 50:50 chance of infecting a normal or deficient cell. Having successfully invaded a G6PD − cell the chances of it completing its growth in that cell are reduced. In the male hemizygote parasites only grow in G6PD − cells and therefore adaptation takes place following several cycles of schizogony *in vivo*. Thus the high frequency of the gene for G6PD − is maintained by the selective advantage against malaria of the female heterozygote specifically related to the dual red blood cell population.

Blood group antigens and malaria invasion

There appears to be no link between ABO blood groups and *P. falciparum* malaria (Facer and Brown, 1979b), although a higher incidence of *P. vivax* malaria in persons of blood group A

has been reported (Gupta and Chowdhuri, 1980). The following represents only a brief overview of parasite invasion in relation to blood group determinants and the reader is referred to two recent publications on the subject (Hadley and Miller, 1988; Mitchell and Bannister, 1988).

Duffy blood group determinants

An outstanding example of how absence of a blood group antigen can protect against infection relates to malaria and the Duffy blood group system. In contrast to the situation with *P. falciparum* and the haemoglobinopathies and enzyme deficiencies where protection is only partial, individuals negative for the Duffy antigens Fy^a and Fy^b are *totally* resistant to infection with *P. vivax*. Thus in West Africa and amongst American blacks derived from these populations, the Fy (a − b −) phenotype predominates (approximately 90% are Duffy negative) and *P. vivax* infection is not encountered (Welch, *et al.*, 1977). Duffy negative individuals do, however, remain susceptible to infection by *P. falciparum*, *P. malariae* and *P. ovale*.

That the resistance to infection by *P. vivax* observed in Fy (a − b −) individuals might be explained by the fact that Fy^a and Fy^b-related antigens act as ligands on the erythrocyte membrane for the *P. virax* merozoite, was first suggested by Miller and colleagues (Miller, *et al.*, 1976). Unfortunately it remains impossible to culture *P. vivax in vitro*, possibly because of the reticulocyte dependence of the parasite. However *P. knowlesi*, the 'monkey equivalent' of *P. vivax* can be grown *in vitro* and, like *P. vivax*, fails to invade human Fy (a − b −) cells and it is likely that both parasites utilize a ligand site(s) associated with Duffy antigens. More recently the Duffy Fy^6 antigen has been implicated in invasion. Fy^6 is present on all Fy (a + b +) human and *Aotus* monkey erythrocytes but is absent on Fy (a − b −) cells. An anti-idiotype made to anti-Fy^6 antibodies was found to effectively bind to *P. knowlesi* merozoites (Barnwell, unpublished observations).

Merozoite invasion of red cells involves three main stages; attachment to the cell, junction formation and interiorization. The data available on *P. knowlesi* and *P. vivax* indicate that there are at least two different receptor-ligand interactions involved in this complex process. One is necessary for attachment and occurs with either Duffy negative or Duffy positive erythrocytes. The second receptor-ligand interaction is required for the other two stages and only occurs with Duffy positive cells. Attempts are currently in progress to identify the *P. knowlesi* proteins involved in this process. A 135 kD protein binds to Duffy-positive human erythrocytes but not to Duffy negative cells (Haynes, *et al.*, 1987) and may represent one parasite receptor for the Duffy ligand.

Glycophorin

Definition of the erythrocyte ligand(s) recognized by *P. falciparum* merozoites is equally, if not more, complex than that described above for *P. vivax*. Several lines of evidence have indicated that the red cell sialoglycoproteins, glycophorins A, B and C are involved and the topic has been extensively reviewed (Hermentin, 1987). Thus trypsin, which cleaves off a large external segment of glycophorin A and C (glycophorin B on the intact cell is insensitive to trypsin degradation) renders erythrocytes largely refractory to *P. falciparum* invasion (Miller, *et al.*, 1977; Perkins, 1981; Pasvol, *et al.*, 1982; Facer, 1983). Glycophorin A-deficient (En(a-)) red cells are similarly partially resistant to invasion (Miller, *et al.*, 1977; Perkins, 1981; Facer, 1983). Furthermore, monoclonal antibodies recognizing defined epitopes on glycophorin, also reduce invasion (Facer, 1984), although the observed effects on invasion may result from a decreased red cell deformability following antibody attachment rather than by a ligand-blocking phenomenon (Pasvol and Wilson, 1989). Nevertheless, glycophorin A cannot be the sole ligand since cells lacking this sialoglycoprotein are still invaded albeit at a reduced rate compared with normal human erythrocytes.

En(a-) cells become even more resistant to invasion following trypsinization, suggesting that glycophorin C contains important epitopes recognized by merozoites (Facer, 1983). The observation that cells deficient in glycophorin C show only 57% of the invasion seen into normal human red cells, endorses this suggestion (Pasvol, Anstee and Tanner, 1984).

The $S^-s^-U^-$ or $S^-s^-U^+$ genotype is present in higher frequencies in Africa, compatible with balanced polymorphism. These cells, which lack glycophorin B, show a 30–60% reduction in the invasion rate by *P. falciparum* merozoites (Facer, 1983). Trypsin treatment of these cells, which removes the N-terminal portions on glycophorin A and C, renders them almost refractory to invasion (Facer, 1983).

Evidence for the Wright b (Wr^b) blood group antigen on glycophorin A as a distinct epitope for invasion, came from the observation that red cells of the only known individual (M.Fr) lacking the Wr^b antigen (but having otherwise normal sialoglycoproteins) were refractory to invasion (Pasvol, *et al.*, 1982). However exhaustive testing of cells from the same donor in a number of laboratories and using different isolates of *P. falciparum*, in fact showed no evidence of resistance to invasion (Facer and Mitchell, 1984; Hermentin, 1987), and thus the specific role of this determinant in invasion is denied.

The sites on glycophorin to which merozoites attach are thought to be the O-linked oligosaccharide side chains, with the active site being sialic acid or containing sialic acid (Hermentin, *et al.*, 1987). However, the situation is not as clear cut as this, since we now know that Tn erythrocytes, which lack both sialic acid and galactose on the O-linked tetrasaccharides, although resistant to most strains of *P. falciparum*, are invaded normally by one strain designated Thai-Tn (Mitchell, *et al.*, 1986). Thus at least two ligands are involved during invasion depending on the parasite strain involved: one is sialic acid and the other remains unknown but is independent of neuraminic acid.

More recently the rare M^kM^k cells which are deficient in both glycophorin A and B, were evaluated for susceptibility to invasion. According to the results obtained with En (a-) and S^-s^- erythrocytes, these cells might have been expected to show almost complete resistance to invasion, but this was not found to be the case (Hadley and Miller, 1988). Thus the data obtained with M^kM^k erythrocytes indicate that red cell components additional to the glycophorins A, B and C, for example band 3, should be investigated as potential ligands. Since the aim of defining the receptor-ligand interaction between parasite and red cell respectively is not only to understand the basic biology of the parasite but also to develop an invasion-blocking vaccine, then the evidence for more than one such interaction has important implications. For example, a vaccine employing a sialic acid-dependent parasite receptor would not be effective against a strain of *P. falciparum* that utilized the sialic acid-independent pathway for invasion.

A variety of parasite proteins have been described which bind either to isolated glycophorin or to glycophorin on intact erythrocytes. These include 140 kD, 70 kD and 35 kD polypeptides (Jungery, *et al.*, 1983), proteins of 155 kD and 130 kD (Perkins, 1984) and, more recently, antigens of 175 kD, 120 kD and 65 kD (Camus and Hadley, 1985). Monoclonal antibodies to both the 155 kD protein and the 195 kD glycoprotein (a major constituent of the merozoite surface membrane) block invasion *in vitro* suggesting that these proteins may be involved in recognition of erythrocytic determinants (Schmidt-Ullrich, *et al.*, 1986).

Finally, a recent report describes a role for the calcium-binding modulator protein, calmodulin, in invasion by *P. falciparum* merozoites (Matsumoto, *et al.*, 1987). Potent calmodulin antagonists inhibited invasion in a dose-dependent manner and also affected the aggregation of calmodulin at the apical end of merozoites. The conclusion was that calmodulin plays an important role during attachment to and/or invasion of the host erythrocyte, possibly through activation of a Ca^{2+} dependent process. The importance of calmodulin during the process of invasion and also its suggested involvement in the development of chloroquine resistance, should become clearer following the recent cloning of the *P. falciparum* calmodulin gene (K. Robson, unpublished observations).

Melanesian ovalocytosis

One common hereditary red cell defect in the lowland (malarious) areas of Papua New Guinea is stomatocytic elliptocytosis or ovalocytosis. An autosomal dominant condition, it is not associated with clinical symptoms or anaemia. As the name of the condition suggests, the red cells of individuals with the trait are oval in shape, presumably because of a red cell cytoskeletal abnormality thought to be an elongated band 3 protein. There is a geographical association between malaria and ovalocytosis, and affected individuals are less commonly infected with *P. vivax* and

P. malariae (Serjeantson, *et al.*, 1977). *In vitro* studies have shown that invasion of ovalocytes by *P. falciparum* and *P. knowlesi* merozoites is greatly reduced (Castelino, *et al.*, 1981; Kidson, *et al.*, 1981; Hadley, *et al.*, 1983; Mohandas, *et al.*, 1984). The latter group also demonstrated by ecktocytometry, that ovalocytes are less deformable than normal erythrocytes. Since *P. falciparum* and *P. knowlesi* do not share any known erythrocyte ligands for invasion, the property of ovalocytes which confers resistance to invasion is therefore likely to be the reduced membrane deformability making merozoite penetration more difficult.

Hereditary pyropoikilocytosis (HPP)

HPP is a disorder closely related to hereditary elliptocytosis (HE) in that it shares the same molecular defect of spectrin and a clinical heterogeneity which is paralleled by differences in the mutant spectrin present. The most common defect, found in about 30% of HE patients and all HPP patients, is an abnormal spectrin dimer (SpD) self-association in which the abnormality is localized on the α_1 domain of spectrin representing the SpD-SpD contact site (Palek, 1985). Several spectrin variants have been described (Palek, 1987) which result in defective SpD-SpD association into tetramers producing an unstable and less deformable cell. The amount of mutant spectrin in the cell and the severity of the spectrin self-association dictates the seriousness of HE and HPP.

In vitro experiments show that HPP cells with the $\alpha 1/74$ mutant spectrin have a variable resistance to invasion by *P. falciparum* (38–71% of the invasion into normal cells; Facer, 1986, 1989; Dhermy, personal communication). The HPP condition is of African origin and this tempts speculation that HPP and the asymptomatic carrier state may confer some protection against the severe effects of falciparum malaria. A recent systematic search for HE and HPP in West Africa has indicated that, interestingly, HE/HPP is ten times more frequent there than in Europe or the USA with the spectrin variants $Sp\alpha_1/64$ and $Sp\alpha_1/46$ predominating (Lecomte, *et al.*, 1988; Dhermy, *et al.*, 1989). It would be of obvious relevance to investigate whether these particular variant cells offer any partial protection against malaria and what the frequency of HE/HPP is in other parts of Africa.

Malaria-induced erythrocyte membrane alterations

Infection of erythrocytes with malaria parasites causes marked molecular alterations in the structure of the erythrocyte membrane integral proteins, glycolipids and phospholipids. The effects of the changes relate to an increase in cell osmotic fragility, increased passive permeability to glucose, changes (induced) in amino acid transport, and decreased ATP-ase dependent Na^+ transport (reviewed by Sherman, 1979).

Phospholipid re-organization

In normal human erythrocytes the phospholipids comprising the plasma membrane are distributed asymmetrically between the bilayer leaflets. This asymmetric distribution results in the exoplasmic leaflet being enriched in phosphatidylcholine (PC) and sphingomyelin (SM) while the cytoplasmic leaflet is enriched in phosphatidylethanolamine (PE) and contains all of the phosphatidylserine (PS). Development of malaria parasites within red cells from the ring to the schizont stage is accompanied by distinct alterations in this red cell transbilayer distribution (Gupta and Mishra, 1981; Schwartz, *et al.*, 1987). Thus in red cells infected with *P. falciparum* (but not *P. knowlesi*) there is a partial loss of the normal asymmetric organization as evidenced by increased amounts of PE and PS and a concurrent decreased amount of PC in the exoplasmic leaflet.

Permselectivity changes

Permselectivity properties of erythrocytes infected with *P. falciparum* are markedly altered, being particularly noticeable in cells containing trophozoites and schizonts as shown using molecular probes to monitor membrane transport (Kutner, *et al.*, 1985). Thus the covalent binding probe, diisothiocyanoditritostilbene disulphonic acid (H_2DIDS; an inhibitor of anion transport), impermeant to normal red cells, becomes markedly permeant to trophozoites and schizonts. Likewise permeation of the fluorescent anion transport substrate NBD-

taurine, measured in the efflux mode, is substantially enhanced in parasitized erythrocytes. Taken together, the data implies that new permeation pathways appear in membranes of malaria infected erythrocytes and that these may originate from the modification of membrane lipids described above.

One new permeation pathway found in malaria-infected erythrocytes relates to the uptake of L-glutamine, an amino acid essential for parasite growth. Normal mature human erythrocytes are relatively impermeable to L-glutamine, the influx of which is partly by diffusion but is mainly controlled by a saturable sodium-dependent process. About 10–15 hours after parasitization, the permeability of the host erythrocyte membrane to L-glutamine is enhanced about 100-fold (Elford, 1986). This modification is a selective process in that the rates of influx of other amino acids such as isoleucine, arginine and glycine remain fairly constant or are slightly increased. One interpretation of these observations is that the parasite is somehow introducing selective pores into the membrane of the host erythrocytes via the insertion of putative L-glutamine receptors. If this were so, then the parasite-induced glutamine receptor would be an ideal target for novel antimalarial compounds.

The uptake of carbohydrates such as glucose and sorbitol increases markedly in parallel with the maturation of the parasite from ring to schizont. The metabolism of glucose in parasitized cells rises some 50–100-fold being accomplished in part by parasite-directed synthesis of a protozon hexokinase with unique kinetic electrophoretic and heat stability properties (Yoshida and Roth, 1987).

One important permselectivity alteration of parasitized erythrocytes relates to the uptake of the antimalarial drug, chloroquine. Interestingly, red cells parasitized with strains of *P. falciparum* resistant to chloroquine, accumulate the drug at a much lower level. The reason for this is uncertain at present although one theory envisages a putative chloroquine pump analogous to the p-glycoprotein on drug-resistant cancer cells, inserted by the parasite into the parasite vacuole membrane and/or erythrocyte membrane, which functions to pump out the passively accumulated chloroquine from the parasitic phagolysosome (Foote, *et al.*, 1989).

Neoantigens, cytoadherence and cerebral malaria

Cytoadherence of *P. falciparum* refers to the ability of erythrocytes infected with the mature asexual stages (trophozoites and schizonts) to attach to endothelial cells lining the blood capillaries. Thus schizonts of *P. falciparum* do not appear in the peripheral circulation but become sequestered within the blood vessels of several organs, most notably in the brain (MacPherson, *et al.*, 1985), the placenta of primigravidae (McGregor, 1978) and the heart capillaries (Merkel, 1946). Cerebral malaria, the most common clinical manifestation of a severe *P. falciparum* infection and carrying a 25% mortality (MacPherson, *et al.*, 1985), is a result of this phenomenon. Infected schizonts cytoadhere to cerebral endothelial cells, thereby obstructing microcirculatory flow and oxygen delivery. There are two possible advantages of cyto-adherence to the parasite; sequestration within an environment of low oxygen tension which is required for full maturation, and as a means of avoiding passage through the spleen. As the parasite matures from ring to schizont, the parasitized erythrocyte becomes progressively less deformable (Lee, *et al.*, 1982) and, as a result, becomes a target for phagocytosis within splenic sinusoids. In addition, the surface of the parasitized erythrocyte is altered with the expression of neoantigens (Howard and Barnwell, 1983; Sherman and Greenan, 1986), thereby promoting phagocytic activity.

For most strains of *P. falciparum* the ability to sequester and cytoadhere is acquired at the same time as the appearance of characteristic knob-like protrusions on the surface of the red cell (Howard, 1988), although there are exceptions as discussed below. Viewed under the electron microscope, knobs appear as 30–40 nm projections comprising electron dense material which decrease in size from the trophozoite to schizont stage whilst increasing in density over the cell (Figure 17.8). The post-mortem material from fatal cases of cerebral malaria demonstrate that attachment to endothelial cells is via contact with the knob processes. The development of an *in vitro* assay for cyto-adherence (Udeinya, *et al.*, 1981) has been an advance in defining strains of parasites for binding potential and for determining the

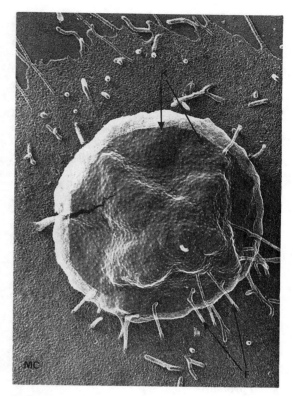

Figure 17.8 Scanning electron micrograph of a *P. falciparum*-infected erythrocyte showing numerous knobs (K) on the surface of the red cell. The schizont is bound to an amelanotic melanoma cell (MC) which filopodia (F) extend and attach to the knobs. Magnification ×17,500 (Photo courtesy of Dr S. Semoff.)

chemical nature of knobs. The assay system utilizes either monolayers of the amelanotic melanoma (C32) cell line or human umbilical cord endothelial cells, both of which express several receptors or 'adhesins' for infected erythrocytes. Using this assay system, strains of *P. falciparum* have been defined as 'knobby' and cytoadherent (K + C +) to distinguish them from the 'knobless' strains which fail to cytoadhere or bind (K − C −; Barnwell, Howard and Miller, 1983). Unfortunately, the situation is more complex than this and there are K − C + strains (Udomsangpetch *et al.*, 1989) and K + C − strains (Udeinya, *et al.*, 1981). This heterogeneity with regards to possession of knobs and cytoadherence does not solely relate to strains adapted to laboratory culture, but is likely to exist within the mixed population of parasites carried by any one infected patient. Indeed the susceptibility to develop cerebral malaria within an individual may relate to the predominance of a strain of parasite with the ability to cytoadhere. A similar situation is also seen in experimental infections of *Aotus* monkeys with *P. falciparum* which have shown that cytoadherence is a major determinant defining parasite virulence since infection with strains which do not cytoadhere in the *in vitro* test are of low virulence in the monkeys (Langreth and Petersen, 1985).

As mentioned above, expression of knobs on *P. falciparum* is not necessarily a prerequisite for cytoadherence. Similarly the schizont-infected red cells of the other human malarias express knobs but fail to sequester, and sequestration of the asexual stages in other malarias (*P. knowlesi*, *P. berghei*, *P. chabaudi*) may also occur in the absence of knobs (Howard, 1988). Thus although knobs are in some malaria parasites connected with cyto-adherence, another associated entity must finally be responsible.

Molecular definition of neoantigens and knob proteins

During maturation of the ring to the early trophozoite stage, new antigens become expressed at the surface of the infected erythro-cyte. Most appear to be anchored to the red cell cytoskeleton and the majority are localized to the knobs as shown by immunelectromicro-scopy (Langreth and Reese, 1979). Human polyspecific IgG from malaria immune donors interacts with these neoantigens expressed on the surface of the red cell to cause agglutination of K + C + schizonts (Leech, *et al.*, 1984). One important observation to emerge from *in vitro* experiments was that malaria-immune human serum had the capacity not only to inhibit cyto-adherence of K + C + cells but also to reverse their attachment (Udeinya, *et al.*, 1983), indicative of a low-affinity interaction. Simi-larly, if monkeys were passively transferred with immune serum, sequestration was reversed and trophozoites and schizonts appeared in the peripheral circulation (David, *et al.*, 1983). Their presence in the circulation was, however, short-lived, presumably because of splenic phagocytosis of the antibody-sensitized infected erythrocytes. The same experiments also demonstrate that this

phenomenon was strain-specific implying that the ligand responsible for cytoadherence was a variant strain-specific antigen or is adjacent to such a molecule so that strain-specific antibodies hinder its interaction with endo-thelial cells via steric hindrance. The apparent variant-specific, trypsin-sensitive nature of the cytoadherence ligand(s) is given credence by the observation that only one of five immunoglobulins (IgGs) from *P. falciparum* immune donors inhibited cytoadherence of the Palo Alto K − C + strain, although all gave positive immunofluorescence with the surface of the infected red cells (Udomsangpetch, *et al.*, 1989). But in the same experiments, a human IgM (K) monoclonal antibody prepared from a malaria-immune donor both stained and inhibited cytoadherence of the K − and a K + (FCR-3 strain) in a dose-dependent manner. Taken together, the results suggested a trypsin-sensitive epitope seen by the mono-clonal antibody which is associated with cyto-adherence of both K + and K − red cells.

The reversal of cytoadherence with immune serum and a monoclonal antibody is clearly relevant to the pathogenesis of falciparum malaria and may explain the propensity of non-immune individuals to develop cerebral malaria. It also suggests a novel approach to treatment although this is confounded by the strain specificity of the phenomenon (Hommel, David and Oligino, 1983).

Data accumulated from several laboratories now indicates that at least ten *P. falciparum* proteins are exported through the red cell cyto-plasm to become components of the erythrocyte membrane in K + infected cells. However only three of these proteins are intimately associated with knobs, viz. the *P. falciparum* histidine rich protein (PfHRP1) and erythrocyte membrane proteins 1 and 2 (PfEMP1 and PfEMP2). All have been reviewed extensively by Howard (1988). A schematic representation of their distribution in the membrane of infected cells is shown in Figure 17.9; PfEMP1 is considered the most likely candidate for cytoadherence. A protein with a molecular weight ranging from 250 to 300 K in different isolates (Leech, *et al.*, 1984) it appears on the surface of K + C + infected erythrocytes but not on K − C − cells (Aley, Sherwood and Howard, 1984). The remaining question was whether K + C − strains expressed the protein. Two clones from the Brazilian isolate (It), K + C + and K + C −,

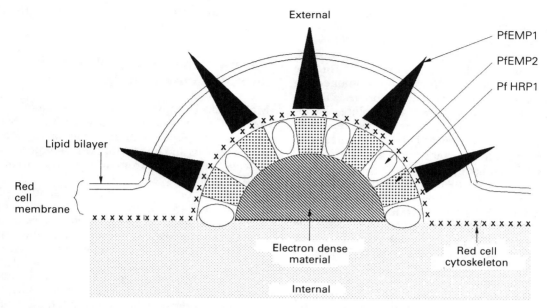

Figure 17.9 Schematic diagram of the infected erythrocyte membrane showing the distribution of knob-associated transported *P. falciparum* proteins

express PfEMP1 molecules of different sizes with the K + C − clone expressing a lower molecular weight protein. Thus, in this case, cytoadherence was correlated with the presence of PfEMP1 of a larger molecular weight (Howard, 1988). The lack of solubility of PfEMP1 in Triton-X but its extraction in sodium dodecyl sulphate (SDS) which disrupts the red cell cytoskeleton, suggests that the protein is attached to the cytoskeleton (Leech, *et al.*, 1984), possibly spectrin which would explain the alteration in deformability of mature infected erythrocytes.

A functionally important molecule such as that involved in cytoadherence might be expected to be structurally and antigenically conserved. However, PfEMP1 is antigenically diverse with the diverse epitope(s) expressed on the external surface of intact infected cells (Leech, *et al.*, 1984). Nevertheless, it is possible that the conserved portion of the molecule resides on another part of the protein also exposed on the cell surface (Howard, 1988).

PfEMP2, also located under the surface membrane of infected cells at knobs, is thought to have a role in knob structure and/or function rather than a direct role in cytoadherence. The PfHRP1 first described in *P. falciparum* by

Kilejian (1984) constitutes part of the electron dense material under knobs and is thus present in K + but not K − strains. This lack of expression in K − parasites is a consequence of a chromosomal rearrangement and deletion of part of the PfHRP1 gene (Pologe and Ravetch, 1986).

Receptors on endothelial cells for parasitized erythrocytes

Current interest resides in three proteins as candidates for the endothelial receptor(s). The first is a molecule of 80 kD designated CD36, present on platelets (where it is known as GPIV), endothelial cells, melanoma cells and monocytes. All these cells mediate cyto-adherence *in vitro*. The monoclonal antibody OKM5 directed against CD36 both inhibits and reverses binding of K + C + and K − C + cells to melanoma and endothelial cells (Ockenhouse, *et al.*; 1989, Udomsangpetch, *et al.*, 1989), indicating that the molecular events involved in both K + C + and K − C + cells are similar or identical. Schizonts from K + C + strains have also been shown to bind to purified platelet-derived CD36 immobilized on plastic (Ockenhouse, *et al.*, 1989).

A second candidate as a receptor is thrombospondin (TSP), a much studied glycoprotein of the α-granules of activated platelets (Howard, 1988). K + C +, but not K + C − parasites, specifically attach to immobilized TSP. Binding to endothelial cells *in vitro* is inhibited by soluble TSP and anti-TSP antibodies. TSP is synthesized and secreted as a soluble extracellular protein by endothelial cells and C32 melanoma cells (Howard, 1988). Asche, *et al.* (1986) have found that soluble TSP can bind to the CD36 antigen.

A third endothelial molecule used as a receptor has recently been identified. A novel cell-adhesion assay using transfected COS cells has shown that the intercellular adhesion molecule-1 (ICAM-1), widely distributed on capillary endothelial cells and inducible by cytokines, is an additional receptor for falciparum schizonts (Berendt, *et al.*, 1989). Thus it can be envisaged that cytoadherence may involve one or more different interactions: (i) TSP alone; (ii) a molecular complex of TSP and CD36; (iii) CD36 alone or (iv) ICAM-1 alone. The first option is unlikely since TSP is synthesized by cells which do not have the capacity to bind to *P. falciparum* schizonts (e.g. fibroblasts) and high concentrations of TSP are required to inhibit cytoadherence. Although CD36 has a widespread distribution on microvascular endothelium, it may not be expressed on all capillary beds where sequestration occurs, especially in the brain (Aikawa, 1988).

To conclude, the general consensus of opinion is that CD36, TSP and ICAM-1 are all contenders as sequestration receptors on endothelial cells. However, the identity of the complementary ligand on the infected erythrocyte surface remains unknown. PfEMP1 is a strong candidate as discussed earlier. The recent cloning and sequencing of a *P. falciparum* gene coding for a protein named thrombospondin related anonymous protein (TRAP) may have relevance to cyto-adherence. This 63 kD protein expressed during late asexual stages of parasite development, shares certain sequence motifs with other well characterized proteins including thrombospondin (Robson, *et al.*, 1988). In addition, TRAP shares with other adhesive glycoproteins the cell recognition signal Arg-Gly-Asp (RGD motif; Pierschbacher and Ruoslahti, 1984). The functional significance of TRAP and its point of insertion into the erythrocyte membrane remains to be determined.

The use of molecular probes for the identification of malaria parasites

Molecular biology has made considerable strides in providing species-specific DNA probes for the identification of malaria parasites within vectors and hosts with the technique now making the transition from the laboratory to the field.

Confirmation of the clinical diagnosis of malaria requires demonstration of parasites in a Giemsa-stained thick or thin blood smear, a technique little improved since its introduction in 1903. This technique, although highly sensitive, is time consuming and requires considerable experience for species differentiation and/or detection of parasitaemia if at low levels. Serum antibodies can be titred out but these do not necessarily indicate a current infection. Thus, during the last decade, several new diagnostic methods have been developed in an attempt to improve standard microscopy. The most promising current approach to diagnosis of active infection involves highly sensitive, species-specific DNA probes for the detection of *P. falciparum* and *P. vivax* (WHO, 1986). Diagnosis, based on the use of a probe containing repetitive sequences of *P. falciparum* DNA, was shown to detect a parasitaemia of 0.001%, less than that, however, of standard microscopy (0.0004%; Franzen, *et al.*, 1984). Given further refinement with regards to increasing sensitivity (perhaps using the polymerase chain reaction (PCR)) and the introduction of non-radioactive markers, the technique could have wider application. For example, besides being standardized for use in diagnosing blood infections, DNA probes could be useful in other areas such as mass screening in epidemiological and vaccination trials, screening of blood in blood banks (where a sensitivity below one parasite/μl or 0.00002% would be required) and detection of parasites within the mosquito (see below). The development and spread of multidrug resistant strains of *P. falciparum* has also stimulated the development of DNA probes to detect resistant isolates (Warhurst, personal communication).

A sensitive and accurate diagnostic test for all

four species of malaria that are pathogenic for man has recently been reported. It involves hybridization of oligonucleotides complementary to species-specific regions of the RNA of the parasite small ribosomal subunit (ssUrRNA) followed by autoradiography (Waters and McCutchan, 1989). rRNA probes were chosen since ribosomal RNA is the most abundant cellular macromolecule and so is a powerful means of microbial detection. Species-specific regions of the ssrRNA genes were obtained and used to generate complementary antisense oligonucleotides within these regions. Using the *P. falciparum* probe, it was possible to detect as little as 13 fg of target and, since a single parasitized cell contains 0.2–1.0 pg per nucleus of RNA target, the detection of parasitaemia is extremely sensitive. The method is thus at least a hundred times more sensitive than the procedure based on hybridization to repetitive DNA molecules, is quantifiable, and provides the first molecular approach to the detection of malaria that is comparable with microscopic identification of parasites. Furthermore the method retains its specificity under conditions of low stringency similar to those that will occur in field diagnosis.

One important aspect of malaria epidemiology involves accurate incrimination of mosquito vectors, and determination of the proportion of infective mosquitoes (known as the sporozoite rate). In many endemic regions the sporozoite rate is very low (<0.1%) making the usual dissection of large numbers of mosquitoes a painstaking process. Moreover, dissection does not permit identification of the species of malarial parasite in the mosquito. DNA hybridization assays using a probe for *P. falciparum* containing 21 base pairs that is repeated several thousand times in the malaria genome has recently been evaluated (Holmberg and Wigzell, 1987). The probe is sufficiently sensitive to detect around 10 pg of *P. falciparum* DNA – roughly equivalent to 500 parasites. Since about 95% of naturally infected mosquitoes are thought to carry at least 500 sporozoites in their salivary glands, the DNA hybridization technique could be useful for detecting anopheline vectors. To date, only a *P. falciparum* probe is available but it is likely that the relevant oligonucleotide probes will be developed in the future for the other species of human malarial parasites.

Conclusions

In this review the major haematologic consequences of malaria have been discussed. Attention has naturally focused on the red cell, how anaemia arises in the course of *P. falciparum* infections in humans, the variable effects on haemopoiesis, and the structural and functional alterations to the erythrocyte induced by the parasite.

There is no question that the high frequency of many of the single gene disorders in the world population, sickle cell anaemia and thalassaemia for example, is due to protection which is afforded to heterozygous carriers against malaria. However, the molecular mechanisms of this protection has been more difficult to define with inconsistency of results from different laboratories. Nevertheless, with the increasing knowledge of red cell physiology and pathology, we should soon be in a position to identify those factors in the red cell and on its surface which may make these genetically variant red cells less attractive to the parasite.

With the current urgent need for a malaria vaccine, ways of interrupting the asexual life cycle of the parasite have been investigated. One obvious way would be to prevent merozoite invasion into red cells thus preventing clinical disease and the various studies have described the importance of the red cell sialoglycoproteins as receptors for the merozoite ligand(s). Identification of those merozoite polypeptides which function as ligands should permit the development of an invasion-blocking vaccine. Likewise a vaccine that would prevent or reverse the life-threatening consequences of *P. falciparum* sequestration within cerebral capillaries is another aim. Such an intervention requires knowledge of those changes on the surface of parasitized red cells which cause them to interact with the vascular endothelium, together with identification of receptor molecules on endothelial cells to which infected erythrocytes attach.

Last, but not least, two major clinical haematological syndromes, namely Burkitt's lymphoma and hyperreactive malaria splenomegaly, in which immune events precipitated by malaria infection have been documented to play a major pathogenetic role, are discussed in the light of recent developments in this area.

Acknowledgements

The author gratefully acknowledges financial support from the Medical Research Council and The Wellcome Trust.

References

Abdalla, S. and Weatherall, D.J. (1982) The direct anti-globulin test in *P. falciparum* malaria. *British Journal of Haematology*, **51**, 415–425

Abdalla, S., Weatherall, D.J., Wickramasinghe, S.N. and Hughes, M. (1980) The anaemia of *P. falciparum* malaria. *British Journal of Haematology*, **46**, 171–183

Aley, S.B., Sherwood, J.A. and Howard, R.J. (1984) Knob-positive and knob-negative *Plasmodium falciparum* differ in expression of a strain-specific malarial antigen on the surface of infected erythrocytes. *Journal of Experimental Medicine*, **160**, 1585–1590

Allison, A.C. (1954) Protection afforded by sickle-cell trait against subtertian malaria infection. *British Medical Journal*, **i**, 290–297

Allison, A.C. (1960) Glucose-6-phosphate dehydrogenase deficiency in red blood cells of East Africans. *Nature*, **186**, 531–543

Asche, A.S., Barnwell, J., Silverstein, R.L. and Nachman, R.L. (1986) Glycoprotein IV is the thrombospondin membrane receptor. *Clinical Research*, **34**, 450A

Aikawa, M. (1988) Human cerebral malaria. *American Journal of Tropical Medicine and Hygiene*, **39**, 3–10

Barnwell, J.W., Howard, R.J. and Miller, L.H. (1983) Influence of the spleen on the expression of surface antigens on parasitized erythrocytes. *Ciba Foundation Symposium*, **94**, 117–136

Bate, C.A.W., Taverne, J. and Playfair, J.H.L. (1988) Malarial parasites induce TNF production by macrophages. *Immunology*, **64**, 227–231

Beale, P.J., Cormack, J.D. and Oldrey, T.B.N. (1972) Thrombocytopenia in malaria with immunoglobulin (IgM) changes. *British Medical Journal*, **1**, 345–349

Berendt, A.R., Simons, D.L., Tansey, J., Newbold, C.I. and Marsh, K. (1989) Intercellular adhesion molecule-1 is an endothelial cell adhesion receptors for *P. falciparum*. *Nature*, **341**, 57–59

Berzins, K., Wahlgren, M. and Perlmann, P. (1983) Studies on the specificity of anti-erythrocyte antibodies in the serum of patients with malaria. *Clinical and Experimental Immunology*, **54**, 313–318

Bhatia, K.K. and Crane, G.G. (1985) HLA and tropical splenomegaly syndrome in the Upper Watut Valley of Papua New Guinea. *Human Immunology*, **13**, 235–242

Bienzle, U., Ayeni, O., Lucas, A.O. and Luzzatto, L. (1972) Glucose-6-phosphate dehydrogenase and malaria. Greater resistance of females heterozygous for enzyme deficiency and males with non-deficient variant. *Lancet*, **i**, 107–110

Brabin, B.J. (1983) An analysis of malaria in pregnancy in Africa. *Bulletin of the World Health Organization*, **61**, 1005–1016

Brockelman, C.R., Wongsattayanont, B., Tan-Ariya, P. and Fucharoen, S. (1987) Thalassaemic erythrocytes inhibit *in vitro* growth of *Plasmodium falciparum*. *Journal of Clinical Microbiology*, **25**, 56–60

Burkitt, D. (1969) Aetiology of Burkitt's lymphoma – an alternative to a vectored virus. *Journal of the National Cancer Institute*, **42**, 19

Byles, A.B. and D'Sa, A. (1970) Reduction of reaction due to iron dextran infusion using chloroquine. *British Medical Journal*, **3**, 625–627

Camus, D. and Hadley, T.J. (1985) A *Plasmodium falciparum* antigen that binds to host erythrocytes and merozoites. *Science*, **230**, 553–556

Cartwright, G.E. and Lee, R. (1975) The anaemia of chronic disorders. *British Journal of Haematology*, **21**, 147

Castelino, D., Saul, A., Myler, P., Kidson, C., Thomas, H. and Cooke, R. (1981) Ovalocytosis in Papua New Guinea – dominantly inherited resistance to malaria. *South-East Asian Journal of Tropical Medicine and Public Health*, **12**, 549–555

Crane, G.G. (1981) Tropical splenomegaly. Part 2: Oceania. Haematology in tropical areas. *Clinics in Haematology*, **10**, 976–982

Crane, G.G. (1986) Hyperactive malarious splenomegaly (Tropical Splenomegaly Syndrome). *Parasitology Today*, **2**, 4–9

David, P.H., Hommel, M., Miller, L.H., Udeinya, I.J. and Oligino, L.D. (1983) Parasite sequestration in *Plasmodium falciparum* malaria: spleen and antibody modulation of cytoadherence of infected erythrocytes. *Proceedings of the National Academy of Sciences, USA*, **80**, 5075–5079

Devakul, K., Harinsuta, T. and Reid, H.A. (1966) ^{125}I-labelled fibrinogen in cerebral malaria. *Lancet*, **ii**, 886–888

Devakul, K., Harinasuta, T. and Kanakakorn, K. (1969) Erythrocyte destruction in *Plasmodium falciparum* malaria: an investigation of intravascular haemolysis. *Annals of Tropical Medicine and Parasitology*, **63**, 317–325

Dhermy, D., Carnevale, P., Blot, I. and Zohoun, I. (1989) Hereditary elliptocytosis in Africa. *Lancet*, **i**, 225

Dutta, P., Pinto, J. and Rivlin, R. (1985) Antimalarial effects of riboflavin deficiency. *Lancet*, **ii**, 1040–1042

Eaton, J.W. and Brewer, G.J. (1974) Pentose phosphate metabolism. In *The Red Blood Cell*, D.M. Surgenor, (ed.), pp. 436–471, Academic Press, New York

Elford, B.C. (1986) L-glutamine influx in malaria-infected erythrocytes: a target for antimalarials? *Parasitology Today*, **2**, 309–312

Essien, E.M. and Ebhota, M. (1981) Platelet hypersensitivity in acute *Plasmodium falciparium* infection in man. *Thrombosis and Haemostasis*, **46**, 547–549

Essien, E.M., Arnout, J., Deckmyn, H., Vermylen, J.B. and Verstraete, M. (1984) Blood changes and enhanced thromboxane and 6-keto prostaglandin F_{1a} production in experimental acute *P. berghei* infection of hamsters. *Thrombosis and Haemostasis*, **51**, 362–385

Facer, C.A. (1980a) Direct Coombs antiglobulin reactions in Gambian children with *P. falciparum* malaria. II. Specificity of erythrocyte-bound IgG. *Clinical and Experimental Immunology*, **39**, 279–288

Facer, C.A. (1980b) Direct Coombs antiglobulin tests in Gambian children with *P. falciparum* malaria. III. Expression of IgG subclass and determination of genetic markers and association with anaemia. *Clinical and Experimental Immunology*, **41**, 81–90

Facer, C.A. (1983) Erythrocyte sialoglycoproteins and *Plasmodium falciparum* invasion. *Transaction of the Royal Society of Tropical Medicine and Hygiene*, **77**, 524–530

Facer, C.A. (1984) Antibodies to red cell glycophorin inhibit invasion by *Plasmodium falciparum* merozoites. *IRCS Medical Science*, **12**, 314–315

Facer, C.A. (1986) The red cell cytoskeleton and invasion by malaria parasites. *Memorias do Instituto Oswaldo Cruz*, **81**, 111–114

Facer, C.A. (1989) Malaria, hereditary elliptocytosis and pyropoikilocytosis. *Lancet*, **i**, 897

Facer, C.A., Bray, R.S. and Brown, J. (1979) Direct antiglobulin reactions in Gambian children with *Plasmodium falciparum* malaria. I. Incidence and class specificity. *Clinical and Experimental Immunology*, **35**, 119–127

Facer, C.A. and Brown, J. (1979a) Incidence of abnormal haemoglobin traits among Gambian children. *Transactions of the Royal Society of Tropical Medicine and Hygiene*, **73**, 309–311

Facer, C.A. and Brown, J. (1979b) ABO blood groups and falciparum malaria. *Transactions of the Royal Society of Tropical Medicine and Hygiene*, **73**, 599–600

Facer, C.A. and Jenkins, G.C. (1989) Abnormal features of peripheral blood films from Gambian children with malaria. *Annals of Tropical Paediatrics*, **9**, 107–111

Facer, C.A. and Mitchell, G.H. (1984) Wr[b] negative erythrocytes are susceptible to invasion by malaria parasites. *Lancet*, **ii**, 758

Facer, C.A. and Playfair, J.H.L. (1989) Malaria, Epstein–Barr virus, and the genesis of lymphomas. *Advances in Cancer Research*, **53**, 33–72

Facer, C.A. and Sangster, J. (1981) Chronic falciparum malaria and anti-I autoantibodies. *Lancet*, **ii**, 1109–1110

Fajardo, L.F. and Tallent, C. (1974) Malarial parasites within human platelets. *Journal of the American Medical Association*, **229**, 1205–1207

Fakunle, Y.M. and Greenwood, B.M. (1976) A suppressor T-cell defect in tropical splenomegaly syndrome. *Lancet*, **ii**, 608–609

Fakunle, Y.M., Greenwood, B.M., Fleming, A.F. and Danon, F. (1979) Tropical splenomegaly syndrome or chronic lymphatic leukaemia? *Tropical Geographical Medicine*, **31**, 353–358

Flatz, G., Pik, C. and Sundharagiati, B. (1964) Malaria and haemoglobin E in Thailand. *Lancet*, **ii**, 385–387

Foote, S.J., Thompson, J.K., Cowman, A.F. and Kemp,

D.J. (1989) Amplification of the multidrug resistance gene in some chloroquine-resistant isolates of *P. falciparum*. *Cell*, **57**, 921–930

Franzen, L., Westin, G., Shabo, R., Aslund, L., Perlmann, H., Persson, T., *et al.* (1984) Analysis of clinical specimens by hybridization with probe containing repetitive DNA from *Plasmodium falciparum*. *Lancet*, **i**, 525

Friedman, M.J. (1979a) Oxidant damage mediates variant red cell resistance to malaria. *Nature*, **280**, 245–247

Friedman, M.J. (1979a) Ultrastructural damage to the malaria parasite in the sickled cell. *Journal of Protozoology*, **26**, 195

Friedman, M.J., Roth, E.F., Nagel, R.L. and Trager, W. (1979) *Plasmodium falciparum*: physiological interaction with the human sickle cell. *Experimental Parasitology*, **47**, 73–80

Frisher, H. and Bowman, J. (1975) Haemoglobin E, an oxidatively unstable mutation. *Journal of Laboratory and Clinical Medicine*, **85**, 531–539

Galili, U., Korkesh, A., Kahane, I. and Rachmilewitz, E.A. (1983) Demonstration of a natural antigalactosyl IgG antibody on thalassemic red cells. *Blood*, **61**, 1258–1264

Golenser, J., Miller, J., Spira, D.T., Navok, T. and Chevion, M. (1983) Inhibitory effect of a fava bean component on the *in vitro* development of *P. falciparum* in normal and glucose-6-phosphate dehydrogenase deficient erythrocytes. *Blood*, **61**, 507–510

Greenwood, B.M. (1987) Asymptomatic malaria infections – do they matter? *Parasitology Today*, **3**, 206–214

Greenwood, B.M. and Fakunle, T.M. (1978) The tropical splenomegaly syndrome: a review of its pathogenesis, in, *The role of the spleen in the immunology of parasitic diseases. Tropical Diseases Research Series*, No. 1, pp. 229–294, Schwabe and Company, Basel

Greenwood, B.M., Herrick, C.R. and Holborrow, E.J. (1970) Speckled antinuclear factor in African sera. *Clinical and Experimental Immunology*, **7**, 75–83

Gregory, C.D., Trusz, T., Edwards, C.F., Tetaud, C., Talbot, M., Caillou, B., *et al.* (1987) Identification of a subset of normal B cells with a Burkitt's lymphoma (BL)-like phenotype. *Journal of Immunology*, **139**, 313–318

Gunapala, D.G., Facer, C.A., Davidson, R. and Weir, W. (1989) *In vitro* analysis of Epstein–Barr virus: host balance in patients with acute *P. falciparum* malaria —1. Defective T-cell control. *Parasitology Research*, **76**, 531–535

Gupta, C.M. and Mishra, G.C. (1981) Transbilayer phospholipid asymmetry in *Plasmodium knowlesi*-infected host cell membrane. *Science*, **212**, 1047–1049

Gupta, M. and Chowdhuri, A.N.R. (1980) Relationship between ABO groups and malaria. *Bulletin of the World Health Organization*, **58**, 913–915

Hadley, T.J. and Miller, L.H. (1988) Invasion of erythrocytes by malaria parasites: erythrocyte ligands and parasites receptors. *Progress in Allergy*, **41**, 49–71

Hadley, T.J., Saul, A., Lamont, G., Hudson, D.E., Miller, L.H. and Kidson, C. (1983) Resistance of Melanesian elliptocytes (ovalocytes) to invasion by *P. knowlesi* and *P. falciparum* parasites *in vitro*. *Journal of Clinical Investigation*, **71**, 780–782

Haldane, J.B.S. (1949) The rate of mutation of human genes, in, *Proceedings of the 8th International Congress of Genetics* pp. 267–273

Haynes, J.D., Klotz, F.W. and Miller, L.H. (1987) A 135 kilodalton receptor molecule from malaria parasites binds to a human erythrocyte ligand associated with Duffy antigens and correlates with invasion. *Clinical Research*, **35**, 615 (A)

Hempelmann, E. and Wilson, R.J.M. (1981) Detection of glucose-6-phosphate dehydrogenase in malarial parasites. *Molecular and Biochemical Parasitology*, **2**, 197

Henle, G. and Henle, W. (1979) The virus as the aetiologic agent of infectious mononucleosis. In *The Epstein–Barr virus*, B.G. Achong, (ed.), pp. 297–320, Springer, Berlin

Hermentin, P. (1987) Malaria invasion of human erythrocytes. *Parasitology Today*, **3**, 52–55

Hill, A.V.S. (1987) Haemoglobinopathies and malaria: new approaches to an old hypothesis. *Parasitology Today*, **3**, 83–85

Hoffmann, S.L., Piessens, W.F., Ratiwayanto, S., Hussein, P.R., Kurniawan, L., Piessens, P.W., *et al.* (1984) Reduction of suppressor T lymphocytes in the tropical splenomegaly syndrome. *New England Journal of Medicine*, **310**, 337–341

Holmberg, M. and Wigzell, H.M. (1987) DNA hybridization assays for detection of malarial sporozoites. *Parasitology Today*, **3**, 380

Hommel, M., David, P.H. and Oligino, L.D. (1983) Surface alteration of erythrocytes in *Plasmodium falciparum* malaria. *Journal of Experimental Medicine*, **157**, 1137–1148

Horstmann, R.D., Dietrich, M., Bienzle, U. and Rasche, H. (1981) Malaria-induced thrombocytopenia. *Blut*, **42**, 157–164

Howard, R.J. (1988) Malarial proteins at the membrane of *Plasmodium falciparum*-infected erythrocytes and their involvement in cytoadherence to endothelial cells. *Progress in Allergy*, **41**, 98–147

Howard, R.J. and Barnwell, J.W. (1983) The roles of surface antigens on malaria-infected red blood cells in evasion of immunity. In *Contempory Topics in Immunology*, **12**, Marchatonis, pp. 127–200, Plenus Press, New York

Inyang, A.L., Sodeinde, O., Okpako, D.T. and Essien, E.M. (1987) Platelet reactions after interaction with cultured *P. falciparum* infected erythrocytes. *British Journal of Haematology*, **66**, 375–378

Jeje, O.M., Kelton, J.G. and Blajchman, M.A. (1983) Quantitation of red cell membrane associated immunoglobulin in children with *Plasmodium falciparum* malaria. *British Journal of Haematology*, **54**, 567–572

Jenkins, G.C. and Facer, C.A. (1985). The haematology of African Trypanosomiasis. In *The Immunology and Pathogenesis of Trypanosomiasis*, I.R. Tizard (ed.), pp. 13–45, CRC Press, Florida

Jungery, M., Boyle, D., Patel, T., Pasvol, G. and Weatherall, D.J. (1983) Lectin-like polypeptides of *P. falciparum* bind to red cell sialoglycoproteins. *Nature*, **301**, 704–705

Kahane, I., Ben Chetrit, E., Shifter, A. and Rachmilewitz, E.A. (1980) The erythrocyte membranes in β thalassaemia. Lower sialic acid levels in glycophorin. *Biochemica Biophysica Acta,* **596**, 10

Kataaha, P.K. (1984) Studies of lymphocyte responsiveness and autoantibody production in human malaria. *PhD Thesis,* University of London, UK

Kataaha, P.K., Facer, C.A. and Holborow, E.J. (1984) *Plasmodium falciparum* products enhance human lymphocyte transformation by Epstein–Barr virus. *Clinical and Experimental Immunology*, **56**, 371–376

Kay, M.M.D., Goodman, S.R. and Sorensen, K. (1983) Senescent cell antigen is immunologically related to band 3. *Proceedings of National Academy of Sciences, USA,* **80**, 1631

Kelton, J.G., Keystone, J., Moore, J., Denomme, G., Tozman, E., Glynn, M., *et al.* (1983) Immune-mediated thrombocytopenia of malaria. *Journal of Clinical Investigation*, **71**, 832–836

Kemp, D.J., Coppel, R.L., Stahl, H.D., Bianco, A.E., Corcoran, L.M., McIntyre, P., *et al.* (1986) Genes for antigens of *Plasmodium falciparum*. *Parasitology*, **91**, S83–S108

Kidson, C., Lamont, G., Saul, A. and Nurse, G.T. (1981) Ovalocytic erythrocytes from Melanesians are resistant to invasion by malaria parasites in culture. *Proceedings of the National Academy of Sciences, USA,* **78**, 5829

Kilejian, A. (1984) The biosynthesis of the knob protein and a 65,000 dalton histidine-rich polypeptide of *Plasmodium falciparum*. *Molecular and Biochemical Parasitology*, **12**, 185–194

Krautrachue, M., Bhaibulaya, K., Klongkamnaunkarn, K. and Harinasuta, C. (1969) Haemoglobinopathies and malaria in Thailand. *Bulletin of the World Health Organization*, **40**, 459–463

Kutner, S., Breuer, W.V., Ginsburg, H., Aley, S.B. and Cabantchik, Z.I. (1985) Characterization of permeation pathways in the plasma membrane of human erythrocytes infected with early stages of *Plasmodium falciparum*. *Journal of Cell Physiology*, **125**, 521–527

Langreth, S.G. and Petersen, E. (1985). Pathogenicity, stability and immunogenicity of a knobless clone of *Plasmodium falciparum* in Colombian owl monkeys. *Infection and Immunity*, **47**, 760–766

Langreth, S.G. and Reese, R.T. (1979) Antigenicity of the infected-erythrocyte and merozoite surface in falciparum malaria. *Journal of Experimental Medicine*, **150**, 1241–1254

Langreth, S.G., Reese, R.T., Motyl, M.R. and Trager, W. (1979b) *Plasmodium falciparum* loss of knobs on the infected erythrocyte surface after long-term cultivation. *Experimental Parasitology*, **48**, 213–219

Lecomte, M-C., Dhermy, D., Gautero, H., Bournier, O., Gautero, G. and Boivin, P. (1988) L'elliptocytose héréditaire en Afrique de l'Ouest: frequence et répartition des variants de la spectrine. *C.R. Academy Science (Paris)*, **306**, 43–46

Lee, M.V., Ambrus, J.L., de Souza, J.M.L. and Lee, R.V. (1982) Diminished red blood cell deformability in uncomplicated human malaria. *Journal of Medicine*, **13**, 479–485

Leech, J.H., Barnwell, J.W., Miller, L.H. and Howard, R.J. (1984) Identification of a strain-specific malarial antigen exposed on the surface of *Plasmodium falciparum*-infected erythrocytes. *Journal of Experimental Medicine*, **159**, 1567–1575

Lenoir, G.M., Preud'homme, J.L., Bernheim, A. and Berger, R. (1982) Correlation between light chain expression and variant translocation in Burkitt's lymphoma. *Nature*, **298**, 474

Lobel, H.O. and Campbell, C.C. (1986) Malaria prophylaxis and distribution of drug resistance. *Clinics in Tropical Medicine and Communicable Diseases*, **1**, 225–243

Lutz, H.U. and Wipf, G. (1982) Naturally occurring auto-antibodies to skeletal proteins from human red cells. *Journal of Immunology*, **128**, 1695–1699

Luzzatto, L. (1979) Genetics of red cells and susceptibility to malaria. *Blood*, **54**, 961–976

Luzzatto, L., Nirachuku-Jarrett, E.S. and Reddy, S. (1970) Increased sickling of parasitized erythrocytes as mechanisms of resistance against malaria in the sickle-cell trait. *Lancet*, **i**, 319–322

Luzzatto, L., Sodeinde, O. and Martini, G. (1983) Genetic variation in the host and adaptive phenomena in *Plasmodium falciparum* infection. *Ciba Foundation Symposium*, **94**, 159–173

MacPherson, G.G., Warrell, M.J., White, N.J., Looareesuwan, S. and Warrell, D.A. (1985) Human cerebral malaria: a quantitative ultrastructural analysis of parasitized erythrocyte sequestration. *American Journal of Pathology*, **119**, 385–401

Malaria Action Programme (1987) *World Health Statistics Quarterly*, **40**, 142–170

Marsh, K. and Greenwood, B.M. (1986) Immunopathology of malaria. *Clinics in Tropical Medicine and Communicable Diseases*, **1**, 91–127

Matsumoto, Y., Perry, G., Schebel, L.W. and Aikawa, M. (1987) Role of calmodulin in *Plasmodium falciparum*: implications for erythrocyte invasion by the merozoite. *European Journal of Cell Biology*, **45**, 36–43

McGregor, I.A. (1978) Topical aspects of the epidemiology of malaria. *Israel Journal of Medical Science*, **14**, 523–536

Merkel, W.C. (1946) *Plasmodium falciparum* malaria. The coronary and myocardial lesions observed at autopsy in two cases of fulminating *P. falciparum* infection. *Archives of Pathology*, **41**, 290–298

Merry, A.H., Looareesuwan, S., Phillips, R.E., Pleehachinda, R., Wattanagoon, Y., Ho, M., *et al.* (1987) Evidence against immune haemolysis in falciparum malaria in Thailand. *British Journal of Haematology*, **67**, 473–478

Miller, J., Golenser, J. and Spira, D.T. (1984) *Plasmodium falciparum*: thiol status and growth in normal and glucose-6-phosphate dehydrogenase deficient human erythrocytes. *Experimental Parasitology*, **57**, 239–247

Miller, L.H., Haynes, J.D., McAuliffe, F.H., Shiroishi, T., Durocher, J.R. and McGinnis, M. (1977) Evidence for differences in erythrocyte surface receptors for the malarial parasites, *P. falciparum* and *P. knowlesi*. *Journal of Experimental Medicine*, **146**, 277–281

Miller, L.H., Mason, S.J., Clyde, D.F. and McGinniss, M.H. (1976) The resistance factor to *P. vivax* in Blacks. The Duffy blood group FyFy. *New England Journal of Medicine*, **295**, 302–304

Mitchell, G.M. (1989) An update on candidate malaria vaccines. *Parasitology*, **98**, S29–S47

Mitchell, G.H., and Bannister, L.H. (1988) Malaria parasite invasion: interactions with the red cell membrane. *Critical Reviews in Oncology and Haematology*, **8**, 255–310

Mitchell, G.H., Hadley, T.J., McGinniss, M.H., Klotz, F.W. and Miller, L.H. (1986) Invasion of erythrocytes by *P. falciparum* malaria parasites: evidence for receptor heterogeneity and two receptors. *Blood*, **67**, 1519–1521

Mohandas, N., Lie-Injo, L.E., Friedman, M. and Mak, J.W. (1984) Rigid membranes of Malayan ovalocytes: a likely barrier against malaria. *Blood*, **63**, 1385

Moss, D.L., Burrows, S.R., Castellino, D., Kane, R., Pope, J.H., Rickinson, A.H., *et al.* (1983) A comparison of Epstein–Barr virus specific T-cell immunity in malaria endemic and non-endemic regions of Papua New Guinea. *International Journal of Cancer*, **31**, 727–732

Motulsky, A.G. (1960) Metabolic polymorphisms and the role of infectious diseases in human evolution. *Human Biology*, **32**, 28–62

Murray, M.J., Murray, A.B., Murray, H.B. and Murray, C.J. (1978) The adverse effect of iron repletion on the course of certain infections. *British Medical Journal*, **2**, 1113–1115

Nagel, R.L., Raventos-Suarez, C., Fabry, M.E., Tanowitz, H., Sicard, D. and Labie, D. (1981) Impairment of the growth of *P. falciparum* in HbEE erythrocytes. *Journal of Clinical Investigation*, **68**, 303–305

Neri, A., Barriga, F., Knowles, D.M., Magrath, I.T. and Dalla-Favera, R. (1988) Different regions of the immunoglobulin heavy chain locus are involved in chromosomal translocations in distinct pathogenetic forms of Burkitt's lymphoma. *Proceedings of the National Academy of Science, USA*, **85**, 2748–2752

Nguyen-Dinh, P. and Parvin, R.M. (1986) Haemoglobin S and *in vitro* chloroquine susceptibility to *Plasmodium falciparum*. *Lancet*, **ii**, 1278

Nussenweig, R.S. and Nussenweig, V. (1985) Development of a sporozoite vaccine. *Parasitology Today*, **1**, 150–152

Ockenhouse, C.F., Tandon, N.N., Magowan, C., Jamieson, G.A. and Chulay, J.D. (1989) Identification of a platelet membrane glycoprotein as a falciparum malaria sequestration protein. *Science*, **243**, 1469–1471

Oppenheimer, S.J. (1989) Iron and malaria. *Parasitology Today*, **5**, 77–79

Oppenheimer, S.J., Higgs, D.R., Weatherall, D.J.,

Barker, J. and Spark, R.A. (1984) Alpha thalassaemia in Papua New Guinea. *Lancet*, **i**, 424–426

Palek, J. (1985) Hereditary elliptocytosis and related disorders. *Clinics in Haematology*, **14**, 45–87

Palek, J. (1987) Hereditary elliptocytosis, spherocytosis and related disorders: consequences of a deficiency or mutation of the membrane skeletal protein. *Blood Reviews*, **1**, 147–168

Pasvol, G., Anstee, D. and Tanner, M.J.A. (1984) Glycophorin C and the invasion of red cells by *Plasmodium falciparum*. *Lancet*, **i**, 907–908

Pasvol, G., Jungery, M., Weatherall, D.J., Parsons, S.F., Anstee, D.J. and Tanner, M.J.A. (1982) Glycophorin as a possible receptor for *Plasmodium falciparum*. *Lancet*, **ii**, 947–950

Pasvol, G., Weatherall, D.J. and Wilson, R.J.M. (1977) Effects of foetal haemoglobin on susceptibility of red cells to *Plasmodium falciparum*. *Nature*, **270**, 171–173

Pasvol, G., Weatherall, D.J. and Wilson, R.J.M. (1978) Cellular mechanisms for the protective effect of haemoglobin S against *P. falciparum* malaria. *Nature*, **274**, 701–703

Pasvol, G. and Wilson, R.J.M. (1982) The interaction of malaria parasites with red blood cells. *British Medical Bulletin*, **38**, 133–140

Pasvol, G. and Wilson, R.J.M. (1989) Red cell deformability and invasion by malaria parasites. *Parasitology Today*, **5**, 215–218

Perkash, A., Kelly, N.I. and Fajardo, L.F. (1984) Enhanced parasitization of platelets by *Plasmodium berghei yoelii*. *Transactions of the Royal Society of Tropical Medicine and Hygiene*, **78**, 451–455

Perkins, M. (1981) Inhibitory effects of erythrocyte membrane proteins on the *in vitro* invasion of the human malarial parasite (*P. falciparum*) into its host cell. *Journal of Cell Biology*, **90**, 563–567

Perkins, M. (1984) Surface proteins of *Plasmodium falciparum* binding to the erythrocyte receptor, glycophorin. *Journal of Experimental Medicine*, **160**, 788–798

Phillips, R.E., Looareesuwan, S., Warrell, D.A., Lee, S.H., Karbwang, J., Warrell, M.J., et al. (1986) The importance of anaemia in cerebral and uncomplicated falciparum malaria: role of complications, dyserythropoiesis and iron sequestration. *Quaterly Journal of Medicine*, **227**, 305–323

Phillips, R.E. and Warrell, D.A. (1986) The pathophysiology of severe falciparum malaria. *Parasitology Today*, **2**, 271–282

Piessens, W.F., Hoffman, S.L., Wadee, A.A., Piessens, P.W., Ratiwayanto, S., Kurniawan, L., et al. (1985) Antibody-mediated killing of suppressor T lymphocytes as a possible cause of macroglobulinaemia in the tropical splenomegaly syndrome. *Journal of Clinical Investigation*, **75**, 1821–1827

Pierschbacher, M.D. and Ruoslaht, E. (1984) Cell attachment activity of fibronectin can be duplicated by small synthetic fragments of the molecule. *Nature*, **309**, 30–33

Polage, L.G. and Ravetch, J.V. (1986) A chromosomal rearrangement in a *P. falciparum* histidine-rich protein gene is associated with the knobless phenotype. *Nature*, **322**, 474–477

Raventos-Saurez, C., Pollack, S. and Nagel, R.L. (1982) *Plasmodium falciparum*: inhibition of *in vitro* growth by desferrioxamine. *American Journal of Tropical Medicine and Hygiene*, **31**, 919–922

Ree, G.H. (1971) C-reactive protein in Gambian Africans with special reference to *P. falciparum* malaria. *Transactions of the Royal Society of Tropical Medicine and Hygiene*, **65**, 574–580

Rickinson, A.B. and Gregory, C.D. (1988) Burkitt's lymphoma. *Transactions of the Royal Society of Tropical Medicine and Hygiene*, **82**, 657–659

Robson, K.J.H., Hall, J.R.S., Jennings, M.W., Harris, T.J.R., Marsh, K., Newbold, C.I., et al. (1988) A highly conserved amino-acid sequence in thrombospondin, properdin and in proteins from sporozoites and blood stages of a human malaria parasite. *Nature*, **335**, 79–82

Rodriguez, M.H. and Jungery, M. (1986) A protein on *Plasmodium falciparum*-infected erythrocytes functions as a transferrin receptor. *Nature*, **324**, 388–391

Rosenberg, E.B., Strickland, G.T., Yang, S-L. and Whalen, G.E. (1973) IgM antibodies to red cells and autoimmune anaemia in patients with malaria. *American Journal of Tropical Medicine and Hygiene*, **22**, 146–151

Roth, E.F., Raventos-Suarez, C., Rinaldi, A. and Nagle, R.L. (1983) Glucose-6-phosphate dehydrogenase deficiency inhibits *in vitro* growth of *P. falciparum*. *Proceedings of the National Academy of Sciences, USA*, **80**, 298–299

Roth, E. and Schulman, S. (1988) The adaptation of *Plasmodium falciparum* to oxidative stress in G6PD deficient human erythrocytes. *British Journal of Haematology*, **70**, 363–367

Roth, E.F., Shear, H.L., Constantini, F., Tanowitz, H.B. and Nagel, R.L. (1988) Malaria in β-thalassaemic mice and the effects of the transgenic human β-globin gene and splenectomy. *Journal of Laboratory and Clinical Medicine*, **111**, 35–41

Santiyanont, R. and Wilairat, P. (1981) Red cells containing haemoglobin E do not inhibit malaria parasite development *in vitro*. *American Journal of Tropical Medicine and Hygiene*, **30**, 541–543

Schmidt-Ullrich, R., Brown, J., Whittle, H. and Peck-Sun, L. (1986) Human-human hybridomas secreting monoclonal antibodies to the Mr 195.000 *Plasmodium falciparum* blood stage antigen. *Journal of Experimental Medicine*, **163**, 179–188

Schwartz, R.S., Olson, J.A., Raventos-Suarez, C., Yee, M., Heath, R.H., Lubin, B., et al. (1987) Altered plasma membrane phospholipid organization in *Plasmodium falciparum*-infected human erythrocytes. *Blood*, **69**, 401–417

Scuderi, P., Sterling, K.E., Lam, K.S., Finley, P.R., Ryan, K.J., Roy, C.G., et al. (1986) Raised serum levels of tumour necrosis factor in parasitic infections. *Lancet*, **ii**, 1364–1365

Seed, T.M. and Krier, J.P. (1980) Erythrocyte destruction - mechanisms in malaria, in *Malaria – vol. 2, Pathology, vector studies and culture*, J.P. Kreir, (ed.), pp. 1–46. Academic Press, New York

Serjeantson, S., Bryson, K., Amato, D. and Bbon, D. (1977) Malaria and hereditary ovalocytosis. *Human Genetics*, **37**, 161–167

Sherman, I.W. (1979) Biochemistry of *Plasmodium* (malarial parasites). *Microbiological Reviews*, **43**, 453

Sherman, I.W. and Greenan, J.R.T. (1986) *Plasmodium falciparum*: regional differences in lectin and cationized ferritin binding to the surface of the malaria-infected human erythrocyte. *Parasitology*, **93**, 17–32

Sherwood, T.A. and Virella, G. (1986) The binding of immune complexes to human red cells: complement requirements and fate of the RBC-bound IC after interaction with phagocytic cells. *Clinical and Experimental Immunology*, **64**, 195–204

Siegel, I., Liu, T.L. and Gleicher, N. (1981) The red cell immune system. *Lancet*, **ii**, 556

Silverman, P.H., Schooley, J.C. and Mahlmann, L.J. (1987) Murine malaria decreases haemopoietic stem cells. *Blood*, **69**, 408–413

Sorensen, P.G., Mickley, H. and Schmidt, K.G. (1984) Malaria-induced thrombocytopenia. *Vox Sanguinis*, **47**, 68–72

Srichaikul, T. (1973) Haematologic changes in human malaria. *Journal of the Thailand Medical Association*, **56**, 658671

Srichaikul, T., Panikbutr, N. and Jeumtrakul, P. (1967) Bone marrow changes in human malaria. *Annals of Tropical Medicine and Parasitology*, **61**, 40–51

Sturchler, D. (1988) How much malaria is there worldwide? *Parasitology Today*, **5**, 39

Sweeney, S. and Facer, C.A. (1988) A study of anti-erythrocyte cytoskeletal autoantibodies in human malaria. *British Journal of Haematology*, **69**, 130

de The, G., Geser, A., Day, N.E., Tukei, P., Williams, E., Beri, D., *et al.* (1978) Epidemiological evidence for causal relationship between Epstein–Barr virus and Burkitt's lymphoma from Ugandan prospective study. *Nature*, **274**, 756–761

Thomasson, D.L., Mansfield, J.M., Doyle, R.J. and Wallace, J.H. (1973) C-reactive protein levels in experimental African trypanosomiasis. *Journal of Parasitology*, **59**, 738

Thurnham, D.I., Oppenheimer, S.J. and Bull, R. (1983) Riboflavin status and malaria in infants in Papua New Guinea. *Transactions of the Royal Society of Tropical Medicine and Hygiene*, **77**, 423–424

Torti, F.M., Dieckmann, B., Beutler, B., Cerami, A. and Ringold, G.M. (1985) A macrophage factor inhibits adipocyte gene expression. An *in vitro* model of cachexia. *Science*, **229**, 867

Trager, W., and Jensen, J.B. (1976) Human malaria parasites in continuous culture. *Science*, **193**, 673–675

Udeinya, I.J., Graves, P.M., Carter, R., Aikawa, M. and Miller, L.H. (1983) *Plasmodium falciparum*: effect of time in continuous culture on binding to human endo-thelial cells and amelanotic melanoma cells. *Experimental Parasitology*, **56**, 207–214

Udeinya, I.J., Schmidt, J.A., Aikawa, M., Miller, L.H. and Green, I. (1981) *Falciparum* malaria-infected erythrocytes specifically bind to cultured human endothelial cells. *Science*, **213**, 555–557

Udomsangpetch, R., Aikawa, M., Berzins, K., Wahlgren, M. and Perlmann, P. (1989) Cytoadherence of knobless *Plasmodium falciparum*-infected erythrocytes and its inhibition by a human monoclonal antibody. *nature*, **338**, 763–765

Usanga, E.A. and Luzzatto, L. (1985) Adaptation of *Plasmodium falciparum*, to glucose-6-phosphate dehydrogenase deficient host red cells by production of parasite-encoded enzyme. *nature*, **313**, 793–795

Vernes, A.J-M., Haynes, J.D., Tang, D.B., Tutdit, E., and Diggs, C.L. (1986) Decreased growth of *P. falciparum* in red cells containing haemoglobin E, a role for oxidative stress, and a sero-epidemiological correlation. *Transactions of the Royal Society of Tropical Medicine and Hygiene*, **80**, 642–648

Waters, A.P. and McCutchan, T.F. (1989) Rapid, sensitive diagnosis of malaria based on ribosomal RNA. *Lancet*, **i**, 1343–1346

Weatherall, D.J. (1983) The haemoglobinopathies. In *Manson's Tropical Diseases*, P.E.C. Manson-Bahr and F.I.C. Apted, (eds), pp. 26–36, Ballière-Tindall, Sussex

Weatherall, D.J. and Abdalla, S. (1982) The anaemia of *P. falciparum* malaria. *British Medical Bulletin*, **38**, 147–151

Weinberg, E.D. (1974) Iron and susceptibility to infectious disease. *Science*, **184**, 952–956

Welch, S.G., McGregor, I.A. and Williams, K. (1977) The Duffy blood group and malaria prevalence in Gambian West Africans. *Transactions of the Royal Society of Tropical Medicine and Hygiene*, **71**, 295–296

Whittle, H.C., Brown, J., Marsh, K., Greenwood, B.M., Seidelin, P., Tighe, H., *et al.* (1984) T-cell control of Epstein–Barr virus is lost during *P. falciparum*, malaria. *Nature*, **312**, 449–450

Wickramasinghe, S.M., Looareesuwan, S., Nagachinta, B. and White, N.J. (1989) Dyserythropoiesis and ineffective erythropoiesis in *Plasmodium vivax* malaria. *British Journal of Haematology*, **72**, 91–99

Willcox, M., Bjorkman, A., Brohult, J., Pehrson, P-O., Rombo, L. and Bengtsson, E. (1983) A case control study in northern Liberia of *Plasmodium falciparum* malaria in haemoglobin S and β-thalassaemia traits. *Annals of Tropical Medicine and Parasitology*, **77**, 239–246

Woodruff, A.W., Andsell, V.E. and Pettitt, L.E. (1979) Cause of anaemia in malaria. *Lancet*, **i**, 1055–1057

World Health Organization (1985) World malaria situation 1983. *World Health Statistical Quarterly*, **38**, 193–231

World Health Organization (1986) The use of DNA probes for malaria diagnosis. *Bulletin of the World Health Organization*, **64m**, 641–652

Yoshida, A. and Roth, E.R. (1987) Glucose-6-phosphate dehydrogenase of malaria parasite *P. falciparum*. *Blood*, **69**, 1528–1530

Yuthauong, Y., Butthep, P., Bunyaratvej, A., Fucharoen, S. and Knusmith, S. (1988) Impaired parasite growth and increased susceptibility to phagocytosis of *P. falciparum* infected alpha-thalassaemia or haemoglobin Constant Spring red blood cells. *American Journal of Clinical Pathology,* **84**, 521–525

Ziegler, J.L. (1973) Cryoglobulinaemia in tropical splenomegaly syndrome. *Clinical and Experimental Immunology,* **15**, 65–78

Ziegler, J.L. and Stuiver, P.C. (1972) Tropical splenomegaly syndrome in a Rwandan kindred in Uganda. *British Medical Journal,* **3**, 79–82

Zouali, M., Druilhe, P., Gentilini, M. and Eyquem, A. (1982) High titres of anti-T antibodies and other haemagglutinins in human malaria. *Clinical and Experimental Immunology,* **50**, 83–91

Zuckerman, A. (1966) Recent studies on factors involved in malarial anaemia. *Military Medicine,* **131** (suppl.), 1201–1216

18

Haematological changes in viral infections and bacterial infections

Barbara A. Bannister

Of all the body tissues the blood is the most readily accessible for cytological examination, biochemical analysis and microbial culture. It is hardly surprising, therefore, that the various elements of the blood have been widely investigated since the earliest awakenings of pathological sciences. Some elements of the blood are unique to the circulation, and are found in the tissues only in abnormal circumstances. Such elements include red blood cells, platelets, IgM and some plasma proteins, particularly metal-carrying proteins such as coeruloplasmin (Shields, *et al.*, 1960). Other elements, particularly neutrophils and eosinophils, spend part of their life-cycle in the blood, or sequestered in the small blood vessels and the spleen, but their ultimate fate is to enter the tissues or to be extruded at mucosal surfaces. Here they undertake their phagocytic functions, and either die in the accompanying inflammatory reaction, or are shed into the environment. The immunoglobulin IgG is the major immunoglobulin of extracellular fluid and like the granulocytes it is delivered into the blood, circulates and functions in it, but probably has an important and final function in the tissues. Finally, there are blood elements which may only be present in the circulation as a small part of their many functions. Many lymphocytes and macrophages probably fall into this category, as they circulate between the blood, the tissues, the lymphatics and the lymphoid structures of the reticulo-endothelial system. These types of cells may have a life-span of several years, only intermittently passing through the circulation. Other lymphocytes probably undergo activation, clonal proliferation, cytotoxic activity and senescence without leaving the lymph nodes. Lymphocyte changes in the bloodstream, therefore, represent only the 'tip of the iceberg' of several overlapping systems of lymphocyte dynamics.

Haematological changes in infection can be seen to represent a range of responses to a pathological insult, involving the blood itself, the general response of the organism to infection, and the immunopathology resulting.

Physicochemical changes in the blood during infection

It has been known for over 50 years that there are large changes in some of the constituents of blood plasma during infection. Changes in immunoglobulin levels, and in the concentrations of iron and iron-binding proteins have been described in other chapters. There remains to be discussed a group of substances the function of which is ill-understood, but which respond suddenly to infections and inflammatory processes.

Acute-reacting proteins

C-reactive protein

The first recognition of a fast-reacting substance was that of C-reactive protein (CRP) by Tillett and Francis (1930). They described the presence of precipitins to a fraction of pneumococci in the serum of patients with acute infection. Although the 'C-function' could be precipitated by normal serum, the titres of precipitins were increased by several hundred times in patients with pneumococcal pneumonia, streptococcal endocarditis, osteomyelitis and rheumatic fever. Titres were not found to be elevated in measles or chickenpox. Studies in man, and particularly in the rabbit, which also has a CRP response, shows that CRP is synthesized in the liver and that the elevated levels of the inflammatory response are due to hugely increased rates of synthesis (Macintyre, Schultz and Kushner, 1983). The function of CRP is not known, but a review by Pepys (1981) puts forward some interesting suggestions. Pepys and others have elucidated the structure of CRP and found it to be a disc-shaped, non-covalently bound pentamer of glycosylated protein sub-units. Its structure is related to the 10-unit double disc of serum amyloid-P. C-reactive protein can bind a variety of substances, using polycation binding sites or Ca^{++} linkage. In its bound form it is a powerful activator of the classical complement pathway, and it may, therefore, have a function as an early non-specific defence against infection.

The stimulus to the prompt rise in CRP is not known, but it may be a part of the general activation of body defences. Merriman, Pulham and Kampschmidt (1975) showed that administration of leucocytic endogenous mediator caused a prompt rise in CRP in rabbits. Whicker, Martin and Dieppe (1980) showed that prostaglandins could stimulate an increase in levels of a number of acute-reacting proteins.

Other acute-reacting proteins

Several plasma proteins show a sharp rise in inflammatory disorders. The most notable of these are haptoglobin (Owen, Better and Hoban, 1960), coeruloplasmin (Pekarek, *et al.*, 1970), α_1 antitrypsin (Ganrot, 1974) and α_1 acid glycoprotein (orosomucoid) (Agostoni and Marasini, 1977). Plasma levels of other proteins, particularly albumin, transferrin and fibronectin tend to fall in acute infections. It has been pointed out by Kampschmidt (1981) that most if not all of these protein responses can be elicited by a large parenteral dose of leucocyte

endogenous mediator, suggesting that they are not a random collection of events but are more likely part of a concerted response to inflammatory stimulation.

The significance of these protein changes is poorly understood; probably different proteins have different effects upon inflammatory responses, as suggested in a review by Powanda and Mayer (1981). Their discussions suggest that both haptoglobin and coeruloplasmin may have a limiting effect on oxidative damage caused by granulocyte activity in the inflammatory response. Haptoglobin-haemoglobin complexes have a peroxidase activity, and coeruloplasmin donates copper to the manufacture of superoxide dismutase. Coeruloplasmin can itself act as a scavenger of oxygen radicals.

It is possible that α_1-acid glycoprotein also has a damage-limiting effect, for it can inhibit platelet aggregation. This could reduce the contribution of platelet products to the inflammatory response, and limit tissue damage caused by platelet-plugging of small blood vessels.

The acute-reacting protein response in infection, though difficult to understand, is highly predictable and can be reproduced experimentally by dosing with known mediators of inflammatory responses. It seems likely that the response is part of a complicated reaction which both promotes local destruction of foreign material, and limits the spread of the resulting inflammation and tissue damage. Its activation in many bacterial diseases but not in most viral conditions; in some inflammatory diseases, such as rheumatic fever and Crohn's disease, but not in others such as ulcerative colitis; and its frequent subsidence in the face of continuing disease, means that it is of limited diagnostic value. Its presence, however, is undeniable and important evidence of reaction to acute inflammation.

The erythrocyte sedimentation rate (ESR)

The ESR is a non-specific indicator of the viscosity of the plasma relative to the red blood cells. Many factors, such as packed cell volume and total plasma protein, have a small effect on the value of the ESR, sometimes additive and sometimes cancelling each other out. Major changes in the ESR are related closely to changes in the concentration of macromolecules such as α and γ macroglobulin, and particularly fibrinogen. These changes are associated with variations in electrical charge on the red blood cell surface. In the presence of increased macromolecule concentrations, red blood cells can aggregate into closely packed groups, and the ESR will increase. The only normal circumstance in which the ESR is elevated is in the second and third trimesters of pregnancy, returning to normal by one month after delivery.

Abnormalities of the ESR are useful indicators of immunological and inflammatory activity. Although in general more intense and widespread pathology tends to cause more elevation of the ESR, this is not always the case, so that the ESR is not diagnostically discriminating. Acute infectious diseases rarely cause the ESR to increase above 40 to 50 mm in 1 hour. Persisting infectious conditions, such as endocarditis, osteomyelitis, abscess formation or widespread tuberculosis may be associated with higher values. The highest values of all are seen in *Mycoplasma pneumoniae* infections and Legionnaire's disease; often then the ESR is 70 to 100 mm in one hour, similar to the levels seen in active collagen disease.

Events associated with infection may oppose the expected elevation of the ESR. The most common of these is a fall in fibrinogen levels, typically seen in disseminated intravascular coagulation (DIC). Even the modest or subclinical type of DIC occurring in early meningococcal disease is sufficient to lower the ESR to one or two mm in one hour. The author has found the ESR to be surprisingly low, even in the normal range, in many cases of extensive cavitating tuberculosis. In these circumstances, there is often a sudden rise in ESR to between 70 and 90 mm per hour when treatment is commenced. The gradual fall in ESR over the next few months then reflects the process of cure.

Finally, in certain cases of fever of unknown origin resulting from drug hypersensitivity, the ESR rises continuously, sometimes reaching 120 or 130 mm per hour by the fifth or sixth week of illness. This is a very unusual feature in infectious diseases, where the ESR is elevated on presentation and varies little unless a complication such as abscess formation causes it to rise further. In a difficult diagnostic situation a rising ESR may be a useful clue to the aetiology of a fever.

Red blood cell changes during infection

Red cell changes occurring as a result of infection are almost exclusively destructive. The only reports of polycythaemia which occur with any regularity in the literature are of those seen in extensive tuberculosis. O'Brien (1954) reviewed 66 cases of severe miliary tuberculosis, two of whom had *polycythaemia vera*. It was not clear whether this was a pre-existing condition or a result of the infection, but a total of 55 of the 66 cases reviewed had definite haematological abnormalities, suggesting that the association may be more than fortuitous.

Direct destruction of red blood cells may be caused by parasitic invasion, as in malaria and in rare cases of babesiosis. These are discussed in Chapter 17. Some bacteria produce toxins which attack components of red-cell membranes; a major example of this is the α-toxin of *Clostridium perfringens*, which is a lecithinase. In *C. perfringens* bacteraemia, or in extensive soft tissue infections intravascular haemolysis is an important component of the disease, and may necessitate large blood transfusions or exchange transfusion. Direct destruction of normal red cells is rare except in these instances.

Some patients' red cells have a pre-existing or acquired abnormality which predisposes them to damage by anoxia, acidosis or immunological attack. The most common of these is deficiency of glucose-6-phosphate dehydrogenase (G6PD), an enzyme necessary for the maintenance of reduced glutathione levels in red blood cells. Cells deficient in G6PD cannot maintain their integrity in the face of hypoxic or chemical stress, a problem which is discussed in Chapter 19.

Immune haemolysis and haemolytic anaemias

By far the commonest red blood cell change causing clinical problems in infectious disease is autoimmune haemolysis. Haemolysis is due to the interaction of antibodies with the red blood cells, usually producing a positive direct antiglobulin (Coombs) test, and resulting either in splenic sequestration and destruction of cells or in complement-mediated intravascular haemolysis. Some of these reactions are drug-dependent, and antimicrobial drugs are common culprits in this group; this is discussed in detail in Chapter 19. A variety of haemolytic syndromes, however, are simply part of the immunopathology of infection. The resulting clinical effects range from minor increases in reticulocyte counts, to sudden onset of severe anaemia and even anaemic heart failure, with or without haemoglobinaemia and haemoglobinuria.

Paroxysmal cold haemoglobinuria

This condition, though rarely resulting in severe anaemia or renal damage, is so spectacular that it was the first immune haemolytic anaemia to be well-documented and investigated. Detailed clinical descriptions of cases in adults and children appeared more than a century ago (Dickinson, 1865; Harley, 1865; Hassal, 1865). Illness always occurred during or soon after severe chilling of the extremities or the whole body. Back pain, mild fever and the passage of dark or black urine were the constant features, and Harley (1865) recognized that the red urine contained no intact red blood cells. Many of the cases were thought to have chronic syphilis, and they suffered repeated attacks. Donath and Landsteiner (1904) described the pathology of the disease. They found a cold antibody in the serum of sufferers. The antibody would bind to red blood cells, in the presence of complement, at temperatures below 15 °C but not at normal body temperature. When the antibody-coated cells and serum were rewarmed to body temperature, the complement system became active and haemolysis promptly occurred. The antibody has subsequently been known as the Donath-Landsteiner antibody.

Later work showed that paroxysmal cold haemoglobinuria (PCH) occurred in a variety of infections, including syphilis, mumps, measles and other viral infections. It is reported rarely in infectious mononucleosis (Wishart and Davey, 1973) and cytomegalovirus infection (Public Health Laboratory Service, Communicable Diseases Surveillance Centre, 1986, unpublished). The antibody was further characterized in 1963 by Levine and co-workers, by Worledge and Rousso and by Hinz, who found it to be a complement-fixing IgG antibody reacting with the recently-described P blood group system.

Those unfortunate enough to suffer from PCH must, therefore, have a combination of the Donath-Landsteiner antibody and the correct P blood group. Since chronic syphilis has become a rarity, PCH is now usually a transient condition occurring late in a viral infection or during convalescence from the acute disease, and disappearing after a few weeks. Avoidance of extreme cold is all that is required to prevent attacks during this time.

Cold haemagglutinins

Nearly one-hundred years after the original descriptions of paroxysmal cold haemoglobinuria, another type of disorder caused by cold autoantibodies in atypical pneumonia cases was described by Peterson, *et al.* (1943) and by Turner (1943). The clinical manifestations associated with these cold agglutinins are very variable, and often appear late in the course of the disease, or during convalescence. Although up to 90 per cent of cases may have detectable cold agglutinins at some stage, very few have clinically detectable problems. A number have a slightly increased mean corpuscular volume, associated with an elevated reticulocyte count. In cold surroundings, or if cold water is applied to a limb, marked acrocyanosis can occur. A modest fall in haemoglobin level may occur during convalescence. Severe anaemia is rare, but does occur, often with an insidious onset. Large-scale intravascular haemolysis is rare indeed.

It can be shown, using anti-IgG and anti-IgM direct autoglobulin tests that the cold agglutinin is an IgM antibody. Dacie suggested in 1962 that it was directed against the I-antigen found on most adult red blood cells, and this has been confirmed by others (Costea, *et al.*, 1966; Feizi and Taylor-Robinson, 1967; Jacobson, *et al.*, 1973). Interestingly, although the antibodies are polyclonal, they all seem to bear kappa light chains (Harboe and Lind, 1966).

The anti-I agglutinins are almost certainly not simply anti-mycoplasma antibodies which cross-react with red-cell antigens. Chanock, *et al.* suggested in 1963 that they were antibodies to infection-modified red cells. Fiezi, *et al.* (1969) showed that neither normal human red blood cells, nor *Mycoplasma pneumoniae* would stimulate the development of cold agglutinins in rabbits, but that human red blood cells pre-incubated with *M. pneumoniae* readily produced in a cold agglutinin response. The red blood cells of patients with mycoplasma pneumonia lose anti-I reactivity (Smith, *et al.*,

1967) as do red blood cells incubated *in vitro* with *M. pneumoniae* (Schmidt, *et al.*, 1965). This suggests that the I-antigen or its expression is altered by the infection, and that the altered antigen may be the stimulus for the anti-I cold agglutinins.

Although anti-I cold agglutinins are relatively common, other cold agglutinins can be detected in other infectious diseases. Calvo, Stein, Kochiva, *et al.* (1965) first described anti-i cold agglutinins with haemolysis in infectious mononucleosis. The patient described also had thalassaemia, and her red blood cells expressed more i-antigenicity than normal red blood cells. Human cord blood erythrocytes strongly express i-antigen and are strongly agglutinated by the infecious mononucleosis cold antibody. However, about 3% of patients with infectious mononucleosis have some evidence of haemolysis, and only about 1 in 20,000 adult individuals have I^-, i^+ red blood cells. Not surprisingly it is now known that the anti-i cold agglutinin, in sufficient titre, can attack red blood cells whatever their Ii antigenic specificity. Antibody reacts with red cells at temperatures below 28 °C and haemolysis proceeds with rewarming as occurs with anti-I cold agglutinins (Worlledge and Dacie, 1969).

Cold agglutinations are recorded occasionally in patients with other bacterial and viral diseases (Lind, Raun and Meller, 1970). When it is considered that many more patients develop agglutinins than have evidence of haemolysis, it seems probable that cold aggutinins are a relatively common concomitant of infectious disease, but rarely come to clinical recognition.

Warm haemagglutinins

The infectious associations of cold haemagglutinins have been well described, probably because the diseases in which they occur last long enough to be recognizable and diagnosable at the time that haematological manifestations occur. The same does not seem to be true for warm agglutinins though rubella is not infrequently recognized as a preceding illness (Ueda, 1985). Many people with warm antibody autoimmune haemolysis give a history of brief feverish illness two or more weeks previously, but too late for cultural or serological diagnosis. Hepatitis B has been an exception to this and is a recognized precursor of haemolysis

(Ting, 1984). It has been estimated by Pirofsky (1976) that up to 40% of patients with warm haemagglutinins have recently recovered from acute infections.

Not all warm immune haemolytic reactions are virally induced. Finland and Curnen (1938) noticed episodes of haemolysis in patients treated with anti-type 14 antisera for pneumococcal pneumonia. It was subsequently found that a disaccharide fragment of type 14 pneumococcal antigen cross-reacted with A B O antigen precursors and particularly with the antigen of blood group A. The type 14 antigen in polyvalent pneumococcal vaccines provokes a sharp rise in titre of anti-A antibodies in blood group O individuals (Boyer, *et al.*, 1981). While this is rarely of any clinical importance, the use of pneumococcal vaccines in pregnant women is not recommended in case of fetal haemolysis in group O mothers with A B O — incompatible pregnancies. Maternal infection with type 14 pneumoccocus could have a similar effect.

Unlike cold agglutinins, which are IgM, the warm-reacting agglutinins are almost always IgG. The antibody-coated cells usually give a positive Coombs reaction, but their antibody load may be very small, requiring enzyme-linked assays or other sensitive tests to demonstrate it. Massive haemolysis is extremely rare, either because insufficient antibody-complement reactions occur on the red cell membrane, or because the IgG is of a class which does not fix complement well. The antibody-coated cells are removed from the circulation by the spleen or other reticuloendothelial organs.

The most common clinical presentation is of anaemia often with splenomegaly, sometimes also with hepatomegaly, fever and lymphadenopathy. The reticulocyte count is raised. It is not known how many cases are transient, but in any series of cases a small minority suffer severe anaemia persisting for many months.

Clinical management of auto-immune haemolytic anaemia

In most cases the anaemia will resolve within three to four weeks after the infection is cured. In patients with minor degrees of haemolysis or anaemia treatment may therefore be expectant. Keeping the patient adequately warm will minimize the effect of cold-reacting antibodies.

In patients with severe or life-threatening haemolysis, emergency treatment can be difficult. The natural tendency is to resort to transfusion, but cross-matching can be complicated in the presence of autoantibodies and transfused blood may be rapidly haemolysed by the patient's plasma antibodies. Cross-matching can be carried out in the presence of cold agglutinins by keeping all reagents and apparatus at 35 to 37°C. Transfusion of warmed blood, or slow transfusion into a large vessel may then be carried out. Exchange transfusion may be an advantage, as IgM antibodies are almost all intravascular, and can be removed by exchange or plasmapheresis. The situation with warm-reacting antibodies is much more difficult, many samples must often be cross-matched to find one which reacts minimally with the offending antibody.

Treatment with corticosteroids will often minimize the continued production of antibody, and make any subsequent cross-matching and transfusion less difficult. After initial high dosage for three or four days, given intravenously if necessary, continued treatment with a smaller oral dose can often be tailed off gradually over four to six weeks.

In patients with persisting severe haemolysis splenectomy may be contemplated. It is important to carry out isotope studies of red-cell sequestration in these cases for, although most IgG-coated cells are sequestered and destroyed in the spleen, very heavily coated cells are also sequestered in large numbers by the liver. In such cases splenectomy may be fruitless.

Platelet abnormalities in infectious diseases

As with the red blood cell count, it is extremely unusual for the platelet count to be highly elevated as a result of infectious disease. In recent literature only one report is to be found: that of a case of secondary syphilis in which a platelet count of over $800 \times 10^9/1$ only returned to normal in the weeks after treatment (Horn, 1985). The major platelet abnormalities of infections are lack of numbers due to consumption or destruction, or lack of function for reasons which are so far poorly understood.

Thrombocytopenia in disseminated intravascular coagulation (DIC)

Disseminated intravascular coagulation is the condition resulting from intravascular activation of the clotting cascade. The cascade may be triggered by a variety of agencies, including endotoxin, immune complexes, thromboxane and other products of vascular endothelial damage, or even by activators released from numerous platelet thrombi. Although two well-recognized associations of DIC are meningococcal septicaemias and septicaemias caused by Gram-negative rods, the condition is not rare in other severe infections, including staphylococcal, pneumococcal and *Haemophilus influenzae* bacteraemic diseases, in severe chickenpox and measles and in malignant malaria. Contrary to expectation, it is not a significant contributor to the haemorrhage of Lassa fever (Cooper, *et al.*, 1982) or of Ebola virus haemorrhagic fever (Fisher-Hoch, *et al.*, 1983) though it does occur in Korean haemorrhagic fever (Greisman, 1970).

Clinical bleeding, except for nosebleeds and moderate oozing from venepuncture sites, is relatively unusual. The features of multiple emboli are common, however, and include anything from petechial lesions in the conjunctiva and skin to large necrotic areas particularly affecting pressure areas or the extremities. In severe cases it is not unusual for thick necrotic sloughs to form on knees, elbows or buttocks, or for digits or joints of digits to be lost. The low platelet count is accompanied by loss of fibrinogen and other factors from the circulation, by prolongation of the prothrombin time and by accumulation of fibrin degradation products in the serum.

Treatment is almost always that of the underlying disease. Anticoagulation is often superfluous in the face of depleted clotting factors, though if platelets and fresh plasma must be given to combat severe haemorrhage, cautious anticoagulation may prevent their being wasted in further intravascular coagulation. Provided that liver and bone marrow function are preserved, the normal clotting process is usually restored within 24 to 48 hours of arresting the primary disease process.

Immune thrombocytopenias in infection

Immune thrombocytopenias are relatively common, particularly in children. Although often called idiopathic thrombocytopenias, in large series over 80% of cases occur within a week or two of an acute feverish illness, often thought or known to be viral (Doan, Bouroncle and Wiseman, 1960; Lusher and Zuelzer, 1966). Implicated infections include Rubella (Morse, Zinkman and Jackson, 1966), mumps (Fama, Paton and Bostock, 1964), measles (Hudson, Weinstein and Chang, 1956), varicella-zoster (Charkes, 1961) and infectious mononucleosis (Sharp, 1969). Over 80% of cases reported are less than eight years old, and all present with purpura. Bleeding occurs in severe cases, and over 60% of the few deaths reported are due to cerebral haemorrhage.

Thrombocytopenia is not exclusively the result of viral diseases, however. It has also been reported in miliary tuberculosis (Proudfoot, *et al.*, 1969) in cat-scratch disease (Belber, Davis and Epstein, 1954) and in *Yersinia enterocolitica* infection (Glud, 1985). Approximately 90% of cases proceed to spontaneous recovery within days or weeks, but the remainder do not recover and have continuing chronic thrombocytopenia.

This thrombocytopenia was shown by a classic cross-infusion study to be caused by a serum factor (Harrington, *et al.*, 1951). Transfused platelets are destroyed almost immediately, and the patient's serum will rapidly destroy normal platelets *in vitro*.

While the peripheral blood contains hardly any platelets, or only a few abnormal giant forms, there are normal or increased numbers of megakaryocytes in the bone marrow. Many of the megakaryocytes are large and active-looking, suggesting intense bone marrow activity in the face of overwhelming peripheral destruction. Anti-platelet antibodies can be demonstrated in many cases in the blood of the patient (Veenhoven, Van der Schand and Nieweg, 1980). It is thought that the main antibody activity is in the form of IgG (Shulman, Marder and Weinrach, 1965). Megakaryocytes from some affected patients also react with IgG. Pizzi, *et al.* (1966) made the interesting observation that in 16 long-standing cases of immune thrombocytopenia, the presence of IgA on megakaryocytes was suggested by anti-IGA staining techniques. This was not so in the two acutely thrombocytopenic cases in their series.

The main bulk of investigation to date suggests that anti-platelet antibodies can be formed during infections, that these adhere to circulating platelets, and that complement lysis and or splenic sequestration destroys the platelets. The rapid destruction of platelets *in vitro* by patient's serum suggests that complement lysis is the important component of platelet destruction. Some workers (Terada, *et al.*, 1966) have used electron microscopy to show that platelets can adsorb influenza viruses, and are probably damaged to them. This raises the possibility that platelets can act as haptens, or that damaged platelet antigens could act as antigens, as in the case with red blood cells. It is also possible that platelets can be involved in 'innocent bystander' reactions, in which immune complexes are adsorbed onto their surface and the ensuing complement activity destroys them. This has been discounted, however, by Poskitt and Poskitt (1985) in the thrombocytopenia of septic conditions. Drugs can sometimes take part in this kind of reaction. The author has seen cases of pseudothrombocytopenia in children with viral infections in which platelets are destroyed in the presence of EDTA-dependent antibodies when collected into EDTA anticoagulant-containing speciment tubes. A patient with no purpura or bleeding then appears to have a profound thrombocytopenia. Fortunately, a blood film made at the bedside from unanticoagulated blood shows normal platelet numbers and structure.

The treatment of immune thrombocytopenia is usually conservative. Platelet transfusions have a limited effect owing to their rapid destruction. Corticosteroids in high doses can help to terminate antibody production within two or three days, and may improve the survival of transfused platelets in the mean time.

In chronic cases, splenectomy offers the chance of at least partial remission, and has been carried out for this purpose since its original success in the early part of the century (Bannister, Wonke and Clendinnen, 1980). A new, non-invasive treatment has more recently become available in the form of high-dose intravenous human immunoglobulin. The way in which this prevents platelet destruction is uncertain. Changes in phagocyte Fc receptors suggest that decreased platelet binding and phagocytosis may be the basis of the increased life-span.

Platelet dysfunction in severe viral infections

A severe defect in platelet aggregation was reported by Fisher-Hoch, *et al.* (1983). They made several haematological studies in monkeys infected with Ebola virus. Platelets lost the ability to aggregate in the presence of collagen, ADP or adrenaline. Normal serum did not correct this failure suggesting that the defect was in the platelets themselves. It was assumed that the defect resulted from previous aggregation and disaggregation of the platelets, producing an 'exhaustion syndrome'. The platelet defect coincided with a failure of prostacyclin production by aortic endothelium. This suggested that prostacyclin deficit led to platelet aggregation, followed by disaggregation and exhaustion.

Unfortunately, further studies, in which infected monkeys were treated with vitamin E, prostacyclin or a thromboxane inhibitor, failed to show any improvement in platelet function. In monkeys recovering from the infection, a prompt return to normal platelet aggregation took place (Fisher-Hoch, *et al.*, 1985). The minimal contribution of disseminated intravascular coagulation to the haemorrhagic state in Ebola infections was confirmed.

A different type of platelet dysfunction has been documented in the tropics. It occurs in children and occasionally young adults, with eosinophilia (Suvatte, *et al.*, 1979). More than half of the patients have evidence of helminth infestation. In most cases, the patient's platelets fail to aggregate on exposure to collagen; occasionally the response to ADP or adrenaline is impaired.

Granulocyte changes in viral and bacterial infections

The granulocytes of the blood are eosinophils, basophils and neutrophils. Discussion in this section will be confined to changes in neutrophils, as the other cell types are little involved in the changes of viral and bacterial infections. Eosinophils are extremely important in parasitic infections, and are mentioned in the relevant chapter of this book.

Neutrophil dynamics, subpopulations and their significance

Before attempting to understand the reactions of the body's neutrophils to infection, it must be made plain that knowledge of the mechanisms of production, distribution and eventual death of neutrophil populations is scanty.

After the neonatal period, neutrophil production is confined to the bone marrow. Radioactive labelling of DNA shows that it takes an average of five days to produce new neutrophils and release them into the blood. Mitotic divisions cease once the cells have reached the metamyelocyte stage and there is then a short maturation period before stab or band forms and early neutrophils enter the circulation (Warner and Athens, 1964).

On entering the circulation, the majority of granulocytes enter a 'marginating pool' of cells which is in close contact with the vascular endothelium (Bierman, *et al.*, 1961). The length of time spent in the vascular compartment seems to be short, averaging less than a day, with a half-life of six or seven hours (Cartwright, Athens and Wintrobe, 1964; Galbraith, Valberg and Brown, 1965). Granulocytes then leave the blood and migrate into the tissues. In their total life span, averaging perhaps eight days (Ottessen, 1954), they do not re-enter the circulation.

The ultimate fate of neutrophils is perhaps to be shed from mucosal surfaces, particularly at sites of inflammation. It is known that large numbers are shed in saliva and urine, and probably also from the digestive tract.

Evidence has recently been accumulating that human neutrophils comprize a number of distinct subpopulations (Gallin, 1984). Using rosette-forming techniques and density-gradient centrifugation it is possible to separate neutrophils with Fc receptors from those without. In normal peripheral blood, half to three-quarters of neutrophils have Fc-receptor (FcR) activity; when neutrophil margination is stimulated, the FcR-positive cells marginate, and the FcR-negatives remain in the circulation. In experimentally-induced abscesses 95% of neutrophils are FcR-positive. There is also evidence that FcR-positive neutrophils exhibit high levels of chemotactic activity. Gallin and other co-workers have also shown that heterogeneity exists when the neutrophil population is characterized by IgA receptors, N-formyl oligopeptide receptors, neutrophil alkaline phosphatase activity and finally by their reaction with monoclonal antibodies. A subpopulation of cells can be defined which bind a monoclonal antibody and also bind N-formyl oligopeptides and exhibit rapid membrane depolarization when activated. It seems likely that when margination of neutrophils takes place, the population exhibiting all of these high levels of activity is the group that marginates.

Neutrophil responses in infection

Changes in the neutrophil count

It is generally stated that the blood neutrophil count rises in acute bacterial infections and is unchanged or reduced in acute viral infections. That this is by no means universally true is well known to those who deal with many infected patients. Intense neutrophilia (15 to 20 × 10^9/1) is usually seen in pneumococcal and *Haemophilus influenzae* disease. More modest counts (12 to 15 × 10^9/1) are the rule in *Streptococcus pyogenes* and Gram-negative invasive diseases. The neutrophil count may be scarcely elevated in the first days of *Staphylococcus aureus* septicaemia, though it usually rises thereafter. In tuberculosis there may be extreme neutrophilia or significant neutropenia. Typhoid fever and acute brucellosis may present with a moderate neutrophilia, but progress within seven to ten days to quite marked neutropenia. Conversely in severe viral conditions with significant tissue damage, a high neutrophilia may develop; this is seen in hepatitis with liver necrosis, in mumps, meningitis and orchitis, and in viral haemorrhagic fevers.

These alterations represent an equilibrium of the minority of neutrophils which circulate in the blood. Factors increasing the blood neutrophil count will be those which release neutrophils from margination, release young neutrophils from the maturation pool in the bone marrow, or increase neutrophil production in the bone marrow. The neutrophil count is decreased by margination of circulating cells and by high rates of destruction of neutrophils or their removal from the circulation, as well as by reduced production in the bone marrow.

It has been shown that stress or severe exercise can release neutrophils from the large marginated pool in the capillary walls, particularly of the spleen and the lung. These effects can be reproduced by injections of adrenaline (Athens, *et al.*, 1961). A further flux of neutrophils from the bone marrow to the blood, can be caused by gluco-corticoid hormones which release granolocytes from the maturation pool (Clemmensen, *et al.*, 1976). Isotope labelling of DNA demonstrates that in acute infections the rate of neutrophil production is increased in the bone marrow (Fliedner, *et al.*, 1964) with labelled neutrophils appearing in the blood in as little as 48 hours. It is possible that neutrophils themselves may regulate bone marrow activity in this respect Broxymeyer and colleages (1980) have shown that FcR-positive neutrophils contain a form of lactoferrin which binds to monocytes and inhibits secretion of granulocyte-macrophage colony-stimulating substances. FcR-negative neutrophils contain a unique proteolytic enzyme which inactivates the effect of lactoferrin.

In contradistinction to all of these neutrophilia-promoting events, injection of endotoxin or of activated complement components causes a rapid fall in the neutrophil count due to increased margination (Gallin, 1984). This may explain the neutropenia which sometimes occurs in severe endotoxic infections.

Direct toxicity may affect neutrophils, though organisms such as the pneumococcus and *Staphylococcus aureus* which are known to produce leucocidins are not often associated with reduced neutrophil counts. The indirect toxicity of interferon for many blood cells via its bone marrow effects may contribute to the neutropenia often seen in severe viral infections (Nissen, *et al.*, 1977), but fortunately its effects are usually transient.

The importance of anti-neutrophil antibodies in infectious diseases is unknown. They are known to occur in haematological malignancies and in auto-immune diseases and therefore seem likely to occur from time to time in infections. They have not, so far, been shown to have a significant role in the response to infection.

Neutrophil activation and neutrophil activity tests

Nitroblue tetrazolium test (NBT test)

This is a test of the oxygen-dependent response of neutrophils which kills ingested organisms.

In the presence of $NADH_2^+$ and an intact electron transport chain, a number of neutrophils in a blood sample can reduce NBT to a dark blue-purple formazan precipitate. This test was used by Park, Firkin and Smithwick (1968) to demonstrate that increased numbers of neutrophils showed this reaction in certain infectious conditions. Normal patients would show a positive NBT test in 3–10% of polymorphs. In sepsis, bacterial meningitis and in systemic candidiasis the percentage of positive cells was increased. A number of workers have used this as a non-specific indicator of bacterial infection (Matsuda, 1975), but it has not gained wide acceptance in this role.

The test can be made more responsive and discriminating by stimulation of the neutrophils with endotoxin or phorbol myristate acetate (Repine, Rasmussen and Whiter, 1979) and has then been used to distinguish bacterial lung infection from colonization in mucoviscidosis sufferers, and to detect bacterial infection in patients with chronic granulocytic leukaemia.

The NBT test is severely impaired in patients with chronic granulomatous disease. These patients' neutrophils will ingest organisms normally, but cannot then mount an oxidative burst to destroy them. Most have an x-linked recessive lack of cytochrome b_{245}, which interrupts the electron transport chain. A few have a defect of neutrophil activation in which phorbol myristate acetate cannot activate the phosphorylation reaction required for the first steps of the response (Segal, 1985). Most patients die from repeated staphylococcal infections, particularly of the reticuloendothelial organs and the blood.

Neutrophil alkaline phosphatase (NAP)

This estimation was first described by Kaplow (1955). The enzyme is found in normal, mature neutrophils, the same population which retreats to the marginating pool when exposed to endotoxin (Gallin, 1984). Margination reduces the NAP-positive neutrophil population of the blood. Release of young neutrophils from the bone marrow, for instance by corticosteroid therapy also reduces it, by diluting the population of mature neutrophils. It is hardly surprising that NAP activity is altered in a large variety of haematological and infectious disorders. Increased NAP activity is seen in many bacterial diseases, but decreased activity is seen

in infectious mononucleosis and viral hepatitis (Lisiewicz, 1980). These correlates are not more helpful however than the total neutrophil count, which they usually parallel.

The measurement of NAP activity found a use in distinguishing leukaemoid reactions (see below), in which NAP activity is high, from true chronic granulocytic leukaemia in which NAP activity is low, unless bacterial infection coexists.

Monoclonal antibody tests

Researchers are now beginning to use monoclonal antibodies as tools for demonstrating the presence or absence of key antigens and receptors on the neutrophil surface. In this way, several patients have been shown to lack a component of the CR_3 receptor, which binds iC3b. These patients had severe impairment of phagocytic and oxidative activity of their neutrophils, and suffered severe, recurrent bacterial sepsis, particularly of soft tissues (Ross, *et al.*, 1985).

Mononuclear cell changes in the blood in viral and bacterial infections

The main mononuclear cells of the blood are the lymphocytes, but lymphocytes are not primarily blood cells. They are to be found in the largest numbers in the lymphoid tissues of the spleen, the lymph nodes, the pharynx and the gut. It is in these sites, rather than in the blood, that lymphocytes usually first encounter foreign antigens and organisms; in these sites they are structurally and functionally integrated with macrophages and can best carry out their classical functions. Even when intense lymphoproliferative activity is going on in these tissues, dividing lymphocytes are extremely seldom seen in the blood (Cooper, 1969).

Changes in blood lymphocyte numbers or activity, therefore, are remote from many of the activities in which lymphocytes are involved. They are a reflection, rather than a true picture, of the state of lymphocyte activation or disorder in the body. This being so it is no surprise that, with few exceptions, absolute lymphocyte numbers are rarely increased or decreased outside the accepted normal range during infections. Wide changes in the percentage of white blood cells which are lymphocytes more often result from the addition or subtraction of large numbers of neutrophils. Marked lymphocyte changes, in morphology, if not in numbers, do occur in some circumstances and these will be discussed.

Viral infections of lymphocytes and other mononuclear cells

Epstein–Barr virus infection

It was shown by Diehl, *et al.* (1968) that herpes-type virus particles could be seen on electron microscopy of cultured human lymphocytes which also showed positive immunofluorescence for Epstein–Barr virus (EBV). It was subsequently shown that some peripheral blood cells of patients contained EBV-determined nuclear antigen (Klein, *et al.*, 1973). The infected cells were found to bear receptors for EBV, and to be B-lymphocytes which expressed immunoglobulin at their surface (Jondal and Klein, 1973).

This infection is not without effect on the B-lymphocytes. They are activated and transformed by it, expressing BLAST-2 and BLAST-1 antigens which predict and follow the morphological changes of blastogenesis (Thorley-Lawson and Mann, 1985).

Measles infection

It was shown by Joseph, Lamport and Oldstone (1975), and by Sullivan, *et al.* (1975) that measles virus could infect human lymphocytes and, to a lesser extent, monocytes. Measles virus antigens are expressed by peripheral blood mononuclear cells in acute measles, but only if the cells are stimulated with phytohaemagglutinin (Hyypia, Korkiamaki and Vainionpaa, 1985). The stimulated cells will release measles virus. Although the infection is silent in unstimulated cells, it is known that these cells have impaired function and secrete interferon. Opposing the action of interferon results in increased virus expression (Jacobson and McFarland, 1982). It is of interest to note that a high proportion of the lymphocytes of patients with subacute sclerosing panencephalitis (SSPE) express measles virus RNA, though very few lymphocytes of normal seropositive adults do this

(Fournier, *et al.* 1985). It has been suggested that persisting measles infection of lymphocytes may be important in the pathogenesis of SSPE.

Measles virus does not exhibit the specificity of EBV. It will infect both B- and T-cells, probably including more than one type of T-cell. The $T_4:T_8$ ratio is unchanged in acute measles.

Respiratory syncytial virus (RSV) infection

The ability of RSV to infect human peripheral blood mononuclear cells *in vitro* was demonstrated by Roberts in 1982. This work was extended to characterize RSV infection of mononuclear leucocytes in children with RSV infections (Domurat, *et al.*, 1985).

Both monocytes and lymphocytes are infected. Virus proteins in the cells of patients were expressed most by atypical or lymphoblastoid cells, which had T-suppressor cell markers. Lymphocytic proliferation in response to mitogens was impaired, and the $T_4:T_8$ ratio was significantly diminished in active infection.

Human immunodeficiency virus (HIV) infection

Infection of T-helper cells by HIV has been well documented following the recognition of the world-wide epidemic of acquired immune deficiency syndrome. It is thought that HIV uses the T_4 antigen as a receptor via which it infects and kills the cell. Considering the tropism of measles virus for blood, mononuclear and brain cells, it is of interest that HIV is thought also to infect brain cells and cervical cells. The question of whether these cells possess T_4 antigen, or an analogue of it, is an intriguing one. Infection with HIV is considered in more detail in Chapter 15.

Atypical lymphocytosis in infectious mononucleosis and other conditions

It was recognized at the beginning of this century that infectious mononucleosis was a disease in which bizarre haematological abnormalities were the rule. It gradually became clear that the abnormal white blood cells seen in the disease were of lymphoid origin, and were not malignant (Carter and Penman, 1969). The limitations of light microscopy and limited staining techniques, made it difficult to study the origins and activities of these cells, but they were easily recognized by their morphological features. All patients with infectious mononucleosis have an atypical blood picture, with at least 20% of mononuclear cells being abnormal. It was soon recognized that cells with the same appearance are seen in other diseases also. Finch (1969) summarized the currently available information, concluding that similar degrees of mononucleosis could occur in viral hepatitis and cytomegalovirus infection. They have also been recorded in parvovirus infections (Schneerson, Mortimer and Vandervelde, 1980). Lower counts occurred in a wide variety of viral infections, atypical pneumonias, tuberculosis, brucellosis, toxoplasmosis and rickettsial infections. Mononucleosis also occurs in some drug reactions, particularly to para-amino salycilic acid and hydantoins, and in infiltrations or intoxications of the reticuloendothelial system. It is not known whether similar populations of mononuclear cells are involved in all of these reactions.

The nature of the atypical lymphocytes in infectious mononucleosis

Although there is no doubt that Epstein–Barr virus (EBV) infects B-lymphocytes, it is difficult to find these infected cells in the peripheral blood of patients. In post-mortem studies, dense infiltration with atypical mononuclear cells is seen in the lymph nodes, tonsils, spleen and in the thymus of young children, but not in the bone marrow. Many mitotic figures are seen in the lymph nodes and thymus. Britton, *et al.* (1978) found that EBV nuclear antigen-positive cells were plentiful in the spleen, tonsils and thymus, but not in the lymph nodes. The infiltration of the lymph nodes contained only cytotoxic cells. It was shown by Scheldon, *et al.* (1973) that most of the circulating atypical lymphocytes were T-cells and, further, that they were probably recently transformed as they were incapable of further response to phytohaemagglutinin stimulation. Svedmyr and Jondal (1975) confirmed that T-cytotoxic cells in infectious mononucleosis were specific for EBV-transformed B-cells. They found that a population of non-specifically cytotoxic cells, distinguishable by the presence of complement receptors, was also present. This double population may accord with the finding of cold

antibodies in infectious mononucleosis to a common antigen expressed by thymocytes and peripheral lymphocytes (Thomas, 1972).

In short, the atypical lymphocytes of the blood in infectious mononucleosis are transformed T-lymphocytes, some of which are specific for EBV nuclear antigen-containing B-cells and some of which have unknown specificity.

The lymphocytosis of pertussis

Unlike the atypical lymphocytosis of infectious mononucleosis, in pertussis there is a large increase in the number of morphologically normal blood lymphocytes. This has been intensively studied by Morse and his colleagues, and by a number of other groups. The lymphocytosis also occurs in mice infected with *Bordetella pertussis*, and this provides a useful model of lymphocyte changes at a time when the western world has enjoyed relative freedom from pertussis epidemics in humans.

It has been recognized for many years that the lymphocytosis is not due to one particular subtype of cell (Morse, 1965) and the availability of immunological techniques, including monoclonal antibodies, has allowed extensive study of the cells involved (Bertotto, *et al.*, 1984). Both B- and T-lymphocytes are involved. Cells expressing CD3, CD4 and CD8 antigens are increased in proportion to those in normal blood, as are T-cells expressing none of these antigens. Radio-labelling studies suggest that the blood lymphocytosis is due to a net shift of cells from lymphoid tissues into the blood (Morse and Reister, 1967a, b). The cells then remain in the blood in large numbers, instead of recirculating back to the lymphoid tissue (Morse and Barron, 1970).

The lymphocytosis is caused by a soluble fraction of *B. pertussis* (Clausen, Munoz and Bergman, 1968) now known to be a filamentous protein substance, originally purified and characterized by Sato and Arai (1972). Purified lymphocytosis-promoting factor (LPF) has been found to be a potent T-cell mitogen in both mice and humans. This effect is not dependent on previous sensitization of the cells to *B. pertussis*, and mainly affects Fc (γ) receptor-negative T-lymphocytes (Morse, *et al.*, 1977; Cläesson, Andersen and Sønderstrup-Hansen, 1978). The clinical significance of these findings is not clear. It is not the author's experience that pertussis alters the effect of concurrent viral or fungal infections, though it does cause temporary depression of the tuberculin response.

The blood and the bone marrow in infection

Infection can depress bone marrow function, or stimulate it to bizarre activity resembling that of leukaemia or other malignancy. Although many of these effects are temporary and disappear with resolution of the infectious process, some of them may be permanent and even fatal. In many instances the pathogenesis of such disorders is little understood, but some recent advances give a hint as to their mechanisms and even a hope of effective therapy.

The leukaemoid reaction

This is a reaction in which very high counts of granulocytes occur in the blood during an infectious process. The total white blood cell count may be astonishingly high, even approaching $10^{12}/1$. The bone marrow, likewise, is packed with granulocytes and shows a high activity of granulocyte precursors. A leukaemoid reaction may be difficult to distinguish from a real case of chronic granulocytic leukaemia, complicated by infection. Two objective criteria can be helpful; one is the absence of the Philadelphia chromosome in leukaemoid reactions, although it is present in the neutrophils in 90% of granulocytic leukaemia cases; the other is the normal or raised neutrophil alkaline phosphatase in leukaemoid reactions (Oswald, 1963), in contrast to granulocyte leukaemias in which it is almost always low.

The most common disease precipitating leukaemoid reactions is tuberculosis (Mills and Townsend, 1937; O'Brien, 1954; Twomey and Leavell, 1965; Proudfoot, *et al.*, 1969). Even so, haematological disorders of many types are reported in tuberculosis, and leukaemoid reactions are far in the minority compared with neutropenia, agranulocytosis and bone marrow aplasia. This is made particularly clear in the series of O'Brien (1954) and Proudfoot, *et al.* (1969). The common factor in patients with leukaemoid reactions is severe miliary disease, often with tubercles detectable in the bone marrow.

The pathogenesis of the condition is not known. Twomey and Leavell (1965) draw attention to the hypercellular reactions in tuberculin-sensitized animals, challenged with further exposure to tuberculin. They postulate a similar mechanism in man. This is of some interest, because there are anecdotal reports of leukaemoid reactions in pneumococcal and meningococcal infections, and in pertussis. Perhaps the powerful antigens and toxins released by these organisms could have a similar effect. Alternatively, a particular type of cell-mediated immunological activity might precipitate the response; recent reports suggest that some lymphocyte subsets may be capable of producing mediators of granulopoiesis (Barr, 1984; Platzer, 1985). Fortunately for the patients, opportunity for clinical research is limited by the disappearance of the leukaemoid reaction when the underlying condition is cured.

The haemophagocytic syndrome

This is a feverish illness in which there is widespread histiocyte proliferation, associated with hepatosplenomegaly and pancytopenia or isolated cytopenias. It was first fully described by Risdall, *et al.* (1979) who presented 19 cases, and distinguished it from the similarly presenting, and malignant, histiocytic medullary reticulosis. Both diseases are characterized by histiocyte infiltration of the reticuloendothelial system with haemophagocytosis, but in histiocytic medullary reticulosis the infiltrate is malignant and the disease is fatal.

Among the 19 original cases of haemophagocytic syndrome, all were children; 14 were taking immunosuppressive therapy of whom 13 had had previous splenectomy. Fourteen of the 19 had diagnostic evidence of recent viral infections, including cytomegalovirus, Epstein–Barr virus, herpes simplex, varicella-zoster and adenovirus. The histiocytic infiltrate affected bone marrow, liver and lymph nodes and consisted of mature, vacuolated cells, some of which contained phagocytosed red blood cells or platelets. The illness resolved clinically within two months in all cases, with a return of the blood count to normal. The histiocytic infiltrate took several weeks longer to clear completely.

Since 1979 several more reports have appeared of two more cases associated with Epstein–Barr virus infection (Wilson, *et al.*, 1981), and one case associated with treated pulmonary tuberculosis (Barnes, *et al.*, 1984). Before the coming of the term 'haemophago-cytic syndrome', Chandra, *et al.* (1975) described two cases with the same clinical and histological features. One had miliary tuber-culosis and one a 'viral infection'. Other agents associated with haemophagocytosis include candidiasis, histoplasmosis, *Escherichia coli*, *Streptococcus pneumoniae* (Risdell, *et al.*, 1984), *Brucella* (Zuazu, *et al.*, 1979) and *Salmonella typhi* (Fame, *et al.*, 1986).

The importance of this syndrome is that, in spite of its alarming presentation, usually with marked pancytopenia and grossly abnormal marrow, its course is usually benign. The temptation to treat the patient with cytotoxic agents must be resisted, for they are not required and the risk of adverse side-effects from their use is high. The bone marrow must be examined critically to ensure that the diag-nosis of malignancy is excluded, and the patient is given supportive therapy until natural recovery occurs.

Aplastic anaemia and infection

Aplastic anaemia in tuberculosis

Aplastic anaemia is one of the many blood disorders associated with severe tuberculosis. It is intermediate in frequency between agranulocytosis and the much rarer leukaemoid reactions (O'Brien 1954; Proudfoot, *et al.*, 1969). Small series of cases are occasionally reported (Evans, DeLuca and Waters, 1952; Medd and Hayhoe, 1955; Zamorano and Thompsett, 1968). In general the patients are seriously ill on presentation, with miliary disease and tubercles in the bone marrow. Medd and Hayhoe (1965) remarked on the lack of cellular infiltrate in the granulomata, but it is not clear whether this was related to the cause of the aplasia or its effect. The four patients with atypical mycobacteria reported by Zamorano and Thompsett are the least fortunate; only one of them had a remission of aplasia with treatment and that patient had a fatal relapse after six months.

The only explanation put forward for the aplasia is that of granulomatous destruction of the bone marrow, but this does not seem entirely reasonable as in many cases the granulomata in the marrow are widely scattered and not large.

Aplastic anaemia in infectious hepatitis

Aplastic anaemia has been recognized as a rare complication of hepatitis for many years. Although the complication is rare, hepatitis is extremely common, so that quite large series of cases are published. Rubin, Gottlieb and Vogel (1968) described 10 cases of their own and reviewed 16 from literature. Rosner (1970) reported one case and noted at least another 55 in world literature. Unlike many virus-associated conditions, post-hepatitis aplasia may not appear for weeks or months after the original illness. When hepatitis B surface antigen tests became available it was soon apparent that aplasia was associated with non-B hepatitis, and it is now thought that almost all cases follow non-A, non-B disease (Zeldis and Dienstag, 1983). Further understanding of the aetiologies of the non-A, non-B hepatitides is necessary before the problem of pathogenesis can be fully addressed.

The presentation of the aplasia is typical, with bleeding, anaemia or infection, pancytopenia on the blood film and acellularity of the marrow. The prognosis is worse than that of many other groups of aplastic anaemias; there is usually no response to corticosteroid or anabolic steroid treatment and even partial remission is extremely rare. Early bone marrow transplantation is considered to be the treat-ment of choice, and multiple transfusions are to be avoided so that anti-blood cell antibodies are not induced (Camitta, *et al.*, 1974).

Red-cell aplasia in infections with parvovirus B19

Human parvovirus B19 is a member of the virus family Parvoviridae. Many parvoviridae have such small genomes that they can only replicate in the presence of other viruses. Parvovirus B19 can invade and infect only those cells which are in the S-phase of mitosis. Rapidly-replicating cells are therefore at most risk, and the red-cell progenitors are particularly affected.

Acute parvovirus B19 infections, including

slapped-cheek syndrome and acute infectious arthritis, are accompanied by transient reticulocytopenia. Patients with congenital haemolytic anaemias rely on a much-increased bone marrow activity to maintain their red blood cell mass in the face of rapid erythrocyte destruction. Even temporary cessation of erythrocyte production can cause an aplastic crisis in these cases. Aplastic crisis in sickle-cell disease was the first clinical consequence of parvovirus B19 infection to be recognized. Fortunately the erythrocyte precursors recover and haematopoiesis returns to normal once the acute infection is determined (Young, 1988).

Immunosuppressed patients who cannot terminate the acute viral infection may suffer from persisting infection of erythrocyte precursors. Cases have been described in which aplastic anaemia persisted for years and parvovirus B19 DNA could be demonstrated in affected cells. Kurtzman, *et al*. (1989) described such a case and reported successful treatment with immunoglobulin.

When a pregnant woman is infected with parvovirus B19 there is a 50% chance of fetal infection. Fetal red-cell precursors are affected in both intramedullary and extramedullary sites leading to temporary aplastic anaemia in the fetus. In the second trimester the fetal red-cell mass usually increases 30-fold or more, so aplasia at this stage can have disastrous effects. Hall (1990) has reviewed the relevant literature, describing the discovery that non-immune fetal hydrops causes significant loss of second-trimester pregnancies in parvovirus B19-infected mothers. The risk of fetal infection and loss can be estimated as approximately 1.5–5%, depending on the epidemiological circumstances of maternal exposure. It is likely that many infected fetuses survive and recover; strategies for the detection and management (e.g. by intrauterine transfusion) of those severely affected are still under discussion.

Mechanisms of aplasia and recent advances in knowledge

Possible ways in which blood cell progenitors can be damaged are many:

1 *Direct infection of progenitors* This has been well described in parvovirus-induced red-cell aplasia. It has also been suggested as a cause of thrombocytopenia in severe systemic viral

infections such as congenital rubella (Zinkha, Medearis and Osborne, 1967) and purpuric varicella (Espinoza and Kuhn, 1974) in which virus particles have been seen in megakaryocytes.

2 *Production of destructive antibodies against progenitors* There is also some compelling evidence for this mechanism. Complement-dependent antibody destruction of stem-cells has been implicated in red-cell aplasia (Krantz, 1973) and in agranulocytosis (Fitchen and Cline, 1980). Antibodies have also been thought responsible for aplastic anaemia (Freedman, Golfand and Saunders, 1979).

3 *Cell-mediated immune mechanisms and interferon* In the last few years it has been recognized that stimulated T-cells suppress normal bone marrow activity, that this activity is probably mediated by interferon, and that it is inhibited by anti-lymphocyte and anti-thymocyte globulin preparations (Zoumbos, 1984). This hypothesis is supported by the finding that both α and γ interferon are toxic for bone marrow cultures (Nissen, *et al.*, 1977), and that antithymocyte globulin can be used successfully to treat aplastic anaemia (Mangan, 1985). Although complete and permanent remission is rare, a number of patients can achieve partial remission on treatment with a combination of corticosteroids, androgens and antilymphocyte preparations.

4 *Mechanisms susceptible to antiviral agents.* A surprising and encouraging discovery that acyclovir can be of benefit in aplastic anaemia was widely publicized by Baciglalupo, Frassoni and Van Lint (1984). They described a case of their own and a published case, both of whom had required repeated transfusions for a year or more in spite of treatment with corticosteroids and immunosuppressive therapy including antilymphocyte globulin. After a 10-day course of acyclovir, both were able to discontinue transfusions. In a later report (Gomez-Almaguer, 1986) two out of five acyclovir-treated patients had similar remissions and another patient had a reduced requirement for transfusion and became able to maintain a neutrophil count above $10^8/l$.

This is a happy note on which to conclude this chapter, which has sought to give an overview of how the blood can reflect so many facets of microbial pathogenetics and human immunopathology. Acyclovir is a fortunate answer to one difficult problem of infection-associated haematological disorders. Many challenging questions still remain.

References

Agostoni, A. and Marasini, B. (1977) Orosomucoid contents of pleural and peritoneal effusions of various etiologies. *American Journal of Clinical Pathology, 67,* 146–148

Athens, J.W., Haab, O.P., Raab, S.O., Mauer, A.M., Ashenbrucker, H., Cartwright, G.E. and Wintrobe, M.M. (1961) Leukokinetic studies IV. The total blood, circulating and marginal granulocyte pools and the granulocyte turnover rate in normal subjects. *Journal of Clinical Investigation, 40,* 989–991

Baciglalupo, A., Frassoni, F. and Van Lint, M.T. (1984) Acyclovir for the treatment of severe aplastic anemia. *New England Journal of Medicine, 310,* 1606

Bannister, B.A., Wonke, B. and Clendinnen, B.G. (1980) Idiopathic thrombocytopenic purpura: a case of particular historic interest. *Journal of the Royal Society of Medicine, 73,* 828–829

Barnes, N., Bellamy, D., Ireland, R., Parsons, V. and Costello, J. (1984) Pulmonary tuberculosis complicated by haemophagocytic syndrome and rifampicin-induced tubulointerstitial nephritis. *British Journal of Diseases of the Chest, 78,* 395–403

Barr, R.D. (1984) Regulation of normal human granulopoiesis *in vitro* by autologous T lymphocyte subsets. *Blood, 64,* 1139–1140

Belber, J.P., Davis, A.E. and Epstein, E.H. (1954) Thrombocytopenic purpura associated with cat-scratch disease. *Archives of Internal Medicine, 94,* 321–325

Bertotto, A., Forenza,. N., Peirone, A.P. Mazzarino, I. and Vaccaro, R. (1984) T-cell subsets in children with pertussis. *Haematologica, 69,* 342–345

Bierman, H.R., Kelly, K.H., Byron, R.L. and Marshall, G.J. (1961) Leukapheresis in man. I. Haematological observations following leucocyte withdrawal in patients with non-haematological disorders. *British Journal of Haematology, 7,* 51–63

Boyer, K.M., Theeravuthichai, J., Vogel, L.C., Orlina, A. and Gotoff, S.P. (1981) Antibody response to group B streptococcus type III and AB blood group antigens induced by pneumococcal vaccine. *Journal of Pediatrics, 98,* 374–378

Britton, S., Andersson-Anvret, M., Gergely, P., Henle, W., Jondal, M., Klein, G., Sandstedt, B. and Svedmyr, E. (1978) Epstein–Barr virus immunity and tissue distribution in a fatal case of infectious mononucleosis. *New England Journal of Medicine, 298,* 89–92

Broxmeyer, H.E., Ralph, P., Bognachi, J., Kinkade, P.W. and Desousa, M. (1980). A subpopulation of human polymorphonuclear neutrophils contains an active form of lactoferrin capable of binding to human monocytes and inhibiting production of granulocyte-macrophage colony

stimulatory activity. *Journal of Immunology, 125,* 903–909

Calvo, R., Stein, W., Kochwa, S. and Rosenfield, R.E. (1965) Acute hemolytic anaemia due to anti-i: frequent cold agglutinins in infectious mononucleosis. *Journal of Clinical Investigation, 44,* 1033

Camitta, B.M., Nathan, D.G., Forman, E.N., Parkman, R., Rappeport, J.M. and Orellana, T.D. (1974) Post-hepatitic severe aplastic anaemia – an indication for early bone marrow transplantation. *Blood, 43,* 473–483

Carter, R.L. and Penman, H.G. (1969) The Early History of Infectious Mononucleosis and its relation to 'Glandular Fever', in *Infectious Mononucleosis,* R.L. Carter and H.G. Penman, (eds), pp. 1–18, Blackwell, Oxford

Cartwright, G.E., Athens, J.W. and Wintrobe, M.M. (1964) The kinetics of granulopoiesis in normal man. *Blood, 24,* 780–785

Chandra, P., Chaudhery, S.A., Rosner, F. and Kagan, M. (1975) Transient histiocytosis with striking phagocytosis of platelets, leukocytes and erythrocytes. *Archives of Internal Medicine, 135,* 989–991

Chanock, R.M., Mufson, M., Somerson, N.L. and Couch, R.B. (1963) Role of Mycoplasma (PPLO) in human respiratory disease. *American Reviews of Respiratory Disease, 88* (suppl.), 218–239

Charkes, N.D. (1961) Purpuric chickenpox: report of a case, review of the literature and classification by clinical features. *Annals of Internal Medicine, 54,* 745–759

Cläesson, M.H., Andersen, V. and Sønderstrup-Hansen, G. (1978) Colony formation by subpopulations of human T lymphocytes. I. effects of phytohaemagglutinin and lymphocytosis – promoting factor from *Bordetella pertussis. Clinical and Experimental Immunology, 34,* 364–373

Clausen, C., Munoz, J. and Bergman, R.K. (1968) Lymphocytosis and histamine-sensitisation of mice by fractions from *Bordetella pertussis, Journal of Bacteriology, 96,* 1484–1487

Clemmensen, O., Andersen, V., Hansen, N.E., Karle, H. and Koch, C. (1976) Sequential studies of lymphocytes, neutrophils and serum proteins during prednisone treatment. *Acta Medica Scandinavica, 199,* 105–111

Cooper, C.G., Gransden, W.R., Webster, M., King, M., O'Mahoney, M., Young, S. and Banatvala, J.E. (1982) A case of Lassa fever: experiences at St. Thomas's Hospital. *British Medical Journal, 285,* 1003–1005

Cooper, E.H. (1969) Experimental studies of the atypical mononuclear cell in infectious mononucleosis, in *Infectious Mononucleosis,* R.L. Carter and H.G. Penman, (eds), pp. 121–145, Blackwell, Oxford

Costea, N., Yakulis, V. and Heller, P. (1966) Light chain heterogeneity of cold agglutinins. *Science, 152,* 1520–1521

Dacie, J.V. (1962) *The haemolytic anaemias.* 2nd edn, p. 530. Grune and Stratton, New York

Dickinson, W.H. (1865) Notes on four cases of intermittent haematuria. *Lancet,* i, 568–569

Diehl, V., Henle, G., Henle, W. and Kohn, G. (1968)

Demonstration of a herpes-group virus in cultures of peripheral leukocytes from patients with infectious mononucleosis. *Journal of Virology,* **2**, 663–669

Doan, C.A., Bouroncle, B.A. and Wiseman, B.K. (1960) Idiopathic and secondary thrombocytopenic purpura: a clinical study and evaluation of 381 cases over a period of 28 years. *Annals of Internal Medicine,* **53**, 861–876

Domurat, F., Roberts, N.J., Walsh, E.E. and Dagan, R. (1985) Respiratory syncytial virus infection of human mononuclear leukocytes *in vitro* and *in vivo. The Journal of Infectious Diseases,* **152**, 895–902

Donath, J. and Lansteiner, K. (1904) Uber paroxysmale Hämoglobinurie. *Münchenen Medizinischen Wochenschrift* **51**, 1590–1593

Espinoza, C. and Kuhn, C. (1974) Viral infection of megakaryocytes in varicella with purpura. *American Journal of Clinical Pathology,* **61**, 203–208

Evans, T.S., Deluca, V.A. and Waters, L.L. (1952) Association between miliary tuberculosis of bone marrow and pancytopenia. *Annals of Internal Medicine,* **37**, 1044–1047

Fama, P.G., Paton, W.B. and Bostock, M.I. (1964) Thrombocytopenic purpura complicating mumps. *British Medical Journal,* **2**, 1244

Fame, T.M., Engelhard, D. and Riley, H.D. (1986) Haemophagocytosis accompanying typhoid fever. *Pediatric Infectious Disease,* **5**, 367–369

Feizi, T. and Taylor-Robinson, D. (1967) Cold agglutinin anti-I and *Mycoplasma pneumoniae. Immunology,* **13**, 405–409

Feizi, T., Taylor-Robinson, D., Shields, M.D. and Carter, R.A. (1969) Production of cold agglutinins in rabbits immunized with human erythrocytes treated with *Mycoplasma pneumoniae. Nature,* **222**, 1253–1256

Finch, S.C. (1969) Laboratory Findings in Infectious Mononucleosis, in *Infectious Mononucleosis,* R.L. Carter and H.G. Penman, (eds), pp. 47–62, Blackwell, Oxford

Finland, M. and Curnen, F.C. (1938) Agglutinins for human erythrocytes in type XIV anti-pneumococcic horse serums. *Science,* **87**, 417–419

Fisher-Hoch, S.P., Platt, G.S., Lloyd, G., Simpson, D.I.H., Neild, G.H. and Barrett, A.J. (1983) Haematological and biochemical monitoring of Ebola infection in rhesus monkeys: implications for patient management. *Lancet,* **2**, 1055–1058

Fisher-Hoch, S.P., Platt, G.S., Neild, G.H., Southee, T., Baskerville, A., Raymond, R.T., Lloyd, G. and Simpson, D.I.H. (1985) Pathophysiology of shock and haemorrhage in a fulminating viral infection (Ebola). *The Journal of Infectious Diseases,* **152**, 887–894

Fitchen, J.H. and Cline, M.J. (1980) Serum inhibitors of myeloporesis. *British Journal of Haematology,* **44**, 7–10

Fliedner, J.M., Cronkite, E.P., Killman, S.A. and Bond, U.P. (1964) Granulocytopoiesis II. Emergence and pattern of labelling of neutrophilic granulocytes in humans. *Blood,* **24**, 683–700

Fournier, J.-G., Tardieu, M., Lebon, P., Robain, O., Posnot, G., Rozenblatt, S. and Bouteille, M. (1985)

Detection of measles virus RNA in lymphocytes from peripheral-blood and brain perivascular infiltrates of patients with subacute sclerosing panencephalitis. *New England Journal of Medicine,* **313**, 910–915

Freedman, M.H., Gelfand, E.W. and Saunders, E.F. (1979) Acquired aplastic anemia. Antibody-mediated haematopoietic failure. *American Journal of Haematology,* **6**, 135–141

Galbraith, P.R., Valberg, L.S. and Brown, M. (1965) Patterns of granulocyte kinetics in health, infection and carcinoma. *Blood,* **25**, 683–684

Gallin, J.I. (1984) Human neutrophil heterogeneity exists, but is it meaningful? *Blood,* **63**, 977–983

Ganrot, K. (1974) Plasma protein pattern in acute infectious diseases. *Scandinavian Journal of Clinical Laboratory Investigation,* **34**, 75–81

Glud, T.K. (1985) Yersinia enterocolitica infection complicated by severe thrombocytopenia resistant to high-dose intravenous immunoglobulin. *Acta Medida Scandinavica,* **217**, 233–234

Gomez-Almagner, D. (1986) More about acyclovir and aplastic anemia. *New England Journal of Medicine,* **314**, 584–585

Greisman, S.E. (1970) Epidemic haemorrhagic fever, in, *Principles of Internal Medicine,* M.M. Wintrobe, G.W. Thorn, R.D. Adams, I.L. Bennett, E. Braunwald, K.J. Isselbacher and R.G. Petersdorf (eds), pp. 1015–1018, McGraw-Hill Book Company, New York

Hall, S.M. (1990) Parvovirus B19 and pregnancy. *Reviews in Medical Microbiology,* **1**, 160–167

Harboe, M. and Lind, K. (1966) Light chain types of transiently-occurring cold haemagglutinins. *Scandinavian Journal of Haematology,* **3**, 269–276

Harley, G. (1865) Notes on two cases of intermittent haematuria: with remarks on their pathology and treatment. *Lancet,* **i**, 568

Harrington, W.J., Hollingsworth, J.W., Minnich, V. and Moore, C.B. (1951) Demonstration of a thrombocytopenic factor in the blood of patients with idiopathic thrombocytopenic purpura. *Journal of Clinical Investigation,* **30**, 646

Hassal, A.H. (1865) On intermittent, or winter, haematuria. *Lancet,* **2**, 368

Hinz, C.F. (1963) Serologic and physiochemical characterisation of Donath–Landsteiner antibodies from six patients. *Blood,* **22**, 600–605

Horn, T.D. (1985) Thrombocytosis in a patient with secondary syphilis. *Archives of Dermatology,* **121**, 1241–1242

Hudson, J.B., Weinstein, L. and Chang, T-W. (1956) Thrombocytopenic purpura in measles. *Journal of Pediatrics,* **48**, 48–56

Hyypiä, T., Korkiamäki, P. and Vainionpää, R. (1985) Replication of measles virus in human lymphocytes. *Journal of Experimental Medicine,* **161**, 1261–1271

Jacobson, L.B., Longstreth, G.F. and Edgington, T.S. (1973) Clinical and immunological features of transient cold agglutinin hemolytic anemia. *American Journal of Medicine,* **54**, 514–521

Jacobson, S. and McFarland, H.F. (1982) Measles virus persistence in human lymphocytes: A role for virus induced interferon. *Journal of General Virology,* **63**, 351–357

Jondal, M. and Klein, G. (1973) Surface markers on human B and T lymphocytes II. Presence of Epstein–Barr virus receptors on B lymphocytes. *Journal of Experimental Medicine,* **138**, 1365–1378

Joseph, B.S. Lampert, B.V. and Oldstone, M.B.A. (1975) Replication and persistence of measles virus in defined subpopulations of human leukocytes. *Journal of Virology,* **16**, 1638–1649

Kampschmidt, R.F. (1981) Leukocytic endogenous mediator/endogenous pyrogen, in *Infection: the physiologic and metabolic responses of the host*, M.C. Powanda and P.G. Canonico, (eds), pp. 55–74, Elsevier, North Holland

Kaplow, L.S. (1955) A histochemical procedure for localising and evaluating leukocyte alkaline phosphatase activity in smears of blood and marrow. *Blood*, **10**, 1023–1029

Klein, G., Svedmyn, E. and Jondal, M. (1976) EBV-determined nuclear antigen (EBNA)-positive cells in the peripheral blood of infectious mononucleosis patients. *International Journal of Cancer*, **17**, 21–26

Krantz, S.B. (1973) Pure red cell aplasia. *British Journal of Haematology*, **25**, 1–12

Kurtzman, G., Frikhofen, N., Kimball, J., Jenkins, D.W., Nienhuis, A.W. and Young, N.S. (1989) Pure red-cell aplasia of ten years duration due to persistent parvovirus B19 infection and its cure with immunoglobulin therapy. *New England Journal of Medicine*, **321**, 519–523

Levine, P., Celano, M.J. and Falkowski, F. (1963) The specificity of the antibody in paroxysmal cold haemoglobinuria (PCH). *Transfusion*, **3**, 278–80

Lind, K., Raun, T.J. and Meller, J. (1970) Occurrences of *Mycoplasma pneumonial* infection in patients hospitalized with acute respiratory illness. *Acta Pathologica et Microbiologica Scandinavica*, **78**, 6–14

Lisiewicz, J. (1980) *Human Neutrophils*, pp. 67–74, Charles Press Publishers Inc., Maryland

Lusher, J.M. and Zuelzer, W.W. (1966) Idiopathic thrombocytopenic purpura in childhood. *Journal of Pediatrics*, **68**, 971–979

Macintyre, S.S., Schultz, D. and Kushner, I. (1983) Synthesis and secretion of C-reactive protein by rabbit primary hepatocyte cultures. *Biochemical Journal*, **210**, 707–715

Mangan, K.F. (1985) Interferon-induced aplasia, recovery after antithymocyte globulin. *American Journal of Haematology*, **19**, 401–413

Matsuda, J. (1975) Studies on NBT-test methodological and clinical significance. *Japanese Journal of Clinical Haematology*, **16**, 599–613

Medd, W.E. and Hayhoe, F.G.T. (1955) Tuberculous miliary necrosis with pancytopenia. *Quarterly Journal of Medicine*, **24**, 351–364

Merriman, C.R., Pulham, L.A. and Kampschmidt, R.F. (1975) Effect of leucocytic endogenous mediator on C-reactive protein in rabbits. *Proceedings of the Society for Experimental Biology and Medicine*, **149**, 782–784

Mills, E. and Townsend, S. (1937) Leukaemoid blood pictures in tuberculosis. *Canadian Medical Association Journal*, **37**, 56–58

Morse, E.E., Zinkman, W.H. and Jackson, D.P. (1966) Thrombocytopenic purpura following rubella infection in children and adults. *Archives of Internal Medicine*, **117**, 573–579

Morse, J.H., Kong, A.S., Lindenbaum, J. and Morse, S.I. (1977) The mitogenic effect of the lymphocytosis promoting factors from Bordetella pertussis on human lymphocytes. *Journal of Clinical Investigation*, **60**, 683–692

Morse, S.I. (1965) Studies on the lymphocytosis induced in mice by *Bordetella pertussis*. *Journal of Experimental Medicine*, **121**, 49–68

Morse, S.I. and Reister, S.K. (1967a) Studies on leukocytosis and lymphocytosis induced by *Bordetella pertussis*. I. Radioautographic analysis of circulating cells in mice undergoing pertussis-induced hyperleukocytosis. *Journal of Experimental Medicine*, **125**, 404–408

Morse, S.I. and Reister, S.K. (1967b) Studies on the leukocytosis and lymphocytosis induced by *Bordetella pertussis*. II. The effect of pertussis vaccine on the thoracic duct lymph and lymphocytes in mice. *Journal of Experimental Medicine*, **125**, 619–628

Morse, S.I. and Barron, B.H. (1970) Studies on the leukocytosis and lymphocytosis induced by *Bordetella pertussis*. III. The distribution of transfused lymphocytes in pertussis-treated and normal mice. *Journal of Experimental Medicine*, **132**, 663–672

Nissen, C., Speck, B., Emadi, G. and Iscove, N. (1977) Toxicity of human leukocyte interferon preparations in human bone marrow cultures. *Lancet*, **1**, 203–204

O'Brien, J.R. (1954) Non-reactive tuberculosis. *Journal of Clinical Pathology*, **7**, 216–225

Oswald, N.C. (1963) Acute tuberculosis and granulocytic disorders. *British Medical Journal*, **2**, 1489–1496

Ottesen, J. (1954) On the age of human white cells in peripheral blood. *Acta Physiologica Scandinavica*, **32**, 75–79

Owen, J.A., Better, F.C. and Hoban, J. (1960) A simple method for the determination of serum heptoglobins. *Journal of Clinical Pathology*, **13**, 163–164

Park, B.H., Firkin, S.M. and Smithwick, E.M. (1968) Infection and nitroblue tetrazolium-reduction by neutrophils. *Lancet*, **2**, 532–534

Pekarek, R.S., Burghen, G.A., Bartelloni, P.J., Calia, F.M., Bostian, K.A. and Beisel, W.R. (1970) The effect of live attenuated Venzuelan equine encephalomyeltitis virus vaccine on serum iron, zinc and copper concentrations in man. *Journal of Laboratory and Clinical Medicine*, **76**, 293–303

Pepys, M.B. (1981) C-reactive protein fifty years on. *Lancet*, **2**, 653–657

Peterson, O.L., Ham, T.H. and Finland, M. (1943) Cold agglutinins (autohaemagglutinins) in primary atypical pneumonias. *Science*, **97**, 167

Pirofsky, B. (1976) Clinical aspects of autoimmune haemolytic anaemia. *Seminars in Haematology,* **13**, 25–38

Pizzi, F., Carrara, P.M., Aldeghi, A. and Eridani, S. (1966) Immunofluorescence of megakaryocytes in the thrombocytopenic purpuras. *Blood,* **27**, 521–526

Platzer, E. (1985) OKT3 monoclonal antibody induces production of colony-stimulating factor(s) for granulocytes and macrophages in cultures of human T lymphocytes and adherent cells. *Journal of Immunology,* **134**, 265–271

Poskitt, J.R. (1985) Thrombocytopenia of sepsis. The role of circulating IgG-containing immune complexes. *Archives of Internal Medicine,* **45**, 891–894

Powanda, M.C. and Mayer, M. (1981) Plasma protein alterations during infection: Potential significance of these changes to host defense and repair systems, in, *Infection: the physiologic and metabolic responses of the host,* M.C. Powanda and P.G. Canonico, (eds), pp. 271–296, Elsevier, North Holland

Proudfoot, A.T., Akhtar, A.J., Douglas, A.C. and Horne, N.W. (1969) Miliary tuberculosis in adults. *British Medical Journal,* **2**, 273–276

Repine, J.E., Rasmussen, R. and Whiter, J.G. (1979) An improved nitroblue tetrazolinin test using phorbol myristate acetate-coated coverslips. *American Journal of Clinical Pathology,* **71**, 582–585

Risdall, R.J., McKenna, R.W., Nesbit, M.E., Krivit, W., Balfour, H.H., Simmons, R.L. and Brunning, R.D. (1979) Virus-associated haemophagocytic syndrome. A benign histiocytic proliferation distinct from malignant histiocytosis. *Cancer,* **44**, 993–1002

Risdall, R.J., Brunning, R.D., Hernandez, J.I. and Gordon, D.H. (1984) Bacteria-associated haemophagocytic syndrome. *Cancer,* **54**, 2968–2972

Roberts, N.J. (1982) Different effects of influenza virus, respiratory syncytial virus, and Sendai virus on human lymphocytes and macrophages. *Infection and Immunity,* **35**, 1142–1146

Rosner, F. (1970) Aplastic anaemia and viral hepatitis. *Lancet,* **2**, 1080

Ross, G.D., Thompson, R.A., Walport, M.J., Springer, T.A., Watson, J.V., Ward, R.H.R., Lida, J., Newman, S.L., Harrison, R.A. and Lachmann, P.J. (1985) Characterisation of patients with an increased susceptibility to bacterial infections and a genetic deficiency of leukocyte membrane complement receptor type 3 and the related membrane antigen LFA-1. *Blood,* **66**, 882–890

Rubin, E., Gottlieb, C. and Vogel, P. (1968) Syndrome of hepatitis and aplastic anaemia. *American Journal of Medicine,* **45**, 88–97

Sato, Y. and Arai, H. (1972) Leukocytosis-promoting factor of *Bordetella pertussis,* purification and characterisation. *Infection and Immunity,* **6**, 899–904

Scheldon, P.J., Papamichail, M., Hernsted, E. and Holborrow, E.J. (1973) Thymic origin of atypical lymphoid cells in infectious mononucleosis. *Lancet,* **i**, 1153–1157

Schmidt, P.J., Barile, M.F. and McGinniss, M.H. (1965)

Mycoplasma (pleuropneumonia-like organisms) and bloodgroup I; associations with neoplastic disease. *Nature,* **205**, 371–372

Segal, A.W. (1985) Variations on the theme of chronic granulomatous disease. *Lancet,* **i**, 1378–1382

Sharp, A.A. (1969) Platelets, bleeding and haemostasis in infectious mononucleosis, in, *Infectious Mononucleosis,* R.L. Carter and H.G. Penman, (eds), pp. 99–110, Blackwell, Oxford

Shields, G.S., Markowitz, H., Cartwright, G.E. and Wintrobe, M.M. (1960) Copper coatings in human subects, in *Metal Binding in Medicine,* M.J. Seven and L.A. Johnson, (eds), pp. 259–264, Lippincott, Philadelphia

Shneerson, J.M., Mortimer, P.P. and Vandervelde, E.M. (1980) Febrile illness due to parvovirus. *British Medical Journal,* **280**, 1580

Shulman, N.R., Marder, V. and Weinrach, R.S. (1965) Similarities between known antiplatelet antibodies and the factor responsible for thrombocytopenia in idiopathic purpura. Physiologic, serologic and isotopic studies. *Annals of the New York Academy of Sciences,* **124**, 499–542

Smith, C.B., McGinniss, M.H. and Schmidt, P. (1967) Changes in erythrocyte I agglutinogen and anti-I agglutinins during *Mycoplasma pneumoniae* infection in man. *Journal of Immunology,* **99**, 333–339

Sullivan, J.L., Barry, D.W., Lucas, S.J. and Albrecht, P. (1975) Measles infection of human mononuclear cells. I. Acute infection of peripheral blood lymphocytes and monocytes. *Journal of Experimental Medicine,* **142**, 773–784

Suvatte, V., Mahasandana, C., Tanphaichitra, V. and Tuchinda, S. (1979) Acquired platelet dysfunction with eosinophilia. Study of platelet function in 62 cases. *Asian Journal of Tropical Medicine and Public Health,* **10**, 358–367

Svedmyr, E. and Jondal, M. (1975) Cytotoxic effector cells specific for B cell lines transformed by Epstein–Barr virus are present in patients with infectious mononucleosis. *Proceedings of the National Academy of Sciences,* **72**, 1622–1626

Terada, H., Baldini, M., Ebbe, S. and Madoff, M.A. (1966) Interaction of influenza virus with blood platelets. *Blood,* **28**, 213–228

Thomas, D.B. (1972) Antibodies to membrane antigen(s) common to thymocytes and a sub-population of lymphocytes in infectious-mononucleosis sera. *Lancet,* **1**, 399–403

Thorley-Lawson, D.A. and Mann, K.P. (1985) Early events in Epstein–Barr virus infection provide a model for B cell activation. *Journal of Experimental Medicine,* **162**, 45–59

Tillett, W.S. and Francis, T. (1930) Serological reactions in pneumonia with a non-protein somatic fraction of pneumococcus. *Journal of Experimental Medicine,* **52**, 561–571

Ting, P.L. (1984) Viral hepatitis B-induced haemolytic anaemia in a patient with normal glucose-6-phosphate dehydrogenase: a case report. *Singapore Medical Journal,* **25**, 360–361

Turner, J.C. (1943) Development of cold agglutinins in a pneumonia. *Nature,* **151**, 419–420

Twomey, J.J. and Leavell, B.S. (1965) Leukaemoid reactions to tuberculosis. *Archives of Internal Medicine,* **116**, 21–28

Ueda, K. (1985) Haemolytic anaemia following post-natally-acquired rubella during the 1975–1977 rubella epidemic in Japan. *Clinical Pediatrics (Philadelphia),* **24**, 155–157

Veenhoven, W.A., Van der Schand, G.S. and Nieweg, H.O. (1980) Platelet antibodies in idiopathic Thrombo-cytopenic purpura. *Clinical and Experimental Immunology,* **39**, 645–651

Warner, H.R. and Athens, J.W. (1964) An analysis of granulocyte kinetics in blood and bone marrow, in leukopoiesis in health and disease. *Annals of the New York Academy of Science,* **113**, 523–536

Whicker, J.T., Martin, J.F.R. and Dieppe, P.A. (1980) Prostaglandin-stimulated increase in acute-phase proteins in man and its failure in systemic sclerosis. *Lancet,* **2**, 1187

Wilson, E.R., Malluh, A., Stagno, S. and Guest, W.M. (1981) Epstein–Barr virus associated haemophagocytic syndrome. *Journal of Pediatrics,* **98**, 260–262

Wishart, M.M. and Davey, M.G. (1973) Infectious mononucleosis complicated by acute haemolytic anaemia with a positive Donath–Landsteiner reaction. *Journal of Clinical Pathology,* **26**, 332–334

Worlledge, S.M. and Rousso, C. (1965) Studies on the serology of paroxysmal cold haemoglobinuria (PCH) with special reference to its relationship with the P blood group system. *Vox Sanguinis,* **10**, 293–297

Worlledge, S.M. and Dacie, J.V. (1969) Haemolytic and other anaemias in infectious mononucleosis, in *Infectious Mononucleosis,* R.L. Carter and H.G. Penman, (eds), pp. 82–98, Blackwell, Oxford

Young, N. (1988) Haematologic and haematopoietic consequences of B19 parvovirus infection. *Seminars in Haematology,* **25**, 159–172

Zamorano, J. and Thompsett, R. (1968) Disseminated atypical mycobacterial infection and pancytopenia. *Archives of Internal Medicine,* **121**, 424–427

Zeldis, J.B. and Dienstag, J.L. (1983) Aplastic anaemia and non-A, non-B hepatitis. *American Journal of Medicine,* **74**, 64–66

Zinkham, W.H., Medearis, D.N. and Osborn, J.E. (1967) Blood and bone-marrow findings in congenital rubella. *Journal of Pediatrics,* **71**, 512–524

Zoumbos, N.C., Djeu, J.T. and Young, N.S. (1984) Interferon is the suppressor of haematopoiesis generated by stimulated lymphocytes *in vitro. Journal of Immunology,* **133**, 769–774

Zuazu, J.P., Duran, J.W. and Julia, A.F. (1979) Haemo-phagocytosis in acute brucellosis. *New England Journal of Medicine,* **301**, 1185–1186

19

The effects of antibiotics on the blood and blood forming tissues

G.C. Jenkins and M.E. Wood

Drugs may adversely affect the blood forming tissues in a variety of ways. The most well recognized of these is depression of the formation of haemopoietic cells in the bone marrow, resulting in pancytopenia. In other examples there may be a single cell line affected, with resulting red cell hypoplasia, leucopenia or thrombocytopenia.

Some agents can cause haemolysis by their interference with the metabolism of the erythrocyte, while others are capable of producing red cell, leucocyte or platelet destruction by inducing an immune response. Cellular maturation and function can be altered by the action of antimetabolites and in some instances there is an associated lupoid reaction.

Haemostasis involves the interaction of vessel wall, platelets and the coagulation cascade. Each of these components may be interfered with by the action of antibiotics, leading to abnormalities in tests and sometimes to clinical bleeding.

In this chapter 'antibiotics' includes antiprotozoal, antiviral, and antifungal agents as well as antibacterial drugs.

Antibiotics affecting cell formation and function

Antibiotics may cause suppression of a single haemopoietic cell line or any combination of the three by a variety of mechanisms, not all of which are as yet fully understood.

Aplastic anaemia and red cell aplasia

Aplastic anaemia is the most extreme form of myelosuppression and is diagnosed when there is peripheral blood pancytopenia together with marrow hypocellularity. In most reports approximately 50% of cases are idiopathic; chloramphenicol is the single commonest identifiable cause, representing up to 35% of cases (Alter, Potter and Li, 1978).

The first report of aplastic anaemia associated with chloramphenicol appeared in 1950 (Rich, Ritterhof and Hoffman) less than two years after the antibiotic first became available. With the appearance of subsequent reports it became apparent that chloramphenicol produces two distinct types of marrow toxicity (Yunis, 1973):

(i) a dose-related reversible marrow suppression involving primarily the red cell series
(ii) a rarer irreversible marrow aplasia.

The dose-related reversible marrow toxicity develops in about 50% of people who are given high doses of the drug, in whom plasma levels are over 25 μg/ml (Scott, et al., 1965). Findings include an increase in serum iron and saturation of transferrin (Rubin, et al., 1958) and the appearance of vacuoles in both the nucleus and cytoplasm of erythroblasts and sometimes also the granulocyte series (Scott, et al., 1965). These changes usually appear between 11 and 28 days after initiation of the antibiotic. The biochemical mechanism of this effect is related to its mode of action as an antibiotic. Chloramphenicol is a potent inhibitor of protein synthesis and in bacteria acts by binding reversibly to the 50S subunit of ribosomes. Experiments *in vitro* and in animals have shown that the drug produces dose-related ultra-structural changes in the mitochondria of bone marrow cells, a mitochondrial respiratory lesion and suppression of the enzyme ferrochelatase. This enzyme, which is located on the inner mitochondrial membrane, is responsible for the last step in the synthesis of haem (Yunis, 1973).

The incidence of idiopathic aplastic anaemia following chloramphenicol is one in 24–40,000 (Alter, Potter and Li, 1978) and it may develop several months to years after exposure to the drug. There is evidence of a genetic predisposition, with the occurrence of blood dyscrasias in both of two sets of twins (Nagao and Mauer, 1969; Nora and Fernback, 1969). This is further supported by *in vitro* work demonstrating an increased sensitivity to chloramphenicol of the marrow cells of parents of affected patients (Yunis, 1973). It has been postulated that a nitrosoderivative of the antibiotic may be the causative agent but the mechanism remains a matter for speculation.

In the developed world the use of chloramphenicol has declined considerably over the past 30 years, however its use topically for ear and eye infections continues and there have been several reports of aplastic anaemia following the use of chloramphenicol eye-drops (Carpenter, 1975; Fraunfelder and Bagby, 1983).

Historically the earliest reports of aplasia related to antimicrobial agents were those associated with the use of the organic arsenicals (mapharsen, neoarsphenamin) to treat syphilis (Loveman, 1932). Numerically however, certain sulphonamides are the next most common antimicrobial agents to be implicated in the aetiology of aplastic anaemia. As with the arsenicals, those sulphonamides which were reported as possible causative agents for the syndrome are no longer in use, having been replaced by more effective and less toxic agents. The same is true for mepacrine (quinacrine), an antimalarial used widely amongst military personnel during the Second World War, in whom there was a significant incidence of aplasia attributed to the drug (Custer, 1946).

It can be difficult to decide which drug is the cause of aplasia when a patient may have been exposed to a number of possible toxic agents; polypharmacy seems sometimes to be an unavoidable feature of modern medical practice. The fact that drug exposure may antedate development of the dyscrasia by many months further complicates the picture. It is also important to differentiate between cases in which there is peripheral pancytopenia with a normocellular or even hypercellular marrow, from true aplastic anaemia. In addition the patient's underlying disease may predispose to pancytopenia, as in the case of fatal aplasia reported following the combination of amphotericin and flucytosine given to treat Cryptococcal meningitis, in a man with untreated multiple myeloma and renal impairment (Bryan and McFarland, 1978).

Other antimicrobial agents which have rarely been associated with the development of aplastic anaemia are streptomycin (Deyke and Wallace, 1946) and tetracycline (Lehrner, Cooke and Enck, 1979).

Pure red cell aplasia In addition to the dose-related marrow suppression caused by chloramphenicol, in which the red cells are primarily affected, other drugs may cause a pure red cell aplasia. There are reports of its occurrence in association with the antituberculous agents Para-amino-salicyclic acid (PAS) and isoniazid (Goodman and Block, 1964).

In a study to determine the aetiology of the anaemia developing during systemic treatment with amphotericin B, Brandriss, *et al.* (1964) found a shortened red cell survival pre-treatment which they attributed to the underlying disease; this was not altered by administration of amphotericin B. Bone marrow examination in seven of the patients while they were anaemic revealed normal erythroid activity in five, hypocellularity in one and 'relative' erythroid hyperplasia in another; they concluded that the anaemia which developed was due to suppression of red cell production in the presence of pre-existing low grade haemolysis.

Other effects upon erythropoiesis

Megaloblastic change in the bone marrow may be caused by some antibiotics whose action in micro-organisms is to inhibit folate metabolism. By inhibiting the enzyme dihydrofolate reductase they block the essential conversion of dihydrofolate to tetrahydrofolate and thus interfere with the production of thymidylate and DNA-thymine.

Trimethoprim produces its bacteriostatic effect as a dihydrofolate reductase inhibitor. It is usually used in a bacteriocidal combination with sulphamethoxazole, which also inhibits folate metabolism at an earlier stage, by blocking the conversion of p-aminobenzoic acid to dihydrofolate. These effects may rarely produce megaloblastic anaemia in a poorly nourished patient, treated for long periods (Girdwood, 1973). Jenkins, *et al.* (1970) reached a similar conclusion but in their series of patients receiving co-trimoxazole there was one individual who also developed quite severe thrombocytopenia, this rapidly responded to systemic folinic acid therapy. As folinic acid is not taken up by bacteria the antibacterial effect of trimethoprim is fully maintained.

Pyrimethamine which is closely related to trimethoprim may have the same effect. However it is unlikely to produce this complication in the doses used to treat malaria or toxoplasmosis, unless the patient is already folate depleted or as not infrequently occurs, the day is given incorrectly.

Pentamidine isoethionate is an antiprotozoal agent which acts by interfering with DNA and folate metabolism with inhibition of RNA and protein synthesis. It has been used intramuscularly, to treat antimony resistant visceral leishmaniasis and more recently in the treatment of *Pneumocystis cariniii* pneumonia (PCP) in HIV infected individuals. However close monitoring is required during therapy because of the high incidence of potentially severe unwanted effects. These include the development of anaemia in at least 21% of patients (Anderson, *et al.*, 1986). The introduction of nebulized pentamidine for the treatment and prophylaxis of PCP has resulted in the elimination of adverse systemic reactions to the drug (Montgomery, *et al.*, 1987) with no loss of efficacy.

The antituberculous drugs isoniazid and cycloserine are recorded as producing megaloblastic anaemia (Klipstein, *et al.*, 1967). Amos and Amess (1983) described three patients with megaloblastic change attributable to acyclovir therapy due to inhibition of DNA polymerase. There were no other haematological effects but they recommended that such patients should be monitored.

Zidovudine (azidothymidine, AZT) is an antiretroviral agent which acts as a thymidine analogue, its triphosphate derivative inhibiting the viral enzyme reverse transcriptase. It also acts as a substrate for DNA polymerase and prevents the addition of further bases to the strand of DNA in host cells; however cellular DNA polymerase is 100 times less susceptible to inhibition than is HIV reverse transcriptase (Yarchoan and Broder, 1987). Use of AZT to treat HIV infection is associated with a number of haematological side-effects, the most common of which is an increase in the mean cell volume, not associated with B12 or folate deficiency (Richman, *et al.*, 1987). Macrocytosis occurs so commonly during AZT therapy that it may be used to monitor compliance. It is not however predictive of the more serious haematological toxicities, anaemia and neutropenia.

About one-third of symptomatic HIV infected individuals treated with AZT will develop anaemia (Richman, *et al.*, 1987). This is dose related, usually develops after six weeks of therapy and improves on withdrawal of the drug (Dournon, *et al.*, 1988). However if full dose treatment is to be continued, the majority of patients will require transfusion to maintain their haemoglobin level. The exact mechanism of the marrow toxicity produced by AZT is uncertain, as pyrimidine metabolism by cells is complex. Bone marrow examination was performed in a few individuals, revealing normal cellularity with a reduction in red cell precursors in some and absent red cell precursors in others whose overall marrow cellularity was reduced (Richman, *et al.*, 1987). In asymptomatic individuals receiving treatment because of a low CD4 count (less than $500/mm^3$), the incidence of anaemia is much less; 6.3% and 1.1% respectively at daily doses of 1500 mg or 500 mg. Transfusion was necessary in 2.0% of those receiving the higher dose (Volberding, *et al.*, 1990). There is more recent evidence that erythropoietin may help to rectify the anaemia produced by AZT (Miles, 1992).

Sideroblastic change in erythropoiesis has been identified with long-term antituberculous therapy in the form of isoniazid (INAH), cycloserine and pyrazinamide. INAH alone or in combination with p-aminosalicylic acid (PAS) rarely causes anaemia, however cycloserine and pyrazinamide readily cause sideroblastic change (Verwilghen, *et al.*, 1965). These drugs cause defects in the haem synthetic pathway.

Chloramphenicol when administered in large doses, or in therapeutic doses to some susceptible individuals, will produce reversible sideroblastic anaemia. The effect is likely to be due to mitochondrial damage in the red cell precursors (see above). More recently Kokkini, *et al.* (1983) described a case of sideroblastic anaemia in a 58-year-old woman after eight days' treatment with lincomycin.

The marrow appearances associated with these drugs are usually reversed after discontinuing them, although it may take several months.

Neutropenia

The β-lactam antibiotics are the antimicrobial agents most commonly associated with neutropenia. Neftel, Hauser and Muller (1985) report an incidence of up to 15% in patients given large doses of any β-lactam for at least 10 days. In the same paper, the associated findings in 140 previously reported cases included eosinophilia (32%), rash (41%), fever (68%); 95% of cases recovered within a week of discontinuing the presumed aetiologic agent. Based upon the appearances of bone marrow 'arrest' (numerous granulocyte precursors and an absence of mature forms) in affected individuals, *in vitro* studies demonstrating a dose dependent inhibition of colony formation and an incidence of relapse on rechallenge of only 31%, the authors propose that a direct toxic effect of the drugs on the bone marrow is responsible for the cytopenia. Other authors have put forward evidence for an immune mechanism of cell destruction. Rouveix, *et al.* (1983) detected leucoagglutinins in eight of nine patients who had developed neutropenia associated with β-lactams and suggest that the neutrophils become sensitized as a result of absorption onto the cell membrane of drug-antibody immune complexes.

Murphy, *et al.* (1983) investigated five patients who developed neutropenia following high dose penicillin for endocarditis and a further two patients (1985) with cephalosporin related neutropenia. In more extensive studies on a patient from the former group, they detected a complement fixing IgG anti-penicillin antibody which reacted with the patient's granulocytes and platelets in the presence of the drug; in the latter two patients they found cephalosporin-dependent anti-neutrophil antibodies. They suggest a hapten-type mechanism for the development of neutropenia, with formation of antibodies against the membrane bound drug. This is very similar to the DAGT positive haemolytic anaemia which is seen with the same agents (see below), and Murphy and colleagues further suggest that the findings of rash, fever and eosinophilia reported by Neftel are compatible with an immune response. Opponents of the immune theory point out the relatively high incidence of antibodies against β-lactam antibiotics, compared with the low rate of occurrence of cytopenia (Neftel, *et al.*, 1986).

There are reports of neutropenia associated with vancomycin and gentamicin. As might be expected, in many cases these drugs have been given in combination with others (particularly β-lactams) for which a causal relationship with neutropenia is well established. In isolated cases however there are either no other causative agents or the temporal relationship is such that vancomycin (Kauffman, *et al.*, 1982) or gentamicin (Chang and Reyes, 1975) appear to be unequivocally implicated.

The commonly used antituberculous agent rifampicin has been associated with leucopenia and in some instances moderate neutropenia (Van Assendelft, 1984), and there are isolated reports of neutropenia in association with isoniazid and ethambutol, including one case in which each of three drugs individually produced a marked fall in the white cell count in the same patient (Jenkins, Williams and Campbell, 1980).

Neutropenia is a recognized side-effect of pentamidine when administered intramuscularly in the treatment of visceral leishmaniasis and Pneumocystis carinii pneumonia. In a historical review of 24 patients treated for PCP, Anderson, *et al.* (1986) found neutropenia in 13%. However when administered by aerosolized inhalation in the treatment or prophylaxis of PCP, pentamidine remains effective with no associated unwanted systemic effects (Montgomery, *et al.*, 1987) (see also anaemia, above).

The use of specific antiretroviral therapies has been shown to reduce significantly the incidence of opportunistic infections, in subjects with AIDS and advanced AIDS-related complex (Fischl, *et al.*, 1987). However bone marrow suppression with the development of anaemia (see above) and neutropenia is a significant toxic effect. Neutropenia occurred in 16% of treated subjects and was more likely to develop in those with more advanced disease, a low CD4 cell count or low vitamin B_{12} level at the start of treatment (Richman, *et al.*, 1987). Concomitant administration of paracetamol was associated with an increased risk of myelosuppression. Although anaemia could be controlled by dose reduction, some patients then went on to develop neutropenia, necessitating withdrawal of therapy. The mechanism by which these toxic effects are produced is unclear though Miles (1992) has recorded that the neutropenia may in some cases respond to therapeutic G-CSF. It is of interest that thrombocytopenia occurs rarely during AZT therapy, indeed an improvement in the platelet count may be seen in those with an immune thrombocytopenia (Richman, *et al.*, 1987).

Cytomegalovirus (CMV) infections are recognized as a major cause of morbidity and mortality in the immunocompromised. The virus lacks the enzyme thymidine kinase and hence acyclovir is ineffective against it. The related compound, 9-(1,3-dihydroxy-2-propoxymethyl guanine) (DHPG) is phosphorylated by cellular enzymes. In its triphosphate form it inhibits viral DNA synthesis by inhibition of viral DNA polymerase and by limitation of viral DNA elongation following its incorporation into that molecule. Phosphorylation appears to be ten-fold more active in virally infected cells and ganciclovir (DHPG) has been shown to bring about an improvement in patients with CMV retinitis or colitis. The most frequently observed adverse reaction during therapy is neutropenia, which appears to be dose related and reversible in the majority of cases (Collaborative DHPG Treatment Study Group, 1986). The mechanism is presumed to be interference with host-cell DNA metabolism. The incidence of neutropenia is between 25–40%, onset usually occurring during the first two weeks of therapy. There have been reports of deaths occurring during neutropenia and careful monitoring is therefore mandatory whilst treatment is in progress.

Amphotericin B, which is known to be toxic to neutrophils *in vitro* (Chunn, Starr and Gilbert, 1977), is rarely associated with neutropenia. There is a report of episodic leucopenia

and neutropenia with recovery over a few hours each time, occurring on three occasions in the same patient over a five-day period, following the administration of amphotericin for disseminated *Candida tropicalis* (Stein and Tolle, 1983).

Certain anthelmintic agents may produce neutropenia when used in high doses; one report suggests an incidence of this complication of 5% with high dose mebendazole, which may be associated with anaemia and thrombocytopenia in some instances (Levin, *et al.*, 1983). The related compound levamisole has found a role as an immunostimulant in the treatment of certain malignancies but its usefulness may be limited by the severe neutropenia which develops in up to 10% of patients (Teerenhovi, *et al.*, 1978). It has been suggested that the drug may trigger the production of autoantibodies to certain neutrophil surface antigens (Thompson, *et al.*, 1980), a mechanism classically described in α-methyl dopa induced haemolytic anaemia.

Other effects upon leucopoiesis

Two cases of eosinophilia have been reported in which there is convincing evidence of it being directly associated with rifampicin treatment (Mungall and Standing, 1978; Lee and Berger, 1980). It rapidly resolved on withdrawing the drug. Eosinophilia of severe degree has also been described following therapy with tetracyclines. Winn, Chatham and Ross (1983) described a case of a leukaemoid reaction with an absolute eosinophil count of $25 \times 10^9/1$ after a course of minocycline, a semi-synthetic derivative of tetracycline. Ho, *et al.* (1979) described two cases of eosinophilia with pulmonary infiltration associated with tetracycline therapy, one of which was minocycline. In all cases the effects disappeared after withdrawing the antibiotics. Eosinophilia was seen in three of 26 patients during treatment with ganciclovir (Collaborative DHPG Treatment Study Group, 1986).

Acute leukaemia may be a rare sequela of chloramphenicol therapy. Over the past thirty years there have been sporadic case reports of its development, with acute non-lymphocytic leukaemia predominating, in patients who already have aplastic anaemia induced by the drug (Brauer and Dameshek, 1967). A recent case-control study from China suggested a significant dose-response relationship between chloramphenicol and both acute lymphocytic leukaemia and acute non-lymphocytic leukaemia in childhood (Ou Shu, *et al.*, 1987). In the same study a similar increase in the risk of development of acute non-lymphocytic leukaemia was observed for the related antibiotic syntomycin.

Thrombocytopenia

A reduction in the platelet count is probably the commonest of the antibiotic induced cytopenias. It may be due to suppression of production, or increased consumption after release of the platelets from the marrow, usually by immune mechanisms.

Hackett, Kelton and Powers (1982) have comprehensively reviewed the subject of drug induced platelet destruction, including possible mechanisms, diagnosis and treatment. They point out that the thrombocytopenia in such cases usually occurs in isolation, whereas drugs causing suppression of platelet production are generally the same agents which produce suppression of all the marrow elements and hence the low platelet count is only part of a pancytopenia. The occurrence of thrombocytopenia in association with megaloblastic change, due to folate deficiency caused by co-trimoxazole has been mentioned above; thrombocytopenia produced in this way may sometimes occur in isolation. It is clearly important to be sure that other causes of a low platelet count have been excluded before the label 'immune destruction' is applied.

As in other drug-induced immune disorders there is almost invariably a history of previous exposure to the drug. The onset is often abrupt and resolution usually occurs within days of discontinuing the causative agent. Elevated levels of platelet associated IgG are consistent with but not diagnostic of the disorder; they are found in a variety of immune thrombocytopenias unrelated to drugs.

Several antibiotics are included amongst the large number of drugs which have been reported as causing a drug-induced thrombocytopenia. However in many instances these are case reports, with insufficient evidence that the drug was the only possible cause of a low platelet count. Four criteria are used by Hackett, Kelton and Powers (1982) in evaluating individual reports: (1) a consistent clinical history; (2) exclusion of other causes; (3) confirmation of the causative agent by an *in vivo* rechallenge; (4) confirmation of the causative agent by an *in vitro* test.

A patient is defined as having drug-induced immune thrombocytopenia if either (1); (2) and (3); (1), (2) and (4); or all four criteria are fulfilled. On this basis they conclude that the following antibiotics which are in common use have caused an immune thrombocytopenia: cotrimoxazole (Barr and Whineray, 1980), methicillin (Schiffer, Weinstein and Wiernik, 1973) and rifampicin (Blajchman, *et al.*, 1970). Quinine and quinidine have more restricted application than these agents but immune thrombocytopenia in association with their use is well documented (Bolton and Young, 1953; Larson, 1953; Weintraub, Perchet and Alexander, 1962). Levamisole, an anthelmintic which is used as an immunostimulant, has been mentioned above as a cause of immune neutropenia; it has also caused immune thrombocytopenia (El-Ghobarey and Capell, 1977). The organic arsenicals (Falconer, Epstein and Mills, 1940) and certain sulphonamides which are no longer in use – sulfathiazole (Hurd and Jacox, 1943) and sulfisoxazole (Hamilton and Sheets, 1978) – also fulfil the criteria laid down by Hackett and colleagues.

It is interesting to note that although many of these agents cause immune destruction of red cells, neutrophils and platelets, drug-dependent antibodies are highly cell specific and only one cell line is usually involved in individual cases. As described elsewhere in this chapter, the actual mechanism of destruction may be due to the attachment on the platelet membrane of a drug-antibody complex which then binds complement, or the drug may form a hapten with molecules on the platelet surface and thus stimulate antibody production. In cases where two cell lines are affected, two separate antibodies may be demonstrated. Chong, *et al.* (1983) describe a patient with neutropenia and thrombocytopenia following quinidine, whose serum contained two quinidine-dependent antibodies, one reacting with platelets and the other with neutrophils.

Although most commonly all three cell lines are affected by an agent causing marrow suppression, isolated thrombocytopenia without evidence of an immune mechanism may occur, in the same way as pure red cell aplasia has been reported occasionally following drugs. Such is the situation in a case report from Chan, Tuazon and Less (1982). They describe a patient with acute leukaemia in remission whose platelet count fell from normal to a low level of $30 \times 10^9/1$ on two occasions associated with the administration of amphotericin for hepatic candidiasis. There was no evidence of peripheral platelet destruction and repeat bone marrow examination showed a marked reduction in megakaryocyte numbers which recovered, as did the platelet count, after the amphotericin was stopped.

Ganciclovir is associated with a reduction in the platelet count below $50 \times 10^9/1$ in up to 20% of subjects, with almost half of these having a count less than $20 \times 10^9/1$ (manufacturer's data). The mechanism is presumably the same as that responsible for the neutropenia seen during treatment with this agent (see above).

A few drugs may cause direct toxic platelet destruction. The antibiotic ristocetin is one of these, producing its effect by inducing aggregation and agglutination of platelets (Gangarosa, Johnson and Ramos, 1960), a phenomenon which is made use of in tests of platelet function.

Immune haemolytic anaemia

This mechanism of haemolysis occurs uncommonly during the use of antibiotic drugs (Table 19.1). Some examples are anecdotal since there is only a single case report in the literature. Clinically the patient may present with a gradual onset of anaemia which is found to be due to extravascular haemolysis, this is typified by the reactions caused by penicillins and cephalosporins. A larger variety of anti-

Table 19.1 Antibiotics and haemolytic anaemia

(1) Producing mostly extravascular haemolysis
    Cephalosporins
    Penicillins

(2) Producing mostly intravascular haemolysis
    Erythromycin
    Isonicotinic acid hydrochloride (INAH)
    P-amino-salicylic acid (PAS)
    Quinine and quinidine
    Rifampicin
    Stibophen
    Streptomycin
    Sulphonamides
    Tetracycline

biotics can be responsible for intravascular haemolysis, when the clinical picture is much more acute and accompanied by haemoglobinaemia.

Penicillin induced haemolysis

First described by Ley, Cahan and Mayer in 1958; considering the vast amount of the penicillins administered, the occurrence of haemolytic anaemia associated with their use is vary rare. There is in fact quite a high incidence of penicillin antibodies in the population and 3% of patients receiving a large dose of penicillin develop a positive Coombs (direct antiglobulin) test. Only a small proportion of these will develop haemolytic anaemia. The occurrence of increased red cell destruction in patients treated with a penicillin depends on two factors:

(i) the coating of the patient's red cells with penicillin. This occurs in most people receiving very large doses, of the order of 12–15 mU/day. The blood level may be enhanced by renal failure or the administration of probenecid

(ii) the ability of the patient to synthesize large amounts of IgG anti-penicillin antibody. This depends on the individual response of the patient (White *et al.*, 1963).

In patients who tend to produce antibodies the drug forms a hapten or conjugates with tissue proteins, on the red cell membrane (where it binds strongly) and also in the serum. In susceptible individuals the hapten acts antigenically to produce antibody against the drug. When a patient receiving large doses of penicillin develops anti-penicillin antibody and the drug is continued, the antibody will react with the drug conjugate adsorbed on the red cell surface resulting in the destruction of the cell (Funicella, *et al.*, 1977).

The haemolysis usually develops in patients who have had previous treatment with and in some cases evidence of previous allergy to the drug. There is most often a fairly rapid fall of haemoglobin with a reticulocytosis and no evidence of bleeding. The cells are destroyed in the spleen. Haemolysis ceases on withdrawal of the drug after a variable period of time, up to several weeks. The Coombs test may remain positive for up to three months. An accompanying leucopenia has been noted in a few cases (see above).

As part of the molecule involved in the reaction is the 6-amino-penicillanic acid nucleus, it follows that this process can be produced by all the penicillins. Most drug-induced antibodies are IgM in character but those producing haemolysis are usually IgG and non-complement binding. Their demonstration *in vitro* requires the presence of penicillin treated cells. There is also cross-reactivity with the cephalosporins, which are chemically related.

Cephalosporin induced haemolysis

The mechanism of cephalosporin induced red cell destruction may be the same as the classical cell-hapten mechanism of penicillin induced haemolysis. There is usually an IgG non-complement binding antibody although, as with penicillin, isolated cases of complement binding antibody with intravascular haemolysis have been reported. A few cases who suffered haemolysis early on exposure to cephalosporins were noted to have a past history of penicillin allergy (Moake, *et al.*, 1978). A positive direct antiglobulin test without evidence of haemolysis was observed in up to three-quarters of the patients taking cephalosporins, particularly those with poor renal function. The positive test develops within one or two days, before an antibody can develop and is due to non-specific adsorption of plasma proteins on the red cell surface. The use of more specific antiglobulin reagents has reduced the incidence of this phenomenon.

Stibophen induced haemolysis

Stibophen is a historic example, first described by Harris (1954), of a drug which produces acute intravascular haemolysis with haemoglobinuria when the drug and an antibody directed against it form a complex, which becomes loosely attached to the red cell membrane. The complex then binds complement, thus increasing the vulnerability of the red cell to haemolysis. This is referred to as the immune-complex mechanism. The antibodies are IgM and complement-binding. As in Harris's original description, the reaction usually arises during a second course of the drug, sensitization having occurred previously. The direct antiglobulin test is positive and depends on the detection of complement. The

indirect antiglobulin test is positive in the presence of the drug. Renal failure may occur.

Other antibiotics which may produce this type of reaction are quinine, quinidine, sulphonamides, p-amino-salicylic acid, isoniazid and rifampicin. Many of these drugs may also immunologically produce thrombocytopenia or neutropenia, either singly or in combination. This particularly applies to quinine and quinidine antibodies (Ziegler, *et al.*, 1979) (see also above). In some instances it has been possible to demonstrate that certain blood group antigens form all or part of the 'target' structure for the drug-antibody complex (Habibi, 1987).

For a number of antibiotics the mechanism by which immune haemolysis is induced is less certain and features of both antibody and immune-complex activity may be present. The following are examples, though their occurrence is very uncommon.

Erythromycin

In 1981, Wong, *et al.* reported a case of severe haemolysis associated with the use of erythromycin in a 21-month-old child. There was quite severe intravascular red cell destruction with impaired renal function and the direct antiglobulin test showed the presence of complement and IgM antibody on the red cells. The child had been treated previously with both penicillin and erythromycin. They were able to demonstrate that the haemolysis was specifically erythromycin induced. The mechanism was more in accordance with a hapten type of reaction, similar to isolated examples of penicillin induced reactions, where there are complement binding IgM or IgG antibodies with intravascular destruction of red cells (Bird, McEvoy and Wingham, 1975; Ries, *et al.*, 1975). This was further supported by the fact that haemolysis ceased immediately upon discontinuation of erythromycin.

Streptomycin is another antibiotic which has been reported on two or three occasions to have induced haemolysis. Letona, *et al.* (1977) described such a case in a 45-year-old man who had been previously treated with the drug for tuberculosis. After comprehensive investigations they concluded that there was strong evidence for a complement-fixing hapten-cell mechanism of red cell destruction, mediated by IgG antibodies. At least some of the breakdown was intravascular. However as in the case described above involving erythromycin, they conceded that an immune-complex mechanism could not be completely ruled out.

Tetracycline provides a further rare example of a drug in which the distinction between a hapten and an immune-complex mechanism is arbitrary and according to Simpson, *et al.* (1985), not entirely appropriate. They described a case of a 43-year-old man who developed intravascular haemolysis with transient renal impairment and they postulated the formation of a tetracycline-lipoprotein complex which generated IgG antibody, invoking both types of mechanism. There was also an associated thrombocytopenia and some evidence to suggest that an intravascular consumptive coagulopathy might be responsible for some of the abnormalities.

Antibiotics causing haemolysis of non-immune type

The majority of drugs causing haemolysis of this type do so only in individuals where the susceptibility is due to an inherited defect in the red cell enzymes. Much more rarely the abnormality is an unstable haemoglobin.

The normal metabolism of the red cell depends partly on the oxidative hexose monophosphate shunt, which relies upon the activity of the enzyme glucose-6-phosphate dehydrogenase (G6PD) to initiate it. Carson, *et al.* (1956) first recognized that subjects deficient in this enzyme were particularly sensitive to antimalarials of the primaquine group and tended to have a variable degree of haemolytic anaemia following their ingestion. The condition is a sex-linked recessive characteristic and therefore most severely expressed in males and homozygous females. The mutant gene occurs more commonly in certain ethnic groups. Thus 12% of American negroes and 10% of Nigerians are affected. it is also present in the Mediterranean, the Indian and the Arab peoples. Other races affected, include Chinese, Malays, Thais, Filipinos and Melanesians, with occasional cases in people of Northern European stock including those from Great Britain. The result of the G6PD deficiency is to shorten the survival of red cells when they are exposed to oxidative stress. This occurs most commonly after the administration of certain drugs. Of the antibiotics, the antimalarials were the first to be found responsible, including quinine and aminoquinolines – primaquine, pamaquine, chloroquine, pentaquine and pyrimethamine. Sulphanilamides are particularly challenging as are nitrofurantoin, chloramphenicol and possibly nalidixic acid.

Oxidative denaturation of the haemoglobin in the red cells occurs, with the production of methaemoglobin and sulphaemoglobin. Further degradation of methaemoglobin produces Heinz bodies within the cells. The resulting haemolytic anaemia is associated with cell fragmentation and basophilic stippling.

A similar tendency to develop haemolysis after exposure to these drugs occurs with deficiencies of other enzymes, such as glutathione reductase, but these are very rare.

Sulphanilamides and aminoquinolines can also produce haemolytic anaemia with Heinz body formation in patients with inherited unstable haemoglobins such as haemoglobin Zurich; these are also rare. In established cases the patient should avoid oxidant drugs (Carrell and Lehmann, 1969).

Dapsone is a sulphone which is used in the treatment of leprosy. In large doses it can cause haemolysis even in subjects with normal red cells.

Antimicrobial agents and haemostasis

There are a variety of ways in which antimicrobial agents may affect haemostasis and such a potentially serious side-effect should not be forgotten.

Abnormalities of platelet function

Thrombocytopenia caused by antibiotics has been dealt with earlier in this chapter, however some of these agents may also induce qualitative changes in platelets.

One of the first reports was of severe and persistent haemorrhage in a patient with renal failure and milder bleeding in two other patients receiving carbenicillin (Lurie, *et al.*, 1970). The bleeding stopped when the antibiotic was discontinued and on the basis of coagulation tests on the patients' plasmas, together with *in vitro* studies, it was initially proposed that the effect was due to interference with the conversion of fibrinogen to fibrin. Subsequent authors pointed out that the doses used by Lurie and his colleagues were considerably in excess of those recommended in renal insufficiency (Gordon, 1970). The significance of a prolonged bleeding time was demonstrated by McClure, *et al.* (1970), in patients with cystic fibrosis and normal renal function being treated with carbenicillin in large doses. They found defective platelet aggregation, particularly in response to ADP and observed that the defect lasted for up to seven days after withdrawal of the antibiotic. The dose response relationship and mechanism of action have been extensively studied using more conventional doses in human volunteers and in animals (Brown, *et al.*, 1974; Johnson, Rao and White, 1978). A loss of the secondary wave of ADP induced platelet aggregation and depression of the primary wave occurs in all subjects, with slightly less consistent abnormalities of epinephrine and collagen induced aggregation. The degree of platelet dysfunction and the rapidity with which it develops are proportional to the dose or serum concentration of antibiotic (Johnson, Rao and White, 1978). In their study of carbenicillin and ticarcillin, prolongation of the bleeding time did not occur until after two to seven days of treatment, with maximum prolongation after three days when normal therapeutic doses were used; the onset was seen sooner with higher drug doses. The effect persisted for between seven and 21 days after withdrawal of the antibiotic, suggesting that megakaryocytes as well as circulating platelets are affected. When the defect is studied *in vitro* much higher concentrations of drug are required to produce the same effect; it has been postulated that activity of a metabolite might explain this discrepancy. The penicilloic acid derivative may be the culprit, acting by blocking receptor sites on the platelet surface.

Although reported most frequently for carbenicillin, prolongation of the bleeding time with abnormal ADP induced platelet aggregation has now been described with several other penicillins including ampicillin (Brown, *et al.*, 1976), azlocillin (Dijkmans, *et al.*, 1980), benzyl penicillin (Andrassy, *et al.*, 1976; Brown, *et al.*, 1976), methicillin (Brown, *et al.*, 1976), nafcillin (Alexander, *et al.*, 1983), piperacillin (Gentry, Jemsek and Natelson, 1981) and ticarcillin (Brown, *et al.*, 1975). Of the cephalosporins, moxalactam (Weitekamp and Aber, 1983) and cephamandole (Custer, Briggs and Smith, 1979) have been reported to cause a similar problem.

Throughout the literature, clinical bleeding due to antibiotic induced platelet dysfunction occurs more commonly in patients with some other predisposing factor such as uraemia, or the concomitant administration of other drugs which interfere with platelet function (Karshmer and Ellman, 1976). There are none the less several reports in which bleeding has occurred in otherwise healthy individuals.

Henoch-Schönlein purpura syndrome

Isolated cases of this syndrome with severe diarrhoea, glomerulonephritis, polyarthritis and purpura rash have been reported following the administration of erythromycin (Handa, 1972), oral ampicillin (Beeching, *et al.*, 1982) and procaine penicillin (Spring, 1951).

Hypoprothrombinaemia

Hypoprothrombinaemia and significant bleeding have been observed in severely ill patients for many years (Ham, 1971; Pineo, Gallus and Hirsh, 1973); an association between the administration of broad spectrum parenteral antibiotics and a vitamin K deficient state has been recognized for a similar time. The vitamin K dependent clotting factors (II, VII, IX and X) are produced in the liver, the final step in their synthetic pathway being a γ-carboxylation of glutamic acid residues on the molecules, which takes place in association with the oxidation of vitamin K to its epoxide form (Figure 19.1). This latter is then reduced again in order that further carboxylation reactions may occur. There are two naturally occurring sources of vitamin K available to man: vitamin K1 (phylloquinone) found in plants and algae and hence derived from the diet; and vitamin K2 (menaquinone) synthesized by colonic microflora, particularly *E. coli* and *bacteroides*. The importance of vitamin K2 in haemostasis has

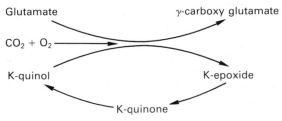

Figure 19.1 The vitamin K epoxyl cycle

been questioned because of doubts about the extent of its absorption from the lower gastro-intestinal tract.

Since the early 1980s, reports of hypopro-thrombinaemia related to parenteral antibiotics have been most commonly associated with the newer cephalosporins; in particular cefamandole (Hooper, Haney and Stone, 1980; Clancy and Glew, 1983), and moxalactam (Pakter, *et al.*, 1982; Conly, *et al.*, 1984).

Two theories have been put forward as to how the defect arises:

(i) inhibition of γ-carboxylation by some part of the antibiotic molecule
(ii) suppression of gut flora causing reduced production of vitamin K2

and there remains controversy as to which of these is more important. In 1982 Neu suggested that the N-methylthiotetrazole (NMTT) side chain which is common to many of these newer cephalosporins, might be responsible for both the 'Antabuse' reaction and hypopro-thrombinaemia associated with their use. *In vitro* experiments have shown that this side chain has a warfarin-like action, inhibiting the vitamin K epoxide reductase enzyme (Lipsky, 1983). The same study failed to show an effect for intact antibiotics bearing the NMTT side chain and it was suggested that *in vivo* degrada-tion of the antibiotic caused release of the NMTT moiety. Others have argued that the concentration of NMTT obtained *in vivo* are much lower than those required to produce inhibition of γ-carboxylation of glutamic acid *in vitro* (Black, Buening and Wolen, 1983) and that compounds which have not been impli-cated in hypoprothrombinaemia proved to be more inhibitive of the reaction than did NMTT (Uotila and Suttie, 1983).

In a comparative study of two different anti-biotic regimes in the empiric treatment of fever, the prothrombin time was more frequently pro-longed and there were more serious bleeding episodes seen in patients given a moxalactam/ticarcillin regime than in those receiving the combination of tobramycin/ticarcillin. This was associated with a greater suppression of bacterial flora in the first group (Conly, *et al.*, 1984). It was postulated therefore that suppres-sion of the flora which produce vitamin K2 was responsible for the hypoprothrombinaemia. There remains however, considerable un-certainty about absorption of the mena-

quinones from the gastrointestinal tract and furthermore, uncertainty about their role in the synthesis of vitamin K dependent clotting factors.

More recent reports have suggested that a sulphydryl (−SH) group within the NMTT side chain may actually be the moiety concerned in inhibition of γ-carboxylation of the K-dependent proteins (Lipsky, 1984). Support for this proposal came from a study by Agnelli, *et al.* (1986) in which ceftriaxone, a newer cephalosporin which bears a −SH group but has no NMTT side chain, produced a similar pro-longation of the prothrombin time and reduction in factor VII activity to cefamandole, while ceftazidime which has neither NMTT nor −SH groups had no effect on either parameter. Whatever is finally found to be responsible for the hypoprothrombinaemia associated with certain cephalosporin antibiotics, there is general agreement that clinically significant bleeding is only seen on severely debilitated and malnourished patients, especially those receiv-ing total parenteral nutrition. It would appear that an acute vitamin K deficiency arises in the context of pre-existing chronic deficiency. In all cases the bleeding tendency can be reversed by the administration of small doses of vitamin K and this should be mandatory in any patient requiring long-term parenteral nutrition.

Other effects of antibiotics on coagulation

Inhibitors of certain coagulation factors can rarely develop as a consequence of antibiotic therapy. These have been reported in associ-ation with penicillin – factor VIII (Green, 1968), streptomycin – Factor V (Crowell, 1975), and isoniazid – Factor XIII (Lorand, *et al.*, 1972).

Finally it must be remembered that anti-biotics can interfere with the control of oral anticoagulants, both potentiating and inhibiting their effect. Nalidixic acid and certain sulphon-amides may compete with warfarin for plasma albumin binding (Potasman and Bassan, 1980; Sioris, Weibert and Pentel, 1980). Metroni-dazole may inhibit hepatic metabolism of the drug, thus increasing its activity (O'Reilly, 1976). Rifampicin, a potent inducer of hepatic microsomal enzymes, may conversely cause increased metabolism and hence reduced activity of anticoagulants; caution on stopping the antibiotic is therefore required.

References

Agnelli, G., Del Favero, A., Parise, P., Guercilini, R., Pasticici, B., Nenci, G.G., et al. (1986) Cephalosporin-induced hypoprothrombinemia: is the N-methylthio-tetrazole side chain the culprit? *Antimicrobial Agents and Chemotherapy,* 29, 1108–1109

Alexander, D.P., Russo, M.E., Fohrman, D.E. and Rothstein, G. (1983) Nafcillin-induced platelet dysfunction and bleeding. *Antimicrobial Agents and Chemotherapy,* 23, 59–62

Alter, B.P., Potter, N.U. and Li, F.P. (1978) Classification and aetiology of the aplastic anaemias. *Clinics in Haematology,* 7, 431–465

Amos, R.J. and Amess, J.A.L. (1983) Megaloblastic haemopoeisis due to acyclovir. *Lancet,* i, 242–243

Andersen, R., Boedicker, M., Ma, M. and Goldstein, E.J.C. (1986) Adverse reactions associated with pentamidine isethionate in AIDS patients: recommendations for monitoring therapy. *Drug Intelligence and Clinical Pharmacy,* 20, 862–868

Andrassy, K., Ritz, E., Hasper, B., Scherz, M., Walter, E., Storch, H., et al. (1976) Penicillin-induced coagulation disorder. *Lancet,* ii, 1039–1041

Barr, A.L. and Whineray, M. (1980) Case report: immune thrombocytopenia induced by cotrimoxazole. *Australian and New Zealand Journal of Medicine,* 10, 54–55

Beeching, N.J., Gruer, L.D., Findlay, C.D. and Geddes, A.M. (1982) A case of Henoch-Schönlein purpura syndrome following oral ampicillin. *Journal of Antimicrobial Chemotherapy,* 10, 479–482

Bird, G.W.G., McEvoy, M.W. and Wingham, J. (1975) Acute haemolytic anaemia due to IgM penicillin antibody in three-year-old child: a sequel to oral penicillin. *Journal of Clinical Pathology,* 28, 321–323

Black, H.R., Beuning, K.K. and Wolen, R.L. (1983) Latamoxef, its side chain, and coagulation. *Lancet,* ii, 1090

Blajchman, M.A., Lowry, R.C., Pettit, J.E. and Stradling, P. (1970) Rifampicin-induced immune thrombocytopenia. *British Medical Journal,* 3, 24–26

Bolton, F.G. and Young, R.V. (1953) Observations on cases of thrombocytopenic purpura due to quinine, sulphamethazine, and quinidine. *Journal of Clinical Pathology,* 6, 320–323

Brandriss, M.W., Wolff, S.M., Moores, R. and Stohlman, F. (1964) Anaemia induced by amphotericin B. *Journal of the American Medical Association,* 189, 663–666

Brauer, M.J. and Dameshek, W. (1967) Hypoplastic anaemia and myeloblastic leukaemia following chloramphenicol therapy. *New England Journal of Medicine,* 277, 1003–1005

Brown, C.H., Bradshaw, M.W., Natelson, E.A., Alfrey, C.P. and Williams, T.W. (1976) Defective platelet function following the administration of penicillin compounds. *Blood,* 47, 949–956

Brown, C.H., Natelson, E.A., Bradshaw, M.W., Williams, T.W. and Alfrey, C.P. (1974) The haemostatic defect produced by carbenicillin. *New England Journal of Medicine,* 291, 265–270

Brown, C.H., Natelson, E.A., Bradshaw, M.W., Alfrey, C.P. and Williams, T.W. (1975) Study of the effects of ticarcillin on blood coagulation and platelet function. *Antimicrobial Agents and Chemotherapy,* 7, 652–657

Bryan, C.S. and McFarland, J.A. (1978) Cryptococcal meningitis: fatal marrow aplasia from combined therapy. *Journal of the American Medical Association,* 239, 1068–1069

Carpenter, G. (1975) Chloramphenicol eye-drops and marrow aplasia. *Lancet,* ii, 326–327

Carrell, R.W. and Lehmann, H. (1969) The unstable haemoglobin haemolytic anaemias. *Seminars in Haematology,* 6, 116–132

Carson, P.E., Flanagan, C.L., Ickes, C.E. and Alving, A.S. (1956) Enzymatic deficiency in primaquine sensitive erythrocytes. *Science,* 124, 484–485

Chan, C.S.P., Tuazon, C.U. and Lessin, L.S. (1982) Amphotericin B induced thrombocytopenia. *Annals of Internal Medicine,* 96, 332–333

Chang, J.C. and Reyes, B. (1975) Agranulocytosis associated with gentamicin. *Journal of the American Medical Association,* 232, 1154–1155

Chen, J-H., Wiener, L. and Distenfeld, A. (1980) Immunologic thrombocytopenia induced by gentamicin. *New York State Journal of Medicine,* 80, 1134–1135

Chong, B.H., Berndt, M.C., Koutts, J. and Castaldi, P.A. (1983) Quinidine induced thrombocytopenia and leucopenia: demonstration and characterisation of distinct anti-platelet and anti-leucocyte antibodies. *Blood,* 62, 1218–1223

Chunn, C., Starr, P. and Gilbert, D. (1977) Neutrophil toxicity of amphotericin B. *Antimicrobial Agents and Chemotherapy,* 12, 226–230

Clancy, C.M. and Glew, R.H. (1983) Hypoprothrombinaemia and bleeding associated with cephamandole. *Lancet,* i, 250

Collaborative DHPG Treatment Study Group, (1986) Treatment of serious cytomegalovirus infections with 9-(1,3-Dihydroxy- 2-propoxymethyl)guanine in patients with AIDS and other immunodeficiencies. *New England Journal of Medicine,* 314, 801–805

Conly, J.M., Ramotar, K., Chubb, H., Bow, E.J. and Louie, T.J. (1984) Hypoprothrombinemia in febrile, neutropenic patients with cancer: association with antimicrobial suppression of intestinal microflora. *Journal of Infectious Diseases,* 150, 202–212

Crowell, E.B. (1975) Observations on a factor-V inhibitor. *British Journal of Haematology,* 29, 397–404

Custer, G.M., Briggs, B.R. and Smith, R.E. (1979) Effect of cefamandole nafate on blood coagulation and platelet function. *Antimicrobial Agents and Chemotherapy,* 16, 869–872

Custer, R.P. (1946) Aplastic anaemia in soldiers treated with atabrine (quinacrine). *American Journal of Medical Science,* 212, 211–224

Deyke, V.F. and Wallace, J.B. (1946) Development of aplastic anaemia during the use of streptomycin. *Journal of the American Medical Association,* 1098

Djikmans, B.A.C., Van der Meer, J.W.M., Boekhout-Mussert, M.J., Zaal-de Jong, M. and Mattie, H. (1980)

Prolonged bleeding time during azlocillin therapy. *Journal of Antimicrobial Chemotherapy*, **6**, 554–555

Dournon, E., Matheron, S., Rozenbaum, W., Gharakhanian, S., Michon, C., Girard, P.M., *et al.* (1988) Effects of zidovudine in 365 consecutive patients with AIDS or AIDS-related complex. *Lancet*, **ii**, 1297–302

El-Ghobarey, A.F. and Capell, H.A. (1977) Levamisole-induced thrombocytopenia. *British Medical Journal*, **2**, 555–556

Falconer, E.H., Epstein, N.N. and Mills, E.S. (1940) Purpura haemorrhagica due to the arsphenamines. Sensitivity in patients as influenced by vitamin C therapy. *Archives of Internal Medicine*, **66**, 319–338

Fischl, M.A., Richman, D.D., Grieco, M.H., Gottlieb, M.S., Volberding, P.A., Laskin, O.L., *et al.* (1987) The efficacy of azidothymidine (AZT) in the treatment of patients with AIDs and AIDS-related complex. *New England Journal of Medicine*, **317**, 185–191

Fraunfelder, F.T. and Bagby, G.C. (1983) Ocular chloramphenicol and aplastic anaemia. *New England Journal of Medicine*. **308**, 1536

Funicella, T., Weinger, R.S., Moake, J.L., Spruell, M. and Rossen, R.D. (1977) Penicillin-induced immuno-haemolytic anaemia associated with circulating immune complexes. *American Journal of Hematology*, **3**, 219–223

Gangarosa, E.J., Johnson, T.R. and Ramos, H.S. (1960) Ristocetin-induced thrombocytopenia: Site and mechanism of action. *Archives of Internal Medicine*, **105**, 83–89

Gentry, L.O., Jemsek, J.G. and Natelson, E.A. (1981) Effects of sodium piperacillin on platelet function in normal volunteers. *Antimicrobial Agents and Chemotherapy*, **19**, 542–533

Girdwood, R.H. (1973) Drug induced megaloblastic anaemia, in, *Blood Disorders Due to Drugs and Other Agents*, R.H. Girdwood, (ed.), pp. 49–82. Excerpta Medica, Amsterdam

Goodman, S.B. and Block, M.H. (1964) A case of red cell aplasia occurring as a result of antituberculous therapy. *Blood*, **24**, 616–623

Gordon, D.H. (1970) Carbenicillin in renal failure. *Lancet*, **ii**, 422

Green, D. (1968) Spontaneous inhibitors of factor VIII. *British Journal of Haematology*, **15**, 57–75

Habibi, B. (1987) Drug-induced immune haemolytic anaemias. *Clinical Immunology and Allergy*, **1**, 343–356

Hackett, T., Kelton, J.G. and Powers, P. (1982) Drug-induced platelet destruction. *Seminars in Thrombosis and Hemostasis*, **8**, 116–137

Ham, J.M. (1971) Hypoprothrombinaemia in patients undergoing prolonged intensive care. *Medical Journal of Australia*, **2**, 716–718

Hamilton, H.E. and Sheets, R.F. (1978) Sulfisoxazole-induced thrombocytopenic purpura immunologic mechanism as cause. *Journal of the American Medical Association*, **239**, 2586–2587

Handa, S.P. (1972) The Schönlein–Henoch syndrome: glomerulonephritis following erythromycin. *Southern Medical Journal*, **65**, 917–920

Harris, J.W. (1956) Studies on the mechanism of a drug-induced haemolytic anaemia. *Journal of Laboratory and Clinical Medicine*, **47**, 760–775

Ho, D., Tashkin, D.P., Bein, M.B. and Sharma, O. (1979) Pulmonary infiltrates with eosinophilia associated with tetracycline. *Chest*, **76**, 33–36

Hooper, C.A., Haney, B.B. and Stone, H.H. (1980) Gastrointestinal bleeding due to vitamin K deficiency in patients on parenteral cefamandole. *Lancet*, **i**, 39–40

Hurd, R.W. and Jacox, R.F. (1943) Thrombocytopenic purpura developing as a complication of sulfa-thiazole and sulfadizine therapy. *Journal of the American Medical Association*, **122**, 296–298

Jenkins, G.C., Hughes, D.T.D. and Hall, P.C. (1970) A haematological study of patients receiving long-term treatment with trimethoprin and sulphonamide. *Journal of Clinical Pathology*, **23**, 392–396

Jenkins, P.F., Williams, T.D.M. and Campbell, I.A. (1980) Neutropenia with each standard antituberculosis drug in the same patient. *British Medical Journal*, **1**, 1069–1070

Johnson, G.J., Rao, G.H.R. and White, J.G. (1978) Platelet dysfunction induced by parenteral carbenicillin and ticarcillin. *American Journal of Pathology*, **91**, 85–106

Karchmer, A.W. and Ellman, L. (1976) Petechiae due to drug-induced platelet dysfuntion. *New England Journal of Medicine*, **295**, 451

Kauffman, C.A., Severance, P.J., Silva, J. and Huard, T.K. (1982) Neutropenia associated with vancomycin therapy. *Southern Medical Journal*, **75**, 1131–1133

Klipstein, F.A., Berlinger, F.G. and Reed, L.J. (1967) Folate deficiency associated with drug therapy for tuberculosis. *Blood*, **29**, 697–712

Kokkini, G., Tsianos, E. and Kappas, A. (1983) Sideroblastic anaemia associated with lincomycin therapy. *Postgraduate Medical Journal*, **59**, 796–798

Larson, R.K. (1953) The mechanism of quinidine purpura. *Blood*, **8**, 16–25

Lee, M. and Berger, H.W. (1980) Eosinophilia caused by rifampicin. *Chest*, **77**, 579

Lehrner, L.M., Cooke, J.H. and Enck, R.E. (1979) Tetracycline-induced aplastic anaemia. *Southern Medical Journal*, **72**, 358–361

Letona, J.M-L., Barbolla, L., Freiyro, E., Bouza, E., Gisanz, F. and Fernandez, M.N. (1977) Immune haemolytic anaemia and renal failure induced by streptomycin. *British Journal of Haematology*, **35**, 561–571

Levin, M.H., Weinstein, R.A., Axelrod, J.L. and Schantz, P.M. (1983) Severe, reversible neutropenia during high-dose mebendazole therapy for Echinococcosis. *Journal of the American Medical Association*, **249**, 2929–2931

Ley, A.B., Cahan, A. and Mayer, K. (1956) A circulating antibody directed against penicillin, in, *Proceedings of the Seventh Congress of the International Society of Blood Transfusion* (Rome, 1958), p. 539, Karger, Basel

Lipsky, J.J. (1983) N-methyl-thio-tetrazole inhibition of the gamma carboxylation of glutamic acid: possible mechanism for antibiotic-associated hypopro-thrombinaemia. *Lancet*, **ii**, 192–193

Lipsky, J.J. (1984) Mechanism of the inhibition of the γ-carboxylation of glutamic acid by N-methylthio-tetrazole-containing antibiotics. *Proceedings of the National Academy of Science USA,* **81**, 2893–2897

Lorand, L., Maldonado, N., Fradera, J., Atencio, A.C., Robertson, B. and Urayama, T. (1972) Haemorrhagic syndrome of autoimmune origin with a specific inhibitor against fibrin stabilizing factor (factor XIII). *British Journal of Haematology,* **23**, 17–27

Loveman, A.B. (1932) Toxic granulocytopenia, purpura haemorrhagica and aplastic anaemia following the arsphenamines. *Annals of Internal Medicine,* **5**, 1238–1252

Lurie, A., Ogilvie, M., Townsend, R., Gold, C., Meyers, A.M. and Goldberg, B. (1970) Carbenicillin-induced coagulopathy. *Lancet,* **i**, 1114–1115

McClure, P.D., Casserly, J.G., Monsier, C. and Crozier, D. (1970) Carbenicillin-induced bleeding disorder. *Lancet,* **ii**, 1307–1308

Miles, S.A. (1992) Haematopoietic growth factors as adjuncts to antiretroviral therapy. *AIDS Research and Human Retroviruses,* **8**, 1073–1080

Moake, J.L., Butler, C.F., Hewell, G.M., Cheek, J. and Spruell, M.A. (1978) Haemolysis induced by Cefazolin and Caphalothin in a patient with penicillin sensitivity. *Transfusion,* **18**, 369–373

Montgomery, A.B., Debs, R.J., Luce, J.M., Corkery, K.J., Turner, J., Brunette, E.N., *et al.* (1987) Aerosolised pentamidine as sole therapy for Pneumocystis carinii pneumonia in patients with acquired immunodeficiency syndrome. *Lancet,* **ii**, 480–483

Mungall, I.P.F. and Standing, V.F. (1978) Eosinophilia caused by rifampicin. *Chest,* **74**, 321–322

Murphy, M.F., Riordan, T., Minchinton, R.M., Chapman, J.F., Amess, J.A.L., Shaw, E.J., *et al.* (1983) Demonstration of an immune-mediated mechanism of penicillin-induced neutropaenia and thrombocytopaenia. *British Journal of Haematology,* **55**, 155–160

Murphy, M.F., Metcalfe, P., Grint, P.C.A., Green, A.R., Knowles, S., Amess, J.A.L., *et al.* (1985) Cephalosporin-induced immune neutropaenia. *British Journal of Heamatology,* **59**, 9–14

Nagao, T. and Mauer, A.M. (1969) Concordance for drug-induced aplastic anaemia in identical twins. *New England Journal of Medicine,* **281**, 7–11

Neftel, K.A., Hauser, S.P. and Muller, M.R. (1985) Inhibition of granulopoiesis *in vivo* and *in vitro* by β-lactam antibiotics. *Journal of Infectious Disease,* **152**, 90–98

Neftel, K.A., Hauser, S.P., Muller, M.R. and Walti, M. (1986) Cephalosporin-induced neutropaenia. *British Journal of Haematology,* **62**, 394–395

Neu, H.C. (1982) The new beta-lactamase-stable cephalosporins. *Annals of Internal Medicine,* **97**, 408–419

Nora, A.H. and Fernbach, D.J. (1969) Acquired aplastic anaemia in children. *Texas Medicine,* **65**, 38–43

O'Reilly, R.A. (1976) The stereoselective interaction of warfarin and metronidazole in man. *New England Journal of Medicine,* **295**, 354–357

Otero, M. and Goodpasture, H.C. (1983) Pulmonary infiltrates and eosinophilia from minocycline. *Journal of the American Medical Association,* **250**, 2602

Ou Shu, K., Tang Gao, Y., Linet, M.S., Brinton, L.A., Nie Gao, R., Jin, F., *et al.* (1987) Chloramphenicol use and childhood leukaemia in Shanghai. *Lancet,* **ii**, 934–937

Pakter, R.L., Russell, T.R., Mielke, C.H. and West, D. (1982) Coagulopathy associated with the use of moxalactam. *Journal of the American Medical Association,* **248**, 1100

Pineo, G.F., Gallus, A.S. and Hirsh, J. (1973) Unexpected vitamin K deficiency in hospitalized patients. *Canadian Medical Association Journal,* **109**, 880–883

Potasman, I. and Bassan, H. (1980) Nicoumalone and nalidixic acid interaction. *Annals of Internal Medicine,* **92**, 571

Rich, M.L., Ritterhoff, R.J. and Hoffman, R.J. (1950) A fatal case of aplastic anaemia following chloramphenicol (chlormycetin) therapy. *Annals of Internal Medicine,* **33**, 1459–1467

Richman, D.D., Rischl, M.A., Grieco, M.H., Gottleib, M.S., Volberding, P.A., Laskin, O.L., *et al.* (1987) The toxicity of azidothymidine (AZT) in the treatment of patients with AIDS and AIDS-related complex. *New England Journal of Medicine,* **317**, 192–197

Ries, C.A., Rosenbaum, T.J., Garratty, G., Petz, L.D. and Fudenberg, H.H. (1975) Penicillin-induced immune haemolytic anaemia – occurrence of massive intravascular hemolysis. *Journal of the American Medical Association,* **233**, 432–435

Rouveix, B., Lassoued, K., Vittecoq, D. and Regnier, B. (1983) Neutropenia due to β lactamine antibodies. *British Medical Journal,* **2**, 1832–1834

Rubin, D., Weisberger, A.S., Botti, R.E. and Storaasli, J.P. (1958) Changes in iron metabolism in early chloramphenicol toxicity. *Journal of Clinical Investigation,* **37**, 1286–1292

Schiffer, C.A., Weinstein, H.J. and Wiernik, P.H. (1973) Methicillin-associated thrombocytopenia. *Annals of Internal Medicine,* **85**, 338–339

Scott, J.L., Finegold, S.M., Belkin, G.A. and Lawrence, J.S. (1965) A controlled double-blind study of the haematologic toxicity of chloramphenicol. *New England Journal of Medicine,* **272**, 1137–1142

Simpson, M.B., Pryzbylik, J., Innis, B. and Denham, M.A. (1985) Haemolytic anaemia after tetracycline therapy. *New England Journal of Medicine,* **312**, 840–842

Sioris, L.J., Weibert, R.T. and Pentel, P.R. (1980) Potentiation of warfarin anticoagulation by sulfisoxazole. *Archives of Internal Medicine,* **140**, 546–547

Spring, M. (1951) Purpura and nephritis after administration of procaine penicillin. *Journal of the American Medical Association,* **147**, 1139–1141

Stein, J.B. and Tolle, S.W. (1983) Episodic leucopenia associated with amphotericin B. *Southern Medical Journal,* **76**, 409–410

Teerenhovi, L., Heinonen, E., Grohn, P., Klefstrom, P., Mehtonen, M. and Thlikainen, A. (1978) High frequency of agranulocytosis in breast-cancer patients treated with levamisole. *Lancet,* **ii**, 151–152

Thompson, J.S., Herbick, J.M., Klasen, L.W., Severson,

C.D., Overlin, V.L., Blaschke, J.W., *et al.* (1980) Studies on levamisole-induced agranulocytosis. *Blood,* **56**, 388–396

Uotila, L. and Suttie, J.W. (1983) Inhibition of vitamin-K dependent carboxylase *in vitro* by cefamandole and its structural analogs. *Journal of Infectious Diseases,* **148**, 571–578

Van Assendelft, A.H.W. (1985) Leucopenia in rifampicin chemotherapy. *Journal of Antimicrobial Chemotherapy,* **16**, 407–408

Verwilghen, R., Reybrouk, G., Collens, L. and Cosemans, J. (1965) Antituberculous drugs and sideroblastic anaemia. *British Journal of Haematology,* **11**, 92–98

Volberding, P.A., Lagakos, S.W., Koch, M.A., Pettinelli, C., Myers, M.W., Booth, D.K., *et al.* (1990) Zidovudine in asymptomatic human immunodeficiency virus infection. *New England Journal of Medicine,* **322**, 941–949

Weintraub, R.M., Pechet, L. and Alexander, B. (1962) Rapid diagnosis of drug-induced thrombocytopenic purpura. *Journal of the American Medical Association,* **180**, 528–532

Weitekamp, M.R. and Aber, R.C. (1983) Prolonged bleeding times and bleeding diathesis associated with moxalactam administration. *Journal of the American Medical Association,* **249**, 69–71

White, J.M., Brown, D.L., Hepner, G.W. and Worlledge, S.M. (1968) Penicillin-induced haemolytic anaemia. *British Medical Journal,* **3**, 26–29

Winn, Chatham, W. and Ross, D.W. (1983) Leukaemoid blood reaction to tetracycline, *Southern Medical Journal,* **76**, 1195–1196

Wong, K.Y., Boose, G.M. and Issitt, C.H. (1981) Erythromycin-induced haemolytic anaemia. *Journal of Paediatrics,* **98**, 647–649

Yarchoan, R., and Broder, S. (1987) Development of anti-retroviral therapy for the acquired immunodeficiency syndrome and related disorders. *New England Journal of Medicine,* **316**, 557–564

Yunis, A.A. (1969) Drug-induced bone marrow injury. *Advances in Internal Medicine,* **15**, 357–376

Yunis, A.A. (1973) Chloramphenicol-induced bone marrow suppression. *Seminars in Hematology,* **10**, 225–234

Ziegler, Z., Shadduck, R.K., Winkelstein, A. and Stroupe, T.K. (1979) Immune haemolytic anaemia and thrombo-cytopenia secondary to quinidine: *in vitro* studies of quinidine-dependent red cell and platelet antibodies. *Blood,* **53**, 396–402

Index